INJURIES AND ILLNESSES IN THE ELDERLY

David L. Kaufman, M.D.
Editor-in-Chief

Mosby

MATTHEW◆BENDER

QUESTIONS ABOUT THIS PUBLICATION?

For questions about the **Editorial Content** appearing in these volumes or reprint permission, please call:

Beverly Lieberman .... 1-800-252-9257 (ext. 2629)
Rina Cascone .... 1-800-252-9257 (ext. 2858)
Outside the United States and Canada please call .... (212) 448-2000

For assistance with shipments, billing or other customer service matters, refer to book code 32338. Please call:

Customer Services Department at .... (800) 426-4545
Outside the United States and Canada, please call .... (314) 872-8370
Fax number .... (800) 535-9935
Outside the United States and Canada, please fax .... (314) 453-4379

LCCN: 97–29279

ISBN: 0–8205–2997–4

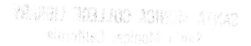

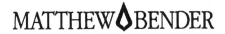

MATTHEW BENDER & CO., INC.
Editorial Offices
2 Park Avenue, New York, NY 10016-5675 (212) 448-2000
201 Mission St., San Francisco, CA 94105-1831 (415) 908-3200

MOSBY-YEAR BOOK, INC.
11830 Westline Industrial Drive
St. Louis, MO 63146
(800) 325-4177; (314) 872-8370

Table of Contents

A COMPLETE SYNOPSIS FOR EACH CHAPTER APPEARS
AT THE BEGINNING OF THE CHAPTER

Preface
Publisher's Editorial Staff
About the Editor-in-Chief

Table of Contents

Table of Contents

Table of Contents

Table of Contents

Table of Contents

Table of Contents

Preface

As our society ages, the health problems of the elderly grow rapidly more complex. Statistics starkly define the dimensions of the challenge: Every 7 seconds, a "baby boomer" turns 50. Today the elderly —those over 65—comprise 12 percent of our population, and the percentage increases daily. In the last 100 years, the life expectancy of the average person has increased by 30 years. As this portion of the population expands dramatically—there are now 76 million baby boomers—their health needs and expectations will explode.

This book approaches the problem in an orderly and comprehensive manner. The major injuries and disorders and the significant diseases of the elderly are carefully defined and described, giving the reader a road map to maneuver through this sometimes daunting territory.

Injuries and Illnesses in the Elderly begins with an outstanding Overview. This first chapter defines the scope and perspective of the book and provides a succinct review of the material. It is followed by 16 chapters that cover the major health problems of the elderly in great detail. Each one deals comprehensively with the material, beginning with the relevant epidemiology and anatomy and progressing to a discussion of etiology, diagnosis, treatment and prognosis.

The book ends with two key chapters: Drug Treatment in the Elderly and Psychological Adaptation to Long-term Care. As our population grows older, the multiple health problems every individual is prey to require increasingly complex medication regimens. In the elderly, pharmacokinetics, drug interactions, medication compliance and adverse effects are enormously important issues that are too often given cursory consideration. This critical chapter is comprehensively written and deserves careful attention. The final chapter, similarly, addresses a vital and somewhat neglected topic: the psychosocial needs of the elderly as they adapt to their deteriorating health, loss of independence and requirements for long-term chronic care. It is an insightful and invaluable chapter.

This volume will appeal to a wide variety of health care providers. Nurses, doctors, physical therapists and other health care staff will find it helpful and clinically relevant. Each chapter has a comprehensive Bibliography, allowing the reader to pursue areas of particular interest.

As we enter the twenty-first century, new discoveries and challenges will confront us. Our elderly population will grow larger and older. Complex social, financial and medical issues will need to be recognized and resolved. Preventive health approaches may prolong our lives, designer drugs may ease our illnesses, innovative treatments may cure or control our disorders. But some things will not change. We will still grow old. The diseases and disorders so carefully described in this book will be with us for a very long time.

David L. Kaufman, M.D.

About the Editor-in-Chief

DAVID L. KAUFMAN, M.D.

David L. Kaufman is a Clinical Assistant Professor of Medicine at New York Medical College, a Faculty Preceptor and a Teaching Attending Physician at St. Vincent's Hospital in Manhattan. He is a Member of the American College of Physicians. Dr. Kaufman is board certified in internal medicine and has been in private practice since 1980. He is active in research, having served as principal investigator on over 15 multicenter studies and co-authored several published papers.

For four years, Dr. Kaufman was the Supervising Attending Physician at the St. Vincent's Walk-in Clinic, where he acquired wide-ranging experience dealing with the acute and chronic medical and social problems of Lower Manhattan's elderly population. He is also a member of St. Vincent's Hospital's renowned team of doctors making house calls to elderly homebound patients.

Publisher's Editorial Staff

Beverly R. Lieberman
Managing Editor

Rina Cascone
Project Editor

CHAPTER 1

OVERVIEW

SCOPE

We in the industrialized world are an aging society. Over the course of the twentieth century, we have added 30 years to our life expectancy, and every year we continue to add another 3 months to that life expectancy. As we age, we develop chronic medical problems. The elderly make up 12 percent of the population, yet they consume 30 percent of all prescription drugs. Cardiovascular disease remains the number-one killer of Americans, but chronic conditions such as osteoporosis, congestive heart failure and diabetes are significant problems in the elderly. The medical problems of the elderly can very quickly become social problems for family members and the community. Hip fractures, Alzheimer's disease, strokes, incontinence and other conditions necessitate removal of the elderly from their homes and subsequent placement with family or in an institution. This move out of well-known surroundings, with its concomitant loss of control, can be traumatic for an older person.

SYNOPSIS

1

1.00   INTRODUCTION

We are an aging society. In 1900, the United States was a nation of relatively young people who died of communicable diseases like tuberculosis, polio, diphtheria, measles and typhoid, all of which we can now treat or prevent. Women often died in childbirth; the causes of heart disease were unknown; cancers claimed victims quickly, checked only by relatively crude surgery. Smoking was not seen as a health risk, but, ironically, several generations of women were protected from its ravages because smoking was seen as "unladylike." By contrast, in the 1990s, four-generation families are common, and active people in their 70s can often be found caring for relatively healthy parents in their 90s. We have added 30 years to our life expectancy in the twentieth century, and every year in the developed world we continue to add 3 months to that life expectancy. By percentage, the fastest-growing demographic group in America is that made up of people over 100. As the 76 million members of the "baby boom" generation continue to age (the largest age cohort in American history; 11,000 "boomers" turn 50 daily), the ranks of our elderly will swell even more dramatically (Lamm, 1997).

Communicable diseases (for, example, acquired immunodeficiency syndrome and tuberculosis) are re-emerging as threats at the end of the twentieth century. However, it is still the more slowly developing, life-style-dependent cardiovascular disease that claims most Americans.

1.10 BONE DISORDERS, TRAUMA AND SURGERY

As the human body ages, the skeleton stops adding minerals and forming new bone; this occurs in individuals in their late 20s to mid-30s. Then after menopause in women, and with advanced age in men, the skeleton loses minerals as well as its underlying fibrous network, leaving bones with a weak, lacy structure. The wrists, hips and vertebrae are especially susceptible to this process of osteoporosis. These skeletal sites are thus the ones most prone to fracture or most likely to be in need of prosthetic replacement in the elderly, leaving the affected individual open to all the risks associated with surgery, anesthesia and immobility and perhaps precipitating either temporary or permanent dependence upon others for help with activities of daily living.

Also with age, joints that in youth were lined with smooth cartilage and connective tissue begin to develop inappropriate mineral deposits, and the cartilage becomes worn. This osteoarthritis is painful and can limit the mobility of the affected joint. The elderly are also prone to rheumatoid arthritis, which often affects peripheral joints symmetrically and can cause great pain and deformity.

1.11 Osteoporosis

Osteoporosis is a metabolic disease characterized by a loss of bone minerals (primarily calcium, but also phosphorus) and of the underlying collagen bone matrix; this occurs throughout the skeleton but especially in the spine, hips and wrists. Spinal fractures cause an affected person (usually a woman) to bend forward, producing the archetypal "dowager's hump." Wrist fractures occur when an osteoporotic person falls and, in reaching out to break the fall, absorbs the shock in the weakened wrist bones. Hip fractures are the most devastating of osteoporosis-associated fractures, for a number of reasons. The person may fall while alone and be unable to get immediate assistance. The surgery to pin or replace the hip and the physical therapy afterward can be enormously stressful (both physically and emotionally) and may precipitate an end to independent living for the affected elderly person.

Not everyone is at equal risk for getting osteoporosis. Women are more at risk than men, and northern Europeans and Asians are more at risk than are people of African descent. Among all groups, thin, small-framed women are more likely to develop the disease than are bigger-boned individuals. Smoking and drinking alcohol increase the risk of osteoporosis, while eating a diet high in calcium and regularly participating in weight-bearing exercise (swimming does not fall into this category) decrease the risk.

Hormone replacement therapy, specifically estrogen replacement, has until recently been the most effective way to prevent osteoporosis in menopausal women and to halt its progression in older, postmenopausal women. No woman is considered too old to receive some benefit from hormone replacement therapy. Long-term hormone therapy (15 to 20 years) has been shown to decrease the risk of hip fracture by about 25 percent and has the added benefit of decreasing the risk of coronary artery disease by 35 percent (Wren, 1992). Recent studies show that hormone replacement therapy starting after age 65 may be equally valuable.

There is now also strong evidence that long-term use of estrogen decreases the risk of and/or delays the onset of Alzheimer's disease (Paganini-Hill and Henderson, 1996). Guidelines issued by the American College of Physicians in 1992 urge all menopausal women, regardless of race, to consider hormone replacement therapy (American College of Physicians, 1992).

A new class of drugs now on the market to treat osteoporosis is the bisphosphonate group; alendronate (Fosamax®) is the one most frequently used for this indication. The bisphosphonates are the first drugs to actually rebuild bone in postmenopausal women rather than to just slow or halt bone loss. This is especially important in elderly women who already have significant osteoporosis and thus are at increased risk of fractures.

Unfortunately, bisphosphonates have some unpleasant (primarily gastrointestinal) side effects. If the drug dissolves in the esophagus instead of the stomach, it can cause ulceration of the esophageal tissue. The patient must sit erect for 30 minutes after taking the drug to prevent any reflux of the drug from the stomach into the esophagus (many elderly people have a loosened cardiac sphincter, the closure at the top of the stomach, and so reflux of gastric contents and attendant heartburn is a common problem). The drug must be taken with a full glass of plain tap water (not juice or mineral water) and must be taken 30 minutes before eating or taking other medications. In the elderly, many of whom take multiple drugs for an array of health problems, anything that makes taking medications more awkward or confusing is a problem, because the patient may stop taking the drug or may take it incorrectly, so that the benefit is lost.

1.12 Arthritis

The word *arthritis* means "joint inflammation." There are two major types: rheumatoid arthritis and osteoarthritis.

Rheumatoid arthritis (RA) is a chronic, multisystem disease with no known cause. The most common feature is inflammation of symmetric peripheral joints. With time, the inflammation causes joint deformities by destruction of cartilage and erosion of bone. In about two thirds of patients the onset is gradual, with fatigue, loss of appetite and generalized weakness coming weeks or months before joint pain. Specific symptoms of pain and swelling usually appear gradually and symmetrically in the hands, wrists, knees and feet. The pain is aggravated by movement.

Rheumatoid arthritis can have a variable course, from mild joint discomfort of brief duration to a progressive disease causing severe pain and joint deformity. Rheumatoid arthritis occurs in about 1 percent of the population. Women are affected three times more often than are men. Eighty percent of patients develop the disease between the ages of 35 and 50, but the prevalence of the disease increases with age, and gender differences are less pronounced in the elderly (Lipsky, 1994).

Therapy for rheumatoid arthritis remains empirical, because the pathogenesis of the disease is not known. Treatment involves first the use of aspirin and other nonsteroidal anti-inflammatory drugs (NSAIDs), such as ibuprofen, and then, if needed, low-dose glucocorticoids (steroids such as prednisone) to control inflammation. Other drugs, such as plaquenil (an antimalarial), are also used. The most common side effects seen with aspirin and the NSAIDs are gastrointestinal upset, erosion and bleeding.

Osteoarthritis is the most common kind of arthritis. It is a degenerative disease of the joints (especially weight-bearing joints) in which cartilage is destroyed and excess bone grows, forming lips and spurs, and impairing function (Thomas, 1993).

The exact cause of osteoarthritis is not known. However, primary osteoarthritis is a normal part of aging and probably results from mechanical wear and tear, metabolic (especially hormonal) changes that occur with aging and genetic factors. Osteoarthritis is not a systemic disease, like rheumatoid arthritis, so not all joints are necessarily affected. The hips and knees, which bear the most weight through life, are most frequently involved.

Diagnosis is made through history, physical examination and x-rays. Symptoms include joint pain (especially after exercise, which is relieved by rest), morning stiffness, aching with changes in the weather, a grating sensation in the joint during motion and limited range of joint motion. Symptoms may begin in middle age and progress over the years. The severity of signs and symptoms increases with poor posture, obesity and occupational stress. X-rays of the affected joint show narrowing of the joint space, cystlike bony deposits in the joint space, joint deformity from degeneration and bony growths in weight-bearing areas.

Treatment of osteoarthritis is primarily symptomatic, not curative. Medications to relieve pain and inflammation include aspirin and an array of nonsteroidal anti-inflammatory drugs such as ibuprofen, indomethacin and fenoprofen. Acetaminophen (Tylenol®) can also be helpful and will not cause the gastrointestinal side effects of the NSAIDs. In some cases, temporary relief can be achieved with corticosteroid injections into the affected joint. Joint stress can be reduced with a back, wrist or knee brace, if necessary.[1]

Hip replacement or knee replacement surgery may be required if the affected joint has deteriorated significantly and pain is severe.[2] Likewise, if disability or pain is severe in the low back, spinal fusion surgery (laminectomy) may be indicated. In a laminectomy, the surgeon removes the disc and one or more of the bony laminae that form the sides of the vertebrae. Then bone chips (usually taken from the hip) are grafted between the vertebral spaces to stabilize the spine.

1.13   Paget's Disease

Paget's disease is a disturbance in the dynamic balance between bone breakdown and bone rebuilding. In normal bone, specialized cells (osteoclasts) continuously break down old bone, while other cells

---

[1] *See also* ch. 6 for further discussion of arthritis in the elderly.

[2] *See also* ch. 3 for further discussion of hip replacement.

(osteoblasts) simultaneously rebuild new bone. It is estimated that in the adult, all the bones are totally replaced every eight years (Krane, 1994).

In Paget's disease, the bone-destroying osteoclasts in one or more parts of the body are too active, breaking down too much bone. The bone-building osteoblasts then cannot keep up with the bone-destroying osteoclasts, and rebuilt bone is weak, deformed, supplied with too many blood vessels and may be larger than the bone it replaced. While the disease can strike many parts of the body, from the skull to the large bones of the leg, the spine and pelvis are two of the most common sites.

It is estimated that 3 to 4 percent of Americans over the age of 45 and up to 8 percent of those over 80 have Paget's disease. The disease is most common in England, where it affects 4.6 percent of the population. Paget's disease is rare in Asia and Africa. In 20 to 30 percent of cases, there appears to be a familial link, though an exact genetic mechanism is not clear. Recent studies point to the role of a so-called slow virus, which becomes active years after the bone becomes infected. An inherited susceptibility to the virus has also been suggested (Krane, 1994).

Paget's disease is usually asymptomatic until severe bone damage has occurred. It may be discovered accidentally when a patient has an x-ray for another problem or when routine blood tests reveal a high level of the enzyme alkaline phosphatase. Alkaline phosphatase is normally produced by bone-forming osteoblasts, and in Paget's disease, they produce it in abnormally large amounts. The bone scan is also a useful tool in diagnosis, because radioactive isotope concentrates in affected bones.

Treatment involves the use of drugs to suppress osteoclasts. The most commonly used drugs are the related hormones calcitonin (given intramuscularly or subcutaneously) and etidronate (given orally), which retard bone resorption. Mithramycin, a cytotoxic (cell-killing) antibiotic usually used as a chemotherapy drug in cancer, is also used to attack osteoclasts. However, mithramycin can also destroy platelets (cells crucial to blood clotting) and damage the kidneys. Nonsteroidal anti-inflammatory drugs such as aspirin, indomethacin and ibuprofen are used to relieve pain in Paget's disease.

A well-tailored exercise program is helpful in maintaining muscle and bone strength as well as joint flexibility. Swimming and brisk walking are preferred activities, providing cardiovascular as well as muscular exercise with a minimum of jarring impact. Surgery is used only for those with severe symptoms who are not helped by conservative therapy, to repair or prevent pathologic fractures, to correct deformities or to relieve neurologic impairment. Joint replacement is difficult because the bonding material (methyl methacrylate) does not set properly on affected bone (Krane, 1994).[3]

1.14   Fractures and Surgical Procedures

Osteoporosis causes weakened bones in the elderly. These weakened bones are prone to fractures with minor trauma—and sometimes without any trauma at all. Unfortunately, the elderly are also prone to falls due to impaired vision, dementia, medications that can affect balance and cause weakness, and circulatory problems, which can cause dizziness. The three areas of the skeleton that are most prone to osteoporotic fractures are the wrists, spine and hips.

Wrist fractures are common in postmenopausal women, most often as a result of reaching out to break a fall. Usually both the radius and the ulna, the two bones in the lower arm, are broken in what is called a Colles' fracture. The bones are realigned (reduced) by a physician, and then a cast or plaster splints are applied to immobilize the fracture for four weeks while it heals.

The spinal fractures that occur in the elderly are called compression fractures. The vertebral bodies—the round bones in between which the intravertebral discs lie—are weakened by osteoporosis and can collapse simply from the weight of supporting the body in an upright position. These fractures, which occur most frequently in the thoracic (chest) and cervical (neck) vertebrae, can be very painful if nearby nerves are involved, but often they occur without symptoms. The affected person loses height and gains what is commonly called a dowager's hump or, in medical parlance, kyphosis. There is no treatment for compression fractures beyond mitigating the underlying osteoporosis to try to prevent further fractures, and good pain management.

Hip fractures are by far the most serious osteoporotic fractures, exerting the greatest impact on the affected person's life. To begin with, the person falls and usually cannot get up again (after an impacted fracture, in which the head of the femur telescopes into the

---

[3] *See also* ch. 5 for further discussion of Paget's disease.

shaft, the person may be unable to walk). If the elderly person lives alone, it can be some time before she or he is rescued.[4]

Once a hip has been fractured, the elderly person often cannot return to living alone after discharge from the hospital. Finding suitable housing either with family or in assisted living facilities then becomes a social work problem.

A hip fracture is almost always repaired by open reduction and internal fixation with a stabilizing rod inserted into the interior of the bone and secured with screws and a metal plate, or by replacing the entire joint with a prosthesis.[5] Pain after surgery can be severe, and the narcotics required to give adequate pain relief can cause confusion in the elderly. (However, pain medication should not be withheld merely to prevent confusion.) The recovery period for hip surgery is substantial, and the elderly person usually requires ongoing physical therapy after discharge to regain the ability to walk independently. The immobility required after surgery can lead to complications such as decubitus ulcers (bed sores) and pneumonia.

The neck of the femur, a common fracture site, does not have a good blood supply. Therefore, nonunion of the bones is a common complication, and avascular (without blood supply) aseptic (not infected) necrosis (death and deterioration) of the head of the femur can also occur after surgery. When the head of the femur—the trochanter—is fractured, these problems do not occur due to the better blood supply in this portion of the bone.

1.20 VASCULAR DISORDERS

Vascular disease, specifically cardiovascular (pertaining to the blood vessels in the heart) disease, remains the number-one killer of Americans. Two terms associated with vascular disease need to be understood: *arteriosclerosis* ("hardening of the arteries") is the more general term and can refer to mineral or fatty deposits in the artery walls. *Atherosclerosis* is the most common form of arteriosclerosis and involves the deposition of fatty materials in artery walls.

Atherosclerosis is caused by the deposition of fatty substances (a varying mixture of cholesterol and other fats, smooth muscle cells and a connective tissue matrix made up of collagen, elastic fibers and large

---

[4] *See also* ch. 2 for further discussion of hip fractures in the elderly.

[5] *See also* ch. 3 for further discussion of hip replacement.

protein/sugar molecules) in clumps called plaques in arterial walls. As a plaque grows within the arterial wall, it forms a fibrous cap over the soft, fatty core and protrudes into the artery, sometimes to the point of total occlusion.

With continued growth, the plaque can no longer be contained within the arterial wall, and the vessel's intima (the smooth, innermost cell layer of the artery) ruptures. The plaque is now termed a "complicated lesion" that may break open, hemorrhage or form a thrombus (clot) on its surface due to increased blood turbulence that initiates platelet clumping. When a plaque's fibrous cap ruptures, spilling fatty substances into the bloodstream, a thrombus often forms. Eighty-five percent of all heart attacks are caused by this process of thrombosis (Frohlich, 1993). As the size of the arterial lumen (hollow inner space) is decreased by the growing plaque, a clot (embolus) floating free in the circulating blood can be snagged by the plaque. Whether it is caused by a snagged embolus or by a thrombus that forms at the site of the plaque, blood flow to distal (downstream) tissues is cut off.

If blood flow is not restored in time, tissue death (infarction) ensues. If the clogged artery is in the heart, a myocardial infarction (heart attack) occurs.[6] If the clogged artery is in the neck or brain, a cerebrovascular accident (CVA or "stroke") occurs.[7]

A vascular disorder that is common in the elderly and that makes all the other vascular disorders worse is hypertension (high blood pressure). As the heart pumps harder against the increased resistance of clogged blood vessels, over time, the heart becomes less efficient, and weak areas (aneurysms) can develop in vessel walls.

The risk factors for vascular disease are familiar: a diet high in fat and cholesterol, lack of exercise, obesity, smoking, uncontrolled diabetes, uncontrolled high blood pressure and a positive family history of vascular disease. Of these risk factors, only a family history of vascular disease is not under the control of the individual.

1.21   Myocardial Infarction

A myocardial infarction (MI) occurs when, due to lack of oxygen, heart tissue dies and the dead cells are replaced by scar tissue, which

---

[6] *See also* ch. 7.

[7] *See also* ch. 8.

is less elastic than normal tissue. When a narrowed coronary artery becomes totally blocked, the muscle downstream of the blockage becomes oxygen-starved and will eventually die (infarct) if circulation is not restored within four to six hours. The more muscle that is served by the affected artery (i.e., the farther "upstream" the blockage occurs), the larger the heart attack; and the larger the heart attack, the more difficult it is for the heart to pump blood properly.

Complications seen after MI include heart failure (the condition in which the heart cannot pump all the blood out of the ventricles with each beat, so blood backs up into the lungs and into the feet and legs), cardiogenic shock (in which cardiac function is so impaired that an adequate blood pressure cannot be maintained), extension of the original MI and pericarditis (inflammation of the pericardium or sac that adheres to the outside of the heart) (Frohlich, 1993).

1.22 Hypertension

Hypertension, or high blood pressure, is an extremely common health problem, affecting approximately a fourth of the adult American population. The prevalence of high blood pressure increases with age and is higher in the African-American population than among whites. Hypertension is a major risk factor for stroke, coronary artery disease, heart failure and kidney disease (Grimm, 1993).

The blood pressure is the amount of pressure generated by the heart both while pumping and at rest. The first number, the systolic blood pressure, represents the amount of pressure generated by the left ventricle during systole, while the heart is pumping blood out to the arterial tree. The second, and lower, number of the blood pressure represents the amount of pressure that remains in the arteries between heartbeats when the heart is filling with blood. Hypertension is arbitrarily defined as a systolic blood pressure greater than or equal to 140 mm Hg (millimeters of mercury) and/or a diastolic blood pressure greater than or equal to 90 mm Hg (a "normal" blood pressure is considered 120 over 80).

Over 95 percent of all cases of hypertension are referred to as "essential" or primary hypertension and have no easily definable cause. Risk factors for hypertension include a family history of hypertension, diabetes, elevated blood cholesterol level, obesity and a sedentary lifestyle, a high-sodium diet, smoking and an elevated alcohol intake. Initial hypertension therapy should be aimed at smoking cessation, alcohol moderation and changing the diet and activity level of the affected person. However, medications may be needed as well, since life-style changes are notoriously difficult to achieve.

Diagnosis is accomplished by simply taking the blood pressure. The heart, kidney and eye can all show the cumulative effects of hypertension, giving the physician an idea of how severely the hypertension has affected body systems. The heart size (as it has to push against greater resistance, the heart muscle will enlarge in an attempt to compensate) and rhythm should be determined. Blood levels of nitrogen wastes normally cleared by the kidneys should also be assessed. The blood vessels at the back of the eye can show increased tortuosity, and small "cotton wool" hemorrhages can also be seen in people with long-standing, significant hypertension.

A wide array of potent drugs is available to effectively treat high blood pressure. Since the 1970s, the death rates from stroke and heart disease have declined dramatically, in part due to better management of hypertension and its risk factors. Diuretics (hydrochlorothiazide, furosemide and others), beta-adrenergic blockers (propranolol, atenolol and others), alpha-adrenergic blockers (doxezocin and others), angiotensin converting enzyme inhibitors (captopril and others), and calcium channel blockers (verapamil and others) are all effective in lowering blood pressure through a number of mechanisms (Frohlich, 1993). Unfortunately, many of these drugs have side effects, from frequent urination to just not feeling very energetic, which tempt patients to skip their medications—which then increases hypertensive problems.

1.23 Congestive Heart Failure

Congestive heart failure is defined as an abnormality of cardiac function in which the ventricles do not deliver adequate blood to the tissues at rest or during normal activity. This is a condition often seen in the elderly because it is caused by long-standing hypertension and by heart muscle malfunction after one or more myocardial infarctions. Many hormonal and anatomic factors can precipitate and then worsen cardiac failure. Most patients develop heart failure due to malfunction of the myocardial cells, valvular heart disease, conduction defects (an irregular or too rapid heart rate will prevent proper pumping of the heart during each beat) or because of stricture of the heart by the surrounding pericardium. The mechanism underlying heart failure can be pressure overload (caused by years of hypertension), volume overload (often precipitated by sodium intake, which causes fluid retention), impaired myocardial contractility (a cardiomyopathy, usually seen in younger people), restricted ventricular filling (caused by abnormally tight valves between the atria and ventricles, the result of rheumatic fever in the past) and loss of functioning myocardium (usually after one or more myocardial infarctions causes large areas of scar tissue in the heart wall) (Frohlich, 1993).

Heart failure can involve either one or both of the ventricles, though the failure usually becomes biventricular eventually. Right-sided heart failure is less serious than left-sided failure. In right-sided failure, venous blood is not entirely pumped out of the right ventricle into the pulmonary artery to go to the lungs. Blood backs up in the venous system, pushing fluid out of the blood vessels and into peripheral tissues, including the legs and the liver. Right-sided failure is relatively easy to diagnose, since these patients are the ones with swollen feet, ankles and legs. This edema starts in the feet and travels up the leg as right ventricular function worsens.

Left ventricular failure affects a person's ability to breathe and robs peripheral tissues of adequate oxygen. Therefore, it is both more uncomfortable and more serious. When blood is not pumped into the aorta from the left ventricle, it backs up into the lungs, pushing fluid into the alveoli, the tiny spaces where gas exchange occurs. The result is shortness of breath (dyspnea), which may only be during exertion but progresses to being present continuously as failure worsens.

In left-sided failure, fluid can be heard in the lungs when the patient is examined by stethoscope. A crackling sound called rales starts in the bottoms (bases) of the lungs and proceeds up the lung fields as failure worsens. Paroxysmal nocturnal dyspnea (PND) is a frightening symptom of left-sided heart failure. The patient may be comfortable when lying down initially. However, during the night, the respiratory center is depressed during sleep, and ventricular function may also be impaired because of reduced stimulation by adrenaline and related hormones. This causes a backup of fluid into the lungs, and the person awakens suddenly with severe air hunger, which is not quickly relieved by sitting up and putting the legs over the bedside.

The goal of treating heart failure is to restore and maintain cardiac output. Rest is important, and sedation (often with a short-acting benzodiazepine such as lorazepam) may be required due to the restlessness that shortness of breath often produces. Dietary sodium (salt) restriction is important to limit the fluid retention sodium causes. Digitalis preparations (digoxin) increase cardiac contractility and improve cardiac output. Diuretics such as hydrochlorothiazide and furosemide are useful in preventing fluid overload and pulling excess fluid out of the lungs and peripheral tissues for excretion through the kidneys. Potassium, an electrolyte required for maintaining a regular heartbeat, is lost in urine and therefore must be prescribed along with diuretics. Medications that dilate peripheral veins (nitroglycerine) and arteries (angiotensin converting enzyme inhibitors) can also be useful in reducing the amount of blood returning to the right side of the heart and in reducing the systemic peripheral resistance against which the heart must pump (Frohlich, 1993).

1.24   Stroke

Cerebrovascular disease is the third leading cause of death in developed countries. It is estimated that in this country, more than 400,000 people are discharged from the hospital each year after having suffered a stroke (also known as a cerebrovascular accident, or CVA). Cerebrovascular disease covers a range of disorders of the blood vessels in the brain; stroke is the acute neurologic injury that results from one of these pathologic processes (Kistler, et al., 1994).

The two broad categories of stroke are *thromboembolic* and *hemorrhagic*. In a thromboembolic stroke, either a blood clot forms on top of a plaque that has ruptured through an artery wall in the brain or in one of the carotid arteries in the neck, or a clot forms in the bloodstream (often in the atria of the heart if they are fibrillating, or beating with a rapid, irregular rhythm). This clot then migrates to the neck or brain, is snagged on an arterial plaque and blocks circulation. In hemorrhagic strokes, an aneurysm (a ballooned-out, weak area of an arterial wall) breaks and bleeds into the rigid, confining space of the skull.

Eighty percent of strokes are thromboembolic, and the remaining 20 percent of strokes are hemorrhagic. The primary risk factors for stroke include hypertension (high blood pressure), hypercholesterolemia (high blood cholesterol levels) and smoking (Kistler, et al., 1994).

The symptoms a person exhibits after a stroke depend upon the area of the brain that has been affected. Symptoms can range from mild weakness to paralysis and coma. Strokes that affect the right side of the brain produce left-sided weakness or paralysis. Strokes that affect the left side of the brain affect the right side of the body and often produce difficulty with speech and/or understanding language (expressive and/or receptive aphasia).

Diagnosis is made with computed tomography (CT) or magnetic resonance (MR) scanning of the brain to determine whether the stroke is of thromboembolic or hemorrhagic origin. Ultrasound of the neck can reveal clotted-off carotid arteries. If the stroke is hemorrhagic and there is active bleeding, emergency surgery is required to relieve pressure.

Initial treatment revolves around preventing another stroke or extension of the existing one. After a thromboembolic stroke, aspirin or warfarin (Coumadin®) is prescribed to anticoagulate the blood and thus prevent inappropriate clot formation. It is important not to make the blood too anticoagulated, so that intracranial and other internal bleeding can be avoided.

The area of damage in the brain is analogous to a bull's-eye: A center of dead cells that will not revive is surrounded by an indeterminately sized area of bruised cells, many of which will regain function. It is impossible to judge initially how much function a person will regain after a stroke. In the initial postinfarction period, the brain swells in reaction to the damage to cells. After roughly a week, the swelling resolves and the patient improves. A person can continue to improve neurologically for up to 18 months after a stroke. After the first few days to a week following a stroke, the emphasis of therapy switches from medical treatment to physical, occupational and speech/cognitive therapy to help the patient regain lost physical and mental functions.[8]

1.30 ALZHEIMER'S DISEASE

Alzheimer's disease, also known as presenile or senile dementia, is an organic (having a definite physical cause) mental disorder in which there is atrophy of the frontal and occipital lobes of the brain. Brain cells (neurons) deteriorate, becoming tangles of tiny fibrils coupled with deposits of a starchlike substance called amyloid.

---

[8] *See also* ch. 8 for a complete discussion of stroke.

Alzheimer's disease can begin at any age but usually develops insidiously in older people, more often in women than in men. It is estimated that from 5 to 15 percent of the population over the age of 65 have Alzheimer's. The condition is characterized by progressive, irreversible memory loss, intellectual deterioration, disorientation, apathy, and speech and gait disturbances. This dementia may also be accompanied by delirium, delusions or depression.

Early in the disease, the affected person may know he is losing his mental abilities and become distressed. However, as the disease progresses, the person becomes unaware of the deterioration (Deckert and Krug, 1993).

The exact cause of Alzheimer's disease is not known, though it has been shown to run in some families, and in these people, it is thought to be associated with chromosome 21. The neurotransmitter (chemical messenger in the brain that transmits nerve impulses) acetylcholine has been implicated in some studies, but there is as yet no clear mechanism to explain how someone gets the disease (Deckert and Krug, 1993). The protective role of estrogen is also currently under investigation. All aspects of Alzheimer's disease are being actively researched, and some drugs currently moving through clinical trials may prove helpful and win the approval of the Food and Drug Administration (FDA), while at least two others—tacrine (Cognex®) and donepezil (Aricept®)—have already been approved.

Since there is no treatment, Alzheimer's disease is currently more a social problem than a medical one. It is distressing for family members to watch a loved one slowly lose all memory, even of family and friends. In addition, people stricken with Alzheimer's usually require institutionalization eventually because they become incontinent, can wander from home and get lost, and may require feeding to obtain adequate nutrition. Nursing home care is expensive, and nursing home beds are not easy to come by in every community.[9]

1.40 SENSORY DISORDERS

With age, our ability to gather information about the world around us decreases. Our senses of sight, hearing, smell and taste can all become diminished. Treatment ranges from curative surgery for

---

[9] *See also* ch. 15 for a complete discussion of Alzheimer's disease.

cataract,[10] to assistive devices (hearing aides) for hearing loss,[11] to work-arounds in the areas of loss of smell and taste.

1.41 Ophthalmologic Problems

Two major eye disorders commonly develop in the elderly: cataracts and glaucoma. A cataract is a clouding or darkening of the lens that normally focuses light on the retina at the back of the eye. When the lens becomes clouded—a cataract-affected lens can range from milky white to dark brown—less light reaches the back of the eye to excite the nerve cells (the rods and cones) in the retina. Vision becomes less acute, and colors are muted. Night vision is affected early on in this process, and cataracts can be the precipitating factor for an elderly person having to stop driving, at least temporarily.

Fortunately, cataracts are easily fixed. Lens replacement surgery is the standard therapy and is performed on an outpatient basis under local anesthesia. An uncomplicated cataract operation usually takes about 20 minutes. One eye is operated on at a time, with surgeries usually separated by a month or two. Complications are uncommon, but macular degeneration (a condition in which the point of maximal acuity on the retina, the macula, loses its nerve cells, leaving the patient with only peripheral vision) can occur after cataract surgery.

Glaucoma is an eye disease characterized by an increase in intraocular pressure that, if it remains untreated, can cause atrophy of the optic nerve and blindness. Intraocular pressure is easily measured by an ophthalmologist or an optometrist with a small instrument called a tonometer that is placed briefly on the eye after anesthetic drops are instilled; normal tonometric readings range from 13 to 22 (Thomas, 1994).

The two types of glaucoma are closed angle and open angle. *Closed angle glaucoma* is caused by a narrowing or closure of the angle in the eye through which aqueous humor, one of the two fluids inside the eye, circulates. This angle closure causes aqueous humor to accumulate in the anterior chamber of the eye, where it is produced. This kind of glaucoma is the least common, and it is usually accompanied by acute eye pain and/or headache. Angle closure glaucoma is considered an ophthalmologic emergency and requires prompt surgery to relieve pressure and prevent blindness.

---

[10] *See also* ch. 11 for further discussion of cataracts.

[11] *See also* ch. 12 for further discussion of impaired hearing in the elderly.

Open angle glaucoma is the most common form of the disease. Its onset is insidious and its cause is unknown, though it does run in families. Unlike angle closure glaucoma, open angle glaucoma is painless. An early symptom of the disease is the appearance of halos around lights. Medications are used to decrease aqueous humor production (acetazolamide, marketed as Diamox® and others). Glaucoma drops (eserine and pilocarpine) are used to keep the pupil constricted, thereby opening the angle as wide as possible. These miotics come in green-topped and -labeled bottles. Eyedrops that dilate the pupil (mydriatics such as atropine) come in red-topped and -labeled bottles. It is vitally important that a glaucoma patient not receive a mydriatic (drops from a red-topped bottle), as dilating the pupil can precipitate angle closure and a dangerous increase in intraocular pressure. If intraocular pressure cannot be controlled medically, a number of surgical procedures can be used to provide an adequate outlet for aqueous humor.[12]

1.42 Auditory Problems

Helen Keller, who was both deaf and blind, is credited with saying that blindness merely isolates a person from things, but deafness isolates a person from other people. This is particularly apt in explaining the effect of hearing loss on the elderly. Hearing loss is very common among the elderly. It interferes with communication, often making even simple conversation an ordeal for the individual and those around her. Dinner with a table full of elderly women in a retirement home dining room is hardly a social experience if no one can understand anyone else. The temptation for the elderly person is to give up attempts at communicating and sink into isolation.

Why do the elderly become hard of hearing? With age, the tympanic membrane (eardrum) becomes thinner and more fibrous, which reduces its ability to transmit sound. In the middle and inner ear, all the structures can degenerate. For example, the three tiny bones there can become calcified, making them less able to transmit vibrations. In the auditory nerve and the brain, transmission and processing are slowed.

The best way to help the elderly person with hearing loss is to have the person evaluated by an audiologist, who will fit the person for a hearing aide either in one or both ears. Hearing aides are not a

---

[12] *See also* ch. 10 for a discussion of glaucoma.

panacea, however. They are expensive, easily lost and, although they will amplify sounds, they cannot correct auditory distortion.[13]

1.43 Smell and Taste

Many older people complain that food no longer has much taste. Studies have shown that in individuals over the age of 60, the taste buds, which control sensing sweet, sour, salt and bitter, tend to atrophy. Also with age, taste cells regenerate more slowly. Many people wear dentures that block the upper palate, and elderly people often take medications that can dry the mouth and affect taste.

The sense of smell, which determines most of what we perceive as taste, is also affected by aging. With age, the olfactory nerve fibers in the brain atrophy, and the number of olfactory nerve cells lining the nose are also significantly reduced (Staab, 1992).

This reduction in an elderly person's ability to smell and taste is important on several levels. From a basic safety standpoint, an elderly person with a reduced sense of smell may not be aware of the smoke of a fire before it is too late to make a safe exit. Probably even more important is that with a reduced sense of taste or smell, food is less appealing. This can lead to poor food intake, weight loss, decreased energy and activity, and then skin breakdown and the development of pressure ulcers (what used to be called bed sores).

Strategies for caregivers to overcome this reluctance to eat in an elderly person include offering frequent small meals, making food visually appealing, including a variety of food textures, adding spices and commercial food flavorings to increase food palatability, limiting alcohol intake because it is an appetite suppressant and providing good oral hygiene to prevent periodontal and gum disease, which can distort food taste or make it offensive (Staab, 1992).

1.50 UROGENITAL DISORDERS

In men, the prostate gland, which aids in the production of semen and surrounds the urethra close to its exit from the bladder, can become problematic with advancing age. Prostate cancer kills 44,000 men annually, with half of new cases being diagnosed among men in their 70s and older.

---

[13] *See also* ch. 12 for a discussion of hearing loss in the elderly.

Benign prostatic hypertrophy is a noncancerous enlargement of the prostate. The cause is unknown, but the disease can lead to a blocking of the urethra. If the condition is left untreated, it can cause bladder infections and kidney failure.[14] In women, advancing age is often accompanied by a progressive loss of bladder control. This incontinence can cause skin breakdown and precipitate removal of an older person from independent living to a more controlled environment.[15]

1.51   Prostate Cancer and Benign Prostatic Hypertrophy

Prostate cancer has become the second leading cause of cancer deaths in adult men, second only to lung cancer. Every year there are 350,000 new cases and 44,000 deaths (Natale, 1997). At first glance, it would seem that a large push to screen men and find the cancer early, analogous to breast cancer screening for women, would be warranted. However, unlike most cancers, prostate cancer is often slow-growing and not aggressive. As a result, there is a wide disparity between the prevalence of the disease in the population and the cancer's mortality. If one took a prostate biopsy of every man at age 50 and examined the specimen in the laboratory, over 30 percent of the samples would show cancer; the number jumps to 60 percent at age 80 (Himsl, 1997). However, a third of all men aged 50 are not fighting for their lives against prostate cancer, and likewise 60 percent of deaths among men aged 80 are not caused by this disease.

The question remains whether all prostate cancer should be aggressively treated. Fifty percent of cases are diagnosed in men who are over the age of 70, when the chances are good that they will die of heart disease or some other illness before the prostate cancer spreads enough to cause death. Added to that is the fact that the treatment can be worse than the disease. Incontinence, impotence, urethra strictures requiring dilatation, acute or chronic inflammation of the bowel and/or bladder, urinary retention, hot flashes, decreased libido, breast development, blood clots and liver toxicity are all complications of prostate cancer therapy. Studies have found that in an estimated 90 to 95 percent of cases, prostate cancer patients receive too much treatment (Himsl, 1997).

Diagnosis of prostate disease is by digital rectal exam and a blood test to determine the level of prostate specific antigen (PSA). In a rectal

---

[14] *See also* ch. 14 for further discussion of male urogenital disorders.

[15] *See also* ch. 13 for a discussion of incontinence.

exam, the physician can feel an increased firmness and change in texture in the prostate. The PSA is a less specific test than its name implies, but an increased PSA level requires investigation. Ultrasonography of the prostate can reveal cancer.

Treatment is determined by the stage of the cancer and how far it has spread. A number of staging systems exist, the simplest of which is the "tumor, node, metastasis" or TNM system. This makes intuitive sense; a tumor that is confined to the prostate is less serious than one that has spread to lymph nodes in the immediate area, which in turn is less serious than a tumor that has spread to bones or other distant spots. The Gleason Grading System looks at the tumor under the microscope and gives a score from 2 to 10 based on the pathologic findings. A high Gleason score is associated with a poor prognosis.

The standard treatment options for prostate cancer include surgery, with or without radiation therapy, and/or hormonal therapy. Surgery and radiation are standard cancer therapies most people understand; surgery cuts out all visible tumor and a safe margin of healthy tissue around it, while radiation is used to kill any cancer cells that might have been missed by the surgery. Hormone therapy is less well understood. Prostate cancer growth is stimulated and cancer cell death is inhibited by male hormones such as testosterone. In hormone therapy, female hormones (luteinizing hormone releasing hormone) or chemicals that block release of male hormones are given to suppress testosterone output and thus suppress tumor growth.

Another, less ominous prostate condition is benign prostatic hypertrophy (BPH, sometimes called hyperplasia). This is a very common condition in men over 50. The prostate enlarges for unknown reasons, and eventually the urethra (the tube leading from the bladder to the outside, which passes through the prostate) may be pinched closed. Symptoms include getting up at night to urinate, a need to urinate often (urinary frequency), a reduction in the force and size of the urinary stream, delay in starting urination, incontinence due to overflow and acute retention requiring catheterization. Chronic bladder inflammation and infection often develop, and as retention increases, urine can back up into the kidneys and cause kidney failure. Benign prostatic hypertrophy can be treated either with medication or by surgical removal of the prostate (Elkins, 1993).

1.52   Incontinence

Urinary incontinence is defined as involuntary loss of urine sufficient to be a problem. Incontinence is a much larger problem among women than among men, starting at an earlier age. The age differential exists primarily because women get pregnant, and pregnancy puts prolonged pressure on the bladder, weakening the supporting pelvic muscles, the bladder neck and the sphincter muscles that control the urinary outlet or meatus. Also, especially in the elderly, the short female urethra from the bladder to the outside allows easier bacterial access and makes women more prone to urinary tract infections (UTIs), which can cause incontinence.

The three kinds of incontinence are stress, urge and overflow. *Stress incontinence* is involuntary loss of urine during coughing, sneezing, laughing or other physical activity. It is caused by intrinsic weakness or deficiency in the sphincter muscle that controls the urinary outlet or by bladder hypermobility. Stress incontinence is by far the most common type, affecting roughly 9 million American women starting as early as the fourth decade of life (American Medical Women's Association, 1997).

Urge incontinence is involuntary loss of urine associated with an abrupt and strong desire to void (urgency). Urge incontinence is usually associated with urinary frequency (often in the presence of a urinary tract infection), and at times, a large amount of urine may be lost suddenly, without warning.

Overflow incontinence is involuntary urine loss due to overdistension of the bladder. The patient may present with constant dribbling or have symptoms of stress or urge incontinence. Elderly men with prostate enlargement often cannot adequately empty their bladder and are prone to overflow incontinence. Many frail, elderly patients have mixed symptoms of both stress and urge incontinence (Agency for Health Care Policy and Research, 1992).

It is important to evaluate urinary incontinence in the elderly, because effective treatments are available, and incontinence can usually be improved. Urge incontinence is often caused by a urinary tract infection, which can be cured with a sulfa drug or broad-spectrum antibiotic in one week to ten days. Stress incontinence can be improved with exercises (Kegel exercises, which alternately tense and relax pelvic floor muscles), medication (anticholinergic/antispasmodic agents and other drugs to relax the bladder and increase its capacity), life-style changes (avoiding alcohol and caffeine, limiting fluid intake before being away from a bathroom and before bed, going to the bathroom on a regular schedule), urethral inserts (the patient inserts a disposable, inflatable device into the urethra and removes it to void, something many elderly may not be able to master), and a variety of surgical options ranging from injecting collagen around the female urethra to add bulk and tighten the urinary outlet, to bladder resuspension (the bladder is sewn up to the abdominal wall) to prostate removal in men (prostatectomy can also cause incontinence through damage to sphincter muscles, so it may not be an ideal solution) (Agency for Health Care Policy and Research, 1992).

Urinary incontinence is often the final straw that gets family attention and precipitates the removal of the elderly person from an independent living arrangement, putting him or her into some level of care, ranging from an assisted living apartment to an outright nursing home. Because of the enormity of life-style change that may be caused by a lack of bladder control, urinary incontinence in a nondemented elderly person requires a careful workup, with discussion of treatment options rather than an assumption that this is a normal part of aging that cannot be helped.

1.60 DIABETES

Diabetes mellitus is a syndrome in which the islets of Langerhans in the pancreas either produce no insulin at all or do not produce enough of the hormone to properly regulate metabolism of carbohydrates, fats and proteins.[16]

Without adequate insulin, the body cannot properly metabolize sugar, and it starts to break down fats for energy. However, the fat metabolism is incomplete, and acids and ketones (relatives of the highly poisonous solvent acetone) begin to build up in the blood. Eventually diabetic coma ensues. Diabetes also has many long-term complications affecting many body systems that can develop even in people whose blood sugar levels are well controlled.

When the pancreas produces no insulin at all, the patient is entirely dependent upon externally supplied insulin (i.e., injections) and is said to have insulin dependent diabetes mellitus (IDDM) or type I diabetes

---

[16] *See also* ch. 9.

(formerly known as juvenile diabetes). Type II diabetes is non-insulin-dependent diabetes mellitus (NIDDM; formerly known as adult onset diabetes). In NIDDM, the pancreas produces some insulin, and the condition can usually be controlled with diet, weight loss and exercise. Oral medication to stimulate insulin release from the pancreas and decrease glucose output by the liver. However, these patients may also require insulin for adequate metabolic control.

The cause of diabetes is unknown, although there seems to be an autoimmune component (in which the patient's own immune system attacks the insulin-producing cells as if they were foreign) in type I diabetes, and both types do run in families. The onset of type I diabetes is usually before the age of 40, though it can arise at any age. Similarly, the onset of type II is usually after age 40, but it also can arise at any age. Most elderly diabetics have type II diabetes, and 60 to 90 percent of people with NIDDM are obese (Frohlich, 1993). Some people with type II diabetes can be entirely free of medication simply by bringing their weight down into the normal range.

Symptoms people experience with the onset of diabetes include excessive thirst (polydipsia), excessive hunger (polyphagia), increased urine output (polyuria) often including getting up at night (nocturia), and weight loss. (Before the discovery of insulin in 1922, hospital kitchens had to be locked to prevent dying diabetics from breaking in and gorging themselves.) Diabetes is diagnosed by a random blood glucose level of greater than 200 mg/dL, a fasting blood glucose level of 140 mg/dL on two separate occasions, a sustained elevated blood glucose level during a standardized glucose tolerance test (Frohlich, 1993), an elevated glycosylated hemoglobin level or a hemoglobin A_1C.

Acute diabetic complications are many. They include ketoacidosis, in which blood levels of ketones are elevated and blood pH is decreased. The patient's breath may smell sweet and vaguely like nail polish remover. In hypoglycemia, there is a decreased level of blood sugar usually as a result of too much inject insulin, too much oral medication and/or not eating while taking glucose-lowering drugs. The person begins to feel shaky; loss of consciousness can be avoided by quick ingestion of a readily available sugar source, such as orange juice with a teaspoon of sugar in it. Nonketotic (without ketones), hyperglycemic (high blood sugar levels), hyperosmolar (the blood is so concentrated with sugar it pulls water out of tissues) coma, recurrent infections, lethargy, muscle weakness and poor wound healing are additional complications of diabetes.

Ketoacidosis, hypoglycemia and nonketotic hyperglycemic hyperosmolar coma can all cause loss of consciousness in the diabetic. The treatment of hypoglycemia—sugar—is the exact opposite of the other two conditions, for which insulin is necessary. Therefore, in the emergency room, when a patient whose history is not known is brought in unconscious from an unknown cause, she or he is given intravenous glucose. Simultaneously a finger-stick glucose reading is obtained and the treatment is adjusted based on that result.

The major chronic complications of diabetes are cataract formation; deterioration of tiny blood vessels in the eyes and kidneys leading to blindness; kidney failure; accelerated atherosclerosis; and deterioration of peripheral motor, sensory and autonomic nerves (especially in a "stocking and glove" distribution on hands and legs). The combination of this peripheral neuropathy and vascular deterioration often produces diabetic foot disease, which can proceed surprisingly quickly and result in the need for amputation (Frohlich, 1993).

The goals in treating diabetes mellitus are to keep the blood glucose levels as near normal as possible (insulin is a vital treatment but not a cure), to prevent acute complications, to maintain ideal body weight and to prevent or minimize chronic diabetic complications (Frohlich, 1993).

1.70 PSYCHOLOGICAL ADJUSTMENTS OF AGING

The psychological adjustments associated with aging are the adjustments required by loss of control and letting go. The elderly lose their spouses, friends and other loved ones; they lose their homes and privacy, the ability to drive, their possessions and their pets. Some people seem to cope with this age-associated loss better than others. Nearly everyone knows of elderly people (often men) who have died within a year of the death of their spouse; they seem to give up and fade away. Yet the majority of elderly people cope well with their grief and the changes in their lives.

Research is being carried out on a number of fronts to try to determine what factors in a person's personality, health and life-style indicate whether they will cope well with the inevitable losses associated with advancing age. Those people who remain engaged in the world seem to do best, but there is a "chicken and the egg" aspect to this, and predicting who will thrive into old age remains difficult to do.[17]

1.80 SPECIAL CONSIDERATIONS OF DRUG THERAPY IN THE ELDERLY

It is estimated that although people over the age of 65 make up only about 12 percent of our population, they take 30 percent of all prescription drugs. The elderly are frequently being treated for multiple chronic diseases at once, such as heart disease, high blood pressure, arthritis, diabetes, osteoporosis and glaucoma. The use of multiple prescription and over-the-counter drugs together (polypharmacy) leaves these elderly people open to adverse drug interactions and confusion over how to take medications (Lepkowsky, 1992).[18]

The elderly also absorb, metabolize and eliminate drugs differently than younger people do. The rate of absorption of oral drugs from the gastrointestinal tract can be slowed by other drugs, by an increased (less acid) gastric pH, by delayed stomach emptying and by decreased (by up to 40 or 50 percent) perfusion of the intestines by blood. As the percentage of body fat increases with age, the body's water content declines. This change means that water-soluble drugs become highly concentrated in the elderly.

Most drugs are broken down by enzymes in the liver, and with age, the liver becomes a less-efficient biotransformation machine. Smoking, other drugs, altered liver blood flow and congestive heart failure can all prolong the amount of time it takes for the liver to metabolize a drug. Most drugs are eliminated from the blood by way of the kidneys, and the functioning of these organs also, due to age or the effects of disease (especially hypertension), can be impaired in the elderly. This means it can take significantly longer than expected for a medication to be cleared from the bloodstream, and that overdosage of drugs is an ever-present danger.

---

[17] *See also* ch. 17 for further discussion of psychological adaptations to the problems of aging.

[18] *See also* ch. 16 for a complete discussion of drug treatment in the elderly.

1.100 BIBLIOGRAPHY

Text References

American College of Physicians, Clinical Efficacy Assessment Project: Guidelines for Counseling Postmenopausal Women about Preventive Hormone Therapy. Ann. Int. Med. 117(12):1038-1041, 1992.

American Medical Women's Association: Understanding Stress Urinary Incontinence. New York: American Medical Women's Association, 1997.

Deckert, G. and Krug, R.: Psychiatry. In: Frohlich, E. (Ed.): Rypins' Clinical Sciences Review, 16th ed. Philadelphia: Lippincott, 1993.

Elkins, R.: Surgery. In: Frohlich, E. (Ed.): Rypins' Clinical Sciences Review, 16th ed. Philadelphia: Lippincott, 1993.

Frohlich, E.: Internal Medicine. In: Frohlich, E. (Ed.): Rypins' Clinical Sciences Review, 16th ed. Philadelphia: Lippincott, 1993.

Grimm, R., Jr.: Public Health and Community Medicine. In: Frohlich, E. (Ed.): Rypins' Clinical Sciences Review, 16th ed. Philadelphia: Lippincott, 1993.

Himsl, K.: Sorting Out the Controversies in Early Prostate Cancer Management. Advances in Colon and Prostate Cancers, Oncology Seminar, SHC Specialty Hospital, Westlake Village, California, April 19, 1997.

Kistler, J., et al.: Cerebrovascular Diseases. In: Isselbacher, K., et al. (Eds.): Harrison's Principles of Internal Medicine, 13th ed. New York: McGraw-Hill, 1994.

Krane, S.: Paget's Disease of the Bone. In: Isselbacher, K.: Harrison's Principles of Internal Medicine, 13th ed. New York: McGraw-Hill, 1994.

Lamm, R.: The Public Client Connection. In: American Institute of Architects: The Client Connection, Annual Meeting CD-ROM. Washington, D.C.: American Institute of Architects, 1997.

Lepkowsky, M.: General Principles of Drug Therapy in the Elderly. In: Lantz, J. (Ed.): Nursing Care of the Elderly. San Diego, Calif.: Western Schools, 1992.

Lipsky, P.: Rheumatoid Arthritis. In: Isselbacher, K.: Harrison's Principles of Internal Medicine, 13th ed. New York: McGraw-Hill, 1994.

Natale, R.: The Future of Advanced Prostate Cancer Management. Advances in Colon and Prostate Cancers Oncology Seminar, SHC Specialty Hospital, Westlake Village, Calif., Apr. 19, 1997.

Paganini-Hill, A. and Henderson, V.: Estrogen Replacement Therapy and Risk of Developing Alzheimer's Disease. Arch. Int. Med. 156(10):2213-2217, Oct. 1996.

Staab, A.: Sensory Changes: Coping and Caregiving Strategies. In: Lantz, J. (Ed.): Nursing Care of the Elderly. San Diego, Calif.: Western Schools, 1992.

Thomas, C.: Taber's Cyclopedic Medical Dictionary, 17th ed. Philadelphia: Davis, 1994.

Urinary Incontinence Guideline Panel: Urinary Incontinence in Adults: Clinical Practice Guideline. AHCPR Pub. No. 92-0038. Rockville, Md.: Agency for Health Care Policy and Research, Public Health Service, U.S. Department of Health and Human Services, Mar. 1992.

Wren, B.: The Menopause. In: Hacker, N. and Moore, J. (Eds.): Essentials of Obstetrics and Gynecology, 2nd ed. Philadelphia: Saunders, 1992.

Additional References

Cooney, L., Jr.: Hip Fracture Outcomes. Arch. Intern. Med. 157(5):485-486, Mar. 10, 1997.

Davidson, H., et al.: Measuring Depressive Symptoms in the Frail Elderly. J. Gerontol. 49(4):159-164, July 1994.

Karlsson, M., et al.: Changes of Bone Mineral Mass and Soft Tissue Composition After Hip Fracture. Bone 18(1):19-22, Jan. 1996.

Kim, S., et al.: Predictors of Perceived Health in Hospitalized Older Persons: A Cross-Sectional and Longitudinal Study. J. Am. Geriatr. Soc. 5(4):420-426, Apr. 1997.

Levi, N.: Early Mortality After Cervical Hip Fractures. Injury 27(8):565-567, Oct. 1996.

Mackenzie, T., et al.: Use of Severity of Illness to Evaluate Quality of Care. Int. J. Qual. Health Care 8(2):125-130, Apr. 1996.

Mackowiak, E.: Adult Urinary Incontinence. Hosp. Pharm. Times 5-16, May 1996.

Nettleman, M., et al.: Predictors of Mortality After Acute Hip Fracture. J. Gen. Intern. Med. 11(12):765-767, Dec. 1996.

Raphael D., et. al.: Frailty: A Public Health Perspective. Can. J. Public Health 86(4):224-227, July-Aug. 1995.

Thomas, M. and Eastwood, H.: Reevaluation of Two Simple Prognostic Scores of Outcome After Proximal Femoral Fractures. Injury 27(2):111-115, Mar. 1996.

U.S. Dept. of Health and Human Services: Acute Pain Management: Operative or Medical Procedures and Trauma. Clinical Practice Guideline. AHCPR Pub. No. 92-0032. Rockville, Md.: Agency for Health for Health Care Policy and Research, Feb. 1992.

CHAPTER 2

HIP FRACTURES IN THE ELDERLY

SCOPE

Of the 280,000 hip fractures that occur in the United States annually, nearly all are suffered by individuals age 65 or older, and the number of hip fractures is continuing to increase. The likelihood of hip fracture increases exponentially with age. This increase is a direct result of age-related changes, the two most significant of which are a loss in postural stability (leading to falls) and decreased bone strength. The implications of a hip fracture in an elderly individual are very serious; they range from loss of mobility and independence to death. Three classifications of hip fractures exist: femoral neck, intertrochanteric and subtrochanteric fractures. Hip fractures are treated with reduction and immobilization, with the specific technique dependent on the nature of the injury and the preinjury status of the patient, and the general course of care tailored to the special considerations necessary for older patients. Previously healthy, oriented patients can regain an active life-style with appropriate treatment; however, despite advances in the field, the prognosis for elderly hip fracture patients in general is poor.

SYNOPSIS

2.100 BIBLIOGRAPHY

2.00 INTRODUCTION

The hip is a ball-and-socket joint formed by the rounded head of the femur, or thighbone, and the acetabulum, the cup-shaped cavity at the side of the pelvis. Although fractures of the acetabulum do occur, they are less common than fractures of the femur and generally result from auto accidents; as a result, they are less of a concern for the elderly population.

Fractures of the hip generally occur in the proximal femur, the topmost portion of the thighbone; hence, "hip fracture" is technically something of a misnomer. This injury can affect the femoral head, the femoral neck, the intertrochanteric region (the area between the trochanters, or bony prominences, near the neck of the thighbone) and the subtrochanteric region. (*See Figure 2–1.*)

Descriptions of hip fractures refer to severity, which ranges from *simple* (a fracture in which the skin above the break is unbroken and the bone is in two parts that are easily reunited) to *comminuted* (a fracture in which there are more than two fragments), and from *compound* (in which a fragment of bone pierces the skin) to closed (in which the skin is unbroken). Descriptions also take into account the location of the break on the femur, which can be *subcapital* (below the head of the femur), *transcervical* (across the neck of the femur); *basal; intertrochanteric* (located between the greater and lesser trochanters of the femur) or *subtrochanteric* (below an imaginary line drawn between the two trochanters).

The choice of treatment will be directly influenced by the severity and location of the fracture (Heithoff and Lohr, 1990). In elderly patients, a simple fracture usually heals in six to eight weeks. More severe fractures, however, may take three or more months to heal completely (Goldstein, 1991).

The hip joint itself is well protected from outside trauma. However, several factors predispose the elderly to fracture of the proximal (closer to the trunk of the body or point of origin) femur, including bone fragility, disease and trauma, primarily falling. The influence of each of these factors increases with age (Jarnlo and Thorngren, 1993).

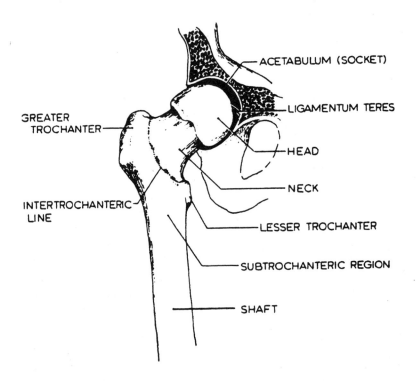

Fig. 2-1. Anatomy of the hip joint.

2.01 Anatomy of the Hip

The hip is the major weight-bearing joint of the body. It is formed by the articulation of the femur (the thighbone) and the acetabulum, a cup-shaped depression at the point where the components of the innominate or hipbone meet within the pelvic girdle. (*See Figure 2–2.*) The innominate bones include the ilium, whose protruding crest is what most people refer to as the hipbone; the ischium and the pubis. Mobility within the joint is made possible by the femoral head, the rounded extension of the femur that is the "ball" to the acetabulum's "socket." The femoral head juts from the femoral epiphysis (the proximal bulge of the femur) by way of the femoral neck.

The angle of the femoral neck makes a limited range of hip motion possible: flexion (bending the knee and raising it) (*see Figure 2–3*), extension (bringing the straight leg back through the plane of the body) (*see Figure 2–4*), abduction (moving the leg out to the side of the

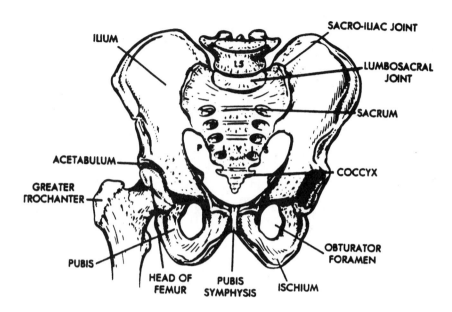

Fig. 2-2. The acetabulum is a cup-shaped depression in the innominate or hipbone, which is formed by the ilium, the ischium and the pubis.

body) (*see Figure 2–5*), adduction (bringing the leg across the midline of the body) (*see Figure 2–6*), and internal and external rotation (twisting the knee in or out from the midline of the body) (*see Figure 2–7*).

The entire joint is reinforced by a tough capsule that extends from the innominate bone to the intertrochanteric region. (*See Figure 2–8.*) The capsule is lined with a thin synovial membrane that secretes a lubricating fluid to facilitate relatively frictionless movement between the cartilaginous ends of the articulating bones.

The joint capsule is reinforced by ligaments, and the entire joint area is supplied by muscles that support the hip and are used to move the lower extremity, including the psoas muscles that originate from the lumbar spine, the iliacus and gluteus medius muscles that arise from the ilium, the obturator muscles that pass from the pelvis to the trochanters, and the adductor and quadriceps muscles of the thigh.

Because the hip joint allows the entire weight of the upper body to be borne upright, its components must be well integrated. When

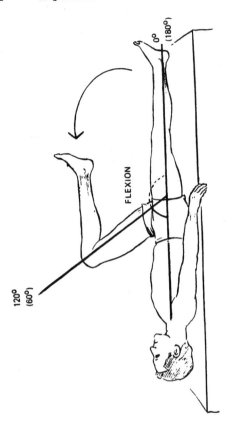

Fig. 2-3. Flexion of the hip is the action of bending the knee and raising it. It is measured by recording the number of degrees in the angle formed between an imaginary line drawn through the raised thigh and one through the horizontal. The normal angle of flexion is 130 degrees measured from the other leg or 60 degrees measured from the trunk.

a muscle is too tight or one of the articulating bones is missing or poorly aligned, this can cause deformities and degenerative changes within the hip and in other parts of the weight-bearing unit, such as the spine, knees and ankles.

2.02   Blood Supply to the Hip

Blood is supplied to the hip via three routes:

- Retinacular (cervical) vessels ascend from an arterial ring around the base of the femoral neck and within the femoral neck in the joint capsule and are routed through the posterior capsule.

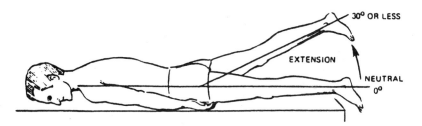

Fig. 2-4. Extension involves bringing the straight leg back through the plane of the body. The angle is measured by hyperextending the leg while the patient lies prone. The normal angle of extension is 30 degrees.

- Medullary vessels are located in the femoral neck.
- Vessels of lesser importance travel through the ligamentum teres (the round ligament of the femur).

The retinacular and medullary arteries are the most important of the three vessel groups, and both can be damaged if a fracture occurs across the femoral neck (Paton, 1988).

2.10 RISK FACTORS AND PREVENTION

Approximately 280,000 hip fractures occur in the United States annually; these fractures occur almost entirely among individuals age 65 or older (Zuckerman, et al., 1993) and are more prevalent in women than men (Jarnlo and Thorngren, 1990). Based on the increasing size of the elderly population, annual hip fracture figures have been projected to be as high as 500,000 per year by the year 2000 (Ochs, 1990).

The increased incidence of hip fracture in the elderly is a direct result of age-related changes, including a loss in postural stability and decreased bone strength (Jarnlo and Thorngren, 1990). Therefore, prevention must focus on reducing the risk of falls and increasing bone strength. Because the hip fracture rate increases exponentially with age, any interventions that lead to postponement possess the potential to reduce incidence substantially.

2.11 Falls

Unlike other age populations, the majority of hip fractures among the elderly occur as a result of moderate trauma, most frequently a

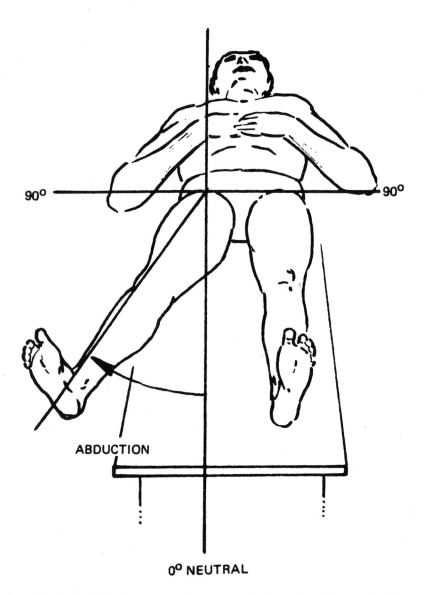

Fig. 2-5. Abduction moves the leg out to the side of the body. The normal range of abduction is 45 degrees from the neutral position (0 degrees).

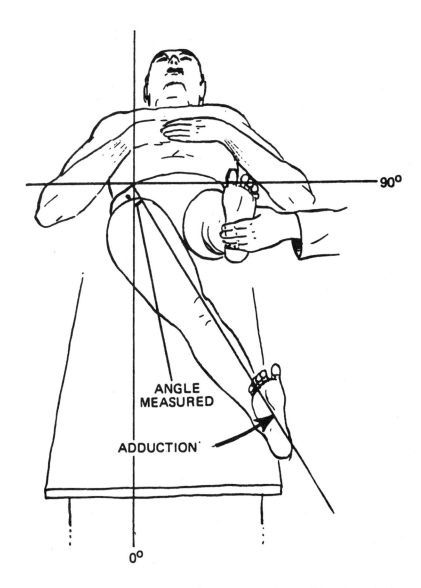

Fig. 2-6. Adduction moves the leg across the midline of the body. The normal range of adduction is 30 degrees from the neutral position (0 degrees).

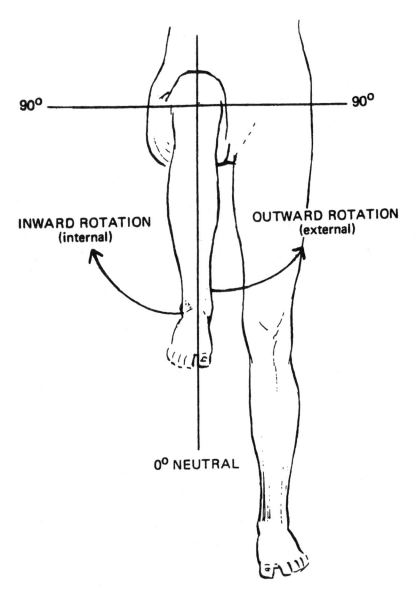

Fig. 2-7. Internal and external rotation are measured with the hip and knee flexed to 90 degrees.

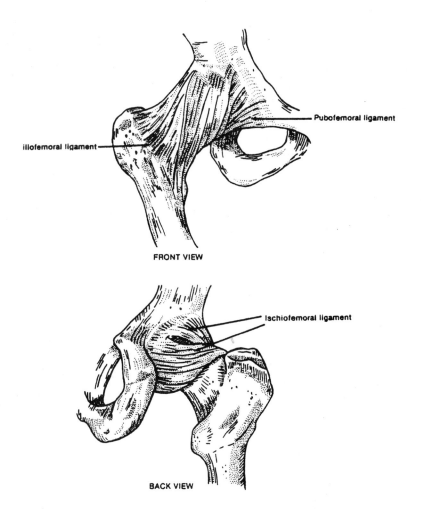

FRONT VIEW

Pubofemoral ligament

Iliofemoral ligament

Ischiofemoral ligament

BACK VIEW

Fig. 2-8. The ligaments of the hip reinforce the joint capsule and help maintain joint stability.

fall from a standing height (Heithoff and Lohr, 1990). Up to 90 percent of hip fractures among the elderly are attributed to such falls (Grisso, et al., 1991). Although all elderly individuals have an increased potential for hip fracture, two groups from opposite ends of the spectrum emerge as being especially at risk: "frequent fallers," who are physically and/or mentally infirm, and active elderly individuals engaged in outside activities such as shopping, walking or dancing. Not all elderly hip fracture patients fit into these bipolar categories, of course, but the delineation is a key one, as it has distinct implications for the expected degree of recovery (Dodson and Seymour, 1992).

Several factors affect the likelihood of fracture as a result of a fall, including bone strength, nature of the fall, protective muscle mass or fat tissue and the ability of the patient to engage in a protective response while falling.

Environmental conditions and structural hazards, such as ice, inadequate lighting, frayed rugs and electrical cords, are involved in as many as half of all falls. By assessing these factors, health care providers can assist the at-risk individual to reduce the likelihood of injury. Preventive interventions may include lowering beds, installing wall-to-wall carpet and providing aids such as grab bars and railings.

Other factors predisposing the elderly to falls include the presence of an acute or a chronic disease, mental or neurologic impairment and abnormalities of gait or balance (Heithoff and Lohr, 1990). In some elderly persons, reduced postural control and muscle strength in the lower extremities have shown improvement with training. By assigning the individual to a program of regular, tailored physical exercises such as walking, gymnastics or household activities, the likelihood of fracture can be reduced. Physical activity has the added benefit of preserving bone mineral content (Elliot, et al., 1992; Jarnlo and Thorngren, 1990).

Visual impairment has also been shown to be a significant factor in predisposing elderly individuals to hip fracture (Felson, et al., 1989). Prevention should include aggressive treatment of ocular disease or impairment (Porter, et al., 1990).

Psychotropic (affecting psychic function or behavior) medications have been consistently associated with a two- to three-fold increase in the risk of falls and hip fractures (Cumming and Klineberg, 1993). As a result, the prevention-minded physician should use such medications only when they are absolutely necessary, in as low a dose as possible, for the shortest possible duration.

Prevention of falls is vital for all elderly individuals. However, because the femoral bone density of many elderly women is considerably below the fracture threshold and measures to prevent further bone loss may be fruitless, reducing the risk of falling is especially important for them (Grisso, et al., 1991).

2.12   Bone Mass and Osteoporosis

Low bone mass is the most critical age-related factor in the increase of hip fractures in the elderly. Eighty percent of all hip fractures are associated with osteoporosis (the gradual loss of bone mass with aging), which correlates directly to several risk factors, including postmenopausal status, low body mass index (weight over height squared), sedentary life-style and physical inactivity, and possibly alcohol and tobacco use (Byyny and Speroff, 1990; Heithoff and Lohr, 1990). In America, white females have a much higher incidence of hip fracture than white males; however, that trend is often reversed in black and Asian populations, with men exhibiting the higher incidence of fracture (Maggi, et al., 1991).

Prevention of bone mass loss must begin early in life, since available treatments can preserve bone mass but not replace lost bone. Studies indicate that by instituting osteoporosis prevention methods for people at 40 to 50 years of age, the incidence of hip fracture in women in their late 80s and 90s can be dramatically reduced (Heithoff and Lohr, 1990). Estrogen replacement therapy has been shown to decrease the likelihood of hip fracture in newly menopausal women, but the benefits of this therapy for women 65 and older are unknown.

Recent studies have indicated that the risk of hip fracture in women can be assessed by measuring the level of circulating undercarboxylated osteocalcin (ucOC). An increase in ucOC reflects changes in the bone matrix (structure) associated with increased fragility (Szulc, et al., 1993).

Although the majority of bone mass loss studies focus on women, recent studies suggest that elderly men with testosterone (male hormone) deficiency are at increased risk for hip fracture, with elderly white men at greatest risk (Stanley, et al., 1991). Carefully monitored hormone replacement therapy is recommended as a preventive measure, using androgen (a hormone responsible for development of male characteristics) (Jackson, et al., 1992).

The use of thiazide diuretics has been supported as a method of enhancing skeletal strength; however, these medications may also result in episodes of orthostatic hypotension (decrease in blood pressure upon assuming erect posture), which creates dizziness and places the patient at an increased risk for falls. Recent studies draw inconsistent conclusions regarding the use of thiazide diuretics for protection against hip fracture (Heidrich, et al., 1991).

Some medications, including anticonvulsants, corticosteroids and replacement thyroid hormones, actually contribute to bone loss and increase the risk of fracture. Therefore, they should be administered with these effects in mind and given only after consideration of alternative therapies.

Artificial fluoridation of water, a common practice in some metropolitan areas, has also been shown to increase the risk of hip fracture in the elderly (Danielson, et al., 1992).

Physical activity has been shown to increase bone mineral density; as a result, it should be prescribed by health care providers in both a preventive and recuperative capacity appropriate to the individual.

2.20 DIAGNOSIS OF HIP FRACTURE

Patients with hip fracture characteristically have a history of a recent fall and seek medical attention because of pain in the region of the hip. The affected leg exhibits shortening, abduction (deviation away from the anatomic midline) and external rotation.[1]

Although they are very unusual, incidents of clinically occult (lacking the presentation of symptoms) hip fractures have been recorded. A delay in the diagnosis of such cases leads to a significant increase in complications and morbidity.[2] A high index of suspicion, including a range-of-motion assessment despite a negative history, and the use of radiographic diagnostic tools are recommended (Lindberg, et al., 1992).

If a fracture is suspected, it should be splinted immediately and traction applied to prevent soft tissue and vascular injury. Great care must be taken to protect the fracture during all patient transfers, during radiography (x-raying and other diagnostic imaging procedures) and while positioning, as additional comminution (splintering into fragments) can compound the problem of fixation (Bray and Templeman, 1988).

An anteroposterior (front-to-back) view of the pelvis and a lateral radiograph should be obtained to confirm the diagnosis, and pathologic (due to a disease rather than trauma) fractures should be ruled out. Computed tomography (CT) can also be used to diagnose traumatic

---

[1] See 2.01 *supra*.

[2] See 2.60 *infra*.

hip fracture. CT scans are useful in detecting loose bone fragments and fractures that may otherwise be overlooked, and as a result, this method can provide additional information when post-traumatic evaluation of the femoral head is difficult. Other modalities, including bone scans and magnetic resonance imaging (MRI), may be used, depending on necessity and their availability.

Some elderly patients are unable to tolerate the supine (lying on the back) traction position required for initial treatment of the injury. In this case, traction is abandoned and the patient is placed in an upright sitting position. Aspiration of the hip joint (removal of fluid through a hollow needle), accomplished with injection of local anesthetic, will lessen swelling and temporarily decrease the pain until the medical team decides if the patient is a good candidate for surgical treatment (Bray and Templeman, 1988).

2.30 PRINCIPLES OF FRACTURE MANAGEMENT

Reduction and immobilization are the primary methods of treatment. The goal is to have the patient mobile as soon as possible.

2.31 Reduction

To restore bone fragments to their normal anatomic position, a fracture is reduced (or "set"). Closed or open (operative) manipulation may be used.

Closed reduction is usually accomplished through manipulation and/or traction. The physician exerts a pulling force on the distal (farther from the point of origin or trunk of the body) fragment and a simultaneous counteraction on the proximal (closer to the point of origin or trunk of the body) fragment until the pieces move into place. Pressure is sometimes used to correct angulation or lateral displacement. Following manipulation, x-rays are taken to confirm that the fragments are in proper alignment.

If traction is used, a continuous pull is placed on the affected part to overcome muscle spasms and achieve reduction. Traction may be the sole means of reduction or a temporary method pending internal fixation.

During open reduction, the fracture site is surgically opened and the bone is placed into its proper position. Generally the fracture fragments are immobilized with internal fixation devices.

2.32 Immobilization

Immobilization is required to maintain the reduction until callus (a mixture of fibrous tissue, cartilage and immature bone) formation or bone healing has occurred. The purpose of immobilization is to hold the fragments together and prohibit movement. The most common methods of hip fracture immobilization involve internal fixation (the use of nails, plates, pins, wires, screws or rods to hold bone fragments together). Spica casts (plaster casts that incorporate the affected limb and a portion of the trunk of the body) are rarely used.

2.33 Internal Fixation

The choice of internal fixation device depends on the preference of the surgeon and the nature of the injury.

The cannulated screw is used primarily to reduce noncomminuted (not fragmented) intracapsular (within the confines of the hip capsule) fractures. These screws are introduced percutaneously (through the skin), which makes them valuable for the treatment of high-risk surgical patients.

Nail devices are also commonly used to stabilize hip fractures. Previously popular types include the Jewett nail, a device that is driven into the femoral neck and head and secured to the femoral shaft with a series of screws, and the Smith-Petersen nail, which operates similarly but requires a side plate for proper fixation.

Sliding nails and compression (condylar) plates are available in several varieties, including the Massie sliding nail, which is no longer used as often as in the past. The Richards compression screw and plate is more commonly used now. After being driven into the femoral head, the sliding screw or nail of these devices can be tightened, theoretically drawing the fracture fragments together and holding them firmly in place.

Prosthetic replacement devices may also be used in hip fracture repair.[3] These include uncemented varieties, which rely on fenestration (openings) and porous surfaces for eventual stabilization due to bony ingrowth, and cemented varieties, which are stabilized with an acrylic cement. The cemented prostheses are the fixation device of choice for intracapsular fractures (those that occur within the joint

---

[3] *See also* ch. 3.

capsule) in patients over the age of 75, as they allow early ambulation and mobility.

2.40 SPECIAL MANAGEMENT CONSIDERATIONS IN THE ELDERLY

Hip fracture in the elderly patient is associated with an increased mortality rate greater than that of the general population (Bredahl, et al., 1992). Age and other contributing factors dictate that comprehensive perioperative evaluation and management are essential in the successful treatment of these patients.

Although the great majority of elderly hip fracture patients are treated with open (operative) surgical procedures, studies of morbidity and mortality after hip fracture have revealed that the potential for complications is serious and that these complications can be divided into two general categories: those related to the injury and its treatment, and those due to co-morbidity (co-existing disease) (Ochs, 1990). Advanced age, dementia and the presence of illness have been identified as increased risk factors for mortality in patients with hip fractures; operative treatment for patients with failing mental ability has been deemed inappropriate by some physicians. Nonoperative treatment of elderly immobile patients has resulted in some reduction of morbidity and mortality; however, providing adequate pain relief and additional nursing care are essential elements of this treatment choice (Wood, et al., 1992).

When surgery is chosen, some controversy exists as to how rapidly it should be performed. Several studies have suggested that surgery within 24 hours is desirable; others suggest that some patients are better served if time is taken to stabilize and/or correct co-existing medical conditions first.

In general, surgical stabilization of the fracture should take place as soon as possible, as otherwise-healthy patients who are operated on within 12 hours of the injury have a higher long-term survival rate and a lower rate of the attendant morbidities that are common to bedridden elderly patients (Parker and Pryor, 1992).

For patients with a poorly controlled, active medical condition, such as congestive heart failure or respiratory compromise, surgery may be intentionally delayed, as preoperative status is an important factor affecting postoperative mortality (Bredahl, 1992).

Some patients (including those with pre-existing medical conditions, dementia and those confined to a nursing home at the time of fracture) are at especially high risk for perioperative complications. Major surgery is costly in physical, mental and financial terms; for these individuals, no appreciable improvement in functional status is achieved, and death within three to six months is probable (Heithoff and Lohr, 1990).

As a result, conservative nonsurgical intervention has been considered as an alternative method of management. Information is limited, but some studies have reported a reduction in mortality and morbidity in patients managed in the nursing home setting rather than transferred to an acute care hospital. In these studies, careful management of pain and skin integrity eliminated major complications, and patients became pain-free after four to six weeks (Ochs, 1990; Wood, et al., 1992).

Current predictors of patients for whom hip fracture treatment should take a nonsurgical form include the following (Heithoff and Lohr, 1990):

- inability to walk three months prior to the fracture;
- low ADL (activities of daily living) status prior to admission;
- a compressed fracture; and
- cancer of the hip.

2.50   CLASSIFICATION AND TREATMENT

Hip fracture locations are classified as being either intracapsular (within the capsule of the hip joint) or extracapsular (outside the capsule). (*See Figure 2–9.*) The fractures themselves are generally divided into three types: femoral neck, intertrochanteric and subtrochanteric (Ochs, 1990; Heithoff and Lohr, 1990). Due to their location within the confines of the hip capsule, femoral neck fractures are characterized as intracapsular; intertrochanteric and subtrochanteric fractures occur just outside the insertion of the hip capsule and are thus characterized as extracapsular. These distinctions are important because the nature of the bone and of the biomechanical stresses varies at each area and, as a result, so do etiology, treatment and recovery.

2.51   Femoral Neck Fractures

The neck of the femur connects the femoral head to the shaft of the bone, is roughly pyramidal in shape and is smaller than the head

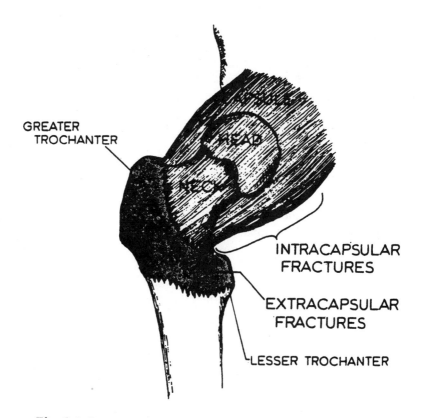

GREATER
TROCHANTER

INTRACAPSULAR
FRACTURES

EXTRACAPSULAR
FRACTURES

LESSER TROCHANTER

Fig. 2-9. Intracapsular and extracapsular fractures. The head and neck of the femur are located inside the joint capsule; the trochanters are outside it.

or the shaft. Considerable controversy exists regarding the treatment of femoral neck fractures. In fact, due to the significant failure rate after primary fixation of these fractures, this type of injury is historically referred to as the "unsolved fracture."

Because the femoral neck and head are enclosed entirely within the joint capsule, they have no periosteum (fibrous outer sheath of bones). In addition, it is common for the arterial blood supply to be interrupted if displacement of fracture fragments occurs. As a result, the serious complication of avascular necrosis (cell death due to decrease or cessation in the blood supply) of the femoral head can occur.[4]

---

[4] *See* 2.70 *infra.*

[1]   Classification

Femoral neck fractures are classified in "Garden stages," as follows:

- Garden stage I is the least severe and is manifested as an incomplete or impacted fracture.
- Garden stage II is complete but nondisplaced.
- Garden stage III is complete and partially displaced.
- Garden stage IV is complete and totally displaced.

[2]   Treatment

Garden stage I and II fractures are most commonly treated with anatomic reduction and stable internal fixation. Patients who seek medical attention with an impacted fracture several weeks after injury and are walking without pain can be treated conservatively, as can patients who represent a high surgical risk, are exhibiting resolution of pain and are able to engage in good range of motion without pain. Internal fixation is recommended for all other patients (Levin, et al., 1989).

It is usually possible to attain multiple pin fixation under spinal or local anesthetic. In order to provide better stability, pinning should be accomplished with several small pins spread into the femoral head (Paton, 1988), although excellent results have been obtained with the use of one large pin (Heithoff and Lohr, 1990).

Conflicting views persist in the treatment of the more severe Garden stage III and IV hip fractures, and few useful criteria exist to assist practitioners in choosing between reduction (manual manipulation to return fracture fragments to their normal anatomic position) and internal fixation, primary hemiarthroplasty (replacement of the femoral head with a prosthesis) or primary total hip arthroplasty. Most physicians base their treatment choices for these fractures on personal experience (Heithoff and Lohr, 1990).

Theoretically, hemiarthroplasty and total hip arthroplasty (partial and total replacement of the hip joint) offer the best opportunities to avoid the complication of nonunion. However, the higher rate of perioperative morbidity and problems with loosening of the components have kept these methods from becoming universally accepted as the treatment of choice. Compared to an infection rate of 0.5 percent for Knowles pinnings, infection in primary prosthetic replacements averages nearly 11 percent (Bray and Templeman, 1988).

[a]   Internal Fixation Methods

A simple procedure that was used often in the past is Knowles pinning, in which multiple pins are advanced from the trochanteric region into the femoral neck and head. Knowles pinning can be performed under local anesthesia and provides reasonable stability. However, weight-bearing precautions must be strictly maintained. In general, touch-down weight-bearing can be initiated two to five days postsurgery; progression to full weight-bearing is delayed for up to three months. Jewitt nails are also used.

The use of a compression screw provides somewhat greater stability and has largely replaced Knowles pinning. Cautious weight-bearing and ambulation can generally be instituted more rapidly using this device than Knowles pinning or Jewitt nailing allows.

The use of sliding nails or compression screws allows compression and stabilization of fracture fragments. In theory, this should provide better contact between the fragments and improve healing, and in reality, modern methods of fixation coupled with good reduction result in union (complete and properly aligned healing of the fracture) in 90 percent of cases and a less than 20 percent rate of occurrence of avascular necrosis; nonetheless, nonunion of femoral neck fractures and avascular necrosis of the femoral head are possibilities. As a result, many surgeons elect to treat Garden III and IV fractures by replacing the joint with a prosthesis. One of two procedures is used: hemiarthroplasty or total hip arthroplasty.

[b]   Hemiarthroplasty

Hemiarthroplasty involves the resection (surgical cutting to remove a portion) of the femoral neck and head, reaming of the femoral canal and placement of a noncemented metallic prosthesis. Many surgeons use the procedure in the treatment of displaced (out of normal anatomic alignment)[5] femoral neck fractures as a matter of course, due to its ability to eliminate the complications of avascular necrosis and nonunion. Regardless of preference, the procedure is recommended in the case of pathologic fractures (due to a disease process rather than trauma) and is absolutely indicated for the surgeon who is unable to achieve a satisfactory stable reduction of a displaced fracture, or in the event of the loss of the reduced position during attempted nailing.

---

[5] *See* 2.52[1] *infra.*

Surgical texts indicate that hemiarthroplasty has the advantage of being stable enough to institute immediate full weight-bearing. However, commonly accepted rehabilitation programs recommend touch-down weight-bearing the day after surgery, with progression to full weight-bearing in six to eight weeks. Total hip precautions (in which motions involving the hip are contraindicated postsurgically) should be observed for three weeks after surgery.

Postoperative dislocation occurs in up to 15 percent of hemiarthroplasties. Dislocation requires treatment involving reduction, prolonged traction, casting or re-operation (Ochs, 1990). It is also common that patients who are active and have a good life expectancy will suffer eventual degeneration of the acetabulum due to cartilage trauma caused by the head of the prosthesis.

[c]   Total Hip Arthroplasty

Degeneration of the acetabulum necessitates revision to a total hip arthroplasty, in which both the femoral head and the acetabular surface are replaced with prosthetic devices. As a result, some sources recommend total hip arthroplasty as the treatment of choice for displaced femoral neck fractures. Other indications for the use of total hip arthroplasty to repair a hip fracture include pre-existing rheumatoid arthritis (Levin, et al., 1989), severe comminution, pathologic fractures and neurologic conditions, including parkinsonism and hemiplegia (partial paralysis) (Bray and Templeman, 1988).

Since the hardware implanted during the total hip arthroplasty must serve as the primary load-bearing structure for the life of the patient, durability of the hardware and cement is of primary concern. Problems most often arise when components loosen as a result of repetitive impact loading. To avoid loosening, some noncemented prostheses are designed to allow the ingrowth of bone. Unfortunately, should this type of prosthesis loosen, the very attribute designed to prevent loosening renders removal of the device very difficult.

Cemented devices are also susceptible to long-term loosening, and the implantation of acrylic cement into the femur may trigger serious, potentially fatal cardiovascular complications in elderly patients with pre-existing cardiac disease and/or hypovolemia (low blood volume) (Tryba, et al., 1991).[6]

---

[6] *See also* ch. 3.

2.52   Intertrochanteric Fractures

The greater and lesser trochanters are bony outgrowths on the upper end of the femur. Intertrochanteric fractures are by definition extracapsular, or outside the hip joint capsule. Almost universally, treatment of intertrochanteric fractures involves some form of internal fixation and an implanted device such as a pin and plate or intramedullary rods (rods that run along the center of the bone and stabilize fracture fragments).

[1]   Classification

A number of systems have been devised, but no generally accepted system of classification for intertrochanteric fractures has been established. In general, intertrochanteric fractures are classified as stable, nondisplaced or unstable. They are considered stable when there is posterior-medial support from the cortical bone (the compact structural element of bone) or the possibility of establishing such support. The degree to which the fractured elements are displaced from their normal anatomic position as well as the extent of comminution (the number of small fragments) are important considerations. (*See Figure 2–10.*)

The Boyd and Griffin system divided fractures into types I through IV. Type I and type II were undisplaced and displaced fractures, respectively. The type III fracture exhibited reverse obliquity (slant),

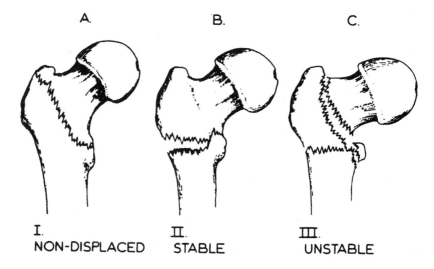

Fig. 2-10. Classification of intertrochanteric fractures.

and a type IV fracture was comminuted and unstable. The Evans system attempted to classify fractures with greater specificity based on stability of the fracture. Further modifications of the Evans system have been developed by both Jensen and Kyle and colleagues (Levin, et al., 1989).

Because unstable intertrochanteric fractures are prone to failure of fixation, classification is important. Because of possible confusion arising from the several classification systems that exist, practitioners must be sure the entire treatment team has a clear understanding of the system in use.

[2]   Treatment

Although methods of fixation for intertrochanteric fractures are similar to those used to repair femoral neck fractures, the procedures for stabilization differ somewhat.

Sliding nails or compression screws are the most commonly used fixation devices. It is important to select a nail or compression screw of a length to permit good purchase in the neck fragment while allowing for the collapse that will occur as the fracture impacts (Levin, et al., 1989). Introducing a device of too great a length may result in late penetration of the femoral head.

Treatment of intertrochanteric fractures by osteotomy (surgical cutting of bone) and medial displacement has been advocated by some authors. This procedure involves the use of femoral osteotomy at the base of the greater trochanter and medial displacement of the femoral shaft, which is then impacted onto a spike fashioned from a portion of the head and neck fragment. A telescoping nail or screw device is then used to secure the fixation at an angle of 150 degrees.

This procedure results in shortening of the limb, and although some shortening can be overcome by abduction (movement away from the midline of the body) of the limb prior to fixation, functional abnormalities remain. As a result, the procedure is not recommended unless the inherent stability of the fixation will strongly affect the patient's prognosis.

Retrograde intramedullary fixation has the ability to stabilize fractures and allow weight-bearing. This is a procedure that involves the insertion of multiple flexible intramedullary pins through a hole in the region of the femur just proximal (closer to the trunk or point of origin) to the medial femoral condyle (smooth, rounded eminence on the end of a bone, which enters into the formation of a joint with another bone), However, it is unsuitable for unstable fractures (Levin, et al., 1989).

[3] Prognosis

Intertrochanteric fracture are usually comminuted (fragmented) and osteoporotic in nature. This makes good anatomic reduction difficult and fixation prone to instability. Patients with intertrochanteric fractures can expect to have delayed ability to bear weight, poorer functional outcome and higher mortality rates than patients with fractures of the femoral neck (Ochs, 1990). However, the vascular supply to the femoral neck and head is rarely disrupted, and the bone in the affected area has a periosteum. As a result, the development of avascular necrosis[7] and nonunion is unlikely.

2.53 Subtrochanteric Fractures

Subtrochanteric fractures occur above the shaft and below an imaginary line drawn between the greater and lesser trochanters. Femoral neck and intertrochanteric fractures make up 97 percent of all proximal femur fractures. The remaining 3 percent are subtrochanteric. The management of these fractures is made difficult by the fact that the region is often under high mechanical stress. In addition, the bone is mainly cortical (lacking periosteum), and comminution is frequent (Levin, et al., 1989; Ochs, 1990).

[1] Classification

The Fielding classification system divides subtrochanteric fractures as follows:

- Type I fractures occur at the level of the lesser trochanter.
- Type II fractures occur from 1 to 2 inches below the upper border of the lesser trochanter.
- Type III fractures occur from 2 to 3 inches below the upper border of the lesser trochanter.

In addition, subtrochanteric fractures have been classified as simple fractures (which may be transverse, oblique or spiral); those with lateral and those with medial butterfly fragments; and those that are comminuted or shattered. (*See Figure 2–11.*)

---

[7] *See 2.70 infra.*

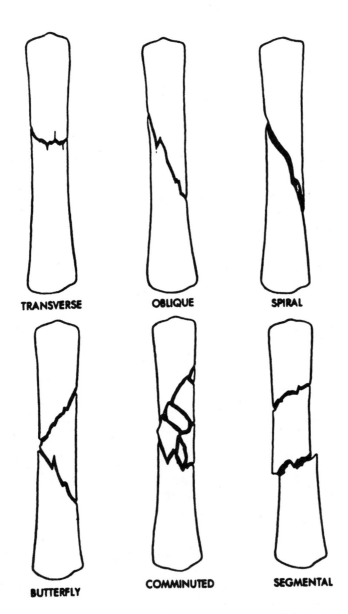

Fig. 2-11. Nomenclature for common types of fractures of the femur.

[2]   Treatment

Due to muscle action, the proximal fragment (closer to the trunk of the body) of a subtrochanteric fracture is frequently abducted (moved away from the midline of the body) and externally rotated, and open reduction[8] and internal fixation[9] are mandatory.

Simple fractures can be reduced and fixation achieved through the use of a lag screw prior to insertion of a condylar plate. When butterfly fragments are present, they should first be reduced and fixed with lag screws, thus converting the fracture to a simple fracture, which is then fixed with a condylar plate.

If a fracture is severely comminuted, the condylar plate should be inserted into the proximal fragment prior to reduction. Fragments should then be repositioned and fixed in an order that is determined preoperatively. Medial cancellous (spongy tissue) bone grafting may be required. A T-shaped plate allowing three cancellous screws to be introduced into the neck may also be useful in treating fractures of this nature.

Intramedullary nails (long nails that run inside the length of the femur) have frequently been used to treat subtrochanteric fractures, and the Zickel nail was for a time seen by some as the internal fixation device of choice (Chapman, 1988). When it is inserted into the femoral head and neck, it offers excellent stability. In cases in which severe comminution is present, additional stabilization achieved through the use of cerclage wiring (a process of encircling fractures with wire) may be required.

If comminution extends into the middle and distal portions of the diaphysis (shaft of the bone), the Grosse-Kempf nail is preferred (Chapman, 1988). Easier to insert by closed methods, this device can be secured distally with screws, giving it the ability to prevent shortening and rotational instability. Once the callus has formed on the bone as a normal part of healing, the fixation can be converted to a dynamic fixation by removing the distal screws, thus exposing the callus to weight-bearing stresses that facilitate union. It should be noted that dynamization (exposure to stress), although it is desirable in many cases, is not necessary to achieve proper union.

---

8 *See* 2.31 *supra.*

9 *See* 2.33 *supra.*

The Grosse-Kempf nail should not be used if the fracture line is not completely below the level of the lesser trochanter.

The Ender nailing technique is another intramedullary system designed specifically with elderly subtrochanteric fracture patients in mind (Ender, 1988). A number of Ender pins (prebent, flexible, solid pins with an oblique tip at one end and an eye in a flange at the other) are inserted at the medial femoral condyle of the knee joint. Two or three nails are introduced from the medial condyle and passed through the medullary canal in the center of the bone to the proximal fragment. One or two nails are then introduced through the lateral condyle into or through the greater trochanter. Enough nails must be used to fully fill the medullary canal, and the nails should create a V-shaped formation in the fracture site, which increases general stability and rotatory stability. This method has varying degrees of popularity among practitioners.

Patients with stable fractures are allowed out of bed one or two days after surgery, and full weight-bearing can be performed with the help of physical therapists.

2.60   COMPLICATIONS

Many complications of hip fractures in the elderly can be avoided or substantially minimized through careful management by the entire health care team. The literature reflects that improved postoperative management has reduced the death rate among hip fracture patients. Despite advances in treatment, however, hip fracture continues to be associated with increased mortality beyond that of the general population (Bredahl, et al., 1992). The one-year mortality rate of 12 to 25 percent over the norm has remained unchanged for a decade (Eiskjaer, et al., 1992; Heithoff and Lohr, 1990).

2.61   Failure

Hip surgery can fail immediately or over time. Immediate failure is generally attributable to infection. Delayed failure is generally attributable to loosening of the fixation device or avascular necrosis (cell death due to decrease or cessation in the blood supply).[10]

---

10 *See* 2.70 *infra.*

Should avascular necrosis occur, the fixation devices are removed. The head of the femur is then removed, and arthroplasty (insertion of an artificial hip joint) is performed.[11]

Naturally the patient who must undergo this process, which is known as revision, will follow a delayed, more conservative course of rehabilitative treatment (Goldstein, 1991).

2.62   Deep Vein Thrombosis and Pulmonary Embolism

Embolic (clot-related) disease occurs following hip fracture at a rate of more than 50 percent (Levin, et al., 1989). Deep vein thrombosis (formation of clots) and pulmonary embolism (migration of a clot to the pulmonary vessels, resulting in blockage and the possibility of respiratory collapse) are extensively studied as complications of hip surgery; however, a consensus does not exist as to what constitutes adequate preventive measures.

The incidence of deep vein thrombosis can be decreased by the delivery of prophylactic anticoagulants (medicines that work to prevent clotting), including aspirin, subcutaneously or intravenously administered heparin, phenindione, warfarin, low molecular weight dextran and heparin with dihydroergotamine; application of external pneumatic compression is also helpful, as it maintains adequate circulation. Despite the evidence supporting the use of low-dose anticoagulants, controversy continues, and many orthopedic surgeons indicate a significant amount of resistance to their use (Ochs, 1990).

2.63   Skin Compromise

Hip fracture patients may be at risk for pressure-related skin breakdown even before they arrive in postoperative care. Tissue damage can occur if the patient was immobile for an extended time prior to treatment, and the condition can be exacerbated by immobility and the hard surfaces encountered during ambulance transfers, emergency room evaluation, and x-ray and other diagnostic procedures.

The literature indicates that anywhere from 20 percent to 70 percent of patients with hip fractures will develop pressure sores (decubitus ulcers). Patients should be evaluated for risk of skin breakdown with appropriate scorable assessment tools, and prevention should include the routine use of egg-crate mattresses and heel protectors, daily skin care and evaluation, and proper hydration and nutrition (Ochs, 1990).

---

[11] See 2.51[2][c] supra.

2.64   Delirium

Thirty percent to 50 percent of patients undergoing surgical repair of hip fractures are in a condition of postoperative confusion. A major cause of morbidity in the elderly, the condition is frequently a response to systemic stressors, including medications, underlying infections and attendant medical conditions. Appropriate treatment and alleviation of the cause are critical; during the period of confusion, patients are at high risk for developing other complications (Ochs, 1990).

2.65   Urinary Complications

Urinary tract infection (UTI) is reported in 10 to 20 percent of hip surgery patients; urinary retention occurs in up to 52 percent.[12] Generally attributed to the use of narcotic analgesics, retention can be combated through the prophylactic use of an indwelling urethral catheter inserted at the time of surgery and retained for 24 hours postoperatively. Use of a catheter for more than 48 hours results in an increase in urinary tract infections (Ochs, 1992).

2.66   Miscellaneous Complications

Infection at the operative site occurs in a small number of patients; of these infections, the majority are superficial and do not affect bone or hardware. Modern surgical techniques and equipment, coupled with the routine perioperative use of broad-spectrum antibiotics, have dramatically improved wound infection rates.

Occasionally hip fracture patients will develop neuropathies (disorders of the nerves) resulting from traction or pressure injuries to peripheral nerves (nerves of the extremities).

The candidate for hip surgery must be evaluated for cardiac status, as the potential for intraoperative hypotension (low blood pressure) exists as a result of two factors:

- the increased incidence of hypotension in patients undergoing spinal anesthesia; and

- the possibility of a significant drop in mean systolic blood pressure due to the introduction of acrylic cement during total hip arthroplasty.

---

12 *See also* ch. 13 for a discussion of urinary tract infection in women and ch. 14 for a discussion of male urogenital problems.

Other potential complications are similar to those associated with general surgery, and pre-, peri- and post-operative assessment and treatment should be delivered appropriately.

2.70 AVASCULAR NECROSIS

Avascular necrosis refers to necrosis, or cell death, that occurs in the absence of infection. It usually occurs in bone when the blood supply to a specific area is disrupted. The hip is the most common site of avascular necrosis, often as a result of hip fracture. When avascular necrosis occurs after a nontraumatic event, it is called idiopathic (primary) necrosis.

Several conditions are associated with avascular necrosis. Those with definite associations include major trauma, Gaucher's disease (a metabolic disorder in which there is an inadequate amount of the enzyme beta-glucosidase in the blood), sickle cell disease (a form of anemia in which the red blood cells assume a crescent or sickle shape rather than being round) and other hemoglobinopathies (diseases characterized by abnormal hemoglobin, the iron-carrying component of blood), and decompression sickness (caused by entering an environment of low atmospheric pressure). Conditions with less certain associations include minor trauma, connective tissue disease, alcoholism, various lipid disorders, gout and hyperuricemia (an excessive level of uric acid in the blood), and high levels of glucocorticoid, whether endogenous (originating within the body), as in Cushing's disease, or exogenous (originating outside the body).

Although the conditions under which avascular necrosis occurs are well known (in most cases it is trauma-related), the etiology remains unknown. Avascular necrosis is probably a result of a combination of mechanical and biological factors.

Avascular necrosis most often occurs in men who are in their 40s and 50s. They have severe chronic pain, usually in one hip; about half of these patients have similar pain in the other hip within several years. Joint motion usually remains good until secondary degenerative arthritis develops. Often a total hip replacement is necessary.

2.71 Mechanisms of Avascular Necrosis and Bone Ischemia

Bone death (necrosis) is always due to ischemia (localized anemia due to a mechanical obstruction of the blood supply). When the blood supply to the bone is cut off (including vascular, fat, marrow, cartilage and bone tissues), it no longer receives adequate oxygen. The ischemia can be due to either an interruption in the arterial supply of blood to the bone or by an occlusion (blockage) within the venous drainage system, resulting in gradual oxygen starvation.

Avascular necrosis is usually found in the bulbous ends of long bones, such as the head or the distal end of the femur (thighbone). The ends of these bones are made of a shell of cortical bone (a thin layer of compact bone) that surrounds a mass of cancellous (spongy) bone that looks like a honeycomb. Cancellous bone is packed with myeloid tissue (derived from or having certain features of bone marrow), fatty marrow and a vascular network that carries blood to and from the tissues. The blood vessels enter and leave this confined space through openings in the periosteum (the thick membrane that covers the surface of a bone) and along the medullary canal (the cavity within the shaft of a long bone where the marrow is contained). Necrosis (tissue death) occurs when the vascular supply is disrupted, either by an outside force (trauma) or the expansion of marrow or another substance within the cavity. Expansion within the nonexpandable space results in an increase in pressure.

It is estimated that bone cells die after 12 to 48 hours without oxygen; marrow fat cells die within five days under the same conditions. However, both physically and radiographically, the bone seems unchanged for some time after its death begins. When visible changes do appear, they are often of two types: failure (collapse) of the dead bone and reparative bone formation. Avascular necrosis is rarely detected on x-rays before six months after onset, but it is usually apparent within two years.

2.72 Factors Associated with Avascular Necrosis

Avascular necrosis is associated with trauma and a variety of disease states and conditions. Bone death often results after severe trauma, fracture and/or dislocation. It is a result of ischemia (inadequate blood supply) secondary to disruption of the blood supply to the bone in these areas. Bone near articular (joint) surfaces seems to be most at risk. The likelihood of avascular necrosis rises with increasing degrees of displacement of the bone (displaced fractures are associated with severe trauma to the surrounding structures).

In dislocations of the femur, avascular necrosis could be due to either arterial insufficiency or venous engorgement. In these cases, the chances of necrosis are increased if reduction (returning the bone to its normal position) is delayed. Necrosis can also occur as a result of internal fixation for certain hip fractures.

2.73 Natural History of Avascular Necrosis

Although avascular necrosis has many etiologies, the natural history is largely the same. Subtle symptoms may precede radiologic changes by several months to two years. Patients rarely seek medical advice in the early stages of disease, however.

When the disease proceeds slowly, the level and frequency of pain and joint dysfunction will suddenly increase. X-rays taken at that time will typically show the crescent sign—an indicator of late disease caused by the collapse of a large segment of the joint surface. Prior to this finding, subtle changes may have been apparent on x-rays. A definite diagnosis can be made through a core biopsy. Most observations and conclusions made about avascular necrosis are based on studies of the hip, the knee and especially the femoral head (the spherical top portion of the thighbone that fits into the hip socket).

The early phases of the disease are characterized by intermittent episodes of pain in the groin, knee, trochanters (two rounded bony prominences at the top of the femur, below the head) or buttock; sometimes the patient limps. X-rays taken at this time are usually normal, but repeated x-rays will reveal diffuse or spotty increases in radiodensity within the femoral head, indicating early collapse. In many patients, the first radiographic evaluation will reveal some collapse. Once either the crescent sign (a cardinal late indicator of disease) or some collapse is noted, disease progression is essentially inevitable.

2.74 Diagnosis

Avascular necrosis can be diagnosed in a number of ways. X-rays, bone scans, computed tomography (CT), magnetic resonance imaging (MRI), intraosseous pressure measurement and intraosseous venograms are all tools used in the staging and diagnosis of avascular necrosis.

[1] X-rays

Radiographic evidence of avascular necrosis varies. After a period of time, microscopic stress fractures develop in the cancellous bone, and as they run together, larger cracks and fissures begin to appear. Often the crescent sign (an indicator of late disease caused by collapse of a large segment of the joint surface) is seen in the dead bone due to a subarticular (under the joint) fracture. Another radiographic sign of bone necrosis is increased bone density in the affected area due to the development of new bone around the dead bone.

Several systems have been proposed for classifying, or staging, avascular necrosis on the basis of radiographic signs. One system includes four stages (Ficat and Arlet, 1980):

- stage I—bone appears normal in x-rays, patient has some symptoms, bone scans are positive;

- stage II—radiographic evidence of disease exists, but joint remains intact;

- stage III—disease is definitely evident on x-rays, there is partial collapse of the head of the bone, the crescent sign, indicating cancellous bone compression, may be observed; and

- stage IV—the disease resembles arthrosis or inflammatory arthritis in x-rays, biopsy needed for definitive diagnosis.

Several other classification systems further subdivide the stages of disease. Although those systems are not as widely used as the four-stage grouping outlined here, further delineation of the various stages may prove to be useful in the future as the number of treatment modalities increases.

[2] Bone Scans

Radionuclide imaging of bone, or bone scans, can often detect avascular necrosis before it is apparent on x-rays. Bone scans with 99mTechnetium-labeled phosphate or phosphate complex (99mTc; bone-seeking radionuclide contrast media) are commonly used in the diagnosis of avascular necrosis. A scan measures the bone's "uptake" of 99mTc, an indication of disease (Bonnarens, et al., 1985).

During stage I of the disease, the bone scan will appear normal or show a slight increase in uptake of contrast medium as the repair process begins. Stage II shows new bone formation and increased blood flow to the area. A large increase in the uptake of 99mTc is evident. Stages III and IV also show increased uptake of 99mTc because of increased cellular activity as the bone ineffectively attempts to repair itself.

Although bone scans can detect disease before the onset of symptoms and before it is detected on x-rays, scans are often used only after radiologic changes have been noticed. Thus, the usefulness of the test as a diagnostic aid is greatly reduced.

[3]   Computed Tomography (CT) and Magnetic Resonance Imaging (MRI)

These two imaging modalities are both used in the diagnosis and staging of avascular necrosis. Often, they can detect the extent of disease more accurately than x-rays and sometimes, in the later stages, they are more accurate than bone scans.

MRI has been the most sensitive method for detecting avascular necrosis (Kursunoglu-Brahme and Resnick, 1990). The advantages of this technique include:

- noninvasiveness;

- lack of ionizing radiation;

- high sensitivity to pathologic bone changes, enabling early detection of changes among asymptomatic patients at risk for developing avascular necrosis; and;

- capability of producing images of equal resolution in all planes.

[4]   Bone Marrow Pressure and Intraosseous Venography

An increase in bone marrow pressure is often a diagnostic sign of avascular necrosis. Such an increase is also predictive of the future development of radiologically apparent disease. Venography, in which a radiopaque substance is injected into a vein in order to observe blood flow, can detect impaired or abnormal drainage patterns in diseased bone.

2.75   Treatment

The treatment plan for avascular necrosis must include consideration of the patients's age, functional demands, body weight, previous surgery, presence of other disease or joint problems and stage of avascular necrosis. Many surgical treatments have been proposed, especially for avascular necrosis of the femoral head, but no one operation has been shown superior. The surgical procedure that is chosen should prevent collapse of the affected bone and, ultimately, degenerative arthritis.

[1] Nonoperative Treatment

Nonoperative treatment is aimed at reducing the stress placed on the affected bone. For example, among patients with femoral head disease, crutches, canes and other non-weight-bearing aids are used. Although most cases of avascular necrosis progress to collapse of the affected bone within three to five years, some reports cite instances in which collapse was prevented with nonoperative treatment. Such cases, however, are unusual (Meyers, 1988).

[2] Biopsy and Core Decompression

A biopsy, combined with other surgical procedures, can be therapeutic if it is performed in the early stages (I or II) of disease. In up to half of the patients treated this way, no further treatment is necessary (Kenzora, 1985). In the United States, this treatment is referred to as a *decompressive core* procedure and can be done with or without bone grafts. In Europe, multiple holes are drilled into the bone, a process called *forage*.

Core decompression with or without autogenous (from the patient's own body) bone grafts or forage procedures are often performed on patients with elevated marrow pressure on the asymptomatic side when clinically apparent disease is present on the opposite side. Success rates of 85 to 90 percent (i.e., the disease does not progress to stage III) have been reported (Meyers, 1988). This finding is significant because between 50 and 80 percent of patients with clinically apparent disease on one side develop disease on the opposite side as well. Why this procedure is successful is unclear, however. Moreover, there is debate as to whether the addition of bone grafts to the core compression surgery is beneficial (Meyers, 1988).

[3] Surgical Procedures Prior to Bone Collapse

A number of surgical procedures have been used to treat stages II and III of disease, including osteotomy (the cutting away of affected bone) and a muscle pedicle graft (a flap of tissue taken from the area of the greater trochanter of the femur and the quadratus femoris muscle of the hip and inserted into a large channel that has been cut in the affected bone). In the long term, the muscle pedicle graft, although it is technically difficult, may be the best procedure for this stage of disease.

[4]   Treatment for Late-stage Disease

Total hip replacement[13] and hip arthrodesis (fusion) are the treatments of choice for late-stage avascular necrosis of the femoral head when the hip joint has already degenerated. The use of artificial replacements in young patients is sometimes discouraged; the incidence of failure is high, due to loosening of the part and other factors that occur within ten years. The search continues for a biological approach to treatment.

2.80   REHABILITATION

The goal of rehabilitation for elderly individuals with hip fractures is to return them to a level of independence and activity equal to that which existed before the injury. The focus of rehabilitation should include not only the ability to walk and perform activities requiring mobility; it should also include the opportunity to live independently, function within the community, participate in social activities and continue other activities as wished (Heithoff and Lohr, 1990).

As noted earlier, great controversy exists in orthopedic medicine regarding the effects on fracture healing of the rate of progression through postoperative stages, including weight-bearing and mobility. Programs of rehabilitation vary depending on the type of institution, the philosophy of its doctors and therapists, and the nature of the patient's injury and course of treatment. Rehabilitation of some patients may involve twice-a-day treatments from a number of different therapists and daily physician evaluation while the patient remains in the hospital; others may go directly home from the hospital after recovering from surgery and receive outpatient care.

The following summary of the treatment of hip fractures has been cited as a general guideline for rehabilitation team members (Goldstein, 1991):

1. Know the type of fracture and internal fixation device, as well as the weight-bearing order.

2. During the first three weeks postoperatively:

---

13 See 2.52[2][c] *supra.*

- Protect the fracture site from unnecessary weight-bearing or rotational forces.
- Begin active assisted exercises in sitting, supine and prone positions, progressing to active independent exercises.
- Begin mobility and training for activities of daily living (ADL) concurrently.

As the fracture stabilizes, the following protocol should be followed:

1. Weight-bearing should progress according to the physician's order.
2. Begin active exercises in standing posture.
3. Customize exercises to include the patient's interests.
4. Discontinue total hip precautions on physician's order.
5. Begin aerobic conditioning.
6. Focus on normal function in mobility and activity of daily living skills.

As the fracture heals, the following guidelines are helpful:

1. Progress to full weight-bearing on physician's order.
2. Normalize gait pattern on all surfaces (with assistive device).
3. Begin proprioceptive (sense of one's position in space) and balance retraining.
4. Teach independence in all activities of daily living, with assistive device.

It is also important not to prescribe unnecessary equipment or exercises.

Philosophies vary among physicians, and a team approach including the orthopedic surgeon, primary care physician, nursing staff and other members of the therapy team is the key to successful rehabilitation of the hip fracture patient.

2.90   PROGNOSIS

Despite advances in surgical, anesthesiology and rehabilitation techniques, hip fractures continue to have a dramatic impact on older individuals. In one six-month study, nearly a fifth of the subjects died after the fracture occurred, and the vast majority of survivors suffered a substantial decline in physical function (Marottoli, 1992). Other studies have shown that 15 to 20 percent of patients with a hip fracture die due to the fracture or complications of it within three months; survivors are frequently severely disabled and may exhibit permanent impairment of function (Byyny and Speroff, 1990).

2.100 BIBLIOGRAPHY

Text References

Bonnarens, F., et al.: Bone Scintigraphic Changes in Osteonecrosis of the Femoral Head. Orthop. Clin. N. Am. 16:697–704, 1985.

Bray, T. J. and Templeman, D. C.: Fractures of the Femoral Neck. In: Chapman, M. W. and Madison, M. (Eds.): Operative Orthopaedics, vol. 1. Philadelphia: Lippincott, 1988.

Bredahl, C., et al.: Mortality After Hip Fracture: Results of Operation Within 12 Hours of Admission. Injury 23(2):83–86, 1992.

Byyny, R. L. and Speroff, L.: A Clinical Guide for the Care of Older Women. Baltimore: Williams & Wilkins, 1990.

Chapman, M. W.: Principles of Intramedullary Nailing. In: Chapman, M. W. and Madison, M. (Eds.): Operative Orthopaedics, vol. 1. Philadelphia: Lippincott, 1988.

Cumming, R. G. and Klineberg, R. J.: Psychotropics, Thiazide Diuretics and Hip Fractures in the Elderly. Med. J. Aust. 158(6):414–417, Mar. 1993.

Danielson, C., et al.: Hip Fractures and Fluoridation in Utah's Elderly Population. J.A.M.A. 268(6):746–748, Aug. 1992.

Dodson, M. E. and Seymour, G.: Surgery and Anaesthesia in Old Age. In: Brocklehurst, J. C., et al. (Eds.): Geriatric Medicine and Gerontology, 4th ed. New York: Churchill Livingstone, 1992.

Eiskjaer, S., et al.: Years of Potential Life Lost After Hip Fracture Among Postmenopausal Women. Acta. Orthop. Scand. 63(3):293–296, June 1992.

Elliot, J. R., et al.: A Comparison of Elderly Patients with Proximal Femoral Fractures and a Normal Elderly Population: A Case Control Study. N.Z. Med. J. 105(944):420–422, Oct. 1992.

Ender, H. G.: Ender Nailing of the Femur and Hip. In: Chapman, M. W. and Madison, M. (Eds.): Operative Orthopaedics, vol. 1. Philadelphia: Lippincott, 1988.

Felson, D. T., et al.: Impaired Vision and Hip Fracture: The Framingham Study. J. Am. Geriatr. Soc. 36:495–500, 1989.

Ficat, R. P. and Arlet, J.: Ischemia and Necroses of Bone. Baltimore: Williams and Wilkins, 1980.

Goldstein, T. S.: Geriatric Orthopaedics. Rockville, Md.: Aspen Publishers, 1991.

Grisso, J. A., et al.: Risk Factors for Falls as a Cause of Hip Fracture in Women. N. Engl. J. Med. 324(19):1326–1331, May 1991.

Heidrich, F. E., et al.: Diuretic Drug Use and the Risk for Hip Fracture. Ann. Intern. Med. 115(1):1–6, July 1991.

Heithoff, K. A. and Lohr, K. N.: Hip Fracture: Setting Priorities for Effectiveness Research. Washington, D.C.: National Academy Press, 1990.

Jackson, J. A., et al.: Testosterone Deficiency as a Risk Factor for Hip Fractures in Men: A Case Control Study. Am. J. Med. Sci. 304(1):4–8, July 1992.

Jarnlo, G. and Thorngren, K.: Background Factors to Hip Fractures. Clin. Orthop. 287:41–49, Jan. 1993.

Kenzora, J. E.: Treatment of Idiopathic Osteonecrosis: The Current Philosophy and Rationale. Orthop. Clin. N. Am. 16:717–726, 1985.

Kursunoglu-Brahme, S. and Resnick, D.: Magnetic Resonance Imaging of the Knee. Orthop. Clin. N. Am. 21:561–572, 1990.

Levin, P. E., et al.: Traumatic Injury to the Lower Limb in Adults. In: Dee, R., et al. (Eds.): Principles of Orthopaedic Practice. New York: McGraw-Hill, 1989.

Lindberg, E. J., et al.: Clinically Occult Presentation of Comminuted Intertrochanteric Hip Fractures. Ann. Emerg. Med. 21(12):1511–1514, Dec. 1992.

Maggi, S., et al.: Incidence of Hip Fractures in the Elderly: A Cross-National Analysis. Osteoporos. Int. 1(4):232–241, Sept. 1991.

Marottoli, R. A., et al.: Decline in Physical Function Following Hip Fracture. J. Am. Geriatr. Soc. 40(9):861–866, Sept. 1992.

Meyers, M. H.: Osteonecrosis of the Femoral Head: Pathogenesis and Long-Term Results of Treatment. Clin. Orthop. 231:51–61, 1988.

Ochs, M.: Surgical Management of the Hip in the Elderly Patient. Clin. Geriatr. Med. 6(3):571–587, Aug. 1990.

Parker, M. J. and Pryor, G. A.: The Timing of Surgery for Proximal Femoral Fractures. J. Bone Joint Surg. 74B(2):203–205, Mar. 1992.

Paton, D. F.: Fractures and Orthopaedics. New York: Churchill Livingstone, 1988.

Porter, R. W., et al.: Prediction of Hip Fracture in Elderly Women: A Prospective Study. Br. Med. J. 301(6753):638–641, Sept. 1990.

Stanley, H. L., et al.: Does Hypogonadism Contribute to the Occurrence of a Minimal Trauma Hip Fracture in Elderly Men? J. Am. Geriatr. Soc. 39(8):766–771, Aug. 1991.

Szulc, P., et al.: Serum Undercarboxylated Osteocalcin is a Marker of the Risk of Hip Fracture in Elderly Women. J. Clin. Invest. 91(4):1769–1774, Apr. 1993.

Tryba, M., et al.: Histamine Release and Cardiovascular Reactions to Implantation of Bone Cement During Total Hip Replacement. Anaesthesist 40(1):25–32, Jan. 1991.

Wood, D. J., et al.: Factors Which Influence Mortality After Subcapital Hip Fracture. J. Bone Joint Surg. 74B(2):199–202, Mar. 1992.

Zuckerman, J. D., et al.: Enhancing Independence in the Older Hip Fracture Patient. Geriatrics 48(5):76–81, May 1993.

Additional References

Drinka, P., et al.: Is Male Hip Fracture a Marker for Low Testosterone in Elderly Male Nursing Home Residents? J. Am. Geriatr. Soc. 41(2):192, Feb. 1993.

Fujiwara, N. K., et al.: Hip Fracture Mortality and Morbidity in Japan: A Cross-Cultural Comparison. Soz. Praventivmed. 38(1):8–14, 1993.

Hayes, W. C., et al.: Impact Near the Hip Dominates Fracture Risk in Elderly Nursing Home Residents Who Fall. Calcif. Tissue Int. 52(3):192–198, Mar. 1993.

Kanis, J. A.: The Incidence of Hip Fracture in Europe. Osteoporos. Int. 3(Suppl 1):10–15, 1993.

Lau, E. M., et al.: Low Bone Mineral Density, Grip Strength and Skinfold Thickness are Important Risk Factors for Hip Fracture in Hong Kong Chinese. Osteoporos. Int. 3(2):66–70, Mar. 1993.

Maitland, L. A., et al.: Read My Hips: Measuring Trochanteric Soft Tissue Thickness. Calcif. Tissue Int. 52(2):85–89, Feb. 1993.

Yamamoto, K., et al.: Risk Factors for Hip Fracture in Elderly Japanese Women in Tottori Prefecture, Japan. Osteoporos. Int. 3 (Suppl 1):48–50, 1993.

CHAPTER 3

TOTAL HIP REPLACEMENT
(ARTHROPLASTY)

SCOPE

Total hip arthroplasty (replacement of both parts of the hip joint with prostheses) is performed on about 800,000 individuals each year, worldwide. This procedure is indicated when more conservative therapies, such as rest and medications, have failed to relieve pain and restore function adequately. The majority of hip replacement operations are performed in older adults whose hips have been damaged by osteoarthritis, either primary or secondary to infection or trauma; fracture; congenital malformation; metabolic or endocrine dysfunction; avascular necrosis or tumor. Hip damage due to rheumatoid arthritis is the second major indication for total hip arthroplasty. The implant may be cemented or press-fit, with or without a porous coating, to the remaining bone of the hip. Whether and what type of arthroplasty should be performed are decided largely on the basis of the hip disease, the patient's age, general medical condition and results of imaging studies to evaluate hip anatomy. The most common complications of total hip arthroplasty are blood clots, infection and failure of the prosthesis.

SYNOPSIS

3.00   INTRODUCTION

The hip, the largest joint in the body, bears the weight of the body during everyday activities such as walking, running and lifting. The key role the hip plays puts this joint at risk of further injury with normal use if the joint is affected by disease or trauma. The importance of the hip to everyday activities also means that individuals with abnormalities of this joint usually experience significant disability due to painful or impaired hip function. Relieving pain and restoring hip joint function thus can contribute notably to a patient's quality of life. To this end, some 800,000 total hip replacement procedures are performed worldwide each year (Herberts, et al., 1995).

The Berlin physician Themistocles Glück is said to have performed the first total hip replacement before the turn of the twentieth century, using an ivory ball-and-socket prosthesis held in place with cement made of colophony (resin), pumice and gypsum. However, the materials used in this and other arthroplasties Glück performed were reported to be readily absorbed, so that the joints failed (McElfresh, 1991). Today a variety of procedures and types of prostheses may be used for surgical treatment of hip problems.

3.01   Anatomy of the Hip

The bones that comprise the hip are the femur (thighbone) and the acetabulum (part of the pelvic bones). The head of the femur, which is shaped roughly like a ball, fits into the cup of the acetabulum, which is like a socket. The hip is thus a ball-and-socket joint, with the ability to move smoothly (when the joint functions normally) over a wide range. *(See Figure 3-1.)*

The hip is a synovial joint, meaning that the surfaces of the two bones that rub against each other are coated with cartilage and lubricated by synovial fluid (secreted by the membrane lining the joint) within a tough fibrous capsule. The movement of the hipbones is powered by muscles and stabilized by ligaments—tough bundles of fiber that stretch across the bones of the joint like stiff rubber bands.

3.02   Evaluation of Hip Function

Hip function may be measured objectively by determining range of motion, discrepancy in leg length and presence of a positive Trendelenburg sign or lurch.

[1]   Range of Motion

Normal joints are able to move (active motion) or to be moved (passive motion) through certain distances in various directions. This movement is called range of motion. Although normally an individual's range of motion decreases somewhat with age, significant limitation is characteristic of joint pathology. *(See Figure 3-2.)*

The hip moves in three anatomic planes (Miller, 1991):

- coronal (as seen looking down on the top of the head): in this plane, the hip can rotate inward 70 degrees and outward 90 degrees;

- sagittal (side view): the hip can flex to 140 degrees and extend to 15 degrees; and

- transverse (face-on view): the hip can abduct (move away from the body) 30 degrees and adduct (move toward the midline) 25 degrees.

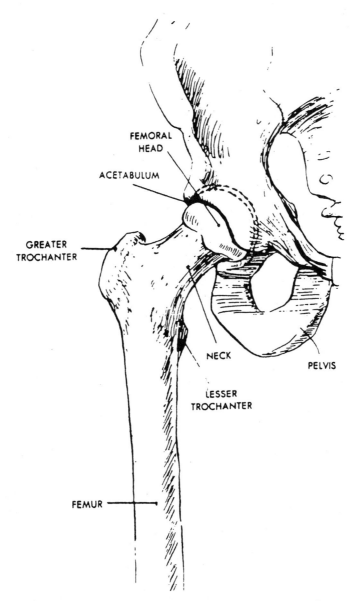

Fig. 3-1. Anatomy of the hip joint. A large cavity called the acetabulum holds the head of the femur. Their articulation forms the ball-and-socket hip joint. Parts of the femur below its head are the neck, the greater and lesser trochanters, and the shaft that descends to the knee.

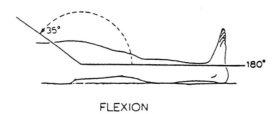

FLEXION

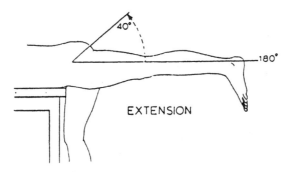

EXTENSION

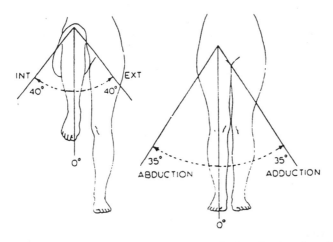

Fig. 3-2. Hip range of motion includes flexion (bending the hip), extension (straightening), abduction (moving the limbs away from the center of the body) and adduction (bringing the limb from a position away from the body back toward its center).

Measurements of the range of hip movement in each direction for everyday activities such as tying shoes and ascending or descending stairs show that most daily tasks require considerable range of motion, particularly in the sagittal plane (Miller, 1991).

[2]   Equality of Leg Length

Chronic hip disease may lead to bone destruction, articulation changes and soft tissue abnormalities that effectively shorten the leg on the affected side. To estimate discrepancy in leg length, the patient is asked to stand straight with legs together. The examiner's hands are placed on the patient's iliac crests (the ridge of bone at the top of the hip, just above and to the side of the buttocks); the hip on the side of the "shorter" leg will be lower. The leg on the affected side may be shorter by an inch or more compared to the normal leg, as a result of progressive hip deformity. Blocks of various heights are placed under the foot on this side until the patient's iliac crests appear to be level.

[3]   Trendelenburg Sign or Lurch

Asking the patient to stand on one leg and then the other can elicit a Trendelenburg sign (an indication of abnormal function of muscles such as the abductor, which are important in stabilizing the hip). In the patient with normal abductor muscle function (a negative Trendelenburg sign), the patient's torso stays centered over the hips and an imaginary line drawn across the tops of the hips stays horizontal when the patient stands on one leg. If the torso stays over the hips but the opposite hip drops when the patient stands on the affected leg, the patient is said to have a positive Trendelenburg sign. *(See Figure 3-3.)* If the hips stay horizontally aligned when the patient stands on the affected leg but the torso shifts over the affected hip, the patient is said to have a Trendelenburg lurch (Petty, 1991a).

3.10   INDICATIONS FOR TOTAL HIP ARTHROPLASTY

The general indication for total hip arthroplasty is severe arthritis (joint inflammation) that causes pain that cannot be adequately relieved by medication. This procedure may also be indicated for patients with unacceptable limitation in joint motion. Such severe arthritis may be due to a variety of conditions.

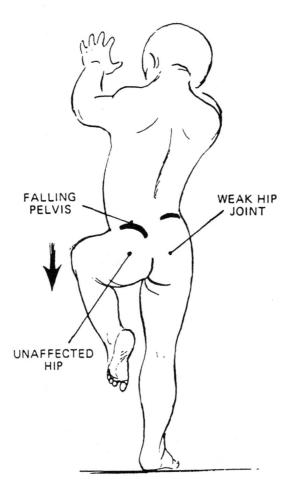

FALLING
PELVIS

WEAK HIP
JOINT

UNAFFECTED
HIP

Fig. 3-3. In a positive Trendelenburg test, the patient's pelvis falls on the unaffected leg when it is lifted from the ground. This indicates a weakness in the hip joint of the opposite leg on which the patient is standing.

3.11 Osteoarthritis

Osteoarthritis is the most frequent diagnosis for which total hip replacement is performed (Herberts, et al., 1995).[1] Changes in the joint that occur with osteoarthritis include changes in cartilage chemistry that lead to pitting, cracking and then erosion of the normally smooth

---

[1] *See also* ch. 6.

surface of the cartilage. This causes the surfaces of the bones to grate instead of glide across one another, which leads to pain with movement. Growth of extra bone (osteophytes) at the edges of the joint space also occurs, and this limits joint motion further.

Osteoarthritis may be secondary to (result from) a variety of traumatic, metabolic, infectious or other conditions, or it may occur without evident predisposing factors (primary osteoarthritis). Changes in the joint characteristic of osteoarthritis can be seen on radiographs of virtually all individuals age 75 years and older worldwide, although symptoms are by no means universal. Women are affected more often than men (Ho and Kammer, 1990).

3.12   Rheumatoid/ Inflammatory Arthritis

The hip can be involved by a variety of inflammatory diseases, of which rheumatoid arthritis is the most common; rheumatoid arthritis is also the second most common reason for hip replacement. Inflammatory types of arthritis are characterized by an immune system reaction, probably related to genetic predisposition and some type of environmental trigger, that results in swelling and damage to tissues. With rheumatoid arthritis, joint cartilage is affected, leading to debilitating changes that occur in young adulthood to middle age. More women than men are affected. Some 10 to 20 percent of patients with rheumatoid arthritis may have hip disease that meets criteria for total hip replacement (Ranawat, et al., 1992).

Although the incidence of hip involvement in rheumatoid arthritis is relatively low, it is often the single most disabling feature of the illness and can progress from onset to the need for surgery in a matter of weeks in some cases. In one series of five patients, protrusion of the acetabulum into the pelvis, which normally progresses at 2 to 3 mm per year in patients with rheumatoid arthritis, occurred over an average of 40 days (Damron and Heiner, 1993). Bilateral (on both sides) involvement and therefore bilateral total hip arthroplasty are usually the case in patients with rheumatoid arthritis (Susman and Clayton, 1992).

Up to half of individuals with ankylosing spondylitis (stiffening of the spine) have clinically significant hip disease, often bilateral (Ranawat, et al., 1992). Protrusion deformities (such as protrusion of the head of the femur and acetabular cup into the pelvic bone), complete ankylosing (fixation by bone) of the hip joints, spine deformities and other changes make evaluation and surgical treatment of these hip problems difficult.

Psoriatic arthritis involves the hips in about 10 percent of cases overall but about 40 percent of those in whom the condition is diagnosed in childhood (Ranawat, et al., 1992).

3.13 Avascular Necrosis

Avascular necrosis (death of tissue due to inadequate blood supply)[2] of the femoral head can occur due to abnormal distribution of stresses in a deformed or an injured joint, or as a complication of corticosteroid drug therapy, which may be prescribed for a variety of conditions, including rheumatoid arthritis and systemic lupus erythematosus (Ranawat, et al., 1992).

3.14 Fracture

Displaced fractures of the head of the femur (thighbone) in elderly persons are a frequent indication for hemiarthroplasty (replacement of the damaged femoral head) or total hip arthroplasty (replacement of the entire joint).[3]

3.15 Metabolic and Endocrine Conditions

Gout and pseudogout—arthritic conditions due to metabolic abnormalities—may cause joint space narrowing and development of cysts under the cartilage of the hip joint that can be seen radiographically. In some cases, crystals in the joint space cause such pain that joint replacement is indicated. However, surgery may precipitate an acute flare of the disease (Ranawat, et al., 1992).

Ochronosis, hemochromatosis and other metabolic conditions can also cause destruction of the joint by deposition of molecules in the joint tissues. Patients with acromegaly (abnormal enlargement of bones due to an endocrine problem) who undergo total hip replacement often need custom implants because of the overly large size of their bones (Ranawat, et al., 1992).

Other diseases of bone metabolism that can lead to the need for hip replacement are osteoporosis (in which the bone becomes brittle), Paget's disease[4] and Gaucher's disease.

---

[2] *See also* ch. 2.

[3] *See also* ch. 2 for a discussion of hip fractures.

[4] *See also* ch. 5.

3.16   Tumors

Tumors in the pelvis (hipbones) are treated by removal of only the part of the pelvis that is affected by the tumor, with reconstruction being performed during the same operation. Only tumors involving the acetabulum (hip portion of the pelvic bones) require significant reconstruction of bone. Options include hip arthrodesis (fusion of the hip joint), grafting of bone and implanting a prosthesis or use of a custom prosthetic pelvis. This last and newest technique option has not been used extensively in the United States (Springfield, 1991).

3.17   Failed Previous Arthroplasty

Operations on the hip constitute trauma to the joint and alter joint function. The benefits of a number of procedures are thus time limited, and total replacement of the joint may be necessary at some time after arthrodesis, subtotal arthroplasty (resection or replacement of part of the joint) (Stulberg and Hupfer, 1991a), osteotomy (reshaping of bone) or an operation to manage infection, traumatic injury or a congenital defect.

3.20   PATIENT EVALUATION FOR HIP REPLACEMENT

Patient factors that need to be considered in the decision for total hip arthroplasty include the patient's general physical condition, general medical condition, level of pain and disability, response to conservative therapy and desired life-style. In addition, patient age is a major concern when considering total hip replacement. Most total hip replacement procedures are performed in older patients, who often have—or are at risk for—a number of medical conditions that may affect the outcome of surgery (Petty, 1991a). Relative contraindications to total hip arthroplasty include sepsis (whole-body infection), neurologic or mental impairment that precludes the patient's ability to control hip movement and multiple previous surgical procedures that have compromised the soft tissues of the hip so that function cannot be restored without extensive bracing (Stulberg and Hupfer, 1991a).

3.21   Symptom Evaluation

The major complaints of individuals with problems in the hip are pain and decreased function of the joint. The patient should be asked to describe the nature of any pain associated with the hip. Qualities of pain to be evaluated include location(s), intensity, duration, type (sharp, dull, aching), triggers for onset and what brings relief. Typically pain caused by hip joint disease is felt in the groin, and it often radiates (spreads) down the front-inside of the thigh, sometimes as far as the knee joint (when pain occurs in the back, a disease of the spine or nerves in the lower back must be excluded). Hip pain may be constant and is usually made worse by movement of the hip and/or by bearing weight on the hip (Petty, 1991a).

Patients with hip disease also usually complain of limitations on activities, either because they cannot move the hip fully or because doing so causes unacceptable pain. Effects of the hip problem on the patient's job performance, leisure activities and activities of daily living should be determined. Some important questions for the patient include (Petty, 1991a):

- Have you had to stop work, change jobs or modify your work activities?
- Do you have trouble dressing, especially putting on stockings and tying shoes?
- Do you have trouble rising from a chair or climbing stairs?
- Do you use a cane or other supportive aid for walking?
- Has your sexual function diminished?
- Have you had to take analgesics (painkillers), narcotics, antiarthritic drugs or other medications to help you continue functioning?
- Have you consulted other physicians about this problem, and if so, what have they advised and what have you tried?

A very important question that should be asked when interviewing a candidate for hip replacement surgery is what the patient expects the surgery to accomplish. If the patient is disabled only for vigorous activities such as running, for example, and expects to be able to return to these activities after surgery, an operation is not indicated, because this type of strenuous activity should be avoided after total hip replacement (Petty, 1991a).

3.22 Medical History

Historic information important to diagnosing the cause of a hip problem and planning hip arthroplasty includes medications the patient has been taking, other medical conditions and previous surgical experiences. Corticosteroid medications, taken to relieve arthritis pain or for another condition, may cause or aggravate hip problems. Alcohol abuse can contribute to hip problems and complicate patient care during and after surgery (Perry, 1991a).

Total hip arthroplasty is an elective (optional) major surgical procedure that may be contraindicated for patients with myocardial infarction (heart attack) in the past six months (because of the much higher rate of another infarction), unstable angina (chest pain due to insufficient supply of blood to the heart), congestive heart failure (inadequate heart function), inadequately controlled high blood pressure, poorly controlled diabetes mellitus (blood glucose level greater than 300 mg/dL) or inadequately treated asthma (Gravenstein, 1991).

3.23 Physical Examination

Observing how the patient moves provides a wealth of information about hip function. As the patient rises from a chair, the examiner should note which moves seem painful and how the patient uses supports. Observation of the patient as he or she stands in front of the examiner may reveal asymmetry in hip height, possibly caused by variations in leg length.[5] If the patient uses a walking aid, he or she should be observed walking both with and without the assistive device. If a limp is present, it could be due to pain, abductor muscle dysfunction (Trendelenburg limp or lurch)[6] or both. A limp helps lessen pain because it involves pivoting the normal side of the body around the affected leg, so as to shorten the time that pressure due to weight-bearing (which causes pain) is put on the affected hip.

Palpation (gentle touching to locate abnormal structures or source of pain) of the hip may reveal a tender, swollen area over the greater trochanter (the knob of bone on the outside of the upper thighbone). This is a sign of trochanteric bursitis (inflammation of the fibrous sac that pads this bone) (Petty, 1991a).

Testing the patient's range of hip motion[7] and evaluating for contracture (abnormal shortening) of hip muscles can also help in diagnosis and planning surgery for a hip problem.

---

[5] *See* 3.02 *supra.*

[6] *See* 3.02[3] *supra.*

[7] *See* 3.02[1] *supra.*

3.24 Laboratory Studies

Laboratory tests may be ordered to diagnose the cause of a hip problem. If the patient is a candidate for surgery, laboratory tests and other procedures will be ordered to evaluate the patient's readiness for surgery and for the presence and severity of conditions that can affect care during and after the total hip arthroplasty. These examinations may include a chest x-ray, an electrocardiogram (EKG) and analyses of blood and urine. If a urinary tract infection is suspected, urine culture or kidney function studies may be performed. Liver function tests may also be indicated for some patients (Petty, 1991a).

Most total hip arthroplasties are performed in elderly patients, who often have poor overall health and nutritional deficiency. Studies have shown that more than a fourth of patients who are scheduled for elective (not emergency) total hip arthroplasty may be malnourished preoperatively. Poor nutritional status can multiply the risk of major wound healing problems significantly and has been associated with increased risk of infection in the urinary tract, lungs and other locations after total hip replacement.

Poor nutritional status and impaired general health are indicated by a recent history of weight loss greater than 10 pounds, a serum albumin (blood protein) level less than 3.4 g/dL or lymphocyte (white blood cell) counts below 1,500 cells/mL. Patients with these indicators of poor health should undergo further evaluation and correction of nutritional deficiency before surgery is scheduled (Petty, 1991a).

3.25 Imaging

Imaging studies are performed before hip arthroplasty to confirm the diagnosis and determine anatomic and functional relationships in the joint. Imaging is also performed postoperatively to follow the course of healing and evaluate possible complications.[8] If measurements will be made on the images to determine sizes and relationships of structures, special attention must be paid to how the patient is positioned and the angle of imaging (Stulberg and Hupfer, 1991a).

Plain radiographs in standard anteroposterior (front-to-back) and lateral (from the side) views may be adequate to evaluate a hip in which primary (initial) total arthroplasty with a cemented prosthesis is planned and no extraordinary conditions are present. Use of such

---

8 *See* 3.70 *infra.*

radiographs alone to make calculations for cementless arthroplasty can result in significant miscalculation, however (Stulberg and Hupfer, 1991a).

Angiography (imaging of arteries), venography (imaging of veins) and intravenous pyelography (imaging of the urinary system) may be indicated before surgery when a device previously implanted in the hip is suspected to have protruded into the pelvis or surgery is expected to extend into the pelvis (Stulberg and Hupfer, 1991a).

Computed tomography (CT), especially with three-dimensional reconstructions or bone models, helps the surgeon visualize abnormal anatomy before it is encountered during the operation. Reconstructions also help the surgeon determine the thickness and configuration of normal bone to anchor prosthetic components. Some imaging centers are able to provide topographic images (reconstructions of the surface appearance of the bones in three dimensions), with the ability to rotate these images to view them in any direction. Such information can be used to design anatomic models of the joints, and they aid in the design of custom prosthetic implants. They also help in planning the steps of a complex reconstruction, including the special equipment and devices that may be needed (Stulberg and Hupfer, 1991a; Heare and Montgomery, 1991).

Magnetic resonance imaging (MRI) provides clear, easily interpreted views of the hip. Abnormalities of bone such as osteonecrosis (dead bone) are well demonstrated by MRI, and these scans can be obtained in any plane desired, which is very important in determining the extent of a tumor or planning for reconstruction or grafting of bone. MRI is thus very helpful in so-called custom arthroplasty, in which bone and soft tissue will be reshaped as well as one or more prosthetic parts implanted. Indications for custom hip arthroplasty would include removal of a tumor and hip replacement to treat congenital hip dysplasia. Gadolinium contrast is used to evaluate arthritis in the hip joint by MRI (Heare and Montgomery, 1991).

When total hip arthroplasty with a cementless prosthesis is planned, "templating" is important to plan the correct position for the implant within the bone: (1) to restore proper length of the involved leg, (2) to place the forces of weight-bearing at the center of the hip, and (3) to restore muscle relationships about the hip. Templating involves measuring distances and angles on various radiographic views to determine where weight-bearing forces are in the individual patient's hip and what changes in anatomy might be made to achieve optimal weight-bearing. When the contralateral (on the opposite side) hip is normal, this hip is often templated first and the hip center on these images used to plan surgery on the abnormal hip. Templating also allows the surgeon to estimate how closely available femoral devices match the patient's femoral anatomy in size and shape (Stulberg and Hupfer, 1991a).

3.30   CHOICE OF SURGICAL PROCEDURE

The appropriate arthroplasty procedure is determined after consideration of the patient's age, physical and medical condition, disease process, expectations and capacity for rehabilitation of function and other factors that are assessed preoperatively. Regardless of the type of surgery decided upon, greater success of the procedure is associated with education and involvement of the patient in the type and goals of surgery and postoperative care (Stulberg and Hupfer, 1991a).

3.31   Total Hip Arthroplasty

Total hip arthroplasty involves replacement of both the acetabular and the femoral components of the hip joint. A very wide variety of prostheses are available for total hip arthroplasty, including all metal, metal with a porous coating and metal with a plastic acetabular liner. Chromium-cobalt alloys are popular; titanium has been found to have poor resistance to abrasion, so it is no longer considered desirable as a material for hip prostheses (Evans, et al., 1993).

Many factors may go into selection of the prosthesis, including the surgeon's knowledge, experience and preference; the patient's size and health; whether primary or revision arthroplasty is planned and whether the operation involves tumor removal (Petty, 1991b).

[1]   Biocompatibility of Prosthetic Materials

Metal hip prostheses were introduced in 1938 by Wiles, who ground stainless steel parts precisely to replace the acetabular and femoral hip joint components. Wiles abandoned hip replacement because the screws and bolts he used to fix the prosthesis in place broke. Soon afterward, however, Bohlman used a chromium-cobalt compound for successful hip replacement. In the 1950s, acrylic compounds came into use for cementing prostheses to bone (McElfresh, 1991).

Today metals and alloys, polymers, ceramics, carbons, and combinations and composites of these types of materials may be used for prostheses to replace joints in the human body. In general, implanted materials that release debris (breakdown products) at concentrations below 100 parts per million (ppm) are tolerated by the body, although some implant locations may be associated with more breakdown because of greater strain on the implant, and some tissues are more sensitive to debris than other tissues. Another factor in tolerableness of foreign materials is how long they are present in the body: longer duration of implantation is associated with greater likelihood of implant breakdown and an adverse reaction to the debris. The goals of research into optimal materials for joint replacement are to identify materials that form stable attachments to living tissues while evidencing minimal biodegradability and wear when implanted (Lemons, 1993).

Debris from breakdown of prosthetic hip parts, whether they are metallic or polymeric, is initially handled the same way: special "scavenger" cells (macrophages or giant cells) phagocytose (ingest) the particles. However, the metals used in prosthetic joints are elements that are normally present in trace amounts in the body, and small concentrations of these metals can generally be processed by the cell. Thus, although some corrosion of metal in the implants occurs, the rate is slow and the process is not considered harmful. In contrast, polymer debris is not broken down by human cells, and some artificial materials may damage cells and cause an inflammatory reaction. Such reactions accounted for notable problems with early hip prostheses that included the polymer Teflon® (Brown and Merritt, 1991).

An issue that may cause concern with implantation of prostheses in the body is carcinogenicity (tendency to cause cancer) of implant particles. Very few tumors have been reported in patients who have received joint replacement implants, and the patient population is one that is already at greater risk of tumor because of advanced age. In addition, animal experiments have pointed to an association between tumor development and implants, but only over a longer life span than older patients would experience with an implant. At present, therefore, it seems that the carcinogenic effects of placing an implant in an older patient are small (Brown and Merritt, 1991).

Finally, a small proportion of patients may be hypersensitive to the materials used in prosthetic implants. About 15 percent of the population is known to be sensitive to one or more of the metals used in stainless steel or cobalt-chromium alloy implants, although the proportion of patients with implants who have observable reactions is much lower. Titanium may also cause allergic reaction in an even smaller proportion of patients. If the patient has had a reaction to a substance (as a result of previous implantation of an orthopedic device or a dental appliance, for example), he or she should not receive a hip prosthesis containing this compound or element (Brown and Merritt, 1991).

[2]   Fixation

Implanted joint prostheses may be fixed in place using bone cement or by one of two uncemented fixation methods: porous fixation or press-fit fixation.

Cemented prostheses, of which the modern variety were developed by Charnley in 1961, are still widely used for hip replacement. The cement material is polymethyl methacrylate (PMMA). PMMA is an acrylic resin that is supplied as a vial of liquid and a bag of powder; when the liquid and powder are mixed, the substance cures by giving off heat. The cement should be manipulated as little as possible while it is curing, because greater handling weakens the final product. Antibiotic powder may be added to the cement powder before mixing (about 4 to 6 g antibiotic per 40 g of bone cement powder), but the final product will have up to 25 percent less mechanical strength (Petty, 1991c).

Bone cement is not adhesive. Thus when PMMA is used to fix a prosthetic hip part in place, the surgeon must prepare surfaces by scraping and reaming to ensure optimal likelihood of tight prosthesis adherence (Petty, 1991c).

Greenfield first described using a *porous* fixation technique in 1909 to stabilize an artificial tooth; clinical use of this technique for hip prostheses dates to around 1970 (Petty, 1991c). Prosthetic hip parts meant for porous fixation have been made of metal, ceramic or polymers, but cobalt-chrome alloy is the most common material. The porous fixation surface consists of a metallic bead coating, a wire coating or a plasma spray applied to the parts of the prosthesis that will contact bone. During implantation of the prosthesis, the closer the porous surface can be brought into contact with bone, the more likely bone is to grow into the porous surface and fix the prosthesis in place. A maximal distance of 2 mm has been recommended, based on experiments in dogs, but 0.5 mm may be the maximum for acetabular components; as the gap decreases, growth increases (Petty, 1991c).

Moore and Bohlman first described using *press-fit* fixation prostheses for the femoral head and shaft in 1943, and over the following 25 years, they designed numerous prostheses for uncemented fixation in the hip. Problems with press-fit prostheses have included loosening and the development of membranes between the prosthesis and bone. Availability of a wider range of sizes, use of improved materials (titanium alloys in addition to alloys of cobalt and chrome) and development of surgical instruments that permit more precise preparation of bone to receive the prosthesis have resulted in more satisfactory results from press-fit fixation of prosthetic hip parts (Petty, 1991c). *(See Figure 3-4.)*

3.32 Bipolar Arthroplasty

Bipolar hip prostheses are most often used to treat a displaced fracture of the femoral (thighbone) neck, although they may also be appropriate for management of arthritis or osteonecrosis, or for revision arthroplasty (Petty, 1991d).

The bipolar prosthesis consists of (1) a femoral head and shaft component that is similar to those of the total hip prosthesis systems, and (2) a two-part acetabular component. The outer shell of the acetabular component is fitted in the acetabular socket, and the inner shell is designed to have some bearing action both with the outer shell and with the prosthetic femoral head. The two-bearing design of the acetabular portion of this prosthesis reflects the observation that in some patients who have undergone replacement of the femoral head and shaft only, cartilage of the acetabulum has gradually eroded, and the experimental finding that articulation of cartilage against metal leads to degeneration of the cartilage. The presence of two concentric bearing surfaces in bipolar prostheses is believed to reduce damaging forces on the acetabulum (Petty, 1991d).

Studies of total hip arthroplasty to treat fracture of the femoral neck have shown better results with bipolar than with fixed-head prostheses for this condition. Bipolar prostheses also give overall excellent results when used to replace hip joints that have been damaged by osteoarthritis. In one series, patients experienced some deterioration in hip

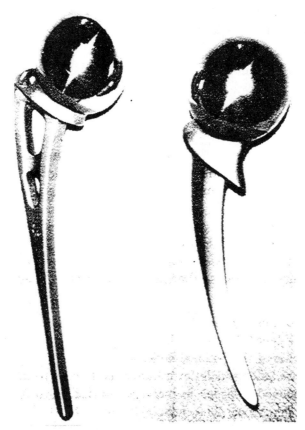

Fig. 3-4. Two of the various types of prostheses used to replace the femoral head. The Austin-Moore prosthesis is on the left and the Thompson prosthesis on the right.

function scores over longer follow-up periods, but the declines were attributed to advancing patient age rather than problems with the prosthesis. In four other series of patients with osteoarthritis who underwent hip replacement with bipolar prostheses, an average of 75 percent had good or excellent hip function an average of four to five years after replacement. In three of these series, pain relief was also excellent; in the fourth study, pain relief was better in patients who had received unipolar prostheses, but the bipolar prostheses gave better range of motion (Petty, 1991d).

Patients with hip disease due to rheumatoid arthritis have also been shown to benefit from total joint replacement with a bipolar prosthesis,

as have those with osteonecrosis. Differences in the degree of improvement with various underlying disease processes may be related to
varying degrees of bearing action that have been measured in the
bipolar prostheses under different loading conditions (applications of
force) (Petty, 1991d).

The complications of bipolar total hip prosthetic implants are the
same as those with unipolar implants. In addition, the bearing action
between the bipolar components may fail, or the bipolar components
may dissociate, both of which occurrences must be treated by open
reduction of the hip and reassembly of the prosthesis or implantation
of a new prosthesis (Petty, 1991d).

3.33 Surface (Double-Cup) Arthroplasty

Because conventional cemented total hip arthroplasty was successful in providing lifelong relief of pain and restoration of function in
elderly patients with arthritis, the procedure began to be performed
in younger patients. Although early results were as successful in
younger as in older patients, after a variable number of years, the
prostheses failed. Because revision (second or later) procedures are
technically more difficult than primary procedures (due to scarring,
bone loss and other alterations in structure during the initial surgery),
a less extensive arthroplasty is usually recommended as the initial
surgical procedure for individuals younger than 40 years old and, in
certain cases, for older individuals as well (Stulberg and Hupfer,
1991a).

The first surface (double-cup) replacement arthroplasty of the hip
was performed in 1961 (McElfresh, 1991). The technique, introduced
specifically to provide pain relief and restore hip joint function to
younger patients, is based on the principle that if joint degeneration
is caused by continued articulation of injured cartilage surfaces,
covering or replacing injured surfaces with smooth articulating surfaces should reverse the process and restore pain-free joint function.
Advantages of this procedure over total hip arthroplasty include
(Amstutz, 1991):

- The femoral head is reshaped rather than removed.
- The femoral shaft and intramedullary canal are left intact.
- There is less disruption of joint biomechanics.
- The less extensive procedure takes less operating time.

- The procedure involves less blood loss.

With surface replacement arthroplasty, however, the acetabulum must be prepared as for total hip replacement, because the new surface applied to the femoral head requires a slightly larger inner diameter of the acetabular component. Nevertheless, this larger diameter has an advantage of its own, in that it distributes pressure over a larger area, thus decreasing pressure over the new articulating surfaces and enhancing joint stability (Amstutz, 1991).

Initially the thinner walls of acetabular cups limited their useful life, but advances in surface replacement materials have led to more durable surfaces and cementless fixation, in turn prolonging the success of these procedures. In one series of 585 resurfacing procedures performed on patients with a mean age of 48 years (range 20 to 67) at the time of surgery, 63 percent of the procedures continued to provide satisfactory pain relief and hip function for 6 to 16 years. Indications for surface replacement in this series included osteoarthritis (44 percent of procedures), avascular necrosis (16 percent), rheumatoid arthritis (including juvenile type, 15 percent), congenital hip dysplasia (9 percent) and post-traumatic arthritis (4 percent) (Amstutz, 1991).

In 86 percent of the cases in this series in which the resurfacing procedure eventually failed (as determined by the need for revision surgery), loosening of the prosthetic surfaces was the cause. Revision surgery showed that osteolysis (breakdown of bone) had occurred as a result of debris between the articulating surfaces and formation of granulation (inflammatory) tissue in the joint. The loosening was often visible on serial radiographs as widening of the joint space followed by migration or shifting of the prosthetic components, similar to changes seen on radiographs after total hip arthroplasty (Amstutz, 1991).

3.40 TOTAL HIP ARTHROPLASTY OPERATIVE PROCEDURE

The patient undergoing total hip arthroplasty should be oriented to the hospital environment before surgery and needs to understand and agree to participate in postoperative care procedures. The use of certain medications most patients use to help relieve arthritis pain is stopped before surgery (Gravenstein, 1991): nonsteroidal anti-inflammatory drugs (NSAIDs) are usually stopped when the patient is told to take nothing by mouth (usually the night before surgery); salicylate preparations (those containing aspirin) are stopped at least a week before surgery.

The night before and the morning of total hip arthroplasty, the patient may shower or bathe with an antibacterial soap. In the operating room, the surgeon assures proper positioning of the patient for the procedure, with the patient lying on the unaffected side, and antibiotic medications are begun to decrease the risk of postoperative infection.

Special precautions during anesthesia for patients with certain medical conditions include (Amstutz, 1991):

- evaluation of anesthesia risk in patients with other conditions such as congestive heart failure in addition to rheumatoid arthritis;

- corticosteroid replacement therapy for those who have received these medications sooner than five days before surgery or who have had a course of corticosteroid therapy within the past 12 months;

- monitoring for arrhythmia (abnormal heartbeats) in patients who have had therapy with diuretic drugs (to promote excretion of fluid) or digoxin (for heart function); and

- careful selection of anesthetic agents for patients who have had recent therapy with certain antidepressant drugs.

The choice of anesthetic technique and agents depends on the preoperative evaluation and the expected length of the procedure. Either general anesthesia or regional anesthesia may be used; regional anesthesia allows the patient to remain conscious and breathing on his or her own, but it fails to give satisfactory analgesia (freedom from the sensation of pain) much more often (in about 10 percent of cases) than happens with general anesthesia. On the other hand, although general anesthesia is uniformly successful in providing analgesia, it requires that the patient undergo ventilation (breathing) by machine, which can cause lung problems. Regional anesthesia and general anesthesia are compared for hip arthroplasty (Gravenstein, 1991) in *Table 3-1*.

Because blood loss is usually significant with total hip arthroplasty, replacement is usual. Patients may be able to receive an autologous transfusion (reinfusion of the patient's own blood), using either blood lost during the operation that is returned by a sterile circuit after washing or units donated by the patient in the weeks before the procedure. Avoiding the use of unknown donor blood brings almost to zero the risk of acquiring human immunodeficiency virus (HIV) infection (although this risk is very low in blood handled and stored in recent years in blood banks); it also decreases the somewhat greater risk of a transfusion reaction (allergic reaction to the donor's blood) and of post-transfusion viral hepatitis, both of which have been estimated to occur in approximately 0.5 percent of transfusions of unknown donor blood (Gravenstein, 1991).

Table 3-1
Comparison of Regional and General Anesthesia
for Total Hip Arthroplasty

Factor	Regional Anesthesia	General Anesthesia
Patient comfort	Patient can help with positioning. Immobility may cause pain/distress.	Position-related injuries possible.
Physiologic changes	Less severe stress response. Lung ventilation/perfusion well maintained.	Greater stress response; not clinically significant. Collapse of lung (atelectasis) on unaffected side more likely.
Blood loss	30-40% less than with general anesthesia.	
Leg vein blood clot (overall rate, 6%)*	Less.	Greater.
Lung blood clot (overall rate, 5%)*	Less.	Greater.

*The risks for blood clots depend upon many factors in addition to type of anesthesia.

3.41 Surgical Approach

Surgical approaches for hip arthroplasty are based on the principle that prostheses cannot be placed to provide long-term success unless the surgeon has a full view of the acetabulum and proximal femur. One of four approaches is usually chosen: anterolateral, direct lateral, transtrochanteric or posterolateral. The approach can also be described in terms of the major muscles that are manipulated to obtain access to the hip joint (Stulberg and Hupfer, 1991b):

- anterolateral—between tensor fasciae latae (one of the muscles that flex the hip) and anterior fibers of the gluteus medius;

- direct lateral—division of the gluteus medius and minimus muscles;

- transtrochanteric—elevation of the gluteus medius and minimus muscles; and

- posterolateral—splitting of gluteus maximus muscle fibers and approach between gluteus maximus and gluteus medius muscles.

A primary consideration for choice of approach is the experience of the surgeon with one or more of the approaches. In addition, various approaches provide advantages and disadvantages, as follows (Stulberg and Hupfer, 1991b).

[1] Anterolateral Approach

The advantages of the anterolateral approach to hip arthroplasty are that it provides excellent exposure of the acetabulum, minimizes disruption of the abductor muscle (the large muscle in the hip that plays a major role in stabilizing this joint) and is less likely to result in hip dislocation. This approach has disadvantages, however, including possible problems with inadequate exposure of the femoral (thighbone) area, leading to suboptimal placement of the femoral component and fracture of the femur during revision (repeat) arthroplasty (Stulberg and Hupfer, 1991b).

The anterolateral approach is begun with an incision that starts about 1 inch down the leg and to the side from the front tip of the superior iliac crest (pelvic bone), then curves to the back of the greater trochanter (the knob of bone on the outside of the thighbone). Blunt retractors (slightly curved metal spatulas) are inserted between the gluteus medius and tensor fasciae latae (two major muscles) and against the abductor muscles to expose the neck of the femur. Care must be taken when placing the retractor blades not to injure the femoral nerve and blood vessels. Also at risk with this approach is the inferior branch of the superior gluteal nerve, but this nerve may be sacrificed if necessary to obtain adequate exposure of the hip joint (Stulberg and Hupfer, 1991b).

Fat over the hip joint capsule is lifted off, and tendons are moved out of the way. Then incisions are made in the joint capsule, and this fibrous covering is pulled aside to expose the bones of the hip joint. These bones are dislocated by flexing the patient's leg (pulling the knee toward the chin) and at the same time pulling the knee up and rotating the leg outward (adduction and external rotation). The head of the femur is lifted free of tissues and resected (removed).

[2]   Direct Lateral Approach

Advantages of the direct lateral approach to hip arthroplasty include excellent exposure of the acetabular area in revision as well as primary procedures, less disruption of the trochanter area (unless cement is used to fix the prostheses) and less likelihood of prosthesis dislocation. Disadvantages of this approach are that it disrupts the abductor muscles (the large muscles stabilizing the hip) and thus can cause a lurching gait after surgery that cannot be corrected with exercises. Furthermore, this approach may not allow for adequate exposure of the femoral and acetabular components during a revision procedure, and it limits the extent to which the leg can be lengthened if this is part of the procedure (Stulberg and Hupfer, 1991b).

The incision for the direct lateral approach to hip arthroplasty begins approximately 2 inches down the patient's leg from the bottom of the greater trochanter, moves up the patient's hip over the greater trochanter and then curves slightly posteriorly. Tissues beneath the skin are retracted (pulled to either side of the incision) to expose the gluteus medius muscle. This muscle and its tendon are divided by electrocautery (application of an electric current to burn apart connecting tissue), and the portions of muscle and tendon are carefully retracted to expose the gluteus minimus muscle, which is divided and retracted similarly. As with the anterolateral approach, the femoral nerve and blood vessels and the inferior branch of the superior gluteal nerve are at risk during this approach to the hip joint and should be protected by using care in placement of incisions and retractors.

Next, a T-shaped incision is made in the joint capsule; the hip is dislocated by flexion, adduction and external rotation; and a femoral neck osteotomy is performed (the head of the thighbone is removed). The joint capsule is cut away from the femur, and the hip end of this bone is freed from other attachments and lifted carefully by a retractor placed beneath the greater trochanter.

After hip arthroplasty by a direct lateral approach, the tendons must be reattached to the femur and the muscles repaired. The gluteus minimus tendon is reattached to the femur first, by suturing (sewing) it to holes drilled in the greater trochanter. The gluteus minimus muscle bundles are then sutured together, to restore preoperative relationships as closely as possible. The gluteus medius tendon is then reinserted, as close as possible to its natural location, and the muscle repaired.

In some cases when this approach was used, the portion of trochanter bone to which tendons had been sutured broke away. A modification to prevent this complication of the direct lateral approach involves severing the portion of greater trochanter with tendon attachments to gain access to the hip joint; after completion of the arthroplasty, the greater trochanter is repaired.

[3] Transtrochanteric Approach

The transtrochanteric approach was developed by Charnley and is the single most versatile approach for hip arthroplasty in general and in particular for total hip arthroplasty when anatomy is complex (usually because of previous surgery). This is because it provides excellent exposure of both parts of the joint and allows the surgeon to adjust muscle tension to changes made during surgery in the length of the femur. However, the duration of surgery and the amount of blood loss are often greater with this approach than with others, and problems are more likely to occur with fixation of the prostheses, which poses greater risk of problems with muscle tension if the prostheses loosen. For these reasons, the transtrochanteric approach is less popular for initial total hip replacement in a patient who is not expected to need substantial reconstruction of the acetabulum or leg lengthening (Stulberg and Hupfer, 1991b).

As with other approaches, the transtrochanteric approach poses risk of injury to the femoral nerve and blood vessels. This approach also poses greatest risk of injury to the sciatic nerve (the large nerve at the back of the hip) by stretching while the hip is flexed, adducted and rotated outward. While the hip is in this position, the knee of the operative leg should be supported.

The incision for the transtrochanteric approach to total hip arthroplasty is a straight line that passes over the greater trochanter. *(See Figure 3-5.)* Tissues under the skin are retracted, and underlying short muscles that rotate the hip (the piriformis, superior gemellus, obturator externus and inferior gemellus) are released (cut from their attachments). The gluteus medius and tensor fasciae latae muscles are then divided, followed by division of the vastus lateralis muscle. Retractors and elevators are applied to pull tissues to either side or up out of the operative area so that the top of the hip joint capsule can be seen. Next, an incision is made longitudinally through the greater trochanter. *(See Figure 3-6.)* The exact location and shape of this incision are variable. A chevron or hemispheric cut is recommended for greater stability when the portion of trochanter is reattached (Stulberg and Hupfer, 1991b).

The severed portion of trochanter is moved out of the way to expose the joint capsule, which is cut open. The hip is dislocated by flexion, abduction and external rotation to expose the acetabulum. *(See Figure 3-7.)*

At the end of hip arthroplasty by a transtrochanteric approach, the greater trochanter is repaired by drilling holes in the lesser trochanter and looping cables through the holes and around the segment of greater trochanter to bind the two portions of bone together. Clamps are then placed on the outside of the bone to clamp the greater trochanter to the neck of the femur.

[4]   Posterolateral Approach

Advantages of the posterolateral approach include excellent exposure of the femoral area for primary arthroplasty and minimal disruption of the abductor muscle (the major-stabilizing muscle of the hip), which promotes early rehabilitation after surgery. The acetabular area is not as well exposed by this approach, however, making inaccurate placement of the acetabular prosthesis a risk. Furthermore, this approach risks fracture of the thighbone if this structure is tightly held in position and not freed sufficiently before manipulation for placement of the femoral prosthesis. Finally, dislocation of the prostheses is more likely with this approach (Stulberg and Hupfer, 1991b).

The incision for a posterolateral approach to hip arthroplasty begins along the shaft of the femur and moves straight up toward the waist as far as the greater trochanter, where it is carried posteriorly in a gentle curve. Tissues under the skin are incised and retracted to expose the gluteus maximus muscle, which is divided by using blunt instruments to separate fibers; the external rotators are divided next, and retraction continues until the joint capsule becomes visible. The hip is then rotated inward so that the back edge of the gluteus medius muscle can be identified.

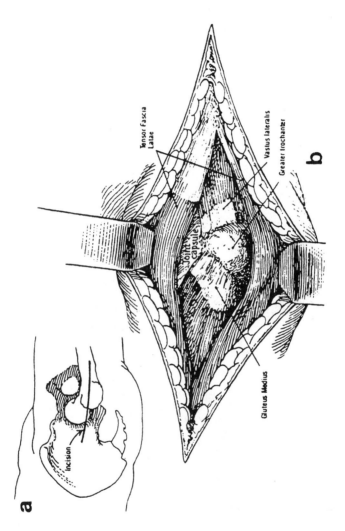

Fig. 3-5. Incision for transtrochanteric approach to total hip arthroplasty (a). In (b), the tensor fascia latae muscles are incised to expose the greater trochanter of the femur.

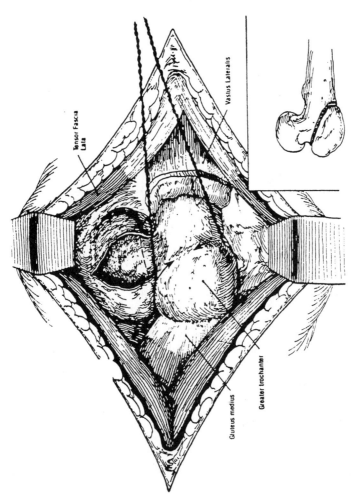

Fig. 3-6. The capsule of the joint is exposed, and the greater trochanter is removed (insert).

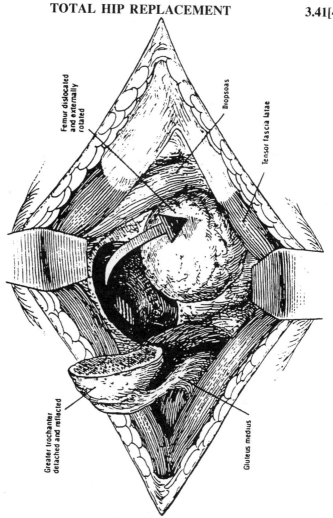

Femur dislocated and externally rotated

Iliopsoas

Tensor fascia latae

Greater trochanter detached and reflected

Gluteus medius

Fig. 3-7. The head of the femur is dislocated from the acetabulum (socket) by flexion, abduction and internal rotation of the leg.

The gluteus medius muscle is carefully pulled forward so that the piriformis tendon and rotator muscles (superior gemellus, obturator internus, inferior gemellus and quadratus femoris) can be seen and severed from their attachments. If the surgeon needs a better view of the joint, the gluteus maximus tendon can be cut before retractors are applied to pull tissues away to expose the hip capsule.

The capsule is cut open and pulled aside to show the bones of the hip. Retractors are placed around the neck of the femur, and the hip is flexed, adducted and rotated outward to pull the femoral head out of the acetabulum. The head of the femur is removed, and the joint capsule is opened more widely if necessary. The femur is then moved anteriorly to expose the acetabulum.

If this approach does not provide sufficient exposure of the acetabulum, it may be converted to a transtrochanteric approach (Stulberg and Hupfer, 1991b).

3.42   Placement of Prostheses

After exposure of the bones of the hip by the surgeon's approach of choice, the acetabular and femoral prostheses are fixed in place, with or without cement.

[1]   Primary Total Hip Arthroplasty with Cemented Prostheses

Standard primary total hip arthroplasty with bone cement begins with removal of the femoral head. This must be done precisely for the prosthesis to fit properly and is preceded by preoperative examination and measurement of distances on radiographic templates of the hip. Intraoperative, measuring devices are used to apply the radiographic measurements to the actual hip. The template measurements may be "translated" to the hip structures intraoperatively by (Petty, 1991e):

- Use of an osteotomy guide—a circular template that has holes or slots at different distances from the reference edge. The template is placed over the femoral head so that the hole corresponding to the neck length selected from preoperative templating is placed over the center of rotation of the femoral head (also determined from preoperative templating); the edge of the guide (where the cut should be made) is aligned perpendicular to the long axis of the femur, at the level of the anterior edge of the greater trochanter.

- Measurement from the anterior extent of the lesser trochanter to the femoral head, as determined by preoperative measurement on templates.

- Determination of thickness of cartilage and bone to be removed from the acetabulum, followed by subtraction of this thickness from the length of the acetabular plus femoral components.

- Placement of fixed markers. The surgeon may want to make the finished joint a particular length, in which case a marker may be placed in the ilium (hipbone) and another in the greater trochanter or hip end of the femur, and the distance measured between the two (with the leg in neutral position and preferably fully extended) before the hip is dislocated. Then any extra length the surgeon has determined is added to this distance, which becomes the reference distance. When prostheses are in place, the hip is reduced (put back in position) and the distance between the markers measured. If the distance is not sufficiently close to that desired, the hip must be dislocated again and adjustments made.

When the femoral head has been removed, the joint capsule is incised further as needed so that it can be fully retracted to expose the acetabulum. Patients with osteoarthritis may have osteophytes (areas of bony overgrowth into the joint capsule), and these should be removed so that the borders of the acetabulum are smooth and as close as possible to normal dimensions. The acetabulum is then prepared for the acetabular prosthesis by reaming, using a drill with hemispheric heads.

Most modern acetabular components intended for cemented fixation are supplied with measured spacers, so the surgeon can determine exactly how much of the acetabulum to ream for the prosthesis and bone cement to fit accurately (Petty, 1991e). When the correct diameter seems to have been reached, the surgeon places the trial prosthesis and evaluates the fit. When the trial prosthesis fits satisfactorily, all soft material is removed from the acetabulum, as are any large bone cysts. The spaces left by the cysts can then be filled in with bone powder and chips collected by reaming; if this material is insufficient, bone can be collected from the resected femoral head and neck to fill in defects.

To promote adherence of bone cement to the acetabular socket, several anchoring holes are drilled in the socket. In addition, the surface may be roughened with the drill, and shallow holes may be drilled in the bone. Just before cement will be applied, a hole is drilled into the socket from above so that a suction tip can be positioned at the top of the socket. Then the socket is cleaned by streams of fluid under pressure (if much bleeding occurs from the acetabular socket, some surgeons use hydrogen peroxide or dilute epinephrine) (Petty,

1991e). Bone cement is mixed and applied to the anchor holes and socket with a syringe. The cement is pressed into the holes and the socket, and then the acetabular component is put in place and held in position under pressure until the cement polymerizes (hardens).

For placement of the femoral component of the hip prosthesis, the femur is first fixed in an appropriate position so it will remain stable during this process. The opening of the femoral canal is squared using a box osteotome (bone cutter). A tapered reamer or flexible reamer is then used to remove material from the femoral canal (middle of the bone). The canal is checked for integrity by inserting a long curved hemostat and tapping the walls; if the wall has been perforated, the perforation is repaired at this time. Special instruments are then used to broach (remove pulp from) the femoral canal to the distance determined preoperatively. If resistance is met, the next smaller size broach is used and a suitably smaller prosthesis is employed, so as not to risk fracturing the femur in trying to insert too large a prosthesis (Petty, 1991e).

A trial prosthesis is placed in the femoral canal, and the hip is reduced (put into anatomic position) to check the fit. If the trial prosthesis is too short, a longer trial prosthesis or neck portion of a modular prosthesis is tried. The motion and stability of the hip are checked with the hip extended and then with the hip flexed; when the length of the reconstructed hip and the fit of the femoral prosthesis in various hip positions has been found satisfactory, the hip is dislocated and the trial prosthesis removed.

The femoral canal is prepared for bone cement fixation of the prosthesis by cleaning with a brush, flushing with liquid and insertion of a plug in the lower end, so that bone cement can be applied under pressure to a limited space. If a defect in the femoral cortex is encountered, the femoral plug may be bone cement inserted with a syringe and allowed to harden before insertion of the fixative, a piece of bone cut from the resected femoral head or a piece of polymer designed for this purpose. Next, the femoral canal is filled with liquid bone cement, and pressure is applied by tapping to encourage intrusion of the cement into the bone of the canal.

The femoral prosthesis is inserted to within 1 cm of final position, and excess bone cement that extrudes with this maneuver is cleared away. The prosthesis is then tapped into final position, and bone cement is allowed to harden.

[2] Primary Total Hip Arthroplasty with Press-Fit Fixation

Press-fit fixation of hip prosthetic components is similar for those with and without porous coatings. Preparation for press-fit fixation is similar to preparation for cemented components except in how fit of the prostheses is determined.

As do cemented prostheses, most press-fit prostheses come with trial components that allow the surgeon to verify that the component fits correctly before the actual prosthesis is inserted. Some prostheses are intended for "line-to-line" fit, so that reaming should provide a space the exact size of the prosthesis. Other prostheses are intended for "interference" fit (the prosthesis is 1 to 2 mm larger than the space that should be prepared by reaming). There is no evidence that one type of fit is better than the other, but the surgeon needs to know which system to use with the intended prosthesis (Petty, 1991e).

Some press-fit acetabular components have spikes intended to be inserted into the bone; if so, a guide is usually provided to help the surgeon drill holes in the correct locations in the acetabular socket. The acetabular socket is cleared of particle debris before insertion of the prosthesis, which is usually accomplished using a guide. The position of the component is checked, and if the cup is intended for screw fixation, holes are drilled and screws inserted. Guides are used for placement of screw holes, to avoid perforating bone and damaging intraperitoneal structures.

The femur is prepared for a press-fit prosthesis by fixing it in position and trimming bone from the lateral femoral neck and medial greater trochanter, if necessary. The femoral canal is reamed and broached (an instrument is inserted to remove a core of pulp) according to the type of prosthesis to be inserted, with the first broach used being several sizes smaller than the expected final canal size. If, as increasingly larger broaches are used, a fracture line appears on the edge of the femur, broaching is stopped and the prosthesis of that size is used. If the crack widens or extends down the femur, a metal band, cable or wire needs to be placed around the femur to preserve the repair (Petty, 1991e).

With the broach of the proper size in place, the trial femoral prosthetic components are placed, the hip is reduced and the length, motion and stability of the reconstruction are evaluated. When final adjustments have been made, the femoral component(s) are seated firmly in place. If a liner is supplied for the acetabular component, this is put in position.

3.43   Wound Closure

When placement of prostheses is complete, the hip is carefully reduced (returned to a position of normal anatomic alignment), and the length and position of the reconstruction are checked once more. Drains are placed in the wound, and it is closed, beginning with reattachment of the short rotator muscles (superior and inferior gemellus, obturator internis and quadratus femoris). These muscles are sutured through holes drilled in the trochanter, with the hip held flexed, adducted and externally rotated as the sutures are tied.

3.50   CONSIDERATIONS FOR PARTICULAR CONDITIONS

Some modifications in procedure and/or choice of prosthesis may be indicated for total hip replacement for patients with certain conditions affecting the hip.

3.51   Congenital Hip Dysplasia

A number of technical difficulties occur with total hip arthroplasty that is performed in adults to treat arthritis due to congenital dysplasia (malformation) of the joint. If the dysplasia is mild, it may be possible to carry out the procedure as for a normal hip but using a small prosthesis. If the dysplasia is severe, however, and in all cases when the hip is dislocated completely, the surgeon needs to watch for the following abnormalities (Petty, 1991e):

- articulation of the femoral head with a false acetabulum several centimeters superior to the true acetabulum and less thickness of acetabular bone than normal in both sockets;

- small femur, requiring a special small or custom-made prosthesis;

- marked upward angling of the head of the femur and acetabulum; and

- muscles, nerves and blood vessels shorter than normal.

It is also likely that patients with severe dysplasia have already undergone previous hip reconstruction surgery, such as acetabular osteotomy (removal of bone), arthroplasty (reconstruction) or femoral osteotomy. Preoperative planning for these patients is particularly challenging and must be done far enough in advance of the operation that special prostheses or other materials can be ordered in a timely manner.

During the operation, the acetabular prosthesis is usually placed in the true socket, unless the false socket has more bone stock. Bone grafts may be necessary to hold the acetabular component, but they have been associated with a high joint failure rate if the prosthesis is not more than two thirds covered by natural bone (Petty, 1991e).

Because it is dangerous to try to stretch muscles, nerves and blood vessels that failed to grow adequately due to hip dysplasia, the femoral portion of hip reconstruction usually requires resecting the femur below the trochanter. This leaves a short, straight femoral shaft, for which a special prosthesis is almost always needed. Alternatively, a segment may be removed from farther down on the femur (step-cut osteotomy). Postoperatively, patients who have tight abductor muscles or who have received bone grafts need extended rehabilitation (Petty, 1991e).

3.52 Rheumatoid Arthritis

Total hip replacement may be indicated for adults with rheumatoid arthritis. The major indication for total hip replacement for adults with rheumatoid arthritis, as with other conditions, is severe hip pain. When knee replacement is also planned, the hip arthroplasty should be performed first. The transtrochanteric approach is appropriate when deformity is severe,[9] and soft tissues must be released carefully to prevent fracture of brittle bone. Bone grafts may be required, and the femur may need to be shortened, as with arthroplasty for congenital hip dysplasia (Petty, 1991e).

3.53 Protrusio Acetabuli

About 20 percent of patients who undergo total hip arthroplasty for rheumatoid arthritis have protrusio acetabuli (acetabulum protruding into the bone of the hip). This condition can also appear in those with Marfan's syndrome and Ehlers-Danlos syndrome (metabolic disorders) (Petty, 1991e). A relatively high proportion of individuals with ankylosing spondylitis (stiffening of the spine) have protrusion deformities (Ranawat, et al., 1992).

---

[9] *See* 3.41[3] *supra.*

Several techniques have been tried to restructure the protruded acetabulum for total hip arthroplasty, including addition of rings, use of enlarged sockets and wire mesh to strengthen the medial (inner) wall. No special treatment is needed for this condition when the following conditions obtain:

1. the protrusio is less than 5 mm;

2. the medial wall is strong; and

3. osteoporosis (brittle bone) is minimal, and the patient has no known collagen or other bone defects.

When this condition does need to be corrected for total hip arthroplasty, bone grafting is preferred because it moves the acetabular component laterally, normalizes the center of rotation of the hip and strengthens the medial wall with a biologic substance (Petty, 1991e).

3.54 Ankylosing Spondylitis

Ankylosing spondylitis is a genetically determined inflammatory joint disease in which the articulations become fused; hip pain may precede lower back symptoms. Patients with this condition who may be candidates for total hip replacement are evaluated on a case-by-case basis. When disease is severe or the patient has had previous hip surgery, special positioning and operative techniques may be needed. When procedures are needed on the ankle and foot, these are done before hip replacement, but if knee replacement is planned, this should wait until after the hip procedure.

The transtrochanteric approach[10] is usually indicated for replacement of these hips, and a small or custom prosthesis is necessary in most cases. If the hip cannot be fully or nearly fully extended, the femur may be shortened, as with replacement for congenital hip dysplasia, and a prosthesis with a longer neck implanted. Cemented fixation may be preferable to press-fit fixation of prostheses for these patients.

Some investigators advocate prophylaxis against heterotopic (out of the normal place) bone development after hip surgery in patients with ankylosing spondylitis, because of the high incidence of this problem among these patients (Ranawat, et al., 1992), but others consider the evidence for prophylaxis equivocal (Petty, 1991e).

---

[10] *See* 3.41[3] *supra.*

3.55 Hip Arthrodesis

When total hip arthroplasty is performed to relieve pain in the patient with hip arthrodesis (fusion of the bones, either due to previous surgery or occurring spontaneously), the transtrochanteric, anterior or posterior approach may be chosen. If the abductor muscles are absent, some surgeons attach the tensor fasciae to the hip end of the femur, and function does not seem lessened without this maneuver. Hip muscle strength may improve for two years or more after total hip arthroplasty in these patients, and unless there is substantial deformity in the hip, the results are nearly as successful as when the procedure is performed for other indications (Petty, 1991e).

3.56 Femoral Osteotomy or Previous Fracture

Total hip replacement is possible, with modifications, in patients who experience pain after proximal femoral osteotomy or healed fracture. Possibilities for managing this situation include the following (Petty, 1991e):

- Standard surgical technique may be possible with a smaller femoral prosthesis, if deformity is minimal; cemented fixation is advised.

- A special prosthesis designed for implantation after femoral osteotomy may be used.

- A custom prosthesis may be used.

- A two-stage reconstruction may be performed, with the osteotomy reversed in the first operation and the joint replaced in the second procedure.

- A second osteotomy may be performed at the same time as total hip arthroplasty.

The chances that the femur will fracture during arthroplasty after femoral osteotomy are higher in direct proportion to the displacement of the osteotomy (that is, the more the angle of the femoral head was changed, the greater the risk of fracture) (Petty, 1991e).

3.57 Previous Arthroplasty

Total hip arthroplasty may be performed to treat pain and dysfunction recurring after partial (resection or cup) arthroplasty.[11] A femoral

---

[11] See 3.33 *supra.*

prosthesis with a longer neck is usually needed in these cases (Petty, 1991e).

3.60   POSTOPERATIVE CARE

Patients recover more rapidly and completely from total hip replacement when the program of postoperative care emphasizes their central role in recovery and education is provided pre-and post-operatively to support them in this role (Petty, 1991f). Attention during the immediate postoperative period focuses on relief of postoperative pain and prevention of complications. Rehabilitation to maximal level of functioning is progressive and usually takes several months.

3.61   Recovery from Surgery

Important aspects of recovery from total hip arthroplasty in the immediate postoperative period are maintaining or restoring blood volume and oxygen-carrying capacity (hemoglobin), achieving pain and infection control, and wound care. Preventing or managing problems with blood clots, particularly venous thrombosis (also called thrombophlebitis), is a particular concern after replacement of the hip joint.

[1]   Usual Postoperative Care

Transfusions may be needed in the first few days after surgery if the patient lost significant amounts of blood during surgery. Drains can usually be removed from the wound by about 24 hours after surgery; they should not remain in place too long, because they offer a portal for infection to enter the hip and inhibit free movement of the joint (Petty, 1991f).

Management of postoperative pain begins in the operating room, with tapering of the narcotic agent if this is given in conjunction with general anesthesia. Patients who have undergone surgery with a regional anesthetic block administered through an epidural (into the space around the spinal column) catheter may be given longer-lasting doses of narcotic, sometimes with another dose of anesthetic, into the same catheter. Other patients may be given narcotic medications intravenously in the recovery room after surgery and then begin *patient-controlled analgesia,* a system that allows the alert and awake patient to deliver small doses of narcotic pain medication at will, intravenously, through a catheter (small plastic tube) placed into a vein (intravenous catheter). When the patient can take fluids by mouth, oral nonsteroidal anti-inflammatory agents can be started and may decrease the need for narcotic medications by half in patients who have undergone total hip arthroplasty (Gravenstein, 1991).

The operated hip is protected and kept in proper position by being placed in balanced suspension (lifted with counterweights) or by placing a special abductor pillow or a regular pillow, carefully positioned, between the legs.

[2]   Venous Thrombosis/Pulmonary Embolism

Some 40 to 60 percent of patients who are 40 years old or more who undergo hip surgery experience venous thrombosis (thromboembolism; a clot in a vein) (Petty and Evarts, 1991). The two most common complications of this condition are deep vein thrombosis (inflammation of a major vein due to a clot) and pulmonary embolism (breathing problems due to a clot in a blood vessel in the lung). The consequences of either can be severe, and pulmonary embolism accounts for death in some 1 to 3 percent of patients undergoing total hip replacement in whom precautions are not taken to prevent thrombosis (Petty and Evarts, 1991).

Thromboembolic complications are more likely in elderly patients, those with decreased mobility, those with a history of blood clotting problems or previous vein surgery and those who are obese; other risk factors include certain inherited blood clotting conditions and other illnesses (such as cancer, stroke or infection) (Petty and Evarts, 1991).

Venous thrombosis may be suspected during physical examination (the condition may be indicated by pain and swelling of the leg and pain in the chest with fever), but these signs are far from diagnostic. Venography and radioactive scanning are most accurate, although radioactive scanning results are skewed by recent surgery in the area being imaged. When the clot is in a major vein, Doppler ultrasonography and venography are the most accurate means to locate the obstruction, and they have the advantage of being noninvasive (Petty and Evarts, 1991).

Pulmonary emboli are best treated by being prevented, because about 80 percent are not suspected until symptoms occur, and about 60 percent of patients who die do so within half an hour of the first symptoms. Preventive therapy includes administration of anticoagulant medication, although this may increase bleeding tendency. If pulmonary embolism is diagnosed, administration of anticoagulant medications is begun immediately to try to prevent the formation of more clots (Petty and Evarts, 1991).

3.62 Rehabilitation

The goal of rehabilitation activities after total hip replacement is to prepare the patient to function maximally in the home and work environments. Based on the needs of these environments, the patient is given instructions about how to perform daily activities, such as walking, with the new hip and provided with exercises to strengthen muscles.

[1] Activities of Daily Living

Most patients can return to their home environment and perform activities of daily living without assistance when they leave the hospital, although they should not be expected to prepare meals or do housework immediately. Those who have multiple problems or other disabilities may need to have a family member or paid help assist them, or they may need to spend some time in a rehabilitation facility (Petty, 1991f).

Physical therapy assessment is performed before the patient with a total hip replacement leaves the hospital. The strength, range of motion and configuration (particularly contractures) of both hips and lower extremities, and the equality of leg length are evaluated. Upper extremity strength and ability to use walking aids also need to be assessed. If the patient may need a cane, crutch or walker postoperatively, he or she should be instructed in its use before surgery and observed for correct use before discharge.

[2] Exercises and Gait Training

Patients should be taught exercises preoperatively that will be used postoperatively to strengthen the leg and hip and increase flexibility. On the first day postoperatively, patients are reminded to begin ankle dorsi and plantar flexion (pulling the foot up and pushing it away), ankle circles, quadriceps and gluteal sets (tightening and releasing the muscles of the thigh and buttocks), alternate lifting of each hip from the bed, and bicycling the knees (moving knees up and down alternately). The second or third day postoperative, the patient adds abduction and increased hip and knee flexion to the exercise routine, and when the quadriceps muscles are strong enough, he or she begins straight-leg raising (Petty, 1991f).

Patients in generally good health preoperatively are able to stand with assistance the day after surgery, and when they can stand comfortably, they are ready to take a few steps with assistance, usually with the support of a walker. Patients whose postoperative pain is managed by epidural administration of a local anesthetic are at increased risk of falls with weight-bearing, because the anesthetic decreases motor activity as well as sensation in the lower limbs. All patients should be assessed for strength and ability to balance while standing before being allowed out of bed. In the approximately 20 percent of patients who have motor block with epidural narcotic, this can be resolved by removing the anesthetic agent from the epidural infusion (Gravenstein, 1991).

A cemented prosthesis is fully fixed during surgery, so patients with this type of prosthesis should not be concerned that exercises or weight-bearing will dislodge the replacement hip. Although some surgeons advocate very gradual weight-bearing to avoid stressing necrotic bone adjacent to the prosthesis, this bone takes months to remodel, and there is no evidence that early weight-bearing affects the duration of a cemented arthroplasty. The only reason to progress gradually is patient comfort—muscles and other tissues affected by surgery will be sore after surgical manipulation and take time to regain strength and flexibility lost due to hip disease (Petty, 1991f).

On the other hand, there is evidence that weight-bearing should proceed more slowly with porous-coated prostheses, because animal studies show that it takes 2 to 3 weeks for bone to begin to grow into the prosthesis, and ingrowth does not plateau until about 12 weeks after implantation. For this reason, it is reasonable to restrict motion between the prosthesis and bone in patients who have porous prostheses, and to restrict weight-bearing when the femoral prosthesis has a porous stem. There is less reason to limit weight-bearing when the acetabular component is porous-coated but the femoral stem is cemented in place (Petty, 1991f).

Gait training after total hip arthroplasty focuses on teaching the patient to walk with equal length of stride for each leg and to place the heel firmly on the floor, extending the knee on the operative side. When both hips were repaired at the same time or very close together, patients are taught to walk with two assists (the "four-point" gait) for greater support. Regular crutches provide greater support, but elbow crutches are easier to maneuver. Once patients can walk safely, they are taught to climb stairs, lifting the unaffected or stronger leg first going up, followed by assists (crutches or canes) and then the affected or less strong leg; going down, the process is reversed.

[3]   Restrictions

Most patients with cemented prostheses and no other disability are able to begin weight-bearing immediately and progress from four-point gait or elbow crutches to cane in two to four weeks. Those with porous-coated femoral stems, however, are advised to limit weight-bearing to a third of body weight for the first six weeks postoperatively, followed by use of a cane in the opposite hand for another six weeks. To prevent lower extremity edema (swelling due to accumulation of fluid) and stiffness, patients should avoid sitting in a chair for more than an hour. Chairs should have seat and arms at heights comfortable for the individual patient to use, and the patient's feet and legs should be supported at hip level most of the time.

Until a fibrous capsule of scar tissue forms around the prosthetic parts several weeks after total hip arthroplasty, the risk of hip dislocation should be decreased by avoiding adduction (movement of the affected leg toward the other leg), and particularly avoiding excessive flexion and internal rotation with this movement. Thus, the patient may cross the ankles but not the thighs, and needs to use caution during certain movements, such as when getting into a vehicle.

Patients who engage in high-impact activities or those that stress a hip joint with prostheses have been found to suffer earlier failure of the joint, so patients are warned about this risk and urged to avoid causing stress or impact pressure on the joint (Petty, 1991f).

Many patients who have sedentary occupations can return to work by six weeks after total hip arthroplasty; those who must lift and carry objects should delay returning to work for three to four months after surgery. However, neither age nor sex has been found to have an effect on the rate or extent of recovery of function, and most patients believe they have recovered fully by three months after the operation, although muscle strength continues to improve for at least six months after surgery. Continued improvement in flexion and abduction can be noted for the first postoperative year, and adduction and rotation can improve over an even longer period (Petty, 1991f).

3.70 COMPLICATIONS

Death has been associated with total hip arthroplasty in 0.4 to 3 percent of cases. These mortality rates are little different from those expected for elderly persons in the populations reported upon, and the major causes of death—venous thrombosis,[12] coronary artery disease, cerebrovascular thrombosis (stroke) and cardiac arrest during the operation—are characteristic of major surgical procedures in general (Petty, 1991g).

Other complications reported after total hip arthroplasty are iatrogenic (surgical) injury to structures such as nerves, heterotopic formation of bone, bone fracture or dislocation and infection. Imaging studies help evaluate the results and complications of arthroplasty.

3.71 Iatrogenic (Surgical) Injury

Major surgery puts nerves, blood vessels and other structures in the operative area at risk of injury.

[1] Nerve Injury

The structures most often injured during total hip replacement surgery are nerves, with injury to the sciatic nerve being reported most often, followed by injury to the femoral nerve and last by injury to the obturator nerve. *(See Figure 3-8.)* Overall incidences of nerve injury have been reported to be between 0.7 and 3.5 percent during primary total hip replacement procedures and up to twice that rate for revision arthroplasties. Nerve injury is more common in women, even after accounting for more frequent difficult operations for congenital hip dysplasia in women compared to men (Petty, 1991g).

Changes in nerve function that are not apparent clinically (to the patient or examiner) occur more often than noticeable nerve injury such as sciatic nerve pain. Possible mechanisms of nerve injury during surgery include stretching, compression, contusion, thermal injury (from bone cement polymerization or cautery), laceration and ischemia (lack of blood to nourish the nerve). Placement and tension of retractors are the most likely causes of nerve injury. The less injury a nerve sustains, the more likely it is to recover function, although burning pain in the nerve often occurs even if sensation and function recover (Petty, 1991g).

---

[12] *See* 3.61[2] *supra.*

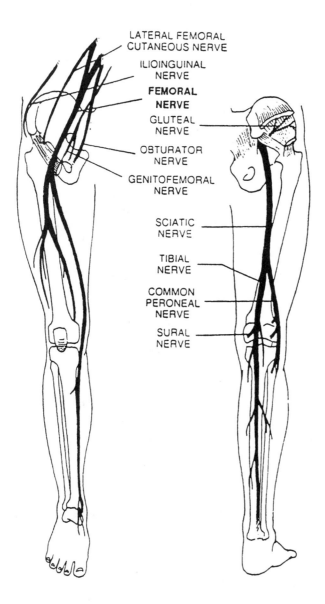

LATERAL FEMORAL
CUTANEOUS NERVE

ILIOINGUINAL
NERVE

**FEMORAL
NERVE**

GLUTEAL
NERVE

OBTURATOR
NERVE

GENITOFEMORAL
NERVE

SCIATIC
NERVE

TIBIAL
NERVE

COMMON
PERONEAL
NERVE

SURAL
NERVE

Fig. 3-8. The femoral nerve in relation to the sciatic, obturator and other nerves of the hip and thigh.

[2] Blood Vessel Injury

Injuries to blood vessels are rare during hip arthroplasty, but they may be severe. As with nerve injury, a major cause of blood vessel damage during surgery is placement or manipulation of retractors. Typical mechanisms by which blood vessels are injured during surgery are similar to those for nerves: laceration (cutting), crushing, thermal injury, compression and tearing. Risk factors are also similar for vascular (blood vessel) and nerve injury: mainly, previous surgery (because it alters normal anatomy) and being female (even considering the greater incidence of total hip arthroplasty in women). In addition, vascular injury is more frequent when the anterior rather than another approach is used, possibly due to placement of retractors (Petty, 1991g).

Brisk bleeding or an unexplained drop in blood pressure may signal the occurrence of intraoperative injury to a blood vessel. The source of the bleeding should be located and the blood vessel repaired, unless it is expendable, in which case both ends should be tied off to stop bleeding. Problems with blood vessels that might appear after surgery include a clot in a vessel, a tear in an artery wall leading to blood leakage or a fistula (abnormal connection between an artery and vein).

[3] Fractures

A fracture (break) may occur in bone or in part of a prosthesis placed during hip arthroplasty. Press-fit prostheses are associated with the highest incidence of intraoperative (during surgery) fractures, occurring in 2.5 percent of primary arthroplasties and nearly three times this rate in revision procedures, compared to only 0.4 percent of cases in which cemented fixation was used (Petty, 1991g). The difference is probably due to use of the largest femoral component that will fit for press-fit fixation, so that the femoral wall may be broken as broaching is carried out assiduously. Congenital defects in the shape or type of bone in the joint and effects of previous surgery are major predisposing factors to bone fracture during surgery. After the operation, patients need to protect the hip joint from added stress by using caution in activities and walking aids to decrease weight-bearing (Petty, 1991g).

Bone fractures may be classified into six categories, depending on their extent and shape. They are also managed differently, depending on their type and severity (Petty, 1991g). Various intraoperative maneuvers are associated with certain types of fracture. For example, a vertical (lengthwise) or spiral fracture of the femur may occur during broaching (removal of material in the core of the thighbone) or insertion of the prosthesis.

3.72   Heterotopic Bone Formation

Heterotopic (extraneous) bone has been reported in various studies to occur after 8 to 90 percent of total hip replacement procedures, but this bone only affects joint function in a reported 1 to 24 percent of cases. Men more often experience this complication than women, as do patients with hypertrophic osteoarthritis (osteoarthritis with overgrowth of tissues), spinal hyperostosis (excess bone in the spine) and those with post-traumatic arthritis. Ankylosing spondylitis and presence of human leukocyte antigen B5 (a genetic marker) are also associated with a higher risk of heterotopic bone formation, and if heterotopic bone forms in one hip after arthroplasty, it is more likely to occur in the same hip or the opposite hip with another arthroplasty (Petty, 1991g).

Some patients with formation of heterotopic bone have pain and a feeling of warmth in the hip; a low-grade fever may also be present. When these symptoms appear two to three weeks after hip arthroplasty, a radiograph may show signs of bone formation, and a bone scan will show marked signs of increased bone activity in the affected area. Patients should limit activity to only that which is comfortable, because increased motion may promote further bone formation.

More advanced stages of heterotopic bone formation are associated with further limitation of joint motion, requiring surgery to remove the excess bone, followed by radiation therapy or administration of the medication indomethacin to prevent repeated formation of heterotopic bone. These measures may also prevent the desirable ingrowth of tissue into porous-coated prosthetic components, however (Petty, 1991g).

3.73   Bone Fracture or Dislocation

Bones may fracture after total hip replacement, at any time from a few days to many years after surgery. Some fractures may be due to major trauma, whereas others occur in association with loosening of the prosthesis. The reported incidence of all types of fractures after total hip replacement is 0.1 percent.

Often, postoperative fractures can be treated by a combination of traction and casting or by bracing, but when bones are also dislocated (higher "grades" of fracture), revision arthroplasty is usually indicated. A rare complication is fracture of the pelvis (the hipbones over the groin) due to fatigue (strain from normal use). This complication causes groin pain that may be so severe that the patient cannot bear weight. Fatigue fractures of the pelvis are more common in patients with rheumatoid arthritis or osteoporosis (Petty, 1991g).

Dislocation of the hip (in which the head of the femur is pulled out of the acetabulum) has been reported to occur after 0.4 to 8 percent of primary total hip replacements, with a higher incidence after revision arthroplasty or surgery among patients with congenital hip dysplasia. Dislocations may be classified according to their cause, as follows (Petty, 1991g):

- type I—the patient puts the hip in a position that cannot be accommodated by the prostheses;
- type II—imbalance of soft tissues during surgery; and
- type III—components not well positioned.

Closed reduction is usually successful in putting the dislocated hip back into position. This procedure is best performed under fluoroscopic (real-time x-ray) guidance; the patient may be given a pain medication or muscle relaxant or both, or receive general anesthetic if the reduction may be difficult. When the hip is back in position, the patient is instructed regarding positions to avoid in order to prevent future dislocation, and a cast or brace may be applied to help the patient avoid these positions while the hip heals (casting or braces are preferable to bed rest for elderly patients, because of the higher risk to general health of immobility in this age group). Exercises to strengthen hip muscles are begun or continued, and usually after four to six weeks, use of the cast or brace can be discontinued. More severe dislocations will need to be reduced surgically (Petty, 1991g).

3.74 Infection

Total joint replacement is performed as an "ultraclean" procedure (Nelson, 1991), meaning that the most stringent precautions are taken to prevent contamination of the wound. In fact, stricter precautions have led to notable decreases in the rate of hip infection after joint replacement. Before antibiotic therapy was used, the rate of infection after hip replacement averaged 11 percent (Petty, 1991g). For a series of operations in which antibiotic medications were administered from shortly before total hip arthroplasty to shortly after surgery, the rate of reported joint infection averaged 1.3 percent, and modern "clean" operating room technique (with unidirectional air flow) has brought the infection rate to an average of 0.7 percent (0.6 percent average when antibiotic therapy is added). Higher incidences of deep wound infection may occur with total hip replacement among patients who have undergone previous hip surgery, had a previous hip infection, have infection elsewhere in the body or who are immunosuppressed (Petty, 1991g).

Infection can become evident months to more than a year after hip replacement surgery. In one series of 2,651 patients who had undergone hip arthroplasty with perioperative antibiotic medication administration, infection was diagnosed in 0.64 percent in the first year of follow-up. Risk factors for infection in this series were diabetes mellitus, failure of a fracture to heal, a break in sterility during the procedure, wound infection or an unhealed wound at the time of discharge from the hospital, postoperative urinary tract infection and difficult rehabilitation from surgery. The hip infections were also found to predispose the patients to later development of septic arthritis (Wymenga, et al., 1992).

A hip infection is also more likely to occur among obese patients (because fat has less adequate blood supply, operative time is prolonged and wound closure is difficult) and those who have been hospitalized longer before hip surgery. Thus, if possible, obese patients should lose weight before surgery (but without compromising their nutritional status). To prevent bacterial "seeding" of the hip after joint replacement, many surgeons also advocate prophylactic antibiotic therapy before dental, genitourinary or gastrointestinal surgery in a patient who has undergone hip arthroplasty (Nelson, 1991).

Treatment for deep hip infection after arthroplasty usually involves the removal of all foreign materials (prosthesis components and bone cement, if used) and their replacement with antibiotic-impregnated space-keeping materials, combined with intravenous administration of antibiotic medications for several weeks before a revision arthroplasty can be performed (Nelson, 1991).

3.75   Osteolysis

Destruction of bone (osteolysis) in the joint has lately emerged as one of the most serious complications of total hip arthroplasty, for both cemented and uncemented prostheses (Herberts, et al., 1995). In this complication, bone cells are destroyed around the implant, earlier and more extensively when the implant is uncemented, and more particularly around the acetabular component.

Osteolysis is not usually symptomatic, and it is difficult to detect in the acetabulum on radiographic images. Cytokines (immune system chemicals) have been associated with the process of bone resorption, which seems to occur more rapidly with larger-size particles.

3.76   Evaluation of Complications

Serial radiologic evaluations are performed after hip arthroplasty to detect infection, prosthesis problems or other complications in the hip.

[1]   Plain Radiography

The radiographic evaluation of hip arthroplasty is based on the set of images obtained preoperatively and a set of plain radiographs obtained soon after surgery; these sets serve as the baseline to evaluate the implantation and any changes that occur subsequently. To obtain comparable results for this purpose, the same size film, same tube-to-film distance, patient-to-film distance and positioning of the patient and x-ray beam should be used each time. Protocols have been developed to evaluate the vector forces in the hip from radiographs taken after implantation of prosthetic parts (Heare and Montgomery, 1991).

Radiographic images taken in series so that anatomy can be compared from one time to the next may show loosening of a cemented hip prosthesis as a lucent (lighter or clear) space between the bone and cement that is 2 mm or more at first and widens on subsequent examinations. These findings do not necessarily correlate with clinical symptoms of loosening, however. Furthermore, narrower gaps are often seen during the first year after implantation of a prosthesis, and these spaces between prosthesis and bone or prosthesis and cement are not associated with symptoms (Heare and Montgomery, 1991).

In addition to indications of prosthetic loosening, plain radiographs can also show signs of other problems, for example:

- joint dislocation or instability;

- fracture of the bone, prosthesis or cement;

- growth of heterotopic (extra) bone; and

- ectopic (located outside the normal area) bone cement.

If heterotopic bone or ectopic cement is damaging soft tissues, these changes may also be evident as swelling on the radiographs (Heare and Montgomery, 1991).

[2]   Aspiration Arthrography

Aspiration arthrography is the most effective way to confirm hip joint infection, a condition that is indicated by hip pain and clinical changes suggestive of infection and no radiographic evidence of joint loosening or malpositioning. For this procedure, the radiologist uses careful sterile technique and radiographic guidance to insert a needle into the joint and withdraw material from the joint space; leaving the needle in place, radiopaque dye (or air, for the patient who may be allergic to dye) is injected to verify that the sample was obtained from the joint space.

If abscesses are evident on radiography or the infection appears to have invaded a bursa (sac filled with fluid that prevents friction as the bones of a joint move), these structures should also be aspirated. Samples are cultured and tested to identify whether and what type of organisms are present.

[3]   Radionuclide Scanning

The results of radionuclide bone scanning can help pinpoint a problem that is suspected from the patient's history, physical examination findings, laboratory test results and other imaging studies. For this test, a radionuclide (a substance that gathers in certain tissues and to which a chemical that shows up on radiologic imaging has been bonded) is injected intravenously.

The most frequently used radionuclide is a phosphate compound labeled with technetium (Tc-MDP). A series of images is obtained immediately after injection, to show Tc-MDP traveling to the hip. A second series of images is obtained right after the first, to show movement of the radioisotope from the blood vessels into the joint. The final set of images is obtained about two to four hours later, to locate blood flow and bone-building activity in the joint, which are marked by concentrations of Tc-MDP.

It is normal for a hip with a prosthesis to show increased uptake of Tc-MDP for about the first year after surgery, but if uptake is increased at subsequent examinations, loosening of the prosthesis or infection in the joint is a possibility. In addition, stress fractures in the bone will take up Tc-MDP, as will heterotopic (excess) bone (Heare and Montgomery, 1991).

The radionuclide gallium may be used to evaluate suspected areas of inflammation or neoplasia (cancer activity) in the hip. Radionuclide scanning with white blood cells labeled with indium (In-WBC) is an excellent way to evaluate suspected infection in the hip or adjacent soft tissues. Various research studies show that the sensitivity (accuracy of identifying infection if it is there) of In-WBC scanning is between 83 and 100 percent, and its specificity (identifying only infection, not mistaking it for another condition) is between 73 and 90 percent. In fact, In-WBC imaging is more sensitive in detecting infection than aspiration arthrography. However, aspiration of the joint is still necessary to obtain a sample for culturing, so that the specific organism can be determined (Heare and Montgomery, 1991).

[4]   Computed Tomography (CT)

Computed tomography scans after joint replacement can be impaired in quality by interference of the metal in the prosthesis, with chromium-cobalt causing the most interference and plastic the least. Although software is available to decrease the impact of these artifacts on computed tomography images, large implants such as are done in the hip are time consuming to image in this fashion. Taking these extra steps to obtain better quality images may be useful, however, when an arthroplasty is planned for the patient's opposite hip or a revision procedure is planned (Heare and Montgomery, 1991).

[5]   Magnetic Resonance Imaging (MRI)

Magnetic resonance imaging (MRI) is important in the preoperative evaluation of hip disease that will be treated by placement of a prosthesis, but it has little use in postoperative evaluation because of the interference caused by the metal prosthesis. The degree of distortion caused by metal is proportional to the strength of the magnetic field used for imaging and the distance of the metal from the area being imaged. Some images of tissues near prostheses have been obtained experimentally using low-field-strength (0.1 to 0.3 tesla) magnets, and these images were considered to be more helpful in diagnosis than computed tomography images of the same area (Heare and Montgomery, 1991).

3.80   REVISION TOTAL HIP ARTHROPLASTY

Failure of a hip arthroplasty procedure is more likely in patients who meet the following criteria (Amstutz, 1991; Herberts, et al., 1995):

- young;
- very active;
- male; or
- with hip disease characterized by loss of bone mass or density (such as avascular necrosis, congenital hip dysplasia or previous hip arthroplasty).

Heavier weight, unilateral hip disease, wide femoral canal and varus position (abnormal turning toward the midline of the body) of the prosthesis have also been correlated with prosthesis loosening (Heare and Montgomery, 1991).

The major considerations for performing a revision (second) total hip arthroplasty are pain and joint loosening. Although these two conditions usually occur together, either alone is possible (Stulberg and Hupfer, 1991).

Radiographic evaluation of a hip that may need revision arthroplasty can determine which parts are loose; it is not necessary to replace the entire prosthesis in many cases when one of the components remains solidly attached. In addition, use of a cemented prosthesis for primary arthroplasty does not dictate that cemented fixation be employed in the revision procedure (Heare and Montgomery, 1991).

3.90   OUTCOME OF TOTAL HIP ARTHROPLASTY

The results of total hip arthroplasty are typically evaluated using scales on which various factors are graded numerically, most often with low numbers representing the worst or least desirable end of the scale. Factors that are evaluated include pain, range of motion and walking. The Harris Hip Rating scale has been widely used in the United States; on this scale, a pain score of 0 is given for severe pain even at rest, and a maximum pain score of 44 is given if the patient has no pain. Function is assessed on a 47-point scale, in categories of activities of daily living (14 points), limp (11 points), walking aids (11 points) and maximum walking distance (11 points); range of motion (5 points) and absence of functional deformity (4 points) are also assessed for a possible final score of 100 for a normal hip. Recently a form was developed and endorsed by orthopedic societies internationally to standardize the reporting of clinical and radiographic results of operations on the hip (Murray, 1993).

Another measure of outcome of total hip arthroplasty is the rate of failure of the prosthesis, determined as the need for revision surgery. On this basis, however, all prostheses eventually fail, considering that 20 years seems to represent the limitation of current hip replacement technology (Schmalzried and Brown, 1995). Furthermore, differences exist in various populations in the indications for primary and revision surgery, making direct comparison of these statistics meaningless as an indication of the success of a technique (Herberts, et al., 1995).

3.91 Fixation

The long-term results of total hip arthroplasty procedures using Charnley prostheses and cemented fixation, as reported in a number of series, showed revision rates of 5 to 14 percent for follow-up periods of 5 to 15 years. Averages for patient pain scores of good to excellent ranged between 78 and 95 percent in these series (Petty, 1991h).

Although up to half of total hip replacements are performed today using cementless fixation, the technique is too new for long-term results to be evident. A number of reports with two-year follow-ups have shown averages of 2 to 37 percent for less than optimal pain scores, 4 to 52 percent for presence of limp and 2 percent for revision of the femoral component (Petty, 1991h).

3.92 Indication for Surgery

The highest proportion of total hip replacement procedures are performed to treat osteoarthritis in elderly patients, with the second highest number being performed in adults with rheumatoid arthritis. Different investigators have reported better results in one or the other group of patients; better results in those with osteoarthritis may be attributable to the likelihood of these patients having a better quality of bone, whereas patients with rheumatoid arthritis could have had better outcomes in other studies because they are less active (Petty, 1991h).

The success rates for one-stage revision procedures for patients with infected prostheses ranged from 75 to 87 percent in several series, and the success rate after the two-stage procedure more popular in the United States has ranged between 60 and 95 percent (Gearen, 1991).

3.100 BIBLIOGRAPHY

Text References

Amstutz, H. C.: Surface Replacement Arthroplasty. In: Petty, W. (Ed.): Total Joint Replacement. Philadelphia: Saunders, 1991.

Brown, S. A. and Merritt, K.: Biocompatibility. In: Petty, W. (Ed.): Total Joint Replacement. Philadelphia: Saunders, 1991.

Damron, R. A. and Heiner, J. P.: Rapidly Progressive Protrusio Acetabuli in Patients with Rheumatoid Arthritis. Clin. Orthop. 289:186-194, 1993.

Evans, B. G., et al.: The Rationale for Cemented Total Hip Arthroplasty. Orthop. Clin. North Am. 24(4):599-610, 1993.

Gearen, P. F.: Results of Revision Total Hip Arthroplasty. In: Petty, W. (Ed.): Total Joint Replacement. Philadelphia: Saunders, 1991.

Gravenstein, N.: Anesthesia for Joint Replacement Surgery. In: Petty, W. (Ed.): Total Joint Replacement. Philadelphia: Saunders, 1991.

Heare, M. M. and Montgomery, W. J.: Imaging of Total Joint Replacement. In: Petty, W. (Ed.): Total Joint Replacement. Philadelphia: Saunders, 1991.

Herberts, P. G., et al.: Revision Hip Surgery: The Challenge. In: Galante, J. O., et al. (Eds.): Total Hip Revision Surgery. New York: Raven Press, 1995.

Ho, G., Jr., and Kammer, G. M.: Osteoarthritis. In: Andreoli, T. E., et al.: Cecil Essentials of Medicine. Philadelphia: Saunders, 1990.

Lemons, J. E.: Keynote Address: Biomaterials for Total Joint Replacements. In: Morrey, B. F. (Ed.): Biological, Material, and Mechanical Considerations of Joint Replacement. New York: Raven Press, 1993.

McElfresh, E.: History of Arthroplasty. In: Petty, W. (Ed.): Total Joint Replacement. Philadelphia: Saunders, 1991.

Miller, G. J.: Biomechanics and Design. In: Petty, W. (Ed.): Total Joint Replacement. Philadelphia: Saunders, 1991.

Nelson, J. P.: Prevention of Postoperative Infections. In: Petty, W. (Ed.): Total Joint Replacement. Philadelphia: Saunders, 1991.

Petty, W.: Total Hip Arthroplasty: Preoperative Evaluation. In: Petty, W. (Ed.): Total Joint Replacement. Philadelphia: Saunders, 1991a.

Petty, W.: Prostheses for Total Hip Arthroplasty. In: Petty, W. (Ed.): Total Joint Replacement. Philadelphia: Saunders, 1991b.

Petty, W.: Fixation Methods. In: Petty, W. (Ed.): Total Joint Replacement. Philadelphia: Saunders, 1991c.

Petty, W.: Bipolar Hip Arthroplasty. In: Petty, W. (Ed.): Total Joint Replacement. Philadelphia: Saunders, 1991d.

Petty, W.: Total Hip Arthroplasty: Operative Technique. In: Petty, W. (Ed.): Total Joint Replacement. Philadelphia: Saunders, 1991e.

Petty, W.: Total Hip Arthroplasty: Postoperative Care and Rehabilitation. In: Petty, W. (Ed.): Total Joint Replacement. Philadelphia: Saunders, 1991f.

Petty, W.: Total Hip Arthroplasty: Complications. In: Petty, W. (Ed.): Total Joint Replacement. Philadelphia: Saunders, 1991g.

Petty, W.: Results of Primary Total Hip Arthroplasty. In: Petty, W. (Ed.): Total Joint Replacement. Philadelphia: W. B. Saunders Company, 1991h.

Petty, W. and Evarts, C. McC.: Thromboembolic Disease. In: Petty, W. (Ed.): Total Joint Replacement. Philadelphia: Saunders, 1991.

Ranawat, C. S., et al.: Total Hip Replacement Arthroplasty in Patients with Inflammatory Arthritis. In: Paget, S. A. and Fields, T. R. (Eds.): Rheumatic Disorders. Boston: Andover Medical Publishers, 1992.

Schmalzried, T. P. and Brown, I. C.: Mechanisms of Prosthetic Hip Joint Failure. In: Galante, J. O., et al. (Eds.): Total Hip Revision Surgery. New York: Raven Press, 1995.

Springfield, D. S.: Joint Reconstruction after Tumor Resection. In: Petty, W. (Ed.): Total Joint Replacement. Philadelphia: Saunders, 1991.

Stulberg, B. and Hupfer, T.: Indications and Preoperative Planning for Total Hip Arthroplasty. In: Petty, W. (Ed.): Total Joint Replacement. Philadelphia: Saunders, 1991a.

Stulberg, B. and Hupfer, T.: Surgical Approaches for Total Hip Replacement. In: Petty, W. (Ed.): Total Joint Replacement. Philadelphia: Saunders, 1991b.

Susman, M. H. and Clayton, M. L.: Management of the Rheumatoid Hip. In: Clayton, M. L. and Smyth, C. J. (Eds.): Surgery for Rheumatoid Arthritis: A Comprehensive Team Approach. New York: Churchill Livingstone, 1992.

Wymenga, A. B., et al.: Perioperative Factors Associated with Septic Arthritis After Arthroplasty: Prospective Multicenter Study of 362 Knee and 2,651 Hip Operations. Acta Orthop. Scand. 63(6):665-671, 1992.

Additional References

Billotti, J., et al.: The Porous-Coated Anatomic (PCA) Total Hip Arthroplasty: A Review of 73 Uncemented Cases with 2-Year Follow Up. Orthopedics 18(1):37–43, Jan. 1995.

Bourne, R. B., et al.: Total Hip Replacement: The Case for Noncemented Femoral Fixation Because of Age. Can. J. Surg. 38 Suppl. 1:S61–S66, Feb. 1995.

Griffiths, H. J., et al.: Total Hip Replacement and Other Orthopedic Hip Procedures. Radiol. Clin. North Am. 33(2):267–287, March 1995.

Harris, W. H.: The Case for Cementing all Femoral Components in Total Hip Replacement. Can. J. Surg. 38 Suppl. 1:S55-S60, Feb. 1995.

Heenan, S. D., et al.: Lymphatic Filling in Arthrography Following Total Hip Replacement. Clin. Radiol. 50(2):90–94, Feb. 1995.

Zicat, B., et al.: Patterns of Osteolysis Around Total Hip Components Inserted with and without Cement. J. Bone Joint Surg. Am. 77(3):432–439, March 1995.

CHAPTER 4

OSTEOPOROSIS

SCOPE

Osteoporosis is a weakening of bones caused by the depletion of calcium, especially from the wrist, spine and hip. Osteoporosis is most often seen in elderly women, who suffer 95 percent of the 1.3 million osteoporosis-related fractures every year. The 250,000 hip fractures that occur yearly are the most serious complication of osteoporosis, with a 34 percent mortality rate within six months of fracture. Type I osteoporosis afflicts women 10 to 15 years after menopause and weakens the trabecular bone, primarily of the distal forearm and vertebral bodies of the spine. Type II affects both men and women over age 70, erodes both cortical and trabecular bone, and is associated with hip fractures. Bone mineral content in any part of the body can now be quantified with dual energy x-ray absorptiometry. Established osteoporosis can be slowed with estrogen and calcium, and the drugs calcitonin, alendronate and etidronate have been shown to stop bone loss and in some cases even add bone mass when given for a year to 18 months.

SYNOPSIS

4.00   INTRODUCTION

Osteoporosis is a metabolic bone disease characterized by a loss of bone minerals (primarily calcium but also phosphorus) and of underlying bone matrix throughout the skeleton, but especially in the spine, hip and wrist. This wasting of bone minerals and matrix makes the affected bone susceptible to fracture with minimal or no trauma.

The American College of Physicians has estimated that there are 1.3 million osteoporosis-related fractures annually, and that 250,000 of those occur in the hip (American College of Physicians, 1990). The lifetime risk of a hip fracture is 15 percent for white women and 5 percent for men. For women, that risk is equal to the combined lifetime risk of developing breast, uterine and ovarian cancer. For men, it is about the same as the risk of developing prostate cancer (National Osteoporosis Foundation, 1989). Among people age 90, a third of all women and a sixth of all men have had a hip fracture (Lyles, 1989).

4.10 NORMAL BONE METABOLISM

Bone is never static. Even after bones stop growing in adolescence, minerals are continually being added to and removed from the skeleton to maintain a constant level of calcium and other minerals in the blood. Calcium, a major constituent of bone, is also an important ion in the contraction of muscles and in blood clotting. Therefore, bone is used as a mineral reservoir, where minerals are deposited and removed as the blood level requires.

Bone is composed of 30 percent minerals, primarily calcium and phosphorus, and 70 percent collagen and other proteins that form the matrix into which the minerals are incorporated. Three calcium regulators (parathyroid hormone, vitamin D and calcitonin) are thought to primarily control the absorption of calcium from the gastrointestinal tract, its deposition into and resorption from bone, and the maintenance of calcium blood levels.

It is the level of calcium in the blood, not the condition of a person's bones, that determines whether calcium is deposited or removed from the skeleton. It is thought that this delicate blood calcium feedback system becomes unbalanced as we age, removing more calcium from bone than can be replaced.

Parathyroid hormone is made by the parathyroid glands (small glands imbedded in the larger thyroid gland in the neck on either side of the trachea, or windpipe). The hormone is released from the parathyroid glands as a large molecule and is activated only when it is broken down in the liver into two parts, one of which is hormonally active, the other inactive. The amount of parathyroid hormone that is secreted is inversely related to the serum calcium level and to the blood level of vitamin D.

Parathyroid hormone increases the serum calcium level in several ways. It actively transports calcium from the skeleton and works with certain enzymes (hydrolytic and lysosomal enzymes) to release calcium from bone. It stimulates osteoclasts (cells that break down bone) and inhibits osteoblasts (cells that build bone). (*See Figure 4–1.*) To further boost blood calcium levels, parathyroid hormone reduces the excretion of calcium ions by the kidneys. It is also thought that in the kidney, parathyroid hormone stimulates the activation of a form of vitamin D that then enhances the absorption of calcium from the intestinal tract. Parathyroid hormone prevents phosphate reabsorption from the kidney tubules into the bloodstream, thereby promoting phosphate excretion. Parathyroid hormone secretion is inhibited by a rise in the blood level of calcium (Wells and Ashley, 1991).

Serum levels of parathyroid hormone increase with age, but it is not clear whether this is the only—or even a major—factor in primary osteoporosis (Lyles, 1989).

Vitamin D increases the absorption of calcium and phosphorus from the intestine, and removes calcium from bone to boost the blood calcium level. Vitamin D may have other, growth-promoting effects, which are not well understood. Vitamin D exists in several forms, but the most physiologically important are vitamins D_2 and D_3. The most active form is vitamin D_3. In the skin, D_3 is made when ultraviolet light transforms a type of cholesterol into the vitamin. The form of vitamin D found in supplements is vitamin D_2 (Wells and Ashley, 1991).

Calcitonin is the third calcium regulator. One of the hormones secreted by the thyroid gland, its actions and effects are believed to be opposite to those of parathyroid hormone. Calcitonin is thought to lower blood calcium levels by inhibiting the removal of calcium from bone and by promoting the urinary excretion of calcium and phosphate.

Calcitonin secretion is stimulated by calcium, pentagastrin (a hormone secreted by the lower portion of the stomach that causes the stomach to secrete hydrochloric acid), beta-adrenergic catecholamines (the "fight or flight" hormones like adrenaline), glucagon (a hormone secreted by the pancreas that increases levels of blood sugar) and cholecystokinin (a hormone secreted by the upper part of the small intestine that stimulates the gallbladder to contract and the pancreas to release digestive enzymes). These hormones are all involved with either digestion of food or avoidance of danger. By stimulating the secretion of calcitonin when adrenaline and glucagon (which mobilizes quick energy to muscles) are released, the body prepares itself to repair bone damage.

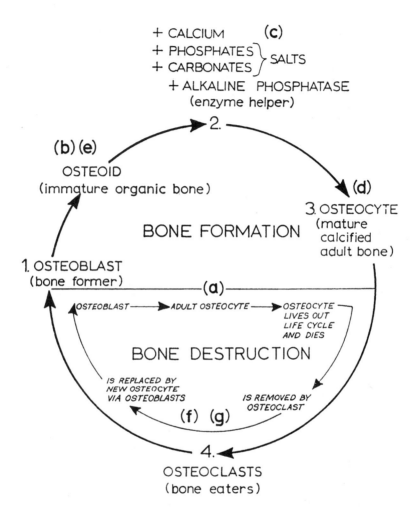

Fig. 4-1. The cycle of bone formation and destruction. The normal cycle (a) takes place through stages 1, 2, 3 and 4. Developmental and deficiency disorders can occur at various points, for example, at (b), osteoporosis (defect in new bone formation); at (c), rickets and osteomalacia (failure of calcification of immature new bone); at (d), Paget's disease (failure to convert immature to mature bone); at (e), osteogenesis imperfecta (excessive immature bone formation); at (f), hyperparathyroidism (excessive resorption of bone, excessive decalcification; also true of osteoporosis); and at (g), osteopetrosis (failure of bone resorption and of conversion to mature bone).

Although calcium blood level is primarily mediated by parathyroid hormone, vitamin D and calcitonin, other hormones also play a part in bone growth and development.

Sex hormones are needed for adequate bone development. Individuals with conditions such as Turner's syndrome or Kleinfelter's syndrome, in which sex hormones are lacking during skeletal growth, do not form adequate amounts of bone. It has also been found that women who are runners and anorexics who stop menstruating have accelerated bone loss in the spine, as if they were postmenopausal (Lyles, 1989).

Thyroid hormone and growth hormone are also needed for proper bone growth and maintenance. However, too much thyroid hormone stimulates bone resorption (absorption back into the body), causing osteoporosis in hyperthyroid people.

As study continues into bone metabolism, more hormones and activating factors are being discovered that have effects on bone, both revealing a vastly more complex series of mechanisms than was previously imagined and pointing to possible future interventions for osteoporosis.

4.20   ETIOLOGY

Ninety percent of the 25 million Americans who are afflicted with osteoporosis are postmenopausal women (Gambrell, 1992). However, the exact mechanisms of osteoporosis are not clear, and indeed, the term "osteoporosis" does not indicate any specific etiologic factor. Clinically the word osteoporosis is a catch-all that denotes any one of a number of conditions (the most common of which occurs in elderly women) that can cause a loss of bone.

Primary osteoporosis—a condition that is not caused by any other disease process or medications—is thought to involve imbalances in the hormones that regulate the removal of calcium and phosphorus from bone and the absorption of these minerals from the intestine. However, the mechanisms are far from clear. As work on these processes continues, more hormones and humoral (blood and lymph) substances, such as interleukin–1, prostaglandins and lymphotoxin, are being found to have effects on bone.

Most osteoporosis experts believe there are two types of primary osteoporosis, though some scientists dispute this theoretical division

(DeLuca and Mazess, 1989). Type I osteoporosis affects women 10 to 15 years after they reach menopause and primarily involves trabecular (spongy; cancellous; a trabecula is one of the needles of bone that extend from the hard, compact outer layer into its cancellous interior) bone, especially in the vertebral bodies of the spine and at the ends of the arm bones. Type II, or senile, osteoporosis occurs in both sexes after the age of 70 but predominates in women by a ratio ranging from 2 to 1 to 3 to 1. Type II affects both cortical (compact, hard bone) and trabecular bone and is thought to cause most hip fractures (Lyles, 1989).

4.21   Primary Osteoporosis

Primary osteoporosis—a condition that is not caused by medications or another disease process—is the most common kind of osteoporosis, comprising 95 percent of cases (Gambrell, 1992). There are thought to be two types of primary osteoporosis. Type I affects postmenopausal women in their 50s and 60s, while type II osteoporosis is found in both sexes after age 70, although women are affected more than men.

Rarely, osteoporosis is found in younger men and women and cannot be traced to a secondary medical cause. This idiopathic (of unknown cause) primary osteoporosis is not well understood.

[1]   Type I

Type I osteoporosis affects primarily trabecular bone and is seen in women 10 to 15 years after menopause, usually in their late 50s and into their 60s.

Trabecular bone, which comprises 20 percent of the adult skeleton, is the spongy (cancellous) bone that forms the interior meshwork of long bones and predominates in the vertebral bodies of the spinal column and at the ends of the forearms. The weakening of trabecular bone causes wrist fractures as well as crush fractures of vertebral bodies, producing the "dowager's hump" (kyphosis) that is often seen in elderly women.

The mechanism of type I osteoporosis is thought to be the following (Lyles, 1989):

1. Decreased amounts of female sex hormones after menopause cause accelerated bone resorption (minerals are taken out of the bone).

2. Increased secretion of parathyroid hormone (the hormone that regulates calcium and phosphorus metabolism) impairs production of calcitriol (a hormone that causes calcium to be absorbed from the intestine), thereby decreasing absorption of calcium from the intestine.

It is not understood why this mechanism does not affect all postmenopausal women equally, and it is possible—even likely—that other mechanisms are at work. The strong link between osteoporosis and estrogen is also not well understood, but estrogen receptors have been found on osteoblasts (the cells that regulate bone development), suggesting an estrogen role in the activation of these bone-forming cells (Lyles, 1989).

[2]   Type II

Type II (senile) osteoporosis weakens both trabecular (spongy, inner) and cortical (hardened, outer) bone and is the form of osteoporosis that is associated with hip fractures. (*See Figure 4–2.*) It is found in both men and women over the age of 70, though women affected by the condition outnumber men by as much as three to one.

As with type I osteoporosis, the cellular and biochemical mechanisms of senile osteoporosis are not well understood. Decreased osteoblast activity and increased secretion of parathyroid hormone are thought to be involved.

A study that compared levels of parathyroid hormone and growth factor binding protein in elderly hip fracture patients and a control group without fractures found that parathyroid hormone levels were significantly higher in the hip fracture group. Also, one serum growth factor binding protein (24/25–kDa insulin-like growth factor binding protein) was found at levels about 2.5 times higher in the hip fracture patients than in the nonfracture group. In vitro (in a test tube), this binding protein has been found to inhibit osteoblast function mediated by two insulin-like growth factors (Rosen, et al., 1992).

4.22   Secondary Causes of Osteoporosis

When osteoporosis is diagnosed, whether as the cause of a fracture, incidentally on an x-ray taken for other reasons or through bone density measurements, there are secondary causes that must be ruled out.

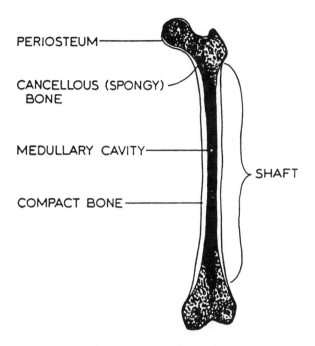

Fig 4-2. Cross section of the femur (thighbone), demonstrating the different areas of bone. Periosteum is the membrane surrounding the bone, from which new bone is formed. Cancellous (spongy; trabecular) bone surrounds the center, or medullary cavity, of the bone. Compact, or cortical, bone is the hardened wall of bone that encloses the cancellous bone.

[1] Cushing's Syndrome

Cushing's syndrome occurs when the level of adrenocorticosteroids (steroid hormones made by the adrenal cortex, the outer layer of the adrenal gland; these hormones are also called glucocorticoids) in the body is increased above normal. This condition can occur naturally when the adrenal cortex produces too much of these hormones, either because of a tumor in the adrenal cortex itself or because the adrenal cortex is overstimulated by hypersecretion of adrenocorticotrophic hormone (ACTH), as a result of a tumor of the anterior pituitary gland or (sometimes) a lung tumor.

The most common cause of Cushing's syndrome, however, is the exogenous (from outside the body) administration of glucocorticoids (drugs like prednisone or hydrocortisone) to treat inflammatory diseases such as ulcerative colitis and arthritis, or to help prevent rejection after organ transplant. Osteoporosis is not the only side effect of adrenocorticosteroid therapy. Others include weight gain and redistribution of fat, fatigue, depression, edema (swelling due to accumulation of fluid), diabetes mellitus, immune system suppression, capillary fragility, excessive hair growth, amenorrhea (discontinuation of menstruation) and impotence. To minimize side effects, these drugs are used for the shortest possible time and then the patient is weaned from them, allowing time for the patient's own adrenal cortex to begin manufacturing hormones again.

Glucocorticoids are thought to cause osteoporosis by inhibiting bone cell division, increasing bone resorption and blocking calcium absorption from the intestine (Lyles, 1989).

Treatment of osteoporosis related to Cushing's syndrome involves treating the tumor that is hypersecreting ACTH or other hormones, or weaning the patient from the steroid drug that is causing the syndrome. Calcium supplementation and exercise are also helpful.

[2]   Other Hormonal Irregularities

Hyperthyroidism—oversecretion of hormones by the thyroid gland in the neck—can also cause osteoporosis. Normal amounts of thyroid hormones are needed for normal bone metabolism, but excessive amounts of these hormones cause calcium to be removed from bones. Hyperthyroidism is caused by Grave's disease (an idiopathic hypertrophy of the thyroid gland) or the presence of a thyroid nodule or tumor (Lyles, 1989).

Hyperparathyroidism also causes osteoporosis. Parathyroid hormone maintains serum calcium levels by stimulating the resorption (removal) of minerals from bone and increasing the absorption of calcium from the intestine. Hyperparathyroidism is usually caused by multiple endocrine neoplasia (cancers or precancerous conditions) that usually involve the pituitary gland and pancreas as well. Treatment involves treating the neoplasia, as well as calcium supplementation.

Hypogonadism in men (decreased secretion of male sex hormones) can also lead to osteoporosis. Androgens have been found to have a role in bone maintenance, and when these hormones are removed, osteoporosis can result. The cause of the hypogonadism—whether it is surgical removal of the testes for cancer, inadequate development as a result of pituitary disorders, or advanced age—should be determined. Administration of exogenous (not produced by the body itself) androgens can stop bone loss.

[3] Immobility

Weight-bearing exercise can maintain bone mass by putting stress on the bones. Likewise, a lack of exercise can hasten the pace of osteoporosis. This is especially seen in the elderly, who often become chair- or bed-bound due to hip fracture, confusion or another medical problem.

Immobility can also lead to the development of pressure sores, pneumonia and thrombophlebitis (blood clots in the calf of the leg), so keeping the elderly up and walking is considered a major priority in geriatric care.

[4] Other Medical and Surgical Conditions

Osteomalacia is an adult disease characterized by decreased bone mineralization; in children, the condition is known as rickets. It is caused by lack of vitamin D. The most common cause in the United States is vitamin D resistance.

Other causes of osteomalacia include disorders of vitamin D metabolism (seen in kidney disease) and vitamin D deficiency (which is rare except in housebound elderly who rarely see the sun and who don't drink vitamin-D-enriched milk). Treatment involves vitamin D replacement either orally or, for patients with malabsorption, intramuscularly (Woodley and Whelan, 1992).

Chronic liver disease and chronic obstructive pulmonary disease have also been associated with osteoporosis, though the mechanisms by which they increase the risk of developing the condition are not clear (Woodley and Whelan, 1992).

Some drugs in addition to adrenocorticosteroids are associated with osteoporosis. These include aluminum compounds, chronic administration of heparin (an injectable anticoagulant) and etidronate and fluoride (drugs that are sometimes used to treat osteoporosis[1] (Woodley and Whelan, 1992). Phenytoin (Dilantin®, an anticonvulsant medication) is associated with osteomalacia.

---

[1] *See* 4.63 and 4.64 *infra.*

Treatment involves using a substitute for the offending drug as well as calcium supplementation.

4.23   Risk Factors for Primary Osteoporosis

Of course, everyone ages, and although all women tend to lose bone after menopause, some women are more at risk for symptomatic osteoporosis than others. Genetic factors, body weight and composition, race, nutritional status, age at menopause and level of physical activity are all thought to contribute to the risk for osteoporosis.

[1]   Demographic and Genetic Factors

White, Asian and Eskimo women are at an increased risk for osteoporosis, compared to black women. This difference in bone mineral density (BMD) among races appears to be present even in children. A study comparing the bone mineral density at a number of skeletal sites in black and white children (mean age 10 years) found that it was significantly greater at all sites in black children than in white children (Bell, et al., 1991).

The mechanism suggested for this effect is that blacks have a greater degree of resistance to the bone-resorbing effects of parathyroid and other hormones. This would allow black people both to lay down more bone to begin with and to lose it less easily later in life (Lyles, 1989).

Low body weight has also been correlated with an increased risk of osteoporosis. This effect was seen in the bone density of the children in the aforementioned study; those of either race who were smaller and thinner had less dense bones (Bell, et al., 1991). A study of patients being treated for rheumatic or lung disease with osteoporosis-promoting glucocorticoid steroid drugs indicated that the most significant correlation with low bone mass at the hip and spine were short height and low weight (Brandli, et al., 1991).

It is known that when a bone is stressed, it will become thicker and stronger. Athletes have wider bones and more cortical bone in limbs that are involved in their particular sport. It has been suggested that the added stress on the bones of obese women caused by supporting their greater weight causes a similar strengthening of their bones (Lyles, 1989).

A study of premenopausal women measured bone density in the femoral neck (angled top portion of the thighbone) and greater trochanter (large bony prominence below the neck of the femur) in relation to lean muscle and fatty tissue. (*See Figure 4–3.*) Femoral neck density increased significantly and linearly for each 30 percent increase in muscle mass. But higher amounts of body fat were found to be protective only when associated with substantial muscle mass (Sowers, et al., 1992).

A positive family history is another risk factor for osteoporosis. Studies of twins suggest that the amount of bone that is initially laid down in the skeleton is genetically determined. These studies show that the bones of identical twins (twins who develop from a single egg and therefore have the same genetic material) are closer in density than those of fraternal twins (who develop from two eggs and are no more closely genetically related than other brothers and sisters) (Lyles, 1989).

The earlier a woman is deprived of estrogen, the earlier osteoporosis occurs (Wren, 1992). This means that women who go into menopause in their late 30s or early 40s develop more serious osteoporosis because they get a "head start" on losing bone over their later-menopause contemporaries. This effect occurs in women with medically induced menopause as well as natural menopause. A 1992 study found that young women with lymphoma (cancer of the lymph system) who experienced chemotherapy-induced menopause were at considerable risk for developing osteoporosis (Ratcliffe, et al., 1992).

[2] Diet and Exercise

Adequate calcium intake (1000 mg per day for premenopausal women and men; 1500 per day for postmenopausal women) can help maintain bone. In order to get this quantity of calcium, supplementation is usually required, because many women avoid dairy products.

Women who exercise regularly but not to excess (one hour of weight-bearing exercise three times weekly is recommended) have been shown to be less prone to osteoporosis than women with a more sedentary life-style (Woodley and Whelan, 1992).

[3] Alcohol, Smoking and Caffeine

Alcohol, smoking and caffeine intake have been associated with an increased risk of osteoporosis (Woodley and Whelan, 1992).

A large study in Boston found a positive relation between caffeine consumption and risk of hip fractures (common with type II osteoporosis) but not forearm fractures (common with type I osteoporosis). The

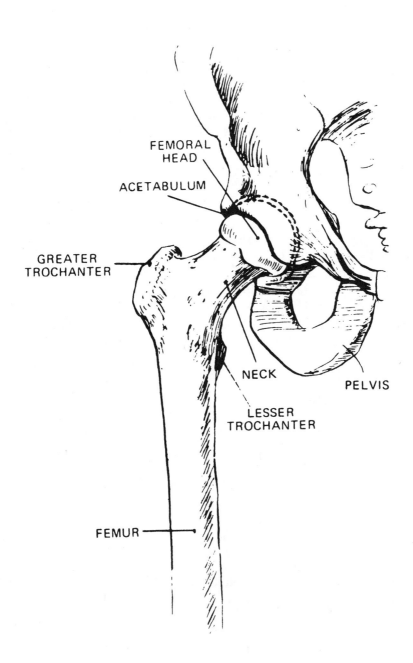

Fig. 4-3. Anterior view of the hip joint.

same study found alcohol to be independently associated with an increased risk of both hip and wrist fractures, with the risk of fractures increasing with the amount of alcohol consumed (Hernandez-Avila, et al., 1991).

How these substances increase the risk of osteoporosis is not known.

4.24   Osteoporosis in Men

Although the vast majority of cases of osteoporosis are seen in postmenopausal women, men's bones do weaken as they age. Men in Western countries have been shown to have greater bone mass than women, though why this effect exists is unclear (Lyles, 1989). However, several reasons are likely—demographic, biochemical and perhaps life-style.

Men do not get type I osteoporosis, the kind seen in women 10 to 15 years after menopause that affects the bones primarily of the spine and wrist. Men do get type II osteoporosis, which develops after age 70, but since women commonly outlive men, there are fewer old men to get the condition.

Also, although bone loss appears to be linked to a decrease in sex hormones in men as well as in women, men experience a gradual lowering in androgens (male sex hormones) as they age, starting at about age 55, rather than the more sudden drop in estrogens (female sex hormones) seen in women at menopause. The rate of bone loss is accelerated during the first years of menopause in women, whereas men do not have an analogous period of increased bone loss.

It is also possible, especially in the current generation of elderly people, that men were more physically active in their youth than women. It is known that lifelong physical activity affects peak bone mass and is instrumental in preventing osteoporosis (Ulrich, 1991). Women in the 1920s through the 1950s were not encouraged to be athletic, and therefore their bones did not become as dense as those of their more active male counterparts.

4.30   DIAGNOSIS AND SCREENING

Diagnosis of osteoporosis has traditionally been made after an osteoporotic fracture has occurred. The physician's job then is to rule out other diseases, especially various malignancies (cancers), and determine whether primary osteoporosis is the cause of the fracture.

However, as the large "baby boom" generation moves into late middle age and interest in all aspects of menopause has begun to rise, pressure has been building for screening methods to identify those who are at risk for osteoporosis.

In 1990, the American College of Physicians (the professional organization of internists) issued a recommendation that all perimenopausal women not be screened (have bone mineral density measurements) for osteoporosis. The rationale for this recommendation was that although preliminary evidence suggests that screening for osteoporosis with bone mass measurements has the potential to reduce the probability of fractures in postmenopausal women, additional evidence, as well as screening and treatment protocols, are needed before widespread screening can begin (American College of Physicians, 1990). Insurance companies still consider absorptiometry "experimental" and will not reimburse patients for its use.

4.31 History and Physical Examination

Osteoporosis is usually diagnosed in an older person when a typical fracture (wrist, spine or hip) has occurred. However, physicians are becoming more proactive in attempting to prevent osteoporosis. Primary physicians are now being urged by the American College of Physicians (American Academy of Physicians, 1992) and the American Academy of Family Physicians (Gambrell, 1992) to encourage all their menopausal patients to consider hormone replacement therapy to prevent osteoporosis and heart disease.

Patients with osteoporosis may be asymptomatic, even with one or more vertebral fractures. When pain occurs, it is usually of two sorts. Pain experienced at the time of fracture is sharp, severe, localized directly over a vertebra and worsened by movement. It may also be spasmodic and radiate into the anterior portions of the abdomen, legs or pelvis. The second sort of pain is a chronic dull aching pain, localized on one or both sides of the midline of the back. Examination may reveal spasm of the back muscles. This pain is worsened by sitting or standing and relieved by lying down. Generalized bone pain is rare in osteoporosis, as are nerve root and spinal cord compressions.

As osteoporosis progresses, height may decrease over a period of months to years due to vertebral compression fractures, most often in the lumbar region. Loss of height is often associated with scoliosis (lateral deviation of the vertebral column).

When an osteoporotic fracture has occurred, the history and physical examination help rule out cancer, osteomalacia, Cushing's syndrome and other secondary causes of osteopenia (weakened bones).[2]

The history should include the patient's osteoporosis risk factors:

- age at menopause;
- race;
- weight and height;
- lifetime physical activity;
- smoking history;
- alcohol consumption;
- medication history; and
- calcium consumption.

Physical examination usually reveals an elderly white or Asian woman (though osteoporosis occurs in all races and should not be ruled out simply because a patient is, for example, African-American) who may otherwise be in good health or may suffer from such chronic conditions as hypertension (high blood pressure), emphysema, diabetes or heart disease. She may have had a wrist fracture in the past, and her spine may show the effects of vertebral crush fractures. Assessment of the hip fracture patient's skin and subcutaneous tissues is important to alert the hospital staff to increased risk of pressure sores.

In a fracture patient, the patient's baseline psychological status should be assessed at the initial examination. When they are hospitalized, elderly people often become confused and disoriented, especially at night. Such a patient may be assumed by hospital staff to have Alzheimer's disease or some other form of senility, when actually, medications such as haloperidol (Haldol®) and efforts to familiarize the patient with the surroundings might greatly improve her or his mental status.

4.32 Laboratory Studies

Only basic laboratory studies are performed when a physician is doing a workup on an osteoporosis patient. A complete blood count and a chemistry panel should be performed.

---

[2] *See* 4.33 *infra.*

Serum calcium and phosphorus levels are normal in osteoporosis. An elevated level in the blood of thyroid stimulating hormone (TSH) would indicate that an overstimulated thyroid may be contributing to bone destruction. Alkaline phosphatase (an enzyme that functions in the mineralization of bone) is normal in osteoporosis except for a brief elevation after a fracture. An elevated alkaline phosphatase level suggests a cause other than primary osteoporosis for weakened bones. If osteomalacia is suspected because of previous gastrointestinal disease or surgery, or if serum chemistry values are abnormal, the version of vitamin D called 25(OH)D should be measured. Serum protein electrophoresis, which separates blood proteins and makes them identifiable, is also considered useful in doing a workup of the osteoporosis patient (Woodley and Whelan, 1992).

Urinalysis is performed to check urine calcium and phosphorus levels. If the level of urine calcium is low, increased levels of parathyroid hormone could be at work destroying bone and decreasing renal calcium excretion.

Bone biopsy can help diagnose the cause of osteoporosis in pre-menopausal women and in men under the age of 65, but it is not considered necessary in the vast majority of osteoporosis patients.

4.33 Radiologic Studies

Although a simple x-ray can detect such osteoporotic complications as vertebral crush fractures or a broken hip, a standard x-ray cannot detect osteoporosis itself until 30 to 40 percent of bone mineral has been lost, and it cannot quantify bone density or distinguish between cortical and trabecular bone (Schurman and Williamson, 1991).

The machines that can determine bone density are much more complex than an x-ray machine. To calculate bone density, radiation (a single beam, or two beams at different speeds) is aimed at the bone, and the machine detects how much radiation is absorbed by the bone. The more radiation absorbed, the more minerals the bone contains. The different forms of this "absorptiometry" (or densitometry) discussed here are variations on this single principle. However, no one method includes all the features required to be entirely satisfactory, and none is able to accurately predict fracture risk, so research is continuing (Greenfield, 1992).

The development of absorptiometers, which can quantify the effects of preventive and therapeutic interventions on the density of bones in both osteoporotic and normal populations, has spurred research and clinical interest in the growing challenge that osteoporosis presents to public health (Schurman and Williamson, 1991).

[1]   Single-Photon Absorptiometry (SPA)

Single-photon absorptiometry was introduced in 1963 and remains in use to measure the bone mineral density of the radius (larger of the two forearm bones). Because there are photons of only one speed, the SPA machine cannot directly differentiate between tissues of different thicknesses, such as bone and muscle. The test is highly precise, widely available and relatively inexpensive (Woodley and Whelan, 1992).

The arm is wrapped in a "tissue equivalent material," while below the arm, there is a source of the radioactive isotope iodine^{125} and above the arm is a sodium iodide detector. The scanner moves across the width of the arm, and photons (energy particles) given off by the radioactive iodine in the source pass through the wrist and are attenuated by tissue before being sensed by the detector. The machine then calculates the difference between the amount of photon attenuation through soft tissue and that through the arm bone. The greater the attenuation, the more calcium is in the bone (Greenfield, 1992).

The duration of the examination is brief, and the absorbed dose of radiation is low.

The major drawback of single-photon absorptiometry is that it can only measure bone density in the wrist and cannot be used on the spine or, more important in terms of morbidity and mortality, on the hip.

[2]   Dual-Photon Absorptiometry (DPA)

Dual-photon absorptiometry uses a radioisotope called gadolinium^{153}, which emits photons at two distinct energy levels. These dual photon energies allow the absorptiometry equipment to distinguish between bone and soft tissue, and the machines (which have gone through several generations) can scan not only the wrist but also the spine, hip and total body.

The total dose of radiation is low, but scanning takes a long time: 25 to 30 minutes for the spine or hip, and up to 70 minutes for the entire body. Dual-photon absorptiometry also is plagued by measurement problems caused by interference from fat, osteophytes (bony outgrowths) and vascular calcifications, which can result in false diagnoses such as calcification of the aorta, degenerative joint disease, severe compression fractures and other disorders (Greenfield, 1992).

[3]   Dual Energy X-ray Absorptiometry (DEXA)

Dual-photon absorptiometers (DPA) are now being replaced with dual energy x-ray absorptiometers. Dual energy x-ray absorptiometry (DEXA) measures bone density in the same manner that DPA does, but the x-ray beams are at a much higher energy level than the photon rays emitted from the dual-photon absorptiometer radioisotope. This greater energy allows DEXA scans to be performed in only a fraction of the time required for DPA scans. A DEXA scan of the hip takes only 4 to 5 minutes, whereas a DPA hip scan takes 25 to 30 minutes (Lunar Corp., 1993).

The radiation dose absorbed from a DEXA scan is low—1 to 3 millirems, or equal to the amount of radiation we absorb from the sun and other natural sources during one week. DEXA machines are precise and produce high-quality images with good resolution.

As with DPA machines, DEXA accuracy is affected by the presence of osteophytes (bony outgrowths), fat and vascular calcifications (Greenfield, 1992).

[4]   Other Techniques

Quantitative computed tomography (QCT) measures bone mineral density in the lumbar spine with computer-enhanced x-rays. The precision (ability to track an individual's response to therapy) is moderate, and the accuracy (ability to quantify severity of osteoporosis) is moderate to poor. The examination takes 10 to 20 minutes, and the absorbed dose of radiation is relatively high. Therefore, QCT has largely been replaced by more accurate and speedy methods.

A different sort of method of total body calcium measurement is under investigation in the United Kingdom but is not in general use. The procedure, known as in vivo neutron activation analysis (IVNAA), involves exposing the patient to a small dose of neutrons, measuring the calcium isotopes that the neutrons induce and then calculating the total amount of calcium in the body. The radiation dose is relatively high with this method, and refinements are being attempted.

Although densitometry can quantify bone mineral density, it cannot evaluate bone strength. Therefore, densitometry is not a good predictor of fracture risk. Evaluation of bone strength has been attempted in the United Kingdom by measuring attenuation of ultrasound through the heel (which is made of trabecular bone); however, this method is still under study (Greenfield, 1992).

4.40 OSTEOPOROTIC FRACTURES OF THE HIP AND THIGH

Fractures occur when osteoporosis has eroded the strength of the femoral neck (at the hip joint) or femoral shaft to the point that the bone breaks with little or no trauma.

It was thought for many years that hip fractures were always a result of a fall or some other, similar type of trauma. This is not an illogical conclusion, since most hip fracture patients are elderly and often have diminished vision, strength and balance. However, it is now thought that often the hip breaks first and causes the fall. This may happen because wear and tear on the osteoporotic hip joint produces micro-fractures, known as stress fractures. The stress fractures in the femoral neck then become a complete fracture following a minor torsional (twisting) injury, which then causes the patient to fall (Iverson and Clawson, 1987).

Femoral shaft fractures are far less common than femoral neck (hip) fractures, because the femoral shaft is protected by the large thigh muscles and is made almost entirely of cortical bone, which is eroded less quickly than the trabecular bone that composes part of the femoral neck. Also, in a fall, the hip is more likely to take the brunt of the force than is the thigh. However, in a motor vehicle accident, fall or other event in which stress is applied to the femur, it can also fracture.

Hip fracture is the most serious complication of osteoporosis, with a 34 percent mortality rate by six months after the fracture (Gambrell, 1992). The incidence of hip fracture doubles every six years after the age of 40 (Lyles, 1989).[3]

Diagnosis of a femoral shaft fracture is confirmed by x-ray examination of the thigh. However, the history of trauma, as well as leg pain and an abnormal position of the upper leg, are also virtually diagnostic.

4.50 TREATMENT OF OSTEOPOROTIC HIP FRACTURES

Treatment of osteoporotic fractures in the hip and thigh is determined by the location of the fracture and the fragility of the remaining

---

[3] *See also* ch. 2 for a complete discussion of hip fracture.

bone. The usual procedure to repair a fractured hip is to perform an open reduction (surgical process in which the broken bone is returned to its normal anatomic position) and internal fixation of the femoral neck with screws or nails and a variety of buttressing plates. However, some hip fractures require almost no treatment, and others require replacement of the hip joint with a prosthesis.

Impacted subcapital fractures do not require surgery because they are not displaced and will heal well if not disturbed. These fractures are treated with skin traction. Skin traction pulls lightly on the hip joint by taping the traction apparatus to the skin (standard traction involves inserting pins into the bone and attaching weights to the pins by ropes). The patient treated with this apparatus must have frequent x-rays of the hip joint to assure that the fracture has not slipped and become displaced (McCollum, 1991). In addition, stabilizing the fracture to enable mobility of the joint is recommended, and bed rest is not encouraged.

In the young, displaced intracapsular hip fractures are repaired with multiple nails (pins) or screws placed through the femoral shaft up into the femoral head. However, in patients with osteoporosis, the femoral shaft is often not strong enough to withstand the pressure of nailing. In these cases, screws are fixed in place with a metal side plate, which is seated down in the bone and provides extra support and impaction for the bone fragments. There are a number of side plates and supportive nailing devices (the Richards apparatus is commonly used), and the choice depends upon the type of fracture and the surgeon's preference.

A stable trochanteric fracture is fixed with screws and a plate (Richards apparatus) and can heal in 12 weeks or less. However, if the trochanteric fracture is comminuted or displaced, a long nail is inserted into the core of the femoral shaft (the medullary canal) and up into the femoral head. These intramedullary nails may have wires that are then wrapped around the bone (a Zickle nail) to provide extra stability to bone fragments. (*See Figure 4–4.*)

A displaced subcapital fracture (in which the head of the femur is broken off) in an elderly person frequently cannot be perfectly reduced (put back into place). In these cases, a prosthetic hip replacement procedure is performed to return the patient to optimal activity as soon as possible. Hip replacements can involve just replacing the head of

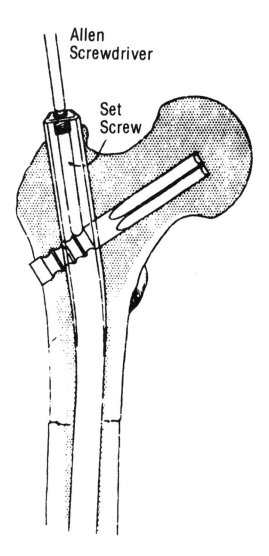

Fig. 4-4. Zickel intramedullary device in place.

the femur, or both the femoral head and the acetabulum (the pelvic portion of the hip joint) can be replaced with a bipolar prosthesis.

During the procedure, the patient's femoral head is removed, and the prosthesis is inserted into the shaft of the femur. The artificial acetabulum of a bipolar prosthesis is then cemented into place in the pelvis.

4.51   Femoral Reduction and Fixation

Femoral fractures, even in osteoporotic individuals, are usually a result of an automobile accident or other major trauma, and there are frequently other serious injuries that require emergency treatment. Briefly, the first, and older, technique is to reduce (realign) the fractured bones with traction while the patient is kept in bed. Pins are attached to the lower bone fragment, and weights are hung by ropes from the pin. This weight, over time, will realign the bones. After the fracture is reduced, then a plaster cast with a moveable metal knee joint is applied. This method requires about ten weeks of hospitalization and puts the patient at risk for pressure sores, pneumonia and the other complications of immobilization.

The second method of treating a femoral fracture, now favored by orthopedic surgeons whether the fracture is compound (open; a condition in which bone has pierced the skin) or closed, is to surgically implant an intramedullary nail (a steel rod that extends the length of the femur) into the core of the bone. (*See Figure 4–5.*) With this internal support, the patient can be mobilized quickly, and the bone can heal without a prolonged period of hospitalization and bed rest.

External fixation, with pins inserted into the bone above and below the fracture and attached to an "outrigger" frame, is not recommended as the sole treatment for femoral fractures. The risk of nonunion, delayed union and poor restoration of knee motion are increased with this method. However, external fixation may be used for a short time if there are extensive soft tissue wounds that must heal before an open reduction procedure and internal fixation with an intramedullary nail can be performed.

Compression plates are also considered less satisfactory than intramedullary nails for treating femoral fractures. As resorption occurs at the fracture site, the rigid plate does not allow normal impaction of bone, resulting in a weaker union. Infection rates are also increased with compression plates (McCollum, 1991).

4.52   Restoring Mobility

Restoring mobility is an essential element in treating osteoporotic fractures and in preventing potentially serious postoperative respiratory, circulatory, mental and skin complications, especially in the elderly.

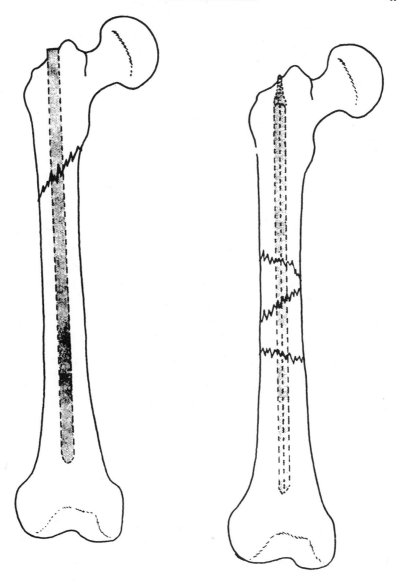

Fig. 4-5. Use of a rod or nail for intramedullary fixation of a simple fracture of the femur (left) and a comminuted fracture (right).

Immobility is known to hasten osteoporosis. A study of patients with spinal cord injuries causing various degrees of paralysis found a strong correlation between the patients' level of physical activity and the patients' bone mineral density; the more mobile the patients were, especially if they were able to stand up regularly, the denser were their bones (Saltzstein, et al., 1992).

Osteoporosis is only one of the serious hazards of immobility. If a person is not gotten up out of bed quickly (at least to sit in a chair, if not walking), pneumonia can develop, due to impaired expansion of the lungs while the individual is lying down. Also, without the normal squeezing of leg muscles on the veins, blood flows sluggishly in the legs, and clots can form. These blood clots can then travel to the lungs, creating a potentially fatal pulmonary embolus.

Skin breakdown, leading to pressure sores (decubitus ulcers; bed-sores), develops easily in frail elderly people, who often have little muscle mass and poor nutritional intake. The longer a patient remains in bed, the greater the chance she will develop one of these difficult-to-control wounds.

In the unfamiliar hospital environment, some elderly patients who are perfectly alert and oriented at home can become confused, especially at night (a condition known as sundowning). This problem is compounded when the elderly patient requires postoperative narcotic pain medication. Early mobilization can help shorten the hospital stay and minimize the disorienting effects of surgery, hospitalization and pain medication.

4.60   OSTEOPOROSIS OF THE SPINE

Patients with osteoporosis of the spine may be asymptomatic, even with one or more vertebral fractures. When pain occurs, it is usually of two sorts. Pain experienced at the time of fracture is sharp, severe, localized directly over a vertebra and worsened by movement. It may also be spasmodic and radiate into the anterior portions of the abdomen, legs or pelvis. The second sort of pain is a chronic, dull aching pain, localized on one or both sides of the midline of the back. Examination may reveal spasm of the back muscles. This pain is worsened by sitting or standing and relieved by lying down. Generalized bone pain is rare in osteoporosis, as are nerve root and spinal cord compressions (Frymoyer, 1988; Avioli and Lindsay, 1990).

As osteoporosis progresses, height may decrease over a period of months to years due to vertebral compression fractures, most often in the lumbar region. Loss of height is often associated with scoliosis (lateral deviation of the vertebral column) (Healey and Lane, 1985).

Decline in height and increased curvature of the lower back lead to an apparent hump in the upper back (kyphosis). The spinal curvature forces the ribs downward so that they come in contact with the iliac crest (hip). Height reduction cannot and does not go any further than this. Such deformity may lead to a forward pelvic tilt, hamstring contractures, stiff ankles and pronated (outwardly rotated) feet.

On vertebral x-rays, there may be accentuation of the vertical trabeculae that conform to the lines of stress in the bone and loss of the horizontal trabeculae. Also, the top and bottom of the vertebrae may be accentuated, even though the cortex may be thinned as a result of greater rarefaction (loss of density) of the main body. However, if osteoporosis is due to adrenal overactivity or exogenous glucocorticoid administration, the upper and lower cortical plates are often truly thickened or eburnated (hardened).

As vertebral bone loss progresses, pressure exerted by the intervertebral discs on the bony vertebrae may cause biconcave compressions or dishing-out of the top and bottom of vertebral bodies. This pattern is called "codfish" vertebrae with "ballooned" intervertebral discs. (*See Figure 4-6.*) There may also be a mushroom-shaped localized intrusion of the material of the disc into the vertebral body, producing what is called a Schmorl's node, although the presence of this finding is not pathognomonic for osteoporosis.

A vertebral index that documents the compression of the vertebral surfaces may be used to determine the degree of bone loss. When the ratio of the minimum vertical thickness to the maximum vertical thickness is less than 80 percent, significant bone loss is assumed to have occurred.

4.61 Spinal Fractures

The eventual result of continued vertebral bone loss is the wedge fracture (a fracture that produces a wedge of bone). Overall, patients who have fractures in the middle or low thoracic vertebrae (T7-T8, T12-L1) have a 98 percent chance of having generalized osteoporosis (Hedlund, et al., 1989; Francis, et al., 1989). (*See Figure 4-7.*) Wedges with apices pointing forward (primarily in the thoracic vertebrae) are

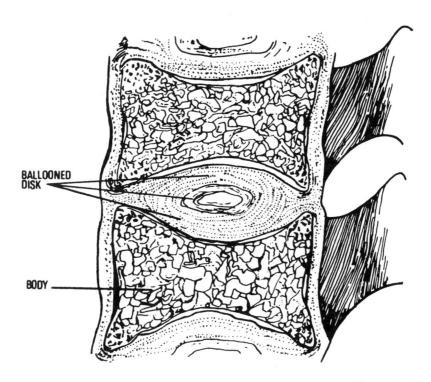

Fig. 4-6. Bone changes associated with osteoporosis. The patient with chronic osteoporosis frequently suffers a ballooning of the intervertebral disk into the vertebral bodies. Because of the change in structural and spatial arrangements this may be a source of low back pain.

typical of osteoporosis, while wedges pointing backward may suggest an underlying bone disease, such as Paget's disease or metastases (Hedlund, et al., 1989). Although its clinical course is different, vertebral osteomyelitis may also present as a compression fracture on x-ray (McHenry, et al., 1988).

4.62   Osteomalacia

The osteoporotic spine may be differentiated from the osteomalacic one by the biconcavity in all vertebral bodies without the Schmorl's nodes characteristic of osteomalacia. However, osteoporosis and osteomalacia may occur simultaneously in the same individual, and Looser's zones (areas of unhealed stress fractures filled with unmineralized osteoid) characteristic of osteomalacia may occur in osteoporotic patients as a result of weakened bone (Hauge, et al., 1988).

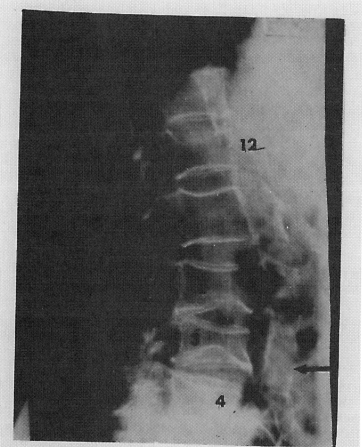

Fig. 4-7. An elderly patient with severe osteoporosis of the vertebrae. The disks have protruded (ballooned) into the soft bone of the vertebral bodies. The bodies of the twelfth thoracic vertebra (T12) and the second and third lumbar vertebrae (L2 and L3) show compression fractures.

4.70 PREVENTION AND TREATMENT OF OSTEOPOROSIS

A woman continues to add bone to her skeleton up until about the age of 30. Between the age of 30 and menopause, there is a period of stasis before bone mineral density begins to be lost with menopause.

Osteoporosis is best treated before it starts, by encouraging girls and young women to maximize the density of their bones while it is still possible. This can be achieved with adequate calcium intake and regular performance of weight-bearing exercise. Then, later in life, bone can be maintained with calcium and vitamin D supplementation, weight-bearing exercise and, perhaps most effectively, hormone replacement therapy. The hormone calcitonin and the anti-osteoclast drug etidronate have also been shown to be beneficial for some patients. Other drugs, such as the thiazide diuretics and bisphosphonates, are also showing promise for treating osteoporosis.

4.71 Hormone Replacement Therapy

Hormone replacement therapy, specifically estrogen replacement, is an effective way to prevent osteoporosis in menopausal women and to halt its progression in older, postmenopausal women. No woman is considered too old to receive some benefit from hormone replacement therapy (Wren, 1992).

Long-term hormone therapy (15 to 20 years) has been shown to decrease the risk of hip fracture by about 25 percent and has the added benefit of decreasing the risk of coronary artery disease by 35 percent. Guidelines issued by the American College of Physicians in 1992 urge all menopausal women, regardless of race, to consider hormone replacement therapy (American College of Physicians, 1992).

Estrogen therapy is not without risks, however. In the 1970s, it was discovered that menopausal women who took unopposed estrogen for 10 to 20 years were at an eight-fold increased risk of developing endometrial cancer (tumor of the uterine lining) (American College of Physicians, 1992). This risk has been reduced to practically zero by combining estrogen with a progestin (a steroid hormone produced by the corpus luteum after ovulation that induces the endometrium to proliferate to prepare for implantation of a fertilized ovum in the second half of the menstrual cycle). Unfortunately, many women find that they cannot tolerate progestin therapy, as they experience bloating, mood changes and other unpleasant side effects (Gambrell, 1992).

It is also known that women taking estrogen alone or combined with progestin for prolonged periods may have an increased risk of breast cancer. The evidence is inconsistent, and the risk with long-term therapy seems increased at most by 2.5 percent (American College of Physicians, 1992). Hormone replacement therapy is contraindicated for women who have had breast cancer themselves, but their first-degree relatives (mothers, daughters, sisters) are no longer advised against this form of treatment (Gambrell, 1992).

For a woman who has had a hysterectomy, unopposed estrogen is prescribed (0.625 mg oral estrogen daily) because she has no uterus to develop cancer. If the woman does have her uterus, there are a number of estrogen/progestin protocols, but two in widespread clinical use are the following (American College of Physicians, 1992):

- estrogen plus cyclic progestin (medroxyprogesterone acetate), 5 to 10 mg orally per day, for 10 to 14 days per month; or

- estrogen plus continuous progestin, at a smaller dose (2.5 mg orally per day).

Under an estrogen/progestin protocol, especially when progestin is given cyclically, a woman is likely to have intervals of vaginal bleeding, which should diminish and will usually stop over the first year of treatment.

The exact mechanisms by which estrogen affects bone are not clear. Estrogen receptors have been found on osteoblasts (cells that help form bone), and estrogen appears to control the function of both osteoclasts (large cells in the bone marrow that act to remove minerals and break down bone) and osteoblasts and therefore influences the rate of calcium absorption and redeposition. Osteoblasts and osteoclasts are continually destroying old bone and building new bone throughout life, but when estrogen is removed, the balance between these two activities is disrupted, and more bone is dismantled than the osteoblasts can replace (Wren, 1992).

Men with severe osteoporosis have been shown to benefit from treatment with androgens (male sex hormones) (Lyles, 1989).

4.72 Weight-Bearing Exercise

Exercise has also been shown to be helpful in building bone mass during youth and maintaining it in later life. Regular walking or other weight-bearing exercise (swimming, for example, is aerobic or oxygen-utilizing and therefore heart-function protective but not weight-bearing) for one hour three times a week has been shown to protect bone mass (Woodley and Whelan, 1992).

A study that compared the effects of low-impact and high-impact exercise on the bone mineral density in the lumbar (lower back) vertebrae of postmenopausal women found no difference between the two groups. The authors concluded that 20 minutes of moderate-intensity low-impact or high-impact exercise performed three days per week is an effective regimen for maintaining bone mineral density among postmenopausal women (Grove and Londeree, 1992). This study has implications for more elderly women, who often cannot tolerate the greater intensity of a high-impact workout.

4.73 Calcium, Vitamin D and Fluoride Supplementation

Calcium intake of 1,000 mg daily in premenopausal women and men and 1,500 mg daily in postmenopausal women is recommended. Adequate calcium intake in postmenopausal women has been shown to slow loss of bone mass (Woodley and Whelan, 1992).

How responsive a postmenopausal woman is to calcium supplementation appears to depend upon how far from menopause she is. A review of controlled clinical trials revealed that among women who are within the first five years of menopause, bone loss from the radius (the larger forearm bone) can be slowed but not halted by added calcium. The spine was found to be unresponsive to even high doses of calcium in these early postmenopausal women. In late postmenopausal women, however, bone loss from both the radius and the spine was slowed with calcium supplementation. The effect of calcium supplements on hip density is not known (Dawson-Hughes, 1991).

The effects of vitamin D and fluoride on the risk for osteoporotic fractures are less clear. A European study found that neither vitamin D nor fluoride had any effect on the risk of hip fracture in women over 50 years of age (Kanis, et al., 1992). Yet another study reported that treatment with calcitriol (a potent metabolite of vitamin D) markedly increased calcium absorption from the intestine and slowed the rate of bone loss in postmenopausal women (Nordin and Morris, 1992).

A 1992 review of available osteoporosis treatments found that calcium and vitamin D supplements were of significant value, especially for elderly people, in whom they even decreased fracture incidence. Fluoride taken in large doses was shown to increase bone density but to have a high rate of side effects and no effect on fracture rates. However, fluoride preparations of lower bioavailability (the extent to which an active drug is absorbed into the general circulation) were better tolerated and decreased fracture rates (Burckhardt, 1992).

Other studies have found fluoride supplementation to be downright dangerous for osteoporosis patients. In one study, fluoride was found to be associated with increased resorption of trabecular bone in some treated patients, and it was concluded that fluoride is a key factor in the pathogenesis of stress fractures, especially in the femoral neck (Orcel, et al., 1990).

Fluoride is thought to cause abnormal bone formation and may protect the spine from osteoporosis while increasing the risk of hip fracture (Weinerman and Bockman, 1990). This conclusion was seconded by another study, which indicated that fluoride therapy may be implicated in the pathogenesis of hip fractures despite a rapid, marked increase in bone mass (Bayley, et al., 1990).

4.74   Other Drug Therapies

Some studies show that estrogen replacement, the primary preventive therapy for osteoporosis,[4] works to preserve bone in individuals only up until about the age of 70. Therefore, the search continues for drugs that will preserve and even replace lost bone later in life. The drugs in the following discussion are currently used in women over 70 and women in whom estrogen replacement is contraindicated, as well as for osteoporotic men (Woodley and Whelan, 1992).

Calcitonin (Calcimar®) is a polypeptide (protein) hormone produced by the thyroid gland and is one of the three major regulators of bone metabolism. Calcitonin lowers the blood calcium level, and thus retards bone loss, by directly suppressing osteoclasts. It also encourages the renal (through the kidneys) excretion of calcium and phosphorus.

Calcitonin stabilizes or increases vertebral bone density for periods of 12 to 24 months, though most patients begin losing bone again after this period, and it is not clear if continuing the treatment after this time is of any use (Woodley and Whelan, 1992). Calcitonin is useful for women who have a high rate of bone turnover or who cannot take estrogen.

Most calcitonin is derived from salmon, and many patients develop resistance to the medication after a year or so of therapy. It is thought that this resistance is due to immune system antibodies that deactivate the foreign hormone. Purified human calcitonin has become available, and although resistance occurs much less frequently with its use, it still happens.

---

[4] *See* 4.71 *supra.*

Calcitonin has relatively mild side effects (nausea, transient flushing and allergic rashes are most common), but because calcium and phosphorus excretion is increased, blood calcium levels should be checked regularly, and the patient should have an adequate calcium intake to replace that lost in urine. Perhaps the biggest drawbacks to calcitonin therapy are that it is expensive and cannot be given orally but can only be administered as an injection.

Etidronate disodium (Didronel®), a pyrophosphate analog (also called a bisphosphonate or diphosphonate), is showing promise for treatment of established osteoporosis. Given in three-month cycles, etidronate has been shown to increase vertebral bone density and to decrease the rate of vertebral fracture (Woodley and Whelan, 1992). A prospective double-blinded placebo-controlled trial demonstrated significant increases in bone mineral density in the hip and spine among individuals in the etidronate-treated group, as well as a 50 percent decrease in the rate of new vertebral fractures in the treated group (Watts, et al., 1990).

Though its exact mechanisms are not clear, etidronate appears to attach to hydroxyapatite (a form of calcium phosphate present with calcium carbonate in bone) crystals in bone and to inhibit both the growth and dissolution of the crystals. The drug also decreases the number of bone-dismantling osteoclast cells. If it is given continuously, etidronate will suppress osteoblasts as well as osteoclasts, and bones will be severely demineralized. When it is used in cycles of 2 weeks on the drug followed by 10 weeks off, etidronate appears to have a synchronizing effect on bone formation. During the drug-free period, bone mineralization occurs with a normal balance between the activity of bone-building osteoblasts and bone-dismantling osteoclasts (Long and Long, 1991).

Although etidronate is widely used to treat osteoporosis in Europe, in this country, it is only approved to treat hypercalcemia associated with malignancy (cancer) and Paget's disease, a chronic inflammatory bone disorder in which bones become thickened and softened in areas of increased but abnormal bone growth. The most common side effects of etidronate are diarrhea and nausea.

Thiazide diuretics (considered mild diuretics, such as hydrochlorothiazide) appear to be associated with decreased bone loss and fewer osteoporotic fractures. Thiazides probably work by reducing the amount of calcium that is lost through the kidneys, which then boosts the blood calcium level and reduces the amount of calcium that is removed from bones (Lyles, 1989). Many elderly people take thiazide diuretics to treat mild to moderate hypertension (high blood pressure) and the edema (swelling due to accumulation of fluid) caused by congestive heart failure. This added benefit of thiazide therapy may encourage physicians to prescribe thiazides instead of other diuretics.

Side effects of thiazides include the following:

- dehydration;
- hypercholesterolemia (increased amount of cholesterol in the blood);
- nausea;
- anorexia (loss of appetite);
- rash;
- gout; and
- increased blood sugar level (hyperglycemia).

A new class of drugs now on the market to treat osteoporosis is the bisphosphonate group; alendronate (Fosamax®) is the one most frequently used for this indication. The bisphosphonates are the first drugs to actually rebuild bone in postmenopausal women rather than to just slow or halt bone loss. This is especially important in elderly women who already have significant osteoporosis and thus are at increased risk of fractures.

Unpleasant (primarily gastrointestinal) side effects include ulceration of the esophageal tissue. The patient must sit erect for 30 minutes after taking the drug to prevent any reflux of the drug from the stomach into the esophagus (many elderly people have a loosened cardiac sphincter, the closure at the top of the stomach, and so reflux of gastric contents and attendant heartburn is a common problem). The drug must be taken with a full glass of plain tap water (not juice or mineral water) and must be taken 30 minutes before eating or taking other medications. In the elderly, many of whom take multiple drugs for an array of health problems, anything that makes taking medications more awkward or confusing is a problem, because the patient may stop taking the drug or may take it incorrectly, so that the benefit is lost.

4.75 Diet and Education

Much research has shown that girls and young women who are physically active and get adequate dietary calcium can minimize their risk for osteoporosis later in life (Lyles, 1989). Women can gain bone mass through their 20s, up until about the age of 30. Along with exercise and calcium intake, use of oral contraceptives ("the pill") has been found to exert a further independent positive effect on bone mass (Recker, et al., 1992).

In a culture that stresses thinness, coupled with the tendency of young people to believe themselves to be indestructible, it can be hard to convince this population to drink milk to prevent a hip fracture late in life. However, increased awareness about osteoporosis and the prevalence of fat-free dairy products, the calcium-enrichment of nondairy drinks, as well as the availability of inexpensive calcium supplements should exert a positive influence on calcium intake in the future.

Exercise, on the other hand, is culturally popular. If a young woman exercises—but not to the point that she stops menstruating, as happens to many long-distance runners, because her bones will begin to deteriorate as if she were menopausal—a young woman can both have the attractive body she desires and strengthen her bones for later in life.

4.100 BIBLIOGRAPHY

Text References

American College of Physicians, Clinical Efficacy Assessment Project: Guidelines for Counseling Postmenopausal Women about Preventive Hormone Therapy. Ann. Int. Med. 117(12):1038–1041, 1992.

American College of Physicians, Clinical Efficacy Assessment Project: Screening for Osteoporosis in Perimenopausal Women. Philadelphia: American College of Physicians, July 13, 1990.

Bayley, T., et al.: Fluoride-Induced Fractures: Relation to Osteogenic Effect. J. Bone Miner. Res. 5(Suppl. 1):S217–222, Mar. 1990.

Bell, N., et. al.: Demonstration that Bone Mass is Greater in Black than in White Children. J. Bone Miner. Res. 6(7):719–723, July 1991.

Brandli, D., et al.: Glucocorticoid-Induced Osteoporosis: A Cross-Sectional Study. Steroids 56(10):518–523, Oct. 1991.

Burckhardt, P.: Treatment of Osteoporosis. Curr. Opin. Rheumatol. 4(3):402–409, June 1992.

Dawson-Hughes, B.: Calcium Supplementation and Bone Loss: A Review of Controlled Clinical Trials. Am. J. Clin. Nutr. 54(1 Suppl.):2748–2808, July 1991.

DeLuca, H. and Mazess, R.: Osteoporosis: Physiological Basis, Assessment, and Treatment. Proceedings of the 19th Steenbock Symposium. Madison, Wisc.: June 5–8, 1989.

Gambrell, R.: Hormone Replacement Therapy Update. American Academy of Family Physicians 1992 Annual Conference, San Diego, Oct. 1992.

Greenfield, M.: Current Status of Physical Measurements of the Skeleton. Med. Phys. 19(6):1349–1357, Nov./Dec. 1992.

Grove, K. and Londeree, B.: Bone Density in Postmenopausal Women: High Impact vs. Low Impact Exercise. Med. Sci. Sports Exerc. 24(11):1190–1194, Nov. 1992.

Hernandez-Avila, G.: Caffeine, Moderate Alcohol Intake, and Risk of Fractures of the Hip and Forearm in Middle-Aged Women. Am. J. Clin. Nutrition 54(1):157–163, July 1991.

Iverson, L. and Clawson, D.: Manual of Acute Orthopedic Therapeutics, 3rd ed. Boston: Little, Brown, 1987.

Kanis, J.: Bone Hypertrophy and Trabecular Generation in Paget's Disease and in Fluoride-Treated Osteoporosis. Bone Miner. 17(3):399–413, June 1992.

Levin, R.: The Prevention of Osteoporosis. Hosp. Pract. (office ed.). 26(5):77, May 1991.

Long, K. and Long. R.: Current Treatment Concepts for Osteoporosis. Nurs. Pract. Forum 2(4):214–215, Dec. 1991.

Lunar Corporation: Personal Communication. Madison, Wisc.: 1993.

Lyles, K.: Osteoporosis. In: Kelley, W. (Ed.): Textbook of Internal Medicine. Philadelphia: Lippincott, 1989.

McCollum, D.: Fractures of the Pelvis, Femur, and Knee. In: Sabiston, D. (Ed.): Textbook of Surgery, 14th ed. Philadelphia: Saunders, 1991.

National Osteoporosis Foundation: Clinical Indications for Bone Mass Measurements. J. Bone Miner. Res. 4(Suppl. 2):1–28, 1989.

Nordin, B. and Morris, H.: Osteoporosis and Vitamin D. J. Cell Biochem. 49(1):19–25, May 1992.

Orcel, P., et al.: Stress Fractures of the Lower Limbs in Osteoporotic Patients Treated with Fluoride. J. Bone Miner. Res. 5(Suppl. 1):S191–S194, Mar. 1990.

Ratcliffe, M., et al.: Bone Mineral Density in Patients with Lymphoma: The Effects of Chemotherapy, Intermittent Corticosteroids and Premature Menopause. Hematol. Oncol. 10(3–4):181–187, May-Aug. 1992.

Recker, R., et al.: Bone Gain in Young Adult Women. J.A.M.A. 268(17):2403–2408, Nov. 1992.

Rosen, C., et al.: The 24/25–kDa Serum Insulin-Like Growth Factor-Binding Protein is Increased in Elderly Women with Hip and Spine Fractures. J. Clin. Endocrinol. Metab. 74(1):24–27, Jan. 1992.

Saltzstein, S.: Osteoporosis in Spinal Cord Injury: Using an Index of Mobility and its Relationship to Bone Density. J. Am. Paraplegia Society 15(4):232–234, Oct. 1992.

Schurman, S. and Williamson, A.: Bone Density Studies: Current Technology. Nurs. Pract. Forum 2(4):246–250, Dec. 1991.

Sowers, M., et al.: Joint Influence of Fat and Lean Body Composition Compartments on Femoral Bone Mineral Density in Premenopausal Women. Am. J. Epidemiol. 136(3):257–265, Aug. 1, 1992.

Ulrich, I.: Osteoporosis. W. V. Med. J. 87(8):347–350, Aug. 1991.

Watts, N., et al.: Intermittent Cyclical Etidronate Treatment of Postmenopausal Osteoporosis. N. Engl. J. Med. 323:73–79, 1991.

Weinerman, S. and Bockman, R.: Medical Therapy of Osteoporosis. Orthop. Clin. North Am. 21(1):109–124, Jan. 1990.

Wells, S., Jr., and Ashley, S.: The Parathyroid Glands. In: Sabiston, D. (Ed.): Textbook of Surgery, 14th ed. Philadelphia: Saunders, 1991.

Woodley, M. and Whelan, A. (Eds.): Manual of Medical Therapeutics, 27th ed. Boston: Little, Brown, 1992.

Wren, B.: The Menopause. In: Hacker, N. and Moore, J. (Eds.): Essentials of Obstetrics and Gynecology, 2nd ed. Philadelphia: Saunders, 1992.

CHAPTER 5

PAGET'S DISEASE OF BONE

SCOPE

Paget's disease of bone, also known as osteitis deformans, is the second most common bone disease affecting older populations. Most likely a result of both hereditary and environmental factors, Paget's disease is identified in the majority of cases by characteristic changes in bone seen on x-rays obtained for other reasons, or an elevated alkaline phosphatase activity on a routine blood test. A course of biphosphonate medication is typically given to halt the disease process. The most common symptoms of advanced disease include hearing loss due to changes in the skull, back pain due to bony compression of the spinal cord or spinal nerves, degenerative arthritis of the hip and problems walking due to involvement of leg bones. Surgery may be needed to relieve symptoms caused by pressure on skull contents, the spinal cord or spinal nerves, or deformed pelvis or lower limbs. A rare although severe complication of Paget's disease is bone cancer, which has a very poor prognosis.

SYNOPSIS

169

5.00 INTRODUCTION

Paget's disease of bone, also called osteitis deformans, was first described by the English physician Sir James Paget in 1876. This disorder has been estimated to be present in 2 to 3 percent of men and women in native English-speaking populations (Singer, 1994) and is believed to be the second most common bone disorder affecting the elderly (Hamdy, 1994).

5.10 PATHOLOGY

In the normal process of bone growth and maintenance, cells called osteoclasts break down old or damaged bone. Cells called osteoblasts then build up new or replacement bone. In Paget's disease of bone, osteoclasts may be larger and have many more nuclei than normal osteoclasts, and they are more active in osteolysis (bone breakdown). Pagetic bone also has more osteoblasts than normal bone, and the collagen fibers that form the framework of bone are irregularly arranged. Over time, foci of Paget's disease in the skull or pelvis spread outward, eventually involving the whole structure. Paget's disease in a long bone usually starts at one end, and the abnormal process forms in a V that slowly advances along the bone. Because pagetic bone is thicker, the bone becomes deformed.

Paget's disease of the skull was present in 34 percent of nearly a thousand older persons (average age 74 years) with Paget's disease, and resultant hearing loss[1] was the most frequent complication

---

[1] *See also* ch. 12 for a discussion of impaired hearing in the elderly.

reported by the group (37 percent) (Gold, et al., 1996). Less often, Paget's disease of the skull leads to vertigo (sensation of whirling in space), tinnitus (ringing in the ears) or headache, or syndromes due to compression of the brain stem, cerebellum or arteries at the back of the skull (basilar and vertebral arteries).

The thoracic (chest) and lumbar (lower back) vertebrae are the most frequently involved by Paget's disease of the spine, which has been reported by 35 percent of elderly patients (Gold, et al., 1996). Enlargement or compression fracture of these bones may cause spinal stenosis (narrowing of the spinal cord space), leading to severe back pain, or compression of a spinal nerve, causing pain along the nerve.

Involvement of the pelvis (in 49 percent of elderly patients) or leg bones (in 48 percent) results in bowed limbs, the second most common complication of Paget's disease of bone in the elderly (reported by 31 percent) (Gold, et al., 1996). The resultant alterations in weight-bearing may lead to degenerative arthritis (inflammation of the joints) and difficulty walking. Sixty-four percent of elderly patients with Paget's disease also report having arthritis[2] (Gold, et al., 1996).

5.20 ETIOLOGY

The tendency to develop Paget's disease seems to be inherited as an autosomal dominant trait with incomplete penetrance (not all individuals who inherit the gene develop the disease), and about a fourth of those with Paget's disease have a relative with the disease (Singer, 1994). Almost all individuals with Paget's disease in a United States survey were Caucasian (Gold, et al., 1996); the disease is uncommon in Japan (Matsukuma, et al., 1995).

Antigens to parts of measles virus and/or respiratory syncytial virus organisms have been found in osteoclasts from pagetic bone (Singer, 1994), indicating that exposure to certain viruses as well as hereditary factors are involved in the development of Paget's disease of bone. The relationship of measles to Paget's disease was strengthened by the results of a case-control study in a French population, in which Paget's disease occurred 2.46 times more often among those with a history of measles than among those without a history of measles. However, a history of mumps (a similar viral disease) did not increase the risk of Paget's disease in this study (Renier, et al., 1996).

---

[2] *See also* ch. 6 for a discussion of arthritis in the elderly.

Some English studies suggest that exposure to dogs increases the risk of Paget's disease (Singer, 1994). In the French case-control study, however, dog ownership did not increase the risk of Paget's disease (Renier, et al., 1996). When the risk of exposure to dogs was more narrowly defined as exposure to canine distemper (a viral disease of the respiratory tract in dogs), a study of 150 patients with Paget's disease and 185 controls showed that the risk of Paget's disease was significantly increased by ownership of a mongrel dog and increased further by ownership of a dog that had not been vaccinated against canine distemper. In this study, ownership of cats or birds also increased the risk of Paget's disease (Khan, et al., 1996).

5.30   EVALUATION

Most cases of Paget's disease are discovered by accident in persons older than 50 undergoing routine radiologic (x-ray) or laboratory studies. Laboratory and radiologic studies are also used to monitor the course of medical therapy and progression of the disease.

5.31   Laboratory Tests

Blood and urine tests may be performed to help diagnose and monitor Paget's disease.

[1]   Serum Markers of Bone Formation

Paget's disease of bone is suspected when routine laboratory testing of a patient's serum (blood) sample shows increased levels of alkaline phosphatase, an enzyme that is found in and released by active osteoblasts—cells that form bone and that are overactive in patients with Paget's disease. Other causes of increased bone formation and thus increased levels of alkaline phosphatase in blood include normal bone growth during childhood, hyperthyroidism (overactive thyroid) and certain types of bone cancer (Mundy and Reasner, 1994).

Alkaline phosphatase levels in blood may also be elevated during pregnancy and, because a form of this enzyme is also produced by the liver, in those with liver disease.

The alkaline phosphatase level correlates well with the stage of Paget's disease, so blood levels of this enzyme are traditionally monitored to follow the effectiveness of drug therapy and progression of the disease. In research studies, bone scan indices of Paget's disease activity correlated best of all with blood levels of propeptide carboxyterminal of type I procollagen (94 percent) (Alvarez, et al., 1997).

[2]   Urine Markers of Bone Resorption

Bone contains collagen, a type of protein that is made up of hydroxyproline and other proteins. When collagen breaks down, its components such as hydroxyproline are released and excreted in the urine. Thus high urine concentrations of hydroxyproline indicate high bone turnover, as occurs with Paget's disease. However, elevated urine hydroxyproline levels also occur with thyrotoxicosis and acromegaly (hormonal disorders). Furthermore, levels vary with dietary intake of gelatin, so patients must be on a gelatin-free diet before testing for the results to accurately reflect collagen turnover (Mundy and Reasner, 1994).

Serial measurements of urine levels of hydroxyproline can be used to monitor treatment of Paget's disease with biphosphonates or calcitonin. When these medications are effective, the urinary hydroxyproline level will start to decrease several weeks before the serum alkaline phosphatase level begins to decline (Mundy and Reasner, 1994).

Another component of collagen that can be measured in urine is deoxypyridinoline. The level of deoxypyridinoline in urine is not affected by diet, but it is increased by any condition that increases the rate of bone resorption, including the postmenopausal period in women (Mundy and Reasner, 1994). Measurement of urinary deoxypyridinoline levels by an enzyme-linked immunoassay (ELISA) technique is faster than the traditional high-performance liquid chromatography method (Robins, et al., 1994).

Other urine markers of bone resorption (collagen breakdown) have been studied. In patients with active Paget's disease, urinary pyridinoline was found to be the most sensitive marker of bone resorption, being increased in 73 percent of the patients; urinary hydroxyproline was increased in 64 percent, and urinary deoxypyridinoline was increased in 60 percent (Alvarez, et al., 1995). In another study, the urinary galactosyl hydroxylysine/creatinine ratio was found to be representative of the activity of Paget's disease and was easier, faster and less costly to monitor—but also less sensitive—than urine levels of hydroxyproline, deoxypyridinolone or alkaline phosphatase (Michalsky, et al., 1995).

The newest techniques for monitoring the success of drug therapy for Paget's disease focus on evaluation of collagen type I telopeptides. Urine concentrations of cross-linked N-telopeptide decreased more after biphosphonate treatment for 10 days than did levels of deoxypyridinoline (measured by two different assays) and about the same as levels of hydroxyproline; in addition, the decrease in the level of N-telopeptide on days 9 and 10 of treatment correlated with the lowest serum alkaline phosphatase activity measured over one year of follow-up (Papapoulos and Frolich, 1996). In another study, the best correlation of a urinary marker with bone scan findings in Paget's disease was found for N-terminal telopeptide (96 percent), followed by deoxypyridinoline (71 percent), pyridinoline (69 percent), C-terminal telopeptide (65 percent) and hydroxyproline (64 percent) (Alvarez, et al., 1997).

5.32   Radiologic Examinations

Paget's disease of bone has a characteristic appearance on radiologic studies that usually leads to the diagnosis without the need to biopsy (sample) the bone. In their early stage, Paget's disease lesions appear radiolucent (less dense than normal). On x-rays of the skull, pagetic foci appear as dark spots, and on x-rays of long bones, as a dark V pointing away from the end of the bone (Singer, 1994).

When Paget's disease has progressed for many years, the involved bone becomes sclerotic (hardened) and appears white on x-rays. Enlarged, white areas of pagetic bone in the skull give it a "cotton-wool" appearance; patients whose skulls have this appearance have probably had Paget's disease of bone since childhood (Singer, 1994). Advanced Paget's disease in the pelvis typically results in a white rim or "brim sign" on x-rays.

Paget's disease involving vertebrae is not usually noticed until the bone is sclerotic, when it is difficult to distinguish from a tumor unless Paget's disease has also resulted in enlargement of the involved vertebra(e). Computed tomography (CT) and magnetic resonance imaging (MRI) are useful in evaluating the spine of patients with back pain that could be due to Paget's or another disease. A bone scan (injection of a radioactive tracer before x-rays are obtained) is often used to visualize pagetic lesions.

5.33   Differential Diagnosis and Co-morbidities

Because many symptoms of advanced Paget's disease of bone, such as hearing loss and arthritis, often occur in the elderly, they may be mistakenly attributed to the aging process (Hamdy, 1994). On the other hand, arthritis does often occur with Paget's disease in older patients (Gold, et al., 1996) or may develop due to pagetic changes in joints. There have also been case reports of Paget's disease accompanied by fibrous dysplasia (displacement of bone due to overgrowth of fibrous tissue in a joint) (Jones, et al., 1996) or ankylosing spondylitis (a form of rheumatoid arthritis affecting the spine) (Peel, et al., 1996). When symptoms cannot be explained by the abnormal bone metabolic process of Paget's disease or do not respond to treatment, another cause should be sought.

5.40 TREATMENT

Because the etiology of Paget's disease is uncertain, treatment can only be aimed at lessening symptoms and preventing progression, not achieving cure. Two types of medication are used to halt or reverse the pagetic process.

5.41 Calcitonin

Calcitonin, a hormone, inhibits osteoclast activity, slowing bone resorption and decreasing abnormal bone formation. Treatment with regular (daily or every other day) subcutaneous (under the skin) injections of 50 units of salmon calcitonin or 0.5 mg of human calcitonin usually decreases serum alkaline phosphatase activity by 50 percent (Singer, 1994). Calcitonin is available as an intranasal spray, and an oral form of calcitonin has been developed. A comparison trial of injectable salmon calcitonin (50 IUs) and injectable (0.2 mg) and oral (20 mg) forms of a calcitonin analogue (similar chemical compound) in patients with Paget's disease found that the three medications provided essentially the same intensity and duration of effect in preventing bone resorption (Devogelaer, et al., 1994).

The side effects of calcitonin injections include nausea and facial flushing, which usually are not severe enough to warrant discontinuation of treatment. In addition, about half of patients treated with salmon calcitonin develop antibodies to this medication and may become resistant to treatment. Fortunately most such patients do well when human calcitonin is substituted. Unfortunately Paget's disease becomes more active within months of discontinuing calcitonin (Singer, 1994).

5.42 Biphosphonates

Biphosphonates or bisphosphonates are chemicals that localize to the surface of bone and, like calcitonin, inhibit bone resorption.

[1] Etidronate

One of the first biphosphonate medications available to treat Paget's disease is disodium etidronate, which is given orally in dosages of 5 to 7.5 mg per kg body weight per day (Key and Bell, 1994) for six months (Singer, 1994). Although disodium etidronate does not heal osteolytic lesions, it is about as effective as calcitonin in relieving symptoms (Singer, 1994). A disadvantage of disodium etidronate is that dosages larger than 5 mg/kg body weight may cause osteomalacia (bone softening) (Singer, 1994; Key and Bell, 1994).

[2] Pamidronate

Pamidronate disodium (APD), a second-generation bisphosphonate that must be given intravenously, has been used for a number of years to inhibit bone resorption in Paget's disease and other hypercalcemic conditions. The drug has not been found to cause osteomalacia. The most frequent side effects of the drug are temporary fever and decrease in lymphocyte concentration (Schweitzer, et al., 1995).

Pamidronate may produce long-term improvement in Paget's disease after a single infusion of 60 mg (Singer, 1994; Chakravarty, et al., 1994; Mazieres, et al., 1996). However, some authorities recommend two 60-mg doses for mild disease and four 60-mg doses for moderate disease (Gutteridge, et al., 1996).

Higher dosages of pamidronate—up to 980 mg total—have been tried for patients who do not respond to lower dosages, and a total of 1.44 to 2.52 g administered over 12 to 42 weeks were used in five patients with Paget's disease that had not remitted with a variety of other treatments. Although all five patients had marked improvement in symptoms and suppression of disease activity, alkaline phosphatase activity returned to the normal range in only one patient, and bone biopsies showed continued pagetic activity in two patients (Cundy, et al., 1996).

Two other studies demonstrated that pamidronate is more effective when used for patients with mild Paget's disease. In the first of these studies, patients with more severe disease had less improvement in symptoms than those with milder disease (Bombassei, et al., 1994).

In the second of these studies, patients received higher total pamidronate dosages for more severe disease, but despite higher dosages, the majority of patients with severe Paget's disease relapsed within two years of treatment (Gutteridge, et al., 1996).

[3] Alendronate

Alendronate, one of the newest bisphosphonates available to treat Paget's disease of bone, may be given intravenously (5 mg/day) for two (Pedrazzoni, et al., 1996) to five (Filipponi, et al., 1994) days. In one study, alendronate led to remission of symptoms and normalization of serum alkaline phosphate levels for a minimum of 12 months in patients given alendronate for relapse after a previous therapy and in those receiving alendronate as initial treatment for newly diagnosed Paget's disease. Moderate, temporary arthromyalgia (joint aching) and fever occurred in half of these patients (Filipponi, et al., 1994). Alendronate may also cause a temporary decrease in lymphocyte count (O'Doherty, et al., 1995).

Oral preparations of alendronate are available. In one study, 20 mg of alendronate taken daily for six months was well tolerated but did not result in disease remission, whereas patients receiving 40 mg per day had significantly more decrease in serum alkaline phosphatase levels but also a notable incidence of gastric and esophageal disturbances (Adami, et al., 1994). In two other studies, however, patients receiving 40 mg per day of alendronate orally for six months tolerated the treatment well and experienced significant improvement in radiologic evidence of disease and normalization of alkaline phosphatase levels (Reid, et al., 1996; Siris, et al., 1996).

[4] Gallium Nitrate

In one study, gallium nitrate, which has potent effects in decreasing resorption of bone, was effective in dosages of 0.25 or 0.5 mg/kg per day by subcutaneous injection for 14 days for patients with advanced Paget's disease that had not responded to prior treatments. Although minor discomfort occurred at the injection site, this did not cause patients to interrupt therapy (Bockman, et al., 1995).

5.50 PROGNOSIS

Progression of Paget's disease may lead to the need for surgery to treat symptoms and may seriously affect patients' quality of life.

5.51 Surgical Procedures

Medical therapy is recommended for as long as three months before surgery to decrease the risk of intraoperative and postoperative bleeding and to prevent hypercalcemia (high blood levels of calcium) that may occur with a long postoperative period of decreased mobility (Singer, 1994).

A neurosurgical operation called occipital decompression may be required when overgrowth of bone in the back of the head (occiput) causes symptoms of pressure on the basilar arteries (major blood vessels serving the back third of the brain). This operation involves removing bone pressing on these vital structures. A similar operation is performed on vertebrae when spinal stenosis (narrowing of the space through which nerves pass) causes symptoms related to compression of the spinal cord or spinal nerves.

Individuals who have severe pain and difficulty walking because of Paget's disease of hipbones usually have their pain relieved by total hip replacement. When pagetic changes in bones of the lower leg cause bowed legs, the resulting abnormalities in weight-bearing can lead to knee or ankle pain. A high tibial osteotomy (surgical reshaping of the tibia, or shinbone) can restore normal weight-bearing, leading to improved walking and relief of pain (Singer, 1994).

A rare complication of Paget's disease is the development of osteosarcoma (bone cancer) in pagetic bone, usually a leg bone. This condition has a very poor prognosis.

5.52 Quality of Life

A survey of a large number of elderly patients with Paget's disease found that only 21 percent felt that their quality of life was very good or excellent; nearly half (47 percent) felt depressed, and 42 percent said that their health was fair or poor (Gold, et al., 1996).

5.100 BIBLIOGRAPHY

Text References

Adami, S.: Effects of Two Oral Doses of Alendronate in the Treatment of Paget's Disease of Bone. Bone 15:415-417, 1994.

Alvarez, L., et al.: Relationship Between Biochemical Markers of Bone Turnover and Bone Scintigraphic Indices in Assessment of

Paget's Disease Activity. Arthritis Rheum. 40(3):461-468, Mar. 1997.

Alvarez, L., et al.: Discriminative Value of Biochemical Markers of Bone Turnover in Assessing the Activity of Paget's Disease. J. Bone Miner. Res. 10(3):458-465, Mar. 1995.

Bockman, R. S.: A Multicenter Trial of Low Dose Gallium Nitrate in Patients with Advanced Paget's Disease of Bone. J. Clin. Endocrinol. Metab. 80(2):595-602, Feb. 1995.

Bombassei, G. J., et al.: Effects of Intravenous Pamidronate Therapy on Paget's Disease of Bone. Am. J. Med. Sci. 308(4):226-233, Oct. 1994.

Chakravarty, K., et al.: A Single Infusion of Bisphosphonate AHPrBP in the Treatment of Paget's Disease of Bone. J. Rheumatol. 2(11):2118-2121, Nov. 1994.

Cundy, T., et al.: High-Dose Pamidronate in the Management of Resistant Paget's Disease. Calcif. Tissue Int. 58(1):6-8, Jan. 1996.

Devogelaer, J. P., et al.: Comparison of the Acute Biological Action of Injectable Salmon Calcitonin and an Injectable and Oral Calcitonin Analogue. Calcif. Tissue Int. 55(1):71-73, July 1994.

Filipponi, P., et al.: Effects of Two Different Bisphosphonates on Paget's Disease of Bone: ICTP Assessed. Bone 15(3):261-267, 1994.

Gold, D. T., et al.: Paget's Disease of Bone and Quality of Life. J. Bone Miner. Res. 11(12):1897-1904, Dec. 1996.

Gutteridge, D. H., et al.: Clinical, Biochemical, Hematologic, and Radiographic Responses in Paget's Disease Following Intravenous Pamidronate Disodium: A 2-Year-Study. Bone 19(4):387-394, Oct. 1996.

Hamdy, R. C.: Paget's Disease of the Bone. Clin. Geriatric Med. 10:719-735, 1994.

Jones, S. M., et al.: Coexisting Polyostotic Fibrous Dysplasia and Paget's Disease. Clin. Exp. Rheumatol. 14(2):187-190, 1996.

Key, L. L., Jr., and Bell, N. H.: Osteomalacia and Disorders of Vitamin D Metabolism. In: Stein, J. H., et al. (Eds.): Internal Medicine, 4th ed. St. Louis: Mosby, 1994.

Khan, S. A., et al.: Paget's Disease of Bone and Unvaccinated Dogs. Bone 19(1):47-50, July 1996.

Matsukuma, S., et al.: Paget Sarcoma of the Cervical Vertebrae: An Autopsy Case Report and Review of the Literature. Pathol. Int. 45(11):885-889, Nov. 1995.

Mazieres, B., et al.: Pamidronate Infusions for the Treatment of Paget's Disease of Bone. Rev. Rhum. Engl. Ed. 63(1):36-43, Jan. 1996.

Michalsky, M., et al.: Galactosyl Hydroxylysine in Assessment of Paget's Bone Disease. Clin. Chim. Acta 234:(1-2):101-108, Jan. 1995.

Mundy, G. R. and Reasner, C. A.: Physiology of Bone and Mineral Homeostasis. In: Stein, J. H., et al.: Internal Medicine, 4th ed. St. Louis: Mosby, 1994.

O'Doherty, D. P., et al.: The Effects of Intravenous Alendronate in Paget's Disease of Bone. J. Bone Miner. Res. 10(7):1094-1100, July 1995.

Papapoulos, S. E. and Frolich, M.: Prediction of the Outcome of Treatment of Paget's Disease of Bone with Biphosphonates from Short-Term Changes in the Rate of Bone Resorption. J. Clin. Endocrinol. Metab. 81(11):3993-3997, Nov. 1996.

Pedrazzoni, M., et al.: Clinical Observations with a New Specific Assay for Bone Alkaline Phosphatase: A Cross-sectional Study in Osteoporotic and Pagetic Subjects and a Longitudinal Evaluation of the Response to Ovariectomy, Estrogens, and Bisphosphonates. Calcif. Tissue Int. 59(5):334-338, Nov. 1996.

Peel, N. F., et al.: Paget's Disease in a Patient with Ankylosing Spondylitis—A Diagnostic Dilemma. Br. J. Rheumatol. 35(10):1011-1014, Oct. 1996.

Reid, I. R., et al.: Biochemical and Radiologic Improvement in Paget's Disease of Bone Treated with Alendronate; A Randomized, Placebo-Controlled Trial. Am. J. Med. 101(4):341-348, Oct. 1996.

Renier, J. C., et al.: An Etiologic Study of Paget's Disease. Rev. Rhum. Engl. Ed. 63(9):606-611, Oct. 1996.

Robins, S. P., et al.: Direct, Enzyme-Linked Immunoassay for Urinary Deoxypyridinoline as a Specific Marker for Measuring Bone Resorption. J. Bone Miner. Res. 9(10):1643-1649, Oct. 1994.

Schweitzer, D. H., et al.: Interleukin-6 and the Acute Phase Response During Treatment of Patients with Paget's Disease with the

Nitrogen-Containing Bisphosphonate Dimethylaminohydroxypropylidene Bisphosphonate. J. Bone Miner. Res. 10(6):956-962, June 1995.

Singer, F. R.: Paget's Disease of Bone. In: Stein, J. H., et al. (Eds.): Internal Medicine, 4th ed. St. Louis: Mosby, 1994.

Siris, E., et al.: Comparative Study of Alendronate Versus Etidronate for the Treatment of Paget's Disease of Bone. J. Clin. Endocrinol. Metab. 81(3):961-967, Mar. 1996.

CHAPTER 6

ARTHRITIS AND RHEUMATIC DISEASES

SCOPE

Rheumatic diseases involve the musculoskeletal system as well as a variety of connective tissues. Musculoskeletal pain and stiffness are the prominent features. Pain, stiffness and joint swelling associated with musculoskeletal disorders may be inflammatory, metabolic, degenerative or combinations thereof. Arthritis involves one or more joints in either a destructive inflammatory process or a noninflammatory mechanical degenerative process. Patients with rheumatic diseases may demonstrate a wide range of signs and symptoms reflecting multiorgan involvement, or they may present with pain and compromised function in a single anatomic area. Major categories of progressive and potentially crippling diseases include rheumatoid arthritis, osteoarthritis, systemic lupus erythematosus, scleroderma, Sjögren's syndrome, the vasculitis syndromes including polyarteritis nodosa, polymyositis and dermatomyositis, and gout. Certain anatomic abnormalities that previously escaped detection can now be identified by newer imaging procedures, including arthroscopy, ultrasonography and magnetic resonance imaging (MRI). New tests must be interpreted in the context of a thorough, comprehensive, multifaceted evaluation.

SYNOPSIS

6.00   DEFINITIONS

"Rheumatism" is an ill-defined and outdated term that in the past was used to describe a number of diseases involving the musculoskeletal system and connective tissue, with musculoskeletal pain and stiffness the prominent features. The term "rheumatic diseases" is a more precise description of these conditions. Arthritis is a classic example of rheumatic disease.

Musculoskeletal diseases are common and can be disabling. Pain, stiffness and joint swelling associated with musculoskeletal disorders may be inflammatory, metabolic, degenerative or a combination of all three. The degree of impact on the patient is determined by the functional interference with daily activities that may result from the disorder.

Treatment of musculoskeletal disorders is based on a correct diagnosis, which may be difficult to determine during the initial stages. In addition, it is important to ascertain whether the patient's problem is urgent, as in acute monoarthritis (involving one joint) due to sepsis or gout, or whether treatment may be postponed until a more complete diagnosis is established (Gordon, 1996).

6.01   Connective Tissue

The connective tissue system is derived from the primordial embryonic mesoderm and its mesenchymal cells. These tissues protect vital organs, facilitate movement and give the body shape and form. The connective tissue system is so widespread that any organ in the body may be involved in rheumatic diseases: the heart (rheumatic fever), the eye (Sjögren's syndrome), the skin (scleroderma), the blood vessel walls (vasculitis) and various organs (systemic lupus erythematosus).

6.02   Origin of Rheumatic Diseases

The origin of rheumatic diseases may be infectious, metabolic, endocrinologic, developmental or inheritable; however, the basic pathogenesis is the same: provoked inflammation. For some rheumatic diseases, the provoking agent is known (e.g., *Streptococci* in rheumatic heart disease; crystals of sodium urate in gout). In many inflammatory diseases, however, such as rheumatoid arthritis or systemic lupus erythematosus, the precise causative agents are unknown.

Rheumatic diseases can result in multiorgan involvement and a series of destructive immunologic events. In general, the term *rheumatic disease* refers to a condition that is both inflammatory and immunologic in nature. In rheumatic disease, the immune system reaction involves attack of the host tissues rather than attack of an invading organism.

6.03   Rheumatology

Rheumatology is a specialty of internal medicine. Initially patients experiencing joint pain and inflammation may consult an internist or an orthopedist, while those experiencing rash or skin thickening as the presenting symptoms often consult a dermatologist. Orthopedists do not treat rheumatic conditions, but they do work closely with rheumatologists.

6.04   Inflammatory and Noninflammatory Arthritis

Arthritis involves one or more joints in either a destructive inflammatory process or a noninflammatory mechanical degenerative process. Inflammatory arthritis may be categorized into four different groups (Hicks and Gerber, 1993):

- inflammatory connective tissue disease, e.g., rheumatoid arthritis;
- inflammatory crystal-induced disease, e.g., gout;
- inflammation induced by infectious agents, e.g., bacterial or fungal arthritis; and
- seronegative spondyloarthropathies, e.g., ankylosing spondylitis.

Noninflammatory arthritis may be categorized as:

- degenerative, e.g., osteoarthritis; or
- metabolic, e.g., lipid storage disease.

Acute painful onset, fever, erythema (reddening) of the skin over the joint or joints involved, warmth over the involved joints and tenderness are clinical features that suggest inflammatory disease. Laboratory and x-ray findings suggesting an inflammatory process include increased peripheral white blood cell count with left shift, elevated erythrocyte sedimentation rate, joint fluid, x-ray demonstration of soft tissue swelling, periositis, bony erosions or uniform cartilage loss (Hicks and Gerber, 1993).

6.10   DIAGNOSTIC WORKUP

Patients with rheumatic diseases may demonstrate a wide range of signs and symptoms reflecting multiorgan involvement, or they may present with pain and compromised function in a single anatomic area. The diversity of the presentation and pathogenesis makes rheumatic diseases difficult to diagnose and classify accurately. Patients with rheumatic conditions may also have more than one diagnostic entity.

Existing classifications used in the diagnosis of rheumatic diseases are based on the recognition of an array of clinical symptoms, patterns of involvement, laboratory findings and disease progression that have been derived from the experiences of various concerned groups, such as the American Rheumatism Association (ARA). Major categories of progressive and potentially crippling rheumatoid diseases include rheumatoid arthritis and its juvenile variant, the spondylarthropathies, systemic lupus erythematosus, scleroderma, Sjögren's syndrome, the vasculitis syndromes, polymyositis and dermatomyositis, and arteritis diseases. These diseases are all identifiable through appropriate testing and diagnostic procedures.

Correct diagnosis of the rheumatic process and optimal management of the patient depends upon the physician's ability to identify the site(s) from which the symptoms arise, ascertain the pathologic process involved, determine the cause of the process and find measures to gauge the activity of the disease so that the appropriate response to treatment can be initiated (Ike and Arnold, 1996). A directed medical history and physical examination is the initial diagnostic procedure, followed by the appropriate laboratory tests, imaging modalities and invasive procedures. The number of specialized procedures applicable to rheumatic diseases continues to grow, and testing for relevant immunologic phenomena becomes more complex as newer tests are developed. Certain anatomic abnormalities that previously escaped detection can now be identified by newer imaging procedures, including arthroscopy, ultrasonography and magnetic resonance imaging (MRI). New tests must be interpreted in the context of a thorough, comprehensive, multifaceted evaluation (Ike and Arnold, 1996).

6.11 Medical History

A wide range of diagnoses are possibilities for patients with musculoskeletal pain and/or dysfunction. The differential diagnosis should first rule out common problems such as bursitis (inflammation of a fluid-filled sac between moving surfaces of a joint). A complete and detailed medical history of the patient's rheumatic complaints should include the anatomic location of the pain and whether it is local or referred; the pattern of occurrence in relation to rest, activity and sleep; the pattern of joint symptoms and involvement—whether it is symmetric, whether it occurs predominantly in upper or lower limbs; the influence of previous and current treatments; systemic symptoms such as weight loss, fatigue, fever and duration of morning stiffness; involvement of skin or eyes; symptoms related to the genitourinary, gastrointestinal and cardiopulmonary organs; muscle pain or weakness; an accurate account and systematic review of all the joints of the body, and the patient's psychosocial history. In addition, the patient's age, gender and occupation are helpful facts (Gordon, 1996).

For example, patients with systemic rheumatic diseases, such as rheumatoid arthritis, usually experience prolonged morning stiffness in multiple symptomatic joints, which decreases as the joints are used, and they may have constitutional symptoms or symptoms of multisystem involvement as well. People with local mechanical problems and osteoarthritis typically experience little morning stiffness, one or a few symptomatic areas, no pain at rest, worsened symptoms after sustained activity and no symptoms or signs of a systemic illness.

The patient's functional ability should be assessed by noting which daily activities have been affected by the condition. A vocational history may be useful in identifying repetitive physical tasks that may need to be modified to aid recovery (Shmerling, et al, 1996).

6.12 Physical Examination

Numerous conditions may result in musculoskeletal emergencies, for example, infection, systemic vaculitis, spinal cord compression, fracture, etc. A delayed diagnosis in these emergency situations may lead to permanent disability and death. Once these have been excluded, an orderly evaluation will distinguish the major diagnostic possibilities (Schmerling, et al., 1996).

The clinical diagnosis of rheumatic disease can usually be made following the history and physical examination. The examination will help distinguish mechanical problems, soft tissue disease and noninflammatory or inflammatory joint disease. Warmth over the joint, joint effusion (leakage of joint fluid) and pain on joint motion are classic indications of synovitis (inflammation of a synovial joint). *(See Figure 6-1.)* Point tenderness, reduced active range of motion and preserved passive range of motion are suggestive of soft tissue disorders. When both active and passive range of motion are limited, soft tissue contracture, synovitis or structural abnormality of the joint are possibilities (Schmerling, et al., 1996).

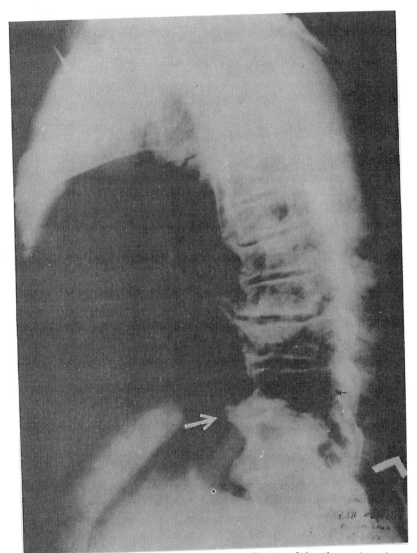

Fig. 6-1. X-rays showing severe osteoarthritis of the thoracic spine. Arrows indicate large spurs projecting from the front margins of the vertebrae.

The physical examination should determine the location and severity of joint pain; assess the presence, absence and severity of tenderness, swelling, joint effusion and warmth; assess the range of motion limitations and functional ability; and determine if inflammatory processes are occurring. Documentation of these findings is important, so that changes can be followed over time (Litman, 1996).

6.13   General Laboratory Tests

The differential diagnosis should be kept in mind, and only those laboratory tests that are most likely to be helpful should be ordered. The results of laboratory tests must be integrated with the clinical findings, as few laboratory test are useful alone in the diagnosis of rheumatic diseases. Most laboratory procedures are an aid in diagnosis and provide a baseline for determining the effectiveness of therapy.

Basic laboratory studies that are not specifically directed at rheumatoid diseases may be ordered as part of the general health assessment. These include a complete blood count (CBC), urinalysis, erythrocyte sedimentation rate (ESR), stool guaiac and automated chemical profile.

Most patients with simple musculoskeletal complaints have self-limiting localized conditions, such as low back pain or tennis elbow, rather than a rheumatic condition. More extensive tests are usually delayed for about six weeks—the average time it takes for these conditions to resolve. Contraindications for delay include significant trauma, severe inflammation of a single joint, systemic illness coupled with trauma or multiple joint involvement. When further testing is indicated, the tests should be based on a particular indication.

6.14   Synovial Fluid Analysis

Examination of the synovial fluid (lubricating substance secreted by the membrane lining the joints) may provide specific information in joint disease and may help differentiate between inflammatory and noninflammatory conditions. A high leukocyte (white blood cell) count is an indication of an inflammatory process.

Examination of synovial joint fluid is mandatory in any patient with undiagnosed arthritis and an associated joint effusion. Gross appearance of the synovial fluid can provide clues to the initial underlying process. Bacterial infections and crystalline arthropathies can be quickly confirmed by microscopic examination of the fluid (Ike and Arnold, 1996).

The white cell count affects the appearance of synovial fluid. Fluid that transmits light and can be read through by holding the tube in front of a printed page usually indicates noninflammatory disorders, most commonly osteoarthritis. Translucent fluid that blurs print is associated with a wide array of inflammatory conditions, such as rheumatoid arthritis. Opaque fluid is usually thick and carries the usual concerns of pus; this is an indication of infection until proven otherwise. Bloody fluid carries a specific differential diagnosis.

Examination of synovial fluid under a polarized light microscope is essential for the diagnosis of crystal-associated arthropathies and should be performed initially on all patients. Reduction of synovial fluid glucose level to less than 50 percent of simultaneous serum measurement may indicate infectious arthritis (Ike and Arnold, 1996).

Timely processing of the joint aspirate tests is important. A delay of as little as five hours can decrease the leukocyte count considerably, and longer delays can lead to inaccurate crystal analysis (Litman, 1996).

6.15   Microbiologic Tests

When the leukocyte count is high, synovial fluid or another biologic specimen is stained and cultured for bacteria, fungi or mycobacterium (e.g., tuberculosis). Identification of a specific pathogen can confirm the diagnosis of infectious arthritis.[1]

6.16   Biopsy

Biopsy of a tissue sample or body fluid can be specific for some connective tissue diseases, such as myositis and vasculitis.

6.17   Rheumatologic Tests

Certain tests are specifically rheumatologic. These include determinations of presence of rheumatoid factor, quantitative studies of immunoglobulins, antinuclear antibody determinations, complement and cryoglobulin studies and measures of circulating immune complexes.

Rheumatoid factors are antigammaglobulins (proteins) found in the sera (blood) of many patients with rheumatoid arthritis. However, in addition to being present in about 80 percent of patients with rheumatoid arthritis, rheumatoid factor can be present in patients with a variety

---

[1] *See* 6.30 *infra.*

of other inflammatory diseases, and about 20 percent of patients with rheumatoid arthritis have a negative rheumatoid factor test result. A rheumatoid factor test should only be ordered for patients showing signs and symptoms of clinically significant rheumatologic disease (Litman, 1996).

Autoantibodies to substances in the cell nucleus are found in patients with a variety of rheumatologic diseases. The antinuclear antibody (ANA) test is sensitive when used to diagnose systemic lupus erythematosus (SLE) and other connective tissue diseases, but it lacks specificity, because many persons who never develop a rheumatologic disorder have a positive antinuclear antibody test result (Litman, 1996). Testing serum for antinuclear antibodies is primarily used in the evaluation of suspected systemic lupus erythematosus (Ike and Arnold, 1996).

6.18 Imaging Studies

Imaging studies are necessary when the physical examination cannot localize the anatomic structure that is causing symptoms. Plain radiographs are helpful in defining the problem and are useful in judging the response to treatment of a chronic process. *(See Figure 6-2.)* They are also relatively inexpensive and widely available. However, the pathologic processes of many rheumatic diseases often occur in structures that require additional or other means of imaging.

When the anatomic structures are complex, as in the spine, or when the areas involved are surrounded by bone, computed tomography (CT) is most valuable. Magnetic resonance imaging (MRI) is the procedure of choice to delineate abnormalities of intra-articular and periarticular soft tissue structures in large joints, although most bony abnormalities are better indicated by plain radiographs or CT (Ike and Arnold, 1996).

6.20 RHEUMATOID ARTHRITIS

Rheumatoid arthritis (RA) is a chronic systemic disorder characterized by inflammation, most commonly involving the synovium (lining membrane) of the peripheral joints. The precise etiology of the disease is unknown, although three areas of inter-related research are most promising: (1) host genetic factors, (2) immunoregulatory abnormalities and autoimmunity, and (3) a triggering or persisting microbial infection (Arnett, 1996).

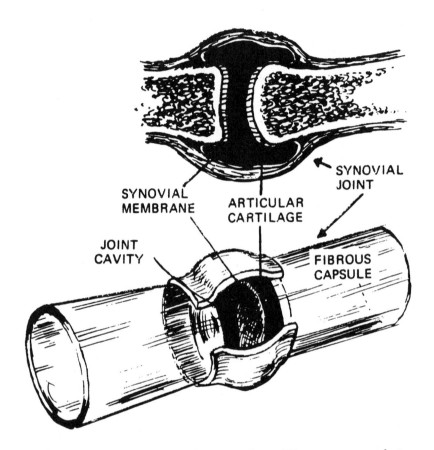

Fig. 6-2. A synovial joint. Rheumatoid conditions can cause degeneration of the synovial lining of a joint and changes in the synovial fluid that inhibit joint function.

It is believed that a genetically susceptible individual develops abnormal or altered IgG (immunoglobulin) antibodies when exposed to an antigen. The body does not recognize the abnormal or altered antibody as part of itself and develops an antibody against it known as rheumatoid factor (RF). RF generates inflammation by aggregating into complexes, and the resulting cartilage damage by inflammation triggers additional immune system responses. This in turn attracts polymorphonuclear leukocytes and produces inflammatory mediators, which contribute to destruction of the joint (Norris, et al., 1995).

6.21 Pathogenesis

The pathogenesis of rheumatoid arthritis is more clearly understood than the etiology of the disease and may be categorized into four stages of progression: The first stage of untreated RA is synovitis from congestion and edema (swelling due to accumulation of fluid) of the synovial membrane and joint capsule. The second stage is marked by the development of proliferating inflammatory tissue (pannus), which invades cartilage and eventually destroys intra-articular and periarticular structures. The third stage is characterized by fibrous ankylosis, or fibrous invasion of pannus and scar formation that occludes joint space. Bone atrophy and malalignment cause deformities, muscle atrophy and imbalance, and may lead to partial dislocations, or subluxations. The fourth stage is characterized by the calcification of fibrous tissue, resulting in bony ankylosis (stiffening) and total immobility (Norris, et al., 1995).

6.22 Diagnostic Criteria

The American College of Rheumatology has defined criteria for the diagnosis of RA. The following criteria are helpful in establishing diagnosis, but it should be noted that failure to meet these criteria, especially during early phases of the disease, does not exclude the diagnosis (Cohen, 1995):

- morning stiffness in and around the joints lasting at least one hour before improvement;
- at least three joint areas with arthritis and tissue swelling;
- arthritis in at least one joint in wrist, metacarpophalangeal (MCP; between the wrist and bones of the hand) joint or proximal interphalangeal joint (PIP; hinge joints between the finger or toe bones);
- symmetric arthritis (in the same joint areas on both sides of the body);
- rheumatoid nodules over bony prominences or extensor surfaces or in juxta-articular regions, observed on examination by a physician;
- abnormal amounts of serum rheumatoid factor; and
- radiographic changes typical of RA.

Although clinical features may suggest RA, firm diagnosis relies on laboratory and other test results, including x-rays, rheumatoid factor test, synovial fluid analysis, serum protein electrophoresis, erythrocyte sedimentation rate, complete blood count and C-reactive protein test (Norris, et al., 1996).

6.23   Clinical Course

Rheumatoid arthritis (RA) is a progressive disease that usually begins insidiously, producing nonspecific symptoms such as fatigue, malaise, anorexia (loss of appetite), persistent low grade fever, weight loss, lymphadenopathy (enlarged lymph nodes) and vague articular symptoms. The course of RA varies considerably; approximately 20 percent of patients improve spontaneously or achieve remission, especially during the first year. However, chronic disease progression and functional deterioration occur in the majority. Approximately 50 percent of RA patients must stop working within ten years of the diagnosis. There is also a higher mortality rate, correlating with the degree of disability and resulting from infections, systemic manifestations and gastrointestinal bleeding or perforation (Ike and Arnold, 1996).

6.24   Pathology

Many organs and structures may be involved in the disease process. The patterns of change are relatively distinct.

[1]   Joint Changes

Although any joint may be involved in the RA process, localized articular symptoms develop frequently in the fingers at the proximal interphalangeal (PIP), metacarpophalangeal (MCP; the joints between the bones of the wrist and the hand) and metatarsophalangeal (MTP; between the bones of the toes and the midfoot) joints, and may extend as well to the wrists, knees, ankles and toes. The fingers may become spindle shaped and deformed from marked edema and congestion in the joints. In active disease, deformities are common. PIP joints may develop flexion (bending) or hyperextension deformities. MCP joints swell dorsally, and instability of the tendons may pull the fingers to the ulnar side (toward the ulna, the large bone of the forearm), a condition called ulnar drift (Norris, et al., 1995). Boutonnière deformities (marked by flexion of the proximal interphalangeal joint, the joint of the finger nearer the knuckle, and hyperextension of the distal interphalangeal joint, nearer the nail) and swan-neck deformities (marked by hyperextension of the finger at the joint nearer the knuckle and flexion of the joint nearer the nail) are also seen. *(See Figure 6-3.)* If the tendons rupture, the individual is unable to extend his or her fingers. Late manifestations may include obliteration of the joint space, fibrous ankylosis (stiffness, or rigidity of a joint resulting from formation of fibrous tissue in the joint capsule and between adjoining joint surfaces of the bones) and cyst formation.

Carpal tunnel syndrome may occur from synovial pressure on the median nerve, causing tingling paresthesias in the fingers. The hands appear foreshortened, and the wrists are swollen or boggy. Changes in the feet are similar to those in the hands.

Changes in the knee are common and may include flexion and varus (bent inward) and valgus (bent outward) deformities. Synovial effusion in the knee joint causes a bulging around the kneecap. Atrophy of the quadriceps and marked joint instability occurs as the soft tissues are destroyed. Late in the disease, an overlay of osteoarthritis, with loss of joint space, subchrondral erosions, cysts and osteophytes (bony protrusions), are common. As the disease progresses, the neck,

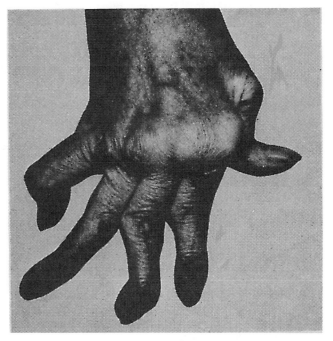

Fig. 6-3. A hand severely affected by rheumatoid arthritis. The second and third fingers show characteristic swan-neck deformity.

shoulders and hips become affected. Neck involvement may result in atlantoaxial subluxation (dislocation of the first two cervical vertebrae), causing spinal cord compression.

[2]   Skin Changes and Rheumatoid Nodules

The most common extra-articular (not in a joint area) occurrence is the gradual appearance of rheumatoid nodules. These appear as subcutaneous, round or oval, nontender masses that vary in size and usually develop on pressure areas, such as the elbows. About 20 percent of patients develop subcutaneous nodules, most commonly over bony prominences, but these may also appear in the bursas (fluid-filled sacs that act as protective pads between adjacent surfaces of moving tissues, such as joints) and tendon sheaths, especially in seropositive patients (Hellmann, 1996).

[3]   Vasculitis

Vasculitis (inflammation of blood vessels) occurs late in the disease process and is a serious sign with a poor prognosis. Skin rashes, nail fold infarcts, ulcerations, splinter hemorrhages, neuropathies (nerve disorders), gangrene and visceral arteritis are the clinical signs. Arteritis causes inflammation, proliferation of the inner lining of the vessel and necrosis (tissue death), all of which can lead to thrombosis (clotting).

[4]   Lung Lesions

Lung problems, such as pleurisy, pleural effusion, intrapulmonary nodules, interstitial pulmonary fibroses and pulmonary hypertension, may occur in some patients with rheumatoid arthritis. Pleural disease, when it is present, is frequently silent clinically (Hellman, 1996).

[5]   Cardiac Lesions

Pericardial disease is the most common cardiac condition in individuals with arthritis, found in approximately 40 percent of patients at autopsy. Clinically evident pericarditis in RA is uncommon (Ike and Arnold, 1996).

Rheumatoidlike nodules may be present in the myocardium (middle, muscular layer of the heart) and heart valves. Valvular insufficiency and myocardial infarction (heart attack) may occur secondary to the inflammatory lesions.

Aortitis is a rare late complication that can result in aortic regurgitation or rupture and is usually associated with evidence of rheumatoid vasculitis elsewhere in the body (Hellman, 1996).

[6] Ocular Disease

Ocular manifestations include keratoconjunctivitis sicca, an inflammation of the membrane that covers the eye and inner eyelid, caused by inadequate tear production. Dryness of the eyes, mouth and other mucous membranes is found in advanced disease.

Sjögren's syndrome (SS), characterized by diminished lacrimal and salivary gland secretion (sicca complex), is the second most common autoimmune rheumatic disorder after rheumatoid arthritis. About 50 percent of patients with SS have confirmed RA and a history of slowly developing sicca complex. The cause of Sjögren's syndrome is unknown (Norris, et al., 1996).

Episcleritis (inflammation of the subconjunctival connective tissue), scleritis (inflammation of the white of the eye) and scleromalacia perforans (degenerative thinning of the eye white) are additional ocular complications associated with rheumatoid arthritis. These conditions usually occur in patients with long-standing disease.

Eye problems in RA patients may be associated with the large doses of medications they take, such as corticosteroids, which can induce cataracts, and gold, which can cause keratopathy (noninflammatory dystrophy of the retina).

[7] Muscle Wasting

Muscle wasting in RA patients may be related to connective tissue disease in muscle, such as inflammatory or chronic myositis, a peripheral neuropathy due to nerve damage caused by the disease, or myopathy (muscle degeneration) or muscle cachexia (wasting) caused by steroids.

6.25 Diagnostic Pitfalls

In the earliest stages, rheumatoid arthritis may be difficult to diagnose, as fatigue, malaise and nonspecific musculoskeletal symptoms are often the presenting features. Although there are defined criteria for the diagnosis of RA, failure to meet these criteria does not exclude the diagnosis (Cohen, 1995).

Considerations in the differential diagnosis of RA are numerous, and the early stages of RA, especially that of acute onset, are more difficult to diagnose than the typical established case (Ike and Arnold, 1996).

A missed diagnosis delays treatment and worsens prognosis; however, hasty and erroneous diagnosis may subject the patient to risky and unnecessary treatment.

6.26 Medical Management

Treatment of established rheumatoid arthritis must be lifelong. Spontaneous disease fluctuations occur with enough frequency to confound the evaluation of therapeutic interventions. In cases showing radiographic erosions, drug therapy is considered by many to be futile, leaving only surgical and physical therapies as options. Treatment of RA occupies nearly half the time of practicing rheumatologists in the United States (McCarty, 1993).

Treatment of RA usually combines anti-inflammatory drug therapy, disease-modifying drug therapy, rest and physical therapy, orthotics and, more recently, patient education.

[1] Nonsteroidal Anti-inflammatory Drugs (NSAIDs)

NSAIDs such as ibuprofen, aspirin and naproxen help suppress inflammation through the inhibition of prostaglandin synthesis. Although these drugs are often effective, they are not truly disease-modifying and may not be sufficient if they are used alone for the treatment of rheumatoid arthritis. The potency and toxicity of NSAIDs differ considerably; they are rarely used in combination due to their potential side effects.

Cost, drug tolerance and compliance are important considerations that must be addressed for each individual. Complications and side effects associated with NSAIDs include dyspepsia and nausea, gastritis, gastric ulceration, frank gastrointestinal bleeding, edema, headache, dizziness and possible aggravation of asthma (Cohen, 1995).

[2] Disease-modifying Drugs

If nonsteroidal anti-inflammatory drugs prove inadequate in controlling the patient's symptoms, disease-modifying drugs may be administered. These drugs control inflammation by interacting with the immune system. They include antimalarials, gold, penicillamine, sulfasalazine and methotrexate.

Some controversy exists concerning the value of these medications for inhibiting disease progression; however, most rheumatologists consider disease-modifying drugs essential in the treatment of aggressive RA, particularly because they are effective in preserving joint function and contribute positively toward the overall prognosis (Cohen, 1995).

All the disease-modifying drugs are associated with potential toxicity, and careful monitoring is mandatory. The potential benefits and toxicities must be evaluated for each individual. Regular evaluation is imperative; improvement is marked by reductions in morning stiffness and palpable synovitis, and improvement in hematologic evidence of disease activity (Cohen, 1995).

Anti-inflammatory drugs should be continued during the administration of disease-modifying drugs, as they have minimal anti-inflammatory or analgesic effects.

[3]   Corticosteroids

Corticosteroids are potent anti-inflammatory drugs that often have a beneficial effect on symptoms associated with rheumatoid arthritis, although they probably do not alter the course of RA and their potential benefit must be weighed against the potential toxicity for each patient. Low-dose corticosteroids—less than 7.5 mg of prednisone or its equivalent—are helpful in treating sustained, debilitating synovitis, especially synovitis involving multiple joints (Cohen, 1995).

If at all possible, corticosteroids should be gradually tapered after six weeks of administration. Toxicity is dependent on both dosage and duration of therapy, and even low-dose corticosteroids have toxic effects. These include cutaneous (skin) changes, osteoporosis, gastrointestinal side effects and fluid retention. Moderate doses are associated with accelerated cataract formation,[2] insomnia, psychosis, glucose intolerance, centripetal obesity, avascular necrosis of bone,[3] increased risk of infection, aggravation of hypertension (high blood pressure), muscle weakness, glaucoma and hyperlipidemia (Cohen, 1995).

---

[2] *See also* ch. 11.

[3] *See also* ch. 2.

[4]   Experimental Therapies

Several experimental therapies are available to patients who are unresponsive to more conventional medications. Monoclonal antibodies directed against T-lymphocyte antigens and receptors, and immunomodulating drugs directed against mediators of inflammation (cytokines) have generated interest as being of potential benefit in RA. Gamma interferon and cyclosporine (an immunosuppressant drug used in transplants) have also been used with some success. Fish oil supplements have been used and have shown some success in providing anti-inflammatory effects. These experimental agents should be used with great care, because clear evidence of their usefulness and safety has not been established (Cohen, 1995).

6.27   Surgical Management

Surgical intervention becomes necessary when other therapeutic modalities fail to relieve the patient's symptoms and restore function. Useful surgical procedures in RA include synovectomies (excision of synovial tissue), arthrodesis (joint fusion), total joint replacements, repair of ruptured tendons and nerve release procedures.

[1]   Synovectomy

Synovectomies are performed on patients with rheumatoid arthritis to relieve pain and inflammation associated with chronic swelling that is unresponsive to medications, to retard the progression of joint destruction (this use is a matter of controversy) and to prevent and retard tendon rupture. The procedure, which is usually performed on the knee, wrist and metacarpophalangeal joint, is not curative, as regrowth of the synovium commonly occurs postoperatively. Major contraindications are very active polyarticular disease, poor general medical condition of the patient, poor motivation of the patient and advanced joint destruction (Hicks and Gerber, 1993).

[2]   Arthrodesis

Although arthrodesis (joint fusion) is performed less today than in the past due to the preference for total joint replacement, it may be the best procedure to eradicate resistant infection that has destroyed significant amounts of bone. The stability provided by this procedure should be permanent. Arthrodesis is usually limited to the wrist, interphalangeal joints of the hand, carpometacarpal joint (between the wrist and the bones of the hand), ankle and subtalar joints, and vertebral bodies.

Arthrodesis may be indicated to relieve persistent joint pain, to provide stability where there is mechanical destruction of a joint and to halt progression of RA. Joints are fused in the most functional position (Hicks and Gerber, 1993).

[3]   Joint Replacement

Joint replacement may be indicated for RA patients when pain persists despite adequate medical and rehabilitative management, when there is loss of critical motion in the involved joint or when there is loss of functional status. The most frequently replaced joints are the hip, knee and metacarpophalangeal joints; others include the wrist, shoulder, elbow, metatarsophalangeal joints and ankle, although in the latter, the procedure has not proven to be very successful. Complications include early or late infection, dislocation, fracture of adjacent bone and wearing out of component parts (Hicks and Gerber, 1993).[4]

[4]   Tendon Surgery

Tendon surgery is common in rheumatic arthritis patients when there is rupture of the extensor tendons, particularly in the fingers, and when release of contracted tendons is required.

6.28   Rehabilitation Treatment

For optimum compliance, rehabilitation therapies require individualized treatment plans that are practical, economical and valued by the patient. Patient and family education is critical.

Rehabilitation therapies may include local and systemic rest periods; passive, active and strengthening exercises; stretching exercises; aquatic therapy; application of heat and cold modalities; and the use of orthotics, such as splints and crutches, spinal orthoses and gait aids. In addition, psychiatric support for both patient and family is often needed, as RA and other rheumatic disorders have a major impact on the patient's mobility, general life-style, self-image, family life, sexuality and work (Hicks and Gerber, 1993).

---

[4] *See also* ch. 3 for discussion of hip replacement.

6.30 INFECTIOUS ARTHRITIS

Infectious (septic) arthritis is a disease of sudden onset that occurs when microorganisms invade the joint cavity, usually as a migration from an infection elsewhere in the body or through an open wound. Acute pain, swelling and heat of one joint, most often the knee, are the most common clinical findings. Other commonly affected sites are the hip, wrist, shoulder and ankle; unusual sites, such as the sterno-clavicular joint of the shoulder or sacroiliac joint of the lower back, can be involved in intravenous drug abusers (Hellman, 1996). Previous damage by trauma or another arthritic disease, or a weakened immune system response due to illness or corticosteroid use, are factors that can predispose a joint to infection.

Although virtually any microorganism can cause infectious arthritis, most infections are caused by a few common agents. In adults, gonococci and staphylococci are the major causes of joint infection. Infection by *Borrelia burgdorferi,* the causative agent of Lyme disease, presents a common diagnostic challenge in endemic areas (Schmid, 1993).

6.31 Pathology

A rapid series of events take place as microorganisms penetrate the joint cavity: the synovial microvasculature dilates, the subsynovial tissue becomes swollen, and the volume of synovial fluid increases dramatically, raising the pressure within the joint capsule. Marked elevation of pressure can induce tamponade (plugging) of subsynovial vessels, which may cause intravascular thrombosis (formation of clots) and ischemia (inadequate supply of blood to a body part), leading to microabscess formation and, in adjacent bone, ischemia and foci of avascular necrosis (Schmid, 1993).

Infectious arthritis occurs in a closed space; the pus-containing by-products of the inflammatory process do not drain. The structures lying within the confines of the synovial-lined capsule or sheath are at the greatest risk, although surrounding soft tissues outside this space are sometimes involved in rare instances of rupture or sinus (cavity) formation. Damage to the synovium of a bursa is reversible, but tendons within the synovial sheath can rupture. At greater risk is the articular cartilage, and destroyed hyaline cartilage cannot be totally or effectively replaced. These anatomic considerations influence the need for drainage, which is especially critical for joints and tendons (Schmid, 1993).

6.32 Clinical Course

Infectious arthritis may present in a variety of ways, both typical and atypical. Approximately 80 to 90 percent of cases are monoarticular (involving one joint), and the knee joint is the one most frequently affected joint (Espinoza, 1996).

Acute septic arthritis begins abruptly. The infected joint feels warm and painful and is distended with fluid. Most patients also experience fever, chills and general malaise. Atypical presentation can occur in patients with a joint damaged by prior disease. Superimposed infection may not be obvious in joints that are chronically painful and swollen.

6.33 Diagnosis

Aspiration (removal of fluid through a needle) and examination of infected joint fluid is a mandatory diagnostic test that should be performed as soon as possible. In the presence of polyarticular involvement, all infected joints should be tapped. Aspiration should be followed by bacteriologic studies, such as stain and culture of synovial fluid, leukocyte count with differential and examination of a wet preparation for crystals. A very high white blood cell count—usually over 100,000 per cubic millimeter—low glucose levels and high protein content are characteristic of bacterial arthritis (Espinoza, 1996).

Other diagnostic measures may include x-rays, which can show typical changes in the joint, and radioisotope joint scans, which may help detect inflammation in less accessible joints (Norris, et al., 1995). *(See Figure 6-4.)*

6.34 Treatment

Antibiotic therapy is promptly started. Penicillin G is effective against most causative agents, including *Neisseria gonorrhoeae.* Nafcillin or ampicillin is recommended for penicillin-G-resistant strains.

Treatment requires constant monitoring through frequent analysis of joint fluid cultures, synovial fluid leukocyte counts and glucose level determinations. A splint helps reduce pain and controls inflammation by immobilization. An attempt to restore range of motion and

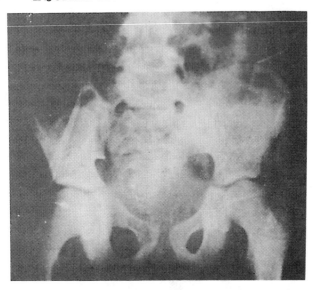

(a)

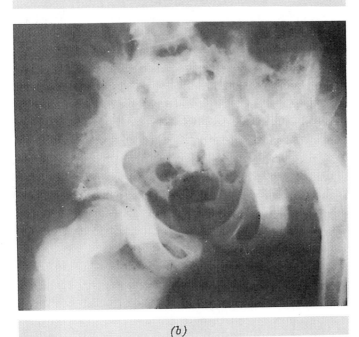

(b)

Fig. 6-4. X-rays taken 11 months apart demonstrate arthritic changes of the left hip. In (a), joint structures are fairly well delineated. Later (b), marked destruction, loss of joint space and ankylosis are evident.

increase muscle strength should be made through passive exercises once the inflammatory process subsides; however, weight-bearing should be deferred until signs of acute inflammation have disappeared. Anti-inflammatory drugs, including aspirin, should be withheld so that joint response to the antibiotics can be correctly assessed. Codeine, propoxyphene or stronger narcotics have no anti-inflammatory properties and may be administered to control pain (Schmid, 1993).

If treatment is prompt and joint function has been normal prior to infection, the prognosis for complete recovery is excellent. Delayed diagnosis is directly related to a poorer outcome. Delaying treatment of any septic joint for more than one or two weeks can lead to permanent damage to cartilage and bone, increased fibrosis and, ultimately, destruction of the normal joint mechanism.

6.40 TRAUMATIC ARTHRITIS

Traumatic arthritis is a descriptive term that used to be given to any joint lesion resulting from acute direct trauma or repeated microtrauma (small, repeated stresses). However, today traumatic arthritis is recognized as a form of osteoarthritis that occurs secondary to joint irregularities caused by traumatic injury. Alterations of joint contour, malalignment of articular surfaces, internal derangement of the joint and injuries to supporting muscles and ligaments can lead to abnormal distribution of pressures and stress on the affected joint and therefore to premature degeneration of joint cartilage.

Blunt, penetrating or repeated trauma, or forced inappropriate motion of a joint or ligament can result in direct traumatic injuries and complications that predispose the individual to the development of traumatic arthritis. Traumatic arthritis caused by repeated microtrauma sometimes occurs in individuals involved in occupations that require repetitive exercise of a specific joint. Examples include tennis or baseball elbow, ballet dancer's toe, housemaid's knee and carpenter's knee.

6.41 Pathogenesis

Traumatically induced changes in the articular (joint) cartilage are often caused by repeated motion and continued use following direct traumatic injury. A second mechanism is the development of fibroplasia, a proliferation of granulation tissue in the synovial membrane or periarticular tissues.

6.42   Clinical Signs and Symptoms

Clinical effects may include swelling, pain, tenderness, joint instability and internal bleeding. Pain and prognosis vary with the individual, but generally patients with strong musculature retain good joint function, although joint activity should be limited. Treatment is the same as for general osteoarthritis.

6.50   OSTEOARTHRITIS

Osteoarthritis is often referred to as degenerative joint disease and sometimes as osteoarthrosis. This "wear and tear" disorder is the leading cause of chronic disability in the United States (Brandt, 1994). Signs of the osteoarthritic process most often appear in individuals in their fifties or older. Because people are usually elderly when symptoms appear, and most elderly individuals have evidence of the osteoarthritic process, it might seem that osteoarthritis is due to aging. However, although the chemical composition of joint cartilage changes somewhat with normal aging, these changes are different from those that occur with osteoarthritis (Brandt, 1994).

6.51   Primary Osteoarthritis

Primary osteoarthritis is a disease for which no predisposing factor such as genetics, infection or trauma can be identified. The idiopathic (with no known cause) variant commonly involves the joints of the hand. Erosive osteoarthritis is another type of primary osteoarthritis that affects the hands, particularly in postmenopausal women (Brandt, 1994).

Involvement of three or more joints by osteoarthritis is called *generalized disease,* and it occurs most often in postmenopausal women (Brandt, 1994). The hands are usually affected first, but the hips, knees, big toe and spine are also often affected. Patients often have episodes of pain and swelling in the involved joints, followed by periods of relief.

6.52   Secondary Arthritis

If a contributing factor can be identified, the osteoarthritis is termed secondary. One or more of several processes may be the cause:

- mechanical problems in the joint, such as congenital malformations or problems due to abnormal development;

- rheumatoid arthritis or another inflammatory disease;
- infection;
- metabolic disorders, such as gout;
- endocrine problems, such as diabetes mellitus; and
- other conditions such as osteonecrosis or hemarthrosis (blood in the joint), for example, in a person with hemophilia.

In cases of secondary osteoarthritis, the cause of the initial damage to the joint cartilage is known. The original insult may be mechanical (as with congenital deformity or trauma), due to release of matrix-damaging proteins because of an immune system problem (as in rheumatoid arthritis) or chemical (as in gout and other crystal deposition diseases). The degenerative process then continues, as described in the next section.

6.53 Pathology of Osteoarthritis

In joints such as the hip, the synovium (joint lining) produces proteins that nourish cartilage—the tough but elastic tissue that covers the articulating ends of the bones of the joint and cushions them. In the joints of older persons without osteoarthritis, synovial cells continue to produce proteins at the same level to keep cartilage in the joint smooth and functioning well. In the normal joint, the flow of nutrients to the cartilage and the deposit of waste from cartilage into the synovial fluid are assisted by slight differences in the articulating surfaces, so that pressure changes with "loading" (weight-bearing) and unloading of the joint compress and release cartilage, something like squeezing and releasing a sponge.

However, concentration of forces in small areas of cartilage, as may happen with a congenital (present from birth) deformity, leads to too much pressure being brought on an area and is thought to be a key factor in cartilage pitting, erosion, eburnation (abnormal conversion of bone into a denser tissue that resembles ivory) and the other processes of osteoarthritis.

Changes have also been identified in the chemistry of a joint with osteoarthritis. In persons with the disease, the normal processes of cartilage metabolism are interrupted, and the cartilage matrix (framework) breaks down.

Two processes have been proposed as causes for osteoarthritis: (1) because there is an underlying defect in the way the cartilage and bone matrix are formed and repaired, they break down with normal use of the joint; or (2) the shape of a particular individual's joint or altered use of the joint puts abnormal pressure on the cartilage at the initial point of erosion, instead of spreading pressure evenly over the joint surface (Brandt, 1994).

6.54   Differential Diagnosis of Osteoarthritis

The clinical feature of osteoarthritis that most clearly distinguishes it from other causes of joint dysfunction is that it is much more prevalent in the elderly than in younger persons. Thus only a fifth of individuals under 45 have radiographic evidence of osteoarthritis, but the incidence rises to a third for those between 45 and 64 and to two thirds (68 percent) for men and women 65 and older (Brandt, 1994). It is often difficult to determine whether a joint problem is osteoarthritis or another disorder, especially in the early stages of disease. Therefore, detailed questioning and a thorough physical examination—and often laboratory testing and imaging studies—are needed to arrive at the correct diagnosis.

[1]   Clinical Signs and Symptoms

Typical complaints of individuals with osteoarthritis are pain and altered function of one or more nonsymmetric joints, most often those of the hips, hands (interphalangeal), knees, spine and big toe. If other joints are affected or symmetric joints are involved, the patient probably has secondary (due to another factor) rather than primary osteoarthritis.

Although the process of osteoarthritis has been identified radiographically in similar proportions of men and women in each age group, the clinician will find differences by sex and other factors among the patients who complain of symptoms of osteoarthritis. Women are more likely to have symptoms of this joint disease. Also, men older than 55 are more likely to have osteoarthritis of the hip, whereas older women more often have pain in the finger joints and base of the thumb (Brandt, 1994).

The pain described by patients with osteoarthritis is a deep ache that is usually worse after use of the joint and relieved by rest. The patient can usually identify the joint that is causing problems, although patients with osteoarthritis of the hip often complain of pain in the groin and thigh, or sometimes in the knee or buttock (Johanson, 1992).

Such "referral" of pain from one area to another is common when the source of pain is deep in the body, as in the hip joint.

In advanced osteoarthritis, pain may be present even at rest, and patients with severe osteoarthritis of the hip often suffer pain at night. Such night pain reflects increased pressure in the bone and indicates a serious problem, such as avascular necrosis (death of tissue due to inadequate blood supply). Osteoarthritis does not cause weight loss, anemia, fatigue or other systemic problems, which are characteristic of rheumatoid (inflammatory) joint diseases.

The stiffness of osteoarthritis has been described as a gelatinous sensation in the joint. In contrast to patients with rheumatoid arthritis, those with osteoarthritis usually experience joint stiffness for less than 30 minutes after arising or a period of immobility.

Physical examination of a joint that is involved by osteoarthritis usually shows swelling, although this is not evident with the hip because it is deep in the body. Crepitus (a crackling sound that is produced when the joint is moved) and limitation in the joint's range of motion are also typical. In advanced disease, the overgrowth of bone and other changes in the joint have caused obvious deformity, often with subluxation (movement of the bones out of alignment); in the hip joint, this deformity may be evidenced by an abnormal gait.

[2] Laboratory Findings

Osteoarthritis does not cause changes in blood values as seen in laboratory tests; specifically, the indicators of immune system function (e.g., erythrocyte sedimentation rate) are normal for the patient's age.

Synovial fluid from a joint affected by osteoarthritis has normal viscosity and yields normal results in the mucin (clotting) test. The concentration of cells in synovial fluid may be increased, but only slightly (fewer than 2,000 cells per cubic millimeter) (Brandt, 1994). In addition, some fragments of cartilage, bone or crystals containing calcium may be seen in the synovial fluid.

[3] Radiology Findings

Typically, radiographs of a joint with osteoarthritis show narrowing of the joint space (the space between the articulating bones), sclerosis (hardening and thus more dense appearance) of the subchondral bone, osteophytes (bone spurs), bone cysts and lack of pronounced osteoporosis (softened bone).

However, radiographic changes or lack of changes do not always correlate well with severity of disease: Patients may have joint pain, and complete erosion of the articular cartilage may be seen on arthroscopy, without any evidence of abnormality in radiographs of the joint. Alternatively, many elderly persons with no symptoms of joint problems have osteophytes, as seen on radiographs of the joint.

6.55   Medical Treatments

Treatment for osteoarthritis is focused on relieving the patient's pain, halting progression of the disease process and maximizing joint function so that disability is decreased.

[1]   Physical Therapies

Pain and changes in joint function may be caused or aggravated by abnormal forces applied to the joint. Since excess weight is a contributing factor to breakdown of cartilage in the hip and joints of the legs, obese patients are encouraged to lose weight in order to decrease strain on these weight-bearing joints. Patients can also decrease strain on foot joints by wearing properly fitted shoes with low heels; supportive running shoes with well-padded soles are ideal.

Patients with osteoarthritis should avoid activities that put strain on affected joints or require repeated use of the joints. If osteoarthritis affects the weight-bearing joints, for example, patients should avoid kneeling or squatting, long periods of standing and impact activities such as jogging. Modifications may be needed in the patient's workplace (for example, to permit sitting instead of standing for long periods) and in the patient's leisure activities (for example, switching from jogging or tennis to swimming or bike riding).

The way a patient uses a joint (body mechanics) can contribute to osteoarthritis. If excess weight or a physical abnormality of the knee or foot joint leads to abnormal movement of the joint, orthotic (corrective) devices may be prescribed. To correct a splay-footed walk, for example, individually fitted wedged insoles for shoes may be prescribed. For osteoarthritis in the hip or knee, patients may use a cane or walking stick in the opposite hand if disease affects one hip or knee only; the cane or stick should reach to the greater trochanter (projection of the femur) when the patient stands erect in normal footwear (Currey, 1988). If disease affects both sides, crutches or a walker may be used for support and to decrease stress on the joints.

Range of motion and strength of a joint affected by osteoarthritis may be improved by exercises. Exercises should be isometric (free movement of muscles) rather than isotonic (such as weight-lifting). Applications of heat to a joint that is affected by osteoarthritis often help relieve pain and improve range of motion. When joints hurt after use, or if heat does not relieve the pain, applications of cold (ice or a similar type of cold pack wrapped in a towel to protect the skin) may be effective.

[2] Pharmacologic Treatments

Current drug therapy for osteoarthritis targets relief of pain; no drugs are known that will halt or reverse the process of cartilage erosion. Nonsteroidal anti-inflammatory drugs (NSAIDs) such as aspirin are the primary treatment for patients with osteoarthritis, even though their joint disease is not basically inflammatory, as it is with rheumatoid arthritis. Analgesic (pain-relieving) dosages of NSAIDs may be as effective as higher dosages, even when some joint swelling is present (Brandt, 1994).

Gastric (stomach) upset is common with regular use of aspirin, even at analgesic dosages, and some patients are sensitive to salicylates (the active ingredient in aspirin). Acetaminophen may be used for pain relief, or another NSAID may be prescribed, although other NSAIDs are typically more expensive than aspirin or acetaminophen.

Corticosteroid drugs are not given systemically (by mouth or intravenously) to treat osteoarthritis, but injections of a glucocorticoid drug into the affected joint may relieve pain and increase function. As when this treatment is used for joints that are affected by rheumatoid arthritis, injections should not be given more often than every four to six months.

6.56 Surgical Treatments

Surgery may be indicated when physical and pharmacologic treatments are ineffective for relieving pain, especially pain at night (usually from the hip). Surgery may halt the progressive and irreversible loss of joint function that would otherwise occur and improves the patient's ability to perform activities of daily living. In planning surgery, physicians take into account the age of the patient and his or her overall activity level as well as the severity of disease.

Total joint replacement (arthroplasty) is the procedure that is most often performed on the hip area. In this procedure, a plastic cup is placed in the socket of the joint, and a metal or metal-and-plastic ball replaces the head and upper end of the femur. Total hip replacement surgery usually provides freedom from pain and good function for many years, and research is resulting in the development of methods that prolong the effectiveness of hip prostheses. Nevertheless, repeat total hip replacement procedures are problematic enough that young patients may undergo arthrodesis (joint fusion) first, with total hip replacement reserved for later.

Arthrodesis is a common procedure that can relieve osteoarthritic pain because it prevents motion. This very effect, however, limits the use of the procedure to situations in which immobility of the joint is the best solution. When it is performed on the hip, it alters the way the patient walks. This leads to abnormal stresses on other joints, with possible alterations in their function. Osteotomy (surgical remodeling of bone), although it was popular in the past, is rarely done now.

6.57 Complications and Prognosis

Possible complications of treatments for osteoarthritis include gastrointestinal irritation from medications to relieve pain, and complications of surgery, including infection, thrombophlebitis (damage of the innermost layer of tissue of a vein resulting from a clot lodged in it), hematoma (accumulation of blood under the skin), abnormal formation of bone, leakage of cement used to anchor the prosthesis, loosening of the prosthesis and subluxation (partial dislocation) or dislocation of the prosthesis.

The severity of pain and disability reported by patients does not correlate very closely with the severity of joint changes demonstrated by radiographic studies. Associations have been found, however, between psychosocial factors and degree of pain. Thus, for the same degree of change on radiographs of the joint, some studies have shown women more likely to complain of pain than men, divorced individuals more so than married persons and those receiving welfare more likely than those who are employed (Brandt, 1994).

Because osteoarthritis is a chronic (lifelong) disease, the patient's attitude and approach to managing the changes brought about by it play a large role in the prognosis. Just as patients differ in their perception of pain, they differ in their ability and willingness to take responsibility for self-care activities such as losing weight, exercising and altering their activities to protect affected joints. The clinician may need also to evaluate and treat possible depression or anxiety occurring in patients with osteoarthritis, particularly those with severe disease (Doherty and Doherty, 1992).

6.60   VASCULITIS SYNDROMES

Vasculitis is a process characterized by inflammation and necrosis (cell death) of blood vessel walls. Many different types of blood vessel disorders have been described in patients with rheumatic disease. The vasculitic syndromes, like other rheumatic disorders, are difficult to classify because they are of idiopathic (unknown) origin.

Vasculitis may occur as the primary process or as a component of another underlying disease. In general, the vasculitic syndromes are thought to result from immunopathogenic mechanisms; however, evidence for this varies among the different syndromes (Rosenwasser, 1996).

6.61   Clinical Presentation

Fever, malaise and weight loss are involved in the typical insidious presentation. Skin rashes, petechia (small red spots on skin), skin ulcerations, peripheral neuropathies and asymmetric arthritis in multiple joints are also common. As the condition involves major organs, new symptoms, such as hypertension (high blood pressure) with renal (kidney) involvement, abdominal pain with gastrointestinal involvement, nausea and vomiting are common. Cardiac involvement occurs late and is manifested by pericarditis, myocarditis and arrhythmias; myocardial infarction secondary to coronary vasculitis may also be observed (Hellman, 1996).

6.62   Diagnosis

Because of the diverse symptoms and the fact that any blood vessel may be involved, diagnosis of vasculitis is difficult. Clinical findings depend on the vessels involved. Laboratory tests indicate a systemic disorder but are nonspecific. Biopsy or angiogram (x-ray of blood vessels) is most helpful in establishing the diagnosis.

6.63   Treatment

Corticosteroids in high doses and immunosuppressive agents are most effective. Patients may experience relapses when the drugs are withdrawn, as well as the side effects commonly associated with long-term corticosteroid use.

6.64 Specific Vasculitis Syndromes

There are several vasculitic syndromes, with diverse clinical and pathologic manifestations. Recent re-examination of clinical, pathologic and immunologic features, as well as patient response to various therapeutic regimens, has resulted in more precise and accurate classification schemes.

The clinical spectrum of vasculitis includes four major groupings: the polyarteritis nodosa group; hypersensitivity vasculitis; granulomatous vasculitides; and other vasculitic syndromes (Rosenwasser, 1996).

[1] Polyarteritis Nodosa

Polyarteritis nodosa is often classified as one of the systemic necrotizing vasculitides. It affects medium to small arteries, especially at bifurcations and branchings. Clinical manifestations are widespread. Early symptoms include fever, weight loss and pain in viscera and/or the musculoskeletal system. The disease involves multiple organs, and clinical manifestations may include renal, gastrointestinal, nervous system, articular and muscular, cardiac, genitourinary, cutaneous and pulmonary signs and symptoms (Rosenwasser, 1996).

The untreated course of polyarteritis nodosa is progressive destruction of vital organs. Without treatment, the five-year survival rate is about 20 percent. Treatment with corticosteroids alone improves the five-year survival rate to about 50 percent. A combined treatment of corticosteroids and immunosuppresive drugs increases the five-year survival rate to 80 to 90 percent (Hellman, 1996).

[2] Hypersensitivity Vasculitis

The hypersensitivity vasculitis group includes disorders thought to represent a hypersensitivity reaction to an antigenic stimulus, such as an infectious agent, a toxin, a foreign or endogenous protein, or a drug.

[3] Granulomatous Vasculitides

Granulomatous vasculitides include Wegener's granulomatosis, a multisystem inflammatory autoimmune disorder involving predominantly the upper and lower respiratory tracts and kidneys. Presentations vary considerably, from mild arthralgias (joint pains), to polymyalgic rheumatic-type symptoms, to rapidly progressive renal and respiratory failure.

The disorder, which was once fatal, is now treated with a combination of cyclophosphamide and prednisone, leading to remission in 75 percent of all patients and improvement in about 90 percent. However, relapses occur in at least 50 percent of those achieving remission, at any time from several months to 15 to 20 years after stopping cytotoxic therapy (Allen, 1996).

Giant cell arteritis and polymyalgia rheumatica are common rheumatic diseases, and although their etiology is unknown and the pathogenesis poorly understood, it is clear that they are closely related. The disorders are characterized by aching and morning stiffness in the shoulder and hip, the proximal (closer to the trunk of the body) extremities, and the neck and torso. Patients will often have fatigue, headaches and proximal muscle weakness. There is usually evidence of inflammation, with an elevated erythrocyte sedimentation rate (ESR) and there may also be a mild anemia. These two illnesses commonly strike individuals after the age of 50, with women affected twice as commonly as men.

No specific therapy exists for these diseases; steroids scan be extremely beneficial but should be tapered as quickly as possible. Saturated potassium iodide, hydroxychloroquine and cimetidine, and high-dose prednisone have been advocated as treatments (Hunder, 1996).

[4]   Other Vasculitic Syndromes

Among the miscellaneous group of vasculitis syndromes are the cutaneous or dermal vasculitides, which affect the small cutaneous vessels. These include erythema nodosum, erythema multiforme and erythema elevatum diutinum.

6.70   OVERLAP CONNECTIVE TISSUE DISEASE

Not infrequently, some patients experience an overlap of various rheumatic syndromes. The focus of attention has been on patients who have overlapping features of systemic lupus erythematosus (SLE), scleroderma and polymyositis. In the recent past, these patients were thought to have a distinct entity, known as mixed connective tissue disease and defined by a specific autoantibody to ribonuclear protein

(RNP). However, with time, in many patients, these manifestations evolve to one predominant disease, such as scleroderma, and many patients with antibodies to RNP have clear-cut SLE. Therefore, "overlap connective tissue disease" is the preferred designation for patients exhibiting features of several rheumatic diseases (Hellman, 1996).

6.71   Clinical Presentation

Nearly all patients with overlap connective tissue disease have multiple joint pain; most have outright arthritis, which may or may not be deforming and erosive. Esophageal abnormalities are common, as are muscle weakness and tenderness. Some patients develop proliferative vascular lesions and involvement of the lungs, heart and nervous system.

6.72   Diagnosis

Studies have shown that this disorder is not an individual clinical entity. Therefore, diagnosis of overlap connective tissue disease involves a general evolution out of the overlap pattern to one of single disease (Nakamura, 1996).

6.73   Treatment and Prognosis

Treatment includes nonsteroidal anti-inflammatory agents for mild disease and corticosteroids and cytotoxic drugs for more serious manifestations. Prognosis is dependent on the complications associated with the evolution of the disease.

6.80   RHEUMATIC FEVER AND RHEUMATIC HEART DISEASE

Rheumatic fever is an inflammatory disease that occurs as a delayed, nonsuppurative sequel to upper respiratory infection with group A streptococci. Although it is classified as a rheumatic disease because of the joint involvement, the importance of this disorder lies in its cardiac involvement, which can lead to rheumatic heart disease, a chronic condition caused by scarring and deformity of heart valves, or death from acute carditis. Although the incidence is highest in children aged 5 to 15 (Massie, 1996), rheumatic fever can occur at any age.

The development of acute rheumatic fever (ARF) requires antecedent infection with group A streptococcus in the upper respiratory tract.

The mechanism by which group A streptococci elicit the connective tissue inflammatory response that constitutes ARF remains unknown (Bisno, 1996). Although streptococcus A has been implicated in the etiology of rheumatic fever, only 0.3 percent of patients with streptococcal infections ever contract rheumatic fever, indicating that other factors such as altered host response must be involved in its development or recurrence (Norris, et al., 1995). It has been suggested that a bacterial allergy or autoimmunity may play a role.

The major significance of rheumatic fever is that in the elderly, it can present as rheumatic heart disease. This diagnosis refers to the long-term sequelae of childhood rheumatic fever. Patients can develop severe valvular heart disease, characterized especially by mitral stenosis and/or mitral regurgitation. These valvular abnormalities can predispose to infection—bacterial endocarditis, cardiac arrhythmias and congestive heart failure.

6.90   GOUT

Gout is a term used to refer to inflammatory arthritis caused by microscopic crystals of monosodium urate monohydrate (MSU) aggregated in various tissues and some organs. The exact cause of *primary* gout is unknown; however, it appears to be associated with a genetic defect in purine (certain chemical compounds, for example, caffeine) metabolism, which results in overproduction of uric acid (hyperuricemia), retention of uric acid or both. *Secondary* gout develops during the course of another disease, most commonly obesity, diabetes mellitus,[5] hypertension, sickle cell anemia or renal disease, and is caused by the breakdown of nucleic acid. Secondary gout may also follow drug therapy (Norris, et al., 1995), such as immunotherapy for leukemia or diuretic therapy for congestive heart failure.

About 90 percent of patients are men over the age of 30; in women, the onset is usually postmenopausal (Hellman, 1996).

6.91   Pathogenesis

The classic indication of gout is an elevated level of uric acid in the body fluids. The precise relationship of hyperuricemia to acute gouty arthritis is not clearly understood, since chronic hyperuricemia is found in people who never develop gout or uric acid stones. Rapid

---

[5] *See also* ch. 9.

fluctuations in serum urate levels are important factors in precipitating acute gout (Hellman, 1996).

6.92   Clinical Picture

Gout is characterized by acute recurrent attacks of arthritis, usually monoarticular, and later by chronic deforming arthritis. A nodular deposit of monosodium urate monohydrate crystals (tophus) in the cartilage, subcutaneous and periarticular tissues, tendon, bone, kidneys or elsewhere is characteristic (Hellman, 1996).

6.93   Gouty Arthritis

Gouty arthritis usually presents with an acute arthritic attack of the lower extremity, which occurs explosively during apparent good health, and usually takes place at night. More than 75 percent of first attacks involve the great toe. The affected joint becomes hot and extremely sensitive and painful, but once the attack subsides, recovery is generally rapid and complete. Attacks often follow physical activity, such as long walks or exercise, or occur after surgery, trauma, alcohol or dietary overindulgence, starvation, infection or the start of hypouricemic drug therapy (Hershfield, 1996).

Although the great toe is most susceptible, the joints of the feet, ankles and knees are also commonly affected. Asymptomatic periods follow the initial attack; later, gouty arthritis can become chronic, with symptoms of progressive functional loss and disability (Hellman, 1996).

6.94   Tophaceous Gout

The progressive inability to dispose of urate may lead to the insidious development of tophaceous crystals in and around joints. These tophi are commonly found in articular and other cartilage, synovia, tendon sheaths, bursae and other periarticular structures, epiphyseal bone, subcutaneous tissues and the kidney interstitium (structural cells). Unlike the acute gouty attack, tophi develop silently and generally evoke little inflammatory response.

Tophi may be detected radiographically in gouty individuals who lack tophi in subcutaneous tissues and who rarely experience acute arthritic attacks. The gradual enlargement of tophi in the joint space results in degeneration of cartilage and subchondral bone, proliferation of synovium and marginal bone, and sometimes fibrous or bony ankylosis (Hershfield, 1996). *(See Figure 6-5.)*

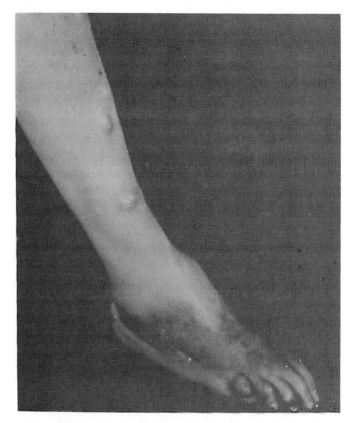

Fig. 6-5. Tophaceous gout in the leg. Nodular tophi appear on the extensor surface of the leg as well as the ankle and foot.

6.95   Renal Disease and Stones

Uric acid kidney stones are found in approximately 5 to 10 percent of patients with gouty arthritis. Uric acid stones are not related to the pathogenesis of gout, and a relationship to renal insufficiency or to the severity of gout has not been established (Hellman, 1996).

Progressive renal failure due to urate nephropathy (kidney disorder) may occur in patients with conditions that cause extreme urate overproduction, such as cancer chemotherapy and certain metabolic disorders. Acute oliguric renal failure can result from bilateral tubular obstruction by uric acid crystals. Control of uric acid levels by maintenance of high alkalinized urine volume, and pretreatment with drug therapy, can help prevent this condition in high-risk patients (Hershfield, 1996).

6.96 Diagnosis and Treatment

The sudden onset of severe inflammatory arthritis, especially in the lower extremity, and the presence of monosodium urate (MSU) crystals in synovial fluid and determination of urinary excretion of urate are confirming diagnostic tests. *(See Figure 6-6.)*

Acute gout must be differentiated from pseudogout, a condition manifested by acute attacks of arthritis in knees and joints and accompanied by calcification of joint cartilage. In pseudogout, nonurate crystals of calcium pyrophosphate are present in the synovial fluid. When gout and pseudogout co-exist, both types of crystals are found in the synovial leukocytes (Hershfield, 1996).

Other disorders that must be differentiated from gout include acute rheumatic fever,[6] rheumatoid arthritis,[7] traumatic arthritis,[8] osteoarthritis,[9] pyogenic arthritis, sarcoid arthritis, cellulitis, bursitis,

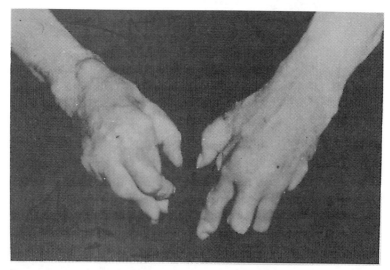

Fig. 6-6. Gouty arthritis in the hands, characterized by nodular enlargement and deformity of the joints.

---

[6] *See 6.80 supra.*

[7] *See 6.20 supra.*

[8] *See 6.40 supra.*

[9] *See 6.27[2] supra.*

tendinitis and thrombophlebitis. Gout can co-exist with any of these conditions (Hershfield, 1996).

Treatment of gout involves treating the acute arthritis first and then the underlying metabolic problem. Nonsteroidal anti-inflammatory drugs (NSAIDs) are the treatment of choice for acute gout; corticosteroids are also effective and usually used to treat patients who are unable to take NSAIDs. Bed rest is important in the management of acute attacks and should continue for about 24 hours after the attack has subsided. Premature activity may result in recurrence. The underlying metabolic problem can be treated with drugs that decrease the production of uric acid (allopurinol) or increase the renal excretion of uric acid (probenecid).

6.100 NEUROGENIC (CHARCOT'S) ARTHROPATHY

Charcot's arthropathy is a chronic progressive degenerative joint disorder resulting from loss or impairment of proprioception (sense of position) and perception of pain and temperature. It has been traditionally associated with tabes dorsalis (syphilitic neuropathy) but is now more frequently seen in diabetic neuropathy, syringomyelia, spinal cord injury, pernicious anemia, leprosy and peripheral nerve injury.

Neurogenic arthropathy usually begins insidiously with swelling, warmth, increased mobility and instability in a single joint or in multiple joints. The specific joint or joints affected can vary: Diabetes usually affects the joints and bones of the feet; tabes dorsalis attacks the large weight-bearing joints, such as the knee, hip, and lumbar and dorsal spine (Charcot spine); syringomyelia attacks the shoulder, elbow and cervical vertebral joint; and neurogenic arthropathy related to intra-articular injection of corticosteroids usually develops in the hip or knee (Norris, et al., 1995).

A patient history of painless joint deformity and underlying primary disease is suggestive of neurogenic arthropathy. X-rays confirm the diagnosis and assess joint damage. Synovial biopsy can reveal bony fragments and bits of calcified cartilage.

Treatment includes immobilization of affected joints, utilization of crutches, splints and braces, and restriction of weight-bearing. Arthrodesis (surgical fusion of the joint) may be necessary to treat severe disease. Amputation may be indicated in severe cases of diabetic neuropathy. However, surgery increases the risk of further damage through nonunion and infection (Norris, et al., 1995).

6.110 AMA EVALUATION OF PERMANENT IMPAIRMENT

The evaluation of impairment resulting from arthritis and rheumatic diseases can be complex and often requires a combination of impairment percentages gleaned from various criteria listed and explained in the American Medical Association's *Guides to the Evaluation of Permanent Impairment* (1993). The impairments are evaluated separately and then combined with other impairment percentages, using the Combined Values Chart. The evaluator must take care to avoid duplication of impairments when other findings, such as synovial hypertrophy, carpal collapse with arthritic changes or limited motion, are present.

Range of motion techniques are of limited value for estimating impairment secondary to arthritis. Most patients are impaired more by pain and weakness secondary to advanced joint surface degeneration but can still maintain functional ranges of motion, while for others, loss of motion is the principle impairment. In the presence of decreased motion, motion impairment percentages are derived separately and combined with arthroplasty or other appropriate impairments.

For most arthritis patients, roentgenographic grading is a more objective and valid method for establishing impairment estimates than physical findings, such as range of motion or joint crepitation (crackling sounds heard upon movement). The best roentgenographic indicator of functional impairment for a patient with arthritis is the cartilage interval or joint space. The hallmark of all types of arthritis is thinning of the articular cartilage, and this correlates well with disease progression.

Impairments related to arthritis are based on standard roentgenograms taken with the patient standing, if possible, and 36 inches from the machine, with the beam at the level of and parallel to the joint surface. The estimate for the patellofemoral joint (between the kneecap and thighbone) is based on a "sunrise view" taken at 40 degrees flexion or on a true lateral view.

Some impairment estimates are assigned more appropriately on the basis of a diagnosis than on the basis of findings of the physical examination. The evaluating physician must determine whether diagnostic or examination criteria best describe the impairment of a specific patient.

6.200 BIBLIOGRAPHY

Text References

Allen, N. B.: Wegener's Granulomatosis. In: Bennett, J. and Plum, F. (Eds.): Textbook of Medicine. Philadelphia: Saunders, 1996.

American Medical Association: Guides to the Evaluation of Permanent Impairment, 4th ed. Chicago: American Medical Association, 1993.

Arnett, F. C.: Rheumatoid Arthritis. In: Bennett, J. and Plum, F. (Eds.): Textbook of Medicine. Philadelphia: Saunders, 1996.

Bisno, A. L.: Rheumatic Fever. In: Bennett, J. and Plum, F. (Eds.): Textbook of Medicine. Philadelphia: Saunders, 1996.

Brandt, K. K.: Osteoarthritis. In: Stein, J. H. (Ed.): Internal Medicine, 4th ed. St. Louis: Mosby, 1994.

Cohen, M.: Rheumatoid Arthritis. In: Rakel, R. (Ed.): Conn's Current Therapy. Philadelphia: Saunders, 1995.

Currey, H. L. F.: Essentials of Rheumatology, 2nd ed. London: Churchill Livingstone, 1988.

Cush, J. and Lipsky, P.: The Spondylarthropathies. In: Bennett, J. and Plum, F. (Eds.): Textbook of Medicine. Philadelphia: Saunders, 1996.

Doherty, M. and Doherty, J.: Clinical Examination in Rheumatology. Aylesbury, England: Wolfe Publishing, 1992.

Espinoza, L.: Infectious Arthritis. In: Bennett, J. and Plum, F. (Eds.): Textbook of Medicine. Philadelphia: Saunders, 1996.

Evans, C. and Robbins, P.: Progress Toward the Treatment of Arthritis by Gene Therapy. Ann. Med. 27:543-546, Oct. 1995.

Gordon, D. A.: Approach to the Patient with Musculoskeletal Disease. In: Bennett, J. and Plum, F. (Eds.): Textbook of Medicine. Philadelphia: Saunders, 1996.

Hanania, E., et al.: Recent Advances in the Application of Gene Therapy to Human Disease. Am. J. Med. 99:537-552, Nov. 1995.

Hellman, D.: Arthritis and Musculoskeletal Disorders. In: Tierney, L., et al.: Current Medical Diagnosis and Treatment. Stamford, Conn.: Appleton and Lang, 1996.

Hershfield, M.: Gout and Uric Acid Metabolism. In: Bennett, J. and Plum, F. (Eds.): Textbook of Medicine. Philadelphia: Saunders, 1996.

Hicks, J. and Gerber, L.: Rehabilitation of the Patient with Arthritis and Connective Tissue Disease. In: DeLisa, J. (Ed.): Rehabilitation Medicine: Principles and Practice. Philadelphia: Lippincott, 1993.

Hunder, G.: Polymyalgia Rheumatica and Giant Cell Arthritis. In: Bennett, J. and Plum, F. (Eds.): Textbook of Medicine. Philadelphia: Saunders, 1996.

Ike, R. and Arnold, J.: Specialized Procedures in the Management of Patients with Rheumatic Diseases. In: Bennett, J. and Plum, F. (Eds.): Textbook of Medicine. Philadelphia: Saunders, 1996.

Johanson, N. A.: Nonoperative Orthopedics. In: Paget, S. A. and Fields, R. R. (Eds.:): Rheumatic Disorders. Boston: Andover Medical, 1992.

Litman, K.: A Rational Approach to the Diagnosis of Arthritis. Am. Fam. Phys.:53:1295-1310, Mar. 1996.

Massie, B.: Heart/Acute Rheumatic Fever and Rheumatic Heart Disease. In: Tierney, L. et al.: Current Medical Diagnosis and Treatment. Stamford, Conn.: Appleton and Lang, 1996.

McCarty, D. J.: Treatment of Rheumatoid Arthritis. In: McCarty, D. and Koopman, W. (Eds.): Arthritis and Allied Conditions: A Textbook of Rheumatology. Malvern, N.Y.: Lea & Febiger, 1993.

Nakamura, R. M.: Clinical and Laboratory Evaluation of Systemic Rheumatic Diseases. In: Henry, J. (Ed.): Clinical Diagnosis and Management by Laboratory Methods. Philadelphia: Saunders, 1996.

Norris, J., et al., (Eds.): Professional Guide to Diseases. Salem: Springhouse Corp., 1995.

Rosenwasser, L. J.: The Vasculitis Syndromes. In: Bennett, J. and Plum, F. (Eds.): Textbook of Medicine. Philadelphia: Saunders, 1996.

Schmerling, R., et al: Guidelines for the Initial Evaluation of the Adult Patient with Acute Musculoskeletal Symptoms. Arthritis Rheum. 39:1-8, Jan. 1996.

Schmid, F.: Principles of Diagnosis and Treatment of Bone and Joint Infections. In: McCarty, D. and Koopman, W. (Eds.): Arthritis and Allied Conditions: A Textbook of Rheumatology. Malvern, N.Y.: Lea & Febiger, 1993.

Thompson, G., et al.: Ankylosing Spondylitis. In: Rakel, R. (Ed.): Conn's Current Therapy. Philadelphia: Saunders, 1995.

CHAPTER 7

HEART DISEASE

SCOPE

Cardiovascular disease remains the primary cause of death in the United States. Some risk factors, such as high cholesterol levels, smoking, obesity, physical inactivity and high alcohol intake, can be modified by changes in diet and life-style. Other risk factors, such as growing older, having a family history of premature heart disease and being of male gender, obviously cannot. Diagnostic methods include exercise stress testing, electrocardiography, echocardiography, x-ray, angiography, computed tomography and various types of radionuclide imaging, such as SPECT and PET. Congenital conditions, such as valve defects, although present from birth, may not be discovered until much later in life. Coronary artery disease often carries the major complications of angina pectoris, myocardial infarction and sudden cardiac death. The four principle objectives in treating heart attack victims are relieving distress, limiting the size of the infarct, reducing heart activity and preventing death from complications. Cardiac arrhythmia may have symptoms of dizziness, fainting, chest pain and difficulty breathing, and is often treated with drugs that themselves may be life threatening. In cardiomyopathy, the cause must be sought for optimum treatment. Respiratory infection may cause exacerbations of chronic cor pulmonale, which is often a result of chronic obstructive pulmonary disease. Numerous drugs can also injure the heart. Heart transplantation is being performed more commonly worldwide, with selection of candidates dependent on often-difficult assessments of a patient's present disability, stability of the disease and likelihood of survival without the operation.

SYNOPSIS

7.00 INTRODUCTION

The cardiovascular system, which comprises the heart and an elaborate system of blood vessels, has two main functions: delivery of oxygen and nutrients to the cells of the body, and removal of the waste products of cellular metabolism, including the gas carbon dioxide. To carry out this function, the heart maintains the blood pressure and blood flow necessary for an adequate supply of blood to be brought to all the tissues and organs.

Diseases of the heart and blood vessels, known collectively as cardiovascular disease, remain the primary cause of death in the United States, despite the fact that from 1980 to 1990, the death rate from these conditions fell by nearly 27 percent. In 1993, officials of the American Heart Association estimated that about 1.5 million Americans experience a heart attack each year and that about 500,000 of these heart attack victims die (Gunby, 1993). In addition, about 50,000 Americans die of heart failure each year (Cohen, 1992).

To appreciate the cardiac system, a basic knowledge of anatomy, physiology and pathophysiology is essential.[1] As well, to understand

---

[1] *See* 7.10 *infra.*

the relationships of disease, injury and other abnormalities, an organized systemic approach to cardiac pathology is necessary.

7.10   ANATOMY AND PHYSIOLOGY OF THE HEART

The heart is situated between the two lungs in the middle of the chest. (*See Figure 7–1.*) About a third of the heart lies to the right of the breastbone, and about two thirds lies to the left of it. The apex of the heart, which is the heart's lower extremity, rests on the upper surface of the diaphragm. The other end of the heart, known as the base, is occupied by the roots of the great vessels that join the heart (the aorta, two venae cavae, the pulmonary artery and four pulmonary veins). Depending on the size and weight of the individual, the heart weighs about 7 to 15 ounces and is about the size of a clenched fist.

7.11   Chambers

The human heart has four chambers: the right atrium and right ventricle, which make up the right side of the heart, and the left atrium and left ventricle, which comprise the left side of the heart. The walls of the chambers are made up primarily of cardiac muscle, a type of muscle that, in its fine structure, resembles skeletal muscle. Unlike skeletal muscle, however, cardiac muscle is not under the control of human will and has the ability to contract rhythmically when stimulated by an electric current.

The left and right atria and the left and right ventricles are separated by the atrial septum and the ventricular septum, respectively. The muscular layers of the atria are separated from those of the ventricles by dense connective tissue that also provides attachment sites for the valves (known collectively as the atrioventricular valves) that close the opening between the atria and the ventricles during ventricular contraction. (*See Figure 7–2.*)

[1]   Atria

The relatively thin-walled atria receive blood returning to the heart through the veins. Their muscles are arranged in two sheets: a superficial one that covers both atria, and an internal one for each individual atrium, with fibers arranged more or less at right angles to those of the superficial sheet.

The atria have three main functions:

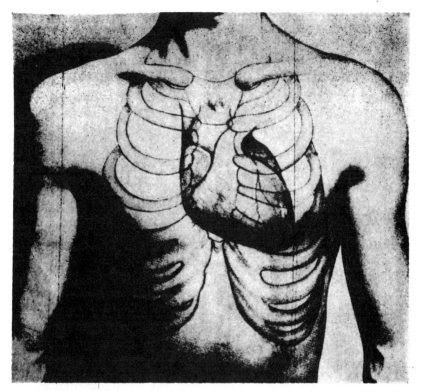

Fig. 7-1. Anterior view of the heart situated in its normal position in the chest.

1. They serve as elastic reservoirs and conduits for blood passing from the veins to the ventricles.

2. They act as "booster" pumps that enhance filling of the ventricles, especially in the setting of underlying heart disease or rapid beating of the heart.

3. Their contraction increases ventricular pressure and decreases atrial pressure, which results in a pressure gradient that causes the atrioventricular valves to close.

When the heart is beating slowly, the pumping action of the atria is relatively minor. At such times, the ventricles fill mainly during the period when the atria and ventricles are not contracting, and venous blood flows into the heart as if the atrium and ventricle were one chamber. At the end of this quiescent period, the atria contract and increase ventricular filling.

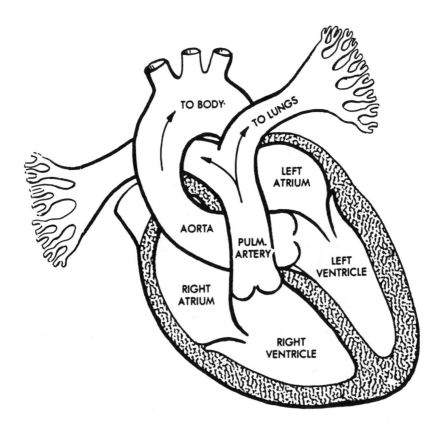

Fig. 7-2. Interior view of the heart, showing the chambers, great vessels and course of blood.

[2]   Ventricles

The ventricles are responsible for most of the weight of the heart. Each ventricle contains three major bands of muscle, and the left ventricle has an additional fourth band. The fibers of the deep layer spiral around the ventricles very gradually, which allows them to function as circular constrictor muscles.

Blood flows into the right ventricle from the right atrium through the tricuspid valve[2] and out again through the pulmonary valve into the pulmonary trunk. Blood enters the left ventricle from the left atrium via the mitral valve and exits through the aortic valve into the aorta.

---

[2] *See* 7.12 *infra.*

When the ventricles contract, all the valves of the heart are closed, causing a buildup of pressure within the heart that causes it to change from an ovoid to a more spherical shape. Eventually the pressure forces the pulmonary and aortic valves to open, and blood flows into the pulmonary artery and the aorta, respectively.

Because the left ventricle pumps blood to the entire body, its wall is two to three times as thick as that of the right ventricle, which delivers blood only to the lungs. When the left ventricle contracts, its volume is reduced by a decrease in the transverse diameter caused by a shortening of the cardiac muscle fibers and by some shortening of the base-apex diameter. Thus, the left ventricle can be thought of as a cylinder that pumps (displaces volume) by decreasing its height and diameter.

When the right ventricle contracts, its free wall is moved toward the ventricular septum by contraction of the spiral muscles. Ejection of blood from the right ventricle is assisted by the left ventricle because, as the constrictor muscles of the left ventricle contract, the curvature of the septum is increased, pulling the free right ventricular wall toward the septum.

[3] Myocardium

The muscular portion of the walls of the chambers of the heart is known as the myocardium. Although the myocardium is composed of distinct cells, each surrounded by a distinct plasma membrane, it functions much like a syncytium (a mass of protoplasm with many nuclei formed by the merging of cells) because of the "tight" junctions between the cells. The tight junctions provide low electric resistance and allow certain ions (electrically charged particles) to pass readily from cell to cell.

There are two general types of myocardial cells: those specialized for generating rhythmic electric impulses, and those specialized for contraction. The latter remain at rest until they are stimulated by an impulse originating elsewhere.

7.12 Valves

Blood flowing through the heart is kept moving in a forward direction by a system of four one-way valves. The cardiac valves open to allow the passage of blood when the chambers contract and then close to prevent blood from flowing backward as the chambers relax.

The valves also help maintain the different pressures in the right and the left sides of the heart that are necessary to ensure that both sides pump equal volumes of blood with each heartbeat.

The two valves that lie between the ventricles and the arteries that supply blood to the pulmonary and systemic systems (the pulmonary valve and the aortic valve, respectively) are called semilunar valves because each consists of three crescent-shaped flaps or leaflets of tissue (cusps).

The valves situated between the ventricles and the atria have not only cusps but also cords of fibrous tissue, called chordae tendineae, that connect the valves to the ventricular walls. When the ventricles contract, small muscles in the ventricular walls that are attached to the cords (the papillary muscles) prevent the cusps of the valves from moving too far backward as they close.

The valve between the right atrium and the right ventricle consists of three cusps and is called the tricuspid valve. The corresponding valve that closes the opening between the left atrium and the left ventricle is called the mitral valve because it is shaped somewhat like the hat, known as a miter, that is worn by Catholic bishops. The mitral valve has only two cusps, and these cusps are thicker than those of the tricuspid valve.

7.13 Endocardium and Pericardium

The chambers of the heart are lined with a smooth, protective membrane called the endocardium. On the outside, the heart and the roots of the great vessels are covered by a fibrous sac known as the pericardium. The inner layer of the pericardium is attached to the heart muscle, and the outer layer is connected by ligaments to the vertebral column, the diaphragm and other structures. The two layers of the pericardium are separated by a thin film of fluid that allows the heart and the inner pericardium to move freely within the outer pericardium.

7.14 Coronary Arteries and Veins

The heart supplies blood to itself through two coronary arteries, so named because together with their branches, they surround the heart like a crown. (*See Figure 7-3.*) The coronary arteries arise from the pockets in the aorta that contain the cusps of the aortic valve and run around the outside of the heart in grooves in the heart muscle. The left coronary artery divides after about 1 inch into an anterior branch and a circumflex branch, and the former usually has a descending branch. The right coronary artery runs downward and to the right over the right ventricle and then curves around to the back of the heart, where it gives off one or more branches to the left ventricle. The right coronary artery also usually gives off a branch near its origin.

Most of the veins of the coronary circulation drain into a cavity called the coronary sinus, which then empties into the right atrium. A few coronary veins drain directly into the cardiac chambers.

7.15 Nerves

The heart is innervated both by fibers from the vagus nerve of the parasympathetic nervous system and by fibers from the sympathetic nervous system. Fibers from the right vagus nerve supply the sinoatrial node of the heart[3] and serve to control the heart rate and the force of atrial contraction. Fibers from the left vagus nerve supply mainly the atrioventricular node. Most of the sympathetic fibers pass to the ventricles, where they function to increase the force of cardiac contraction, but the atria also receive sympathetic innervation.

The heart also has sympathetic pain receptors that respond to myocardial ischemia (lack of oxygen in the myocardium) and other stimuli. Like other visceral sensations, heart pain is poorly and variably localized and may be indistinguishable from pain originating in the great vessels or the pericardium.

7.16 Conduction System

The electric signals that regulate the rhythmic contraction and relaxation of the heart originate in a microscopic bundle of specialized myocardial cells called the sinoatrial node (SA node; sometimes called simply the sinus node) and travel through a network of fibers referred to as the cardiac conduction system. The sinoatrial node, which sometimes is referred to as the cardiac pacemaker, is located at the junction of the superior vena cava (the uppermost of the two large veins that bring blood to the heart from the body) and the right atrium. Any portion of the myocardium can generate electric impulses, but normally the impulses originate in the sinoatrial node.

Electric impulses from the sinoatrial node are conducted through muscle fibers of the two atria to the atrioventricular node (AV node),

---

[3] *See* 7.16 *infra.*

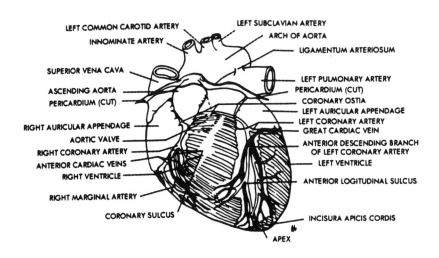

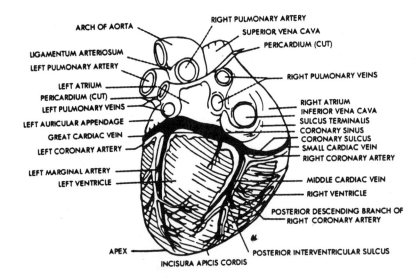

Fig. 7-3. Anterior (top) and posterior (bottom) views of the heart and coronary vessels.

which is located in the posterior portion of the atrial septum near the base of the tricuspid valve. The atrioventricular node delays the conduction of the impulse from the sinoatrial node by about 140 milliseconds, which allows the atria to contract shortly before the ventricles and thereby act as booster pumps in the manner described earlier.[4]

From the atrioventricular node, the impulses travel along fibers called the bundle of His, which divides into a left bundle branch and a right bundle branch at the top of the ventricular septum. These branches divide again to become the Purkinje fibers, which carry the impulses to all parts of the left and right ventricular myocardium. It takes the impulse only about 40 milliseconds to travel from the atrioventricular node to the ventricles (Ross, 1992).

7.17 Cardiac Cycle

The cardiac cycle consists of two phases, diastole and systole, which together last about one second. During diastole, which occupies about two thirds of the cardiac cycle, the ventricles of the heart are relaxed. Systole is the phase during which blood is ejected from the heart as the ventricles contract.

The cardiac cycle is arbitrarily considered to begin with atrial contraction. During diastole, the sinoatrial node generates an electric impulse, generally measuring less than one millionth of an ampere, that causes the atria to contract. In this phase, the tricuspid and mitral valves are open and blood is propelled from the atria into the relaxed ventricles. When the impulse reaches the ventricles, they contract, and systole begins.

During systole, the blood pressure created by the contracting ventricles closes the tricuspid and mitral valves, and, shortly afterward, the pressure inside the ventricles increases to the point that the pulmonary and aortic valves are forced open and blood is ejected into the pulmonary artery and the aorta. As the ventricles relax again, blood backs up in the pulmonary artery and the aorta, creating a pressure that re-closes the pulmonary and aortic valves. The pressure in the relaxed ventricles is now lower than that in the atria; the tricuspid and mitral valves open again, and the cardiac cycle repeats itself.

The dull, prolonged "lub" sound heard over the beating heart, which is known as the first heart sound, corresponds to the closure of the

---

[4] *See* 7.11 *supra.*

tricuspid and mitral valves at the beginning of systole. The shorter and sharper second heart sound, the "dupp" of the heartbeat, is created primarily by the closure of the pulmonary and aortic valves.

7.18   Heart Rate, Cardiac Output and Stroke Volume

In the average resting adult, the sinoatrial node creates 100 electric impulses a minute, which results in the heart going through 100 full cardiac cycles per minute. The number of cardiac cycles—or beats— gone through in a unit of time is referred to as the heart rate. For example, on examination, the heart rate of the average person just described would be found to be 70 beats per minute.

Generally the performance of the heart increases as physical fitness increases. This means that the heart of a fit person can deliver an adequate supply of blood to the tissues while beating slower than the heart of an untrained person. The heart rate of a well-trained athlete at rest may be as low as 35 beats per minute, or half the average rate of the general population. For the athlete, a low heart rate poses no danger, but in an untrained individual, a heart that is beating too slowly may not provide enough blood to the brain and other vital organs.

The amount of blood pumped by the heart in one minute is called the cardiac output. The average cardiac output of a person at rest is about 6 or 7 liters. When the body needs an increased blood supply—as it does during exercise, for example—the heart generally increases its output by beating faster. This mechanism of increasing cardiac output is limited, however, because, after a certain heart rate has been reached, the chambers do not have time to fill properly, and cardiac pumping becomes less efficient.

Cardiac output is determined not only by the rate at which the heart is beating but also by the amount of blood ejected by the ventricles with each contraction. This amount is referred to as the stroke volume. Usually with each contraction, the ventricles eject about half the blood they contain, which is about 3 ounces in the average person at rest.

7.19   Arterial Blood Pressure

The pressure exerted by the blood on the walls of the arteries is referred to as the arterial blood pressure. Blood pressure usually is expressed indirectly as the number of millimeters of mercury (mmHg) in a glass column needed to exert the same pressure. The average systolic atrial blood pressure of young male adults at mental and physical rest in a sitting position is about 120 mmHg; the corresponding average diastolic pressure is about 80 mmHg. Slight variations in systolic pressure of between 5 and 10 mmHg occur over the course of a day, with the peak pressure occurring in the afternoon and the lowest level occurring in the early hours of the morning.

Several factors acting together determine the arterial blood pressure: the pumping action of the heart, the peripheral vessel resistance, the viscosity of the blood in the arterial system, the amount of blood in the arterial system and the elasticity of the arterial walls.

[1] Pumping Action of the Heart

The pumping action of the heart affects arterial blood pressure through the amount of blood ejected by the left ventricle into the aorta. This amount is expressed as the cardiac output or the stroke volume multiplied by the heart rate. When blood is forced into the already filled arterial system, it normally cannot escape from the system at the same rate as it is pumped in, so the arterial walls become more stretched, and the blood pressure rises.

[2] Peripheral Resistance

Peripheral resistance depends on the caliber of the small vessels, primarily that of the arterioles but also that of the capillaries and the small arteries and veins. Most of the peripheral resistance of the body comes from the vessels of the skeletal muscle and those of the abdominal viscera.

The effect of the caliber of the small vessels on arterial blood pressure is illustrated by the following example: Stimulation of the great splanchnic nerve, which innervates the rings of muscle fibers in the walls of the small vessels of the viscera, causes them to constrict, which, in turn, reduces outflow from the arterial system. The arterial blood pressure then rises until it becomes high enough to overcome the resistance and restore peripheral flow. Arterial pressure remains elevated as long as the resistance persists. Dilation of the small visceral vessels has the opposite effect: a reduction in peripheral resistance and a decline in arterial blood pressure.

[3] Viscosity of the Blood

The greater the viscosity or thickness of a liquid, the greater the pressure needed to force it along a length of narrow tube in a given time. If the pressure remains constant, the greater the viscosity, the longer will be the time required for the liquid to pass along the tube. This property depends on the frictional (or internal) resistance between the parts of the fluid itself, that is, the degree to which the molecules or particles of the liquid cohere.

On average, blood is five times more viscous than water. Its viscosity is due in part to the proteins suspended in it and in part to the red and white blood cells. Changes in the concentration of protein or number of cells in the blood alter the blood's viscosity. Like peripheral resistance, the viscosity of the blood affects arterial blood pressure mainly at the site of the arterioles. As blood viscosity increases, the driving pressure must increase if flow through the arterioles is to remain constant.

[4]   Quantity of Blood in the Arterial System

In any closed system of rigid tubes, pressure can develop only after the system is filled to capacity. The arterial walls are not rigid but distensible and elastic. They are stretched by the blood they contain because they are actually overfilled while the blood is circulating normally. The greater the extent of overfilling, the greater the arterial blood pressure. Loss of blood, as in a hemorrhage, or a loss of some of the fluid portion of the blood, as in prolonged vomiting or diarrhea, results in a reduction in blood pressure.

[5]   Elasticity of the Vessel Walls

The elasticity of the arterial walls allows them to maintain a pressure during contraction of the ventricles, and that permits them to maintain a nearly uniform rate of flow through the capillaries. If the vessel walls were rigid, each beat of the heart would create pressure in the system, and the pressure would fall to zero after each systole. Thus the elastic recoil of the arterial walls acts as a subsidiary pump that drives the blood onward in a continuous stream between heartbeats.

7.20   RISK FACTORS IN HEART DISEASE

Scientific studies performed in many countries have provided solid evidence that certain factors make it more likely that a person will develop heart disease (Friedewald, 1992). These elements, the so-called risk factors, are classified as modifiable or unmodifiable. Hypercholesterolemia (excess cholesterol in the blood), the use of tobacco products, high blood pressure and diabetes mellitus are the major potentially modifiable risk factors in the development of heart disease. Other potentially remediable factors include obesity, physical inactivity, certain psychosocial and behavioral factors and high alcohol intake. Unmodifiable risk factors include growing older, being male and having a family history of premature heart disease.

7.21   Hypercholesterolemia

Cholesterol is a fatlike substance found in the blood and other body fluids and tissues that serves as a building block in the synthesis of bile acids and certain hormones. A higher than normal concentration of cholesterol in the blood, a condition referred to as hypercholesterolemia, has been shown in numerous studies to be correlated with coronary artery disease.

Cholesterol in the blood is transported by substances known as lipoproteins. The cholesterol transported by low-density lipoproteins (the so-called bad cholesterol) has been found to be associated with coronary artery disease, whereas that transported by high-density lipoproteins (the so-called good cholesterol) is negatively (inversely) correlated with coronary artery disease, that is, the higher the concentration of high-density lipoprotein, the lower the risk (Tribble and Krauss, 1993). This may explain some of the difference in risk for coronary artery disease found between men and women, because women have higher average levels of high-density lipoprotein.

Hypercholesterolemia has traditionally been defined as a total (good and bad) plasma cholesterol level that exceeds that of 95 percent of persons in the same age group and of the same sex. By this definition, 200 milligrams of cholesterol per deciliter of plasma or more is a high level for a person under the age of 20, but a high level for a woman over the age of 55 is 295 milligrams per deciliter or more (Farmer and Gotto, 1992). Because studies have shown that there is still a risk of coronary artery disease at levels in this range, the National Cholesterol Education Program now defines a plasma cholesterol level of less than 200 milligrams per deciliter as desirable, concentrations ranging from 200 to 240 milligrams per deciliter as borderline high, and levels of 240 milligrams per deciliter as high (Berkow and Fletcher, 1992).

The results of risk factor intervention studies in which total blood cholesterol levels were reduced to as low as 182 milligrams per deciliter show that the risk of coronary artery disease continues to fall as the cholesterol level falls, at least down to that level. Other clinical studies, moreover, have provided strong evidence that even in persons who subsequently develop coronary artery disease, lowering blood cholesterol concentrations lowers the morbidity and mortality of the disease (Friedewald, 1992).

7.22   Hypertension

Hypertension (high blood pressure) is a risk factor for the development of heart disease that extends across race, gender and age categories. In the United States, hypertension usually is defined as a systolic blood pressure equal to or greater than 140 mmHg or a diastolic blood pressure of 90 mmHg or greater. High blood pressure frequently co-exists with other risk factors, and along with hypercholesterolemia may have a synergistic effect in the development of coronary artery disease. It is estimated that 58 million people in the United States may have hypertension (Friedewald, 1992).

Epidemiologic studies have shown not only that there is a positive relationship between hypertension and coronary artery disease but that there is no blood pressure below which the risk remains constant or disappears. Thus, within physiologic limits, the lower a person's blood pressure, the lower his or her level of risk for coronary artery disease.

7.23   Use of Tobacco

The use of tobacco products has been established as a major risk factor in patients already prone to the development of heart disease. A number of studies have shown that cigarette smokers have about twice the risk of developing coronary artery disease as nonsmokers, and that the risk increases with the number of cigarettes one smokes and the length of time one has smoked. It also has been shown that passive smoking (breathing the tobacco smoke of others) is associated with an increased risk of coronary artery disease (Glantz, et al., 1991; Farmer and Gotto, 1992; Steenland, 1992).

Tobacco use may interact with other risk factors. The use of tobacco products, for example, may accelerate the process of atherosclerosis (the formation of plaques within the arteries that narrow the arteries and cause their walls to thicken and become less elastic), and heavy smokers have been found to have lower levels of high-density lipoprotein and higher levels of low-density lipoprotein than nonsmokers.[5]

The inhalation of tobacco smoke by nonsmokers causes an immediate rise in blood pressure, but chronic smokers tend to have lower blood pressure than nonsmokers, a phenomenon that may be associated with the fact that smokers tend to have lower body weight than nonsmokers. The inhalation of tobacco smoke also affects blood clotting factors and other hematologic factors that may play a role in the development of atherosclerosis and coronary artery disease.

The nicotine absorbed through the lungs with the use of tobacco products has been shown to increase coronary artery tone and to increase vasoconstriction in patients with coronary artery disease. This increased vasoconstriction may result in an imbalance between the oxygen supply to the heart and the heart's demand for oxygen.

After smoking cessation, the increased risk of coronary artery disease decreases rapidly with time. In one study, it was found that smokers who quit smoking lowered their risk of myocardial infarction within 2 years of quitting (Friedewald, 1992). It has been estimated that about 40 percent of the risk is eliminated within 5 years of discontinuation of smoking, although it usually takes several more years for a former smoker's risk to fall to that of a person who has never smoked (Friedewald, 1992). Some studies have found that even after 20 years, many former smokers still have an increased risk of coronary artery disease (Farmer and Gotto, 1992).

7.24   Diabetes Mellitus

Diabetes mellitus (a metabolic disease in which the ability to oxidize carbohydrates is lost, usually due to poor pancreatic function)[6] is well established as a risk factor for coronary artery disease, and cardiovascular diseases are the major cause of death in diabetic patients. In addition, diabetes frequently co-exists with other risk factors for heart disease, such as hypercholesterolemia and hypertension, which are more prevalent in the diabetic population than the healthy population.

It is not known how diabetes mellitus increases a patient's chances of developing coronary artery disease, but possible contributing factors include diabetes-associated hyperglycemia (excess glucose in the

---

[5] *See* 7.21 *supra.*

[6] *See also* ch. 9.

blood), which inhibits the formation of certain important linkages in proteins, and dyslipoproteinemia (the presence of abnormal lipoproteins in the blood). The hyperinsulinemia (excess insulin in the blood) that is sometimes present in diabetic patients may pose an additional risk by increasing the synthesis of cholesterol and the proliferation of arterial smooth muscle cells, factors that contribute to atherosclerosis.

It presently is a matter of controversy whether controlling the elevated blood glucose levels of diabetics lowers their risk of heart disease, but there is widespread agreement that co-existing risk factors, such as hypertension, obesity and smoking, must be controlled or eliminated in these patients.

7.25 Obesity

Definitions of obesity vary considerably and are arbitrary. The condition frequently is defined as a body weight that is 20 percent above ideal body weight. Ideal body weight, in this definition, is the weight associated with the lowest mortality rate in persons of the same age and body build who are applying for life insurance. Many physicians prefer to define obesity on the basis of body weight index. A person's body weight index is calculated by dividing his or her weight in kilograms by the square of his or her height in meters (kg/m^2). Other definitions describe obesity in terms of the thickness of skin folds measured with calipers at various locations on the body.

Regardless of the definition, obesity has been found to correlate positively with total blood cholesterol concentration and negatively with high-density-lipoprotein level, and there is a strong epidemiologic association between obesity and hypertension. It is not known, however, whether obesity acts to increase the risk of coronary artery disease by elevating blood pressure and blood cholesterol concentration or whether it constitutes an independent risk factor. Regardless of the actual role of obesity in the development of atherosclerotic complications, weight reduction with the goal of approaching the ideal weight should be encouraged in patients who have this risk factor.

It is not only obesity per se but the distribution of fat in the body that is an important element in the development of coronary artery disease. The so-called waist-hip ratio (the abdominal circumference divided by the hip circumference), for example, has been found to be associated with risk. In men, coronary artery disease is correlated with high relative abdominal fat distribution (often defined as a waist-hip ratio of 0.86 or greater), regardless of whether the men are obese. In women, deposition of fat within the abdomen constitutes a greater risk for the development of coronary artery disease than obesity alone. Thus a masculine distribution of fat (more fat in the abdominal area than on the hips) increases the risk of heart disease in both men and women, and the waist-hip fat ratio appears to be a more significant predictor than the total degree of obesity.

7.26 Physical Inactivity

The role of physical inactivity in the development of heart disease is a matter of some debate in the medical community. Epidemiologic studies show an association between a sedentary life-style and heart disease, but no definite cause-and-effect relationship has been established. As people begin to exercise regularly, their body weight usually falls, their blood pressure is more likely to be normal, their cholesterol values are more apt to be at a desirable level and they frequently discontinue the use of tobacco, all of which makes it difficult to isolate physical inactivity as a risk factor. The question of whether physical inactivity is an independent risk factor for heart disease probably has little clinical relevance when the ability of exercise to modify other risk factors of heart disease is taken into consideration.

7.27 Psychosocial and Behavioral Factors

There is a correlation between depression, anxiety and neuroticism and coronary artery disease. It has been difficult, however, to establish a statistical link between myocardial infarction and these emotional factors. One mechanism that could account, at least in part, for the association between chronic emotional stress and coronary artery disease is the increase in the release of epinephrine (adrenaline) by the adrenal glands that occurs in stressful situations. Epinephrine increases blood pressure and heart rate, stimulates the heart muscle and increases cardiac output.

[1] Occupational Factors

Job stress, role ambiguity in the workplace, lack of autonomy on the job, job change, unemployment and retirement are factors that have been studied as possible risk factors for coronary artery disease. Clinical studies have revealed little statistical evidence that these occupational factors play a role in the development or exacerbation of heart disease. One well-designed study, however, has shown a correlation between job stress (high psychosocial demands associated with little latitude in decision making) and two factors frequently associated with heart disease, namely, hypertension and increased left ventricular mass (Farmer and Gotto, 1992).

[2]   Type A Personality

Persons with a "type A" personality are characterized by ambition, competitiveness, a sense of urgency and a high degree of disturbance by environmental factors. This is in contrast to people with a "type B" personality, who are more passive and less disturbed by environmental factors. The possibility of a correlation between type A personality and coronary artery disease has been examined in a number of studies. In several of these, subjects with type A personalities have been found to suffer angina pectoris (typically, chest, left arm and shoulder pain caused by contraction of the coronary arteries)[7] at least twice as often as type B subjects, but long-term survival data have not shown a correlation between type A personality and the frequency of fatal myocardial infarction (Farmer and Gotto, 1992).

[3]   Educational Level and Socioeconomic Status

There appears to be an inverse statistical relationship between educational level and both high blood pressure and death from coronary artery disease. These differences probably are due to life-style differences: the higher the level of education and socioeconomic status, the more likely a person is to behave in ways (exercising, controlling weight and not smoking, for example) that lower his or her incidence of heart disease.

7.28   High Alcohol Intake

The effects of alcohol (the alcohol contained in alcoholic beverages is ethyl alcohol) on the heart are very complex. High alcohol intake may be associated with cardiomyopathy (disease of the muscular wall of the heart) in the absence of coronary artery disease, and it is well established that excessive alcohol consumption can contribute to high blood pressure. In some individuals, binge drinking appears to cause cardiac arrhythmia (irregular heartbeat), even when there are no other signs of heart disease. It is not clear, however, whether moderate alcohol intake has a positive correlation with these conditions.

---

[7] *See* 7.42 *infra.*

The protective role against heart disease that some investigators have attributed to alcohol is still a matter of controversy. It is known that alcohol raises high-density-lipoprotein levels, but it is not clear whether this change correlates with a decrease in the prevalence or extent of coronary artery disease. There appears to be a negative correlation between the daily consumption of small (one or two drinks a day) or moderate (three to five drinks a day) amounts of alcohol and atherosclerosis of the coronary arteries. Heavy drinking, however, has been found to be positively associated with coronary artery disease and myocardial infarction. It generally is not recommended that patients begin drinking alcohol as a means of preventing heart disease.

7.29 Male Gender

Coronary artery disease is much less common in women before menopause (menopause occurs in most women at age 48 to 50 years) than in men of the same age, and the difference between men and women is the greatest between the ages of 35 and 44 years. After menopause, the prevalence of coronary artery disease in women gradually approaches that in men.

Because the process of atherosclerosis does not appear to differ between men and women, and because the risk factors associated with the development of coronary artery disease are more or less the same for both sexes, it seems probable that the difference in the prevalence of coronary artery disease in men and women is due to relative differences in their levels of the hormones estrogen and testosterone. When males enter puberty, their blood testosterone concentrations increase, whereas puberty in females is marked by an increase in circulating estrogen levels. Until puberty, high-density-lipoprotein levels are about the same in males and females, but at puberty, the effect of testosterone causes them to decline in males. As women undergo natural menopause, their blood levels of high-density lipoprotein gradually decline, which increases the likelihood of the development of coronary atherosclerosis. Although the advisability of estrogen replacement therapy in postmenopausal women is still a matter of debate—partly because of the potential for an increased risk of breast and endometrial cancer—there is a negative correlation between such treatment and the severity of coronary artery disease.

7.30   DIAGNOSIS OF HEART DISEASE

Generally the diagnosis of heart disease begins with the simplest, least expensive and least invasive procedures, and progresses to more sophisticated, expensive and invasive techniques only if they are necessary. Procedures that fall into the former category include the medical history, the physical examination, electrocardiography, roentgenography (x-ray examination), echocardiography and exercise stress testing. The more sophisticated techniques include radionuclide imaging, single photon emission computed tomography (SPECT), positron emission tomography (PET), computed tomography (CT), magnetic resonance imaging (MRI), cardiac catheterization and cardiac angiography.

The sections that follow describe the various diagnostic procedures in the order in which they might logically be performed to provide an accurate and complete diagnosis of heart disease. It is very unlikely that all of them would be used in any one patient. Many patients with heart disease require only one or two tests to confirm a diagnosis made on the basis of the medical history and the physical examination.

A complete cardiac diagnosis, as defined by the New York Heart Association, must reveal the following (Braunwald, 1992):

- Etiology—Is the disease congenital, hypertensive, ischemic or rheumatic?

- Anatomic abnormalities—Are chambers enlarged? Are valves affected? Is the pericardium involved? Has there been a myocardial infarction?

- Physiologic disturbances—Is arrhythmia present? Is there evidence of heart failure or of myocardial ischemia?

- Extent of functional disability—How strenuous is the physical activity required to elicit symptoms?

7.31   Medical History

The interviews with the patient and/or the patient's family that provide the medical history should elicit information about a family history of heart disease, the presence of risk factors[8] and the presence of the symptoms of heart disease. The symptoms of heart disease include chest pain or discomfort, weakness and fatigability, hypotension (low blood pressure), syncope (fainting), dyspnea (abnormal

---

[8] *See* 7.20 *supra.*

shortness of breath), cyanosis (bluish discoloration of the skin and/or mucous membranes) and cardiac arrhythmia. Heart function may be adequate when a person is at rest but inadequate during exertion. Therefore, the occurrence of symptoms such as chest pain or dyspnea only during physical activity is a sign that heart disease may be present.

Dyspnea and chest pain or discomfort may be caused by a variety of conditions other than heart disease. Whether heart disease is responsible for these symptoms can frequently be determined by a detailed physical examination. In some cases, a determination of their causes requires more specialized diagnostic procedures.[9]

7.32 Physical Examination

An appropriate physical examination of the cardiovascular system includes taking the patient's blood pressure in both arms with the patient in both the supine and upright positions, timing the patient's heart rate for one minute, careful examination of the optic fundi (the back portions of the interior of the eyeballs) and the vessels of the retinas of the eyes for evidence of hypertension, and examination of the legs for swelling. A complete physical examination also includes palpation of the arterial pulses in the arms and legs to determine the adequacy of blood flow, evaluation of the pulses of the carotid arteries and the jugular veins, palpation (feeling with the fingers) of the motions of the heart, and cardiac auscultation (listening to the heart with the aid of a stethoscope).

7.33 Diagnostic Tests

The variety of diagnostic tests used to confirm the presence of heart disease are discussed herein.

[1] Electrocardiography

One of the simplest techniques used by physicians to detect and diagnose heart disease is electrocardiography. Millions of electrocardiographic examinations are performed each year in health care facilities of all types, including doctors' private offices. Electrocardiography is noninvasive, requires little time (usually only about five minutes), entails no risk to the patient and is relatively inexpensive. The technique is useful primarily in the detection of myocardial

---

[9] *See* 7.33 *infra.*

infarction (old or current), the detection and definition of arrhythmia and the detection of hypertrophy (thickening) of the walls of the heart.

The electrocardiograph (the machine used to perform electrocardiography) produces an electrocardiogram (EKG), which is a graph of the electrical activity of the heart. The electrical impulses originating in the working myocardial cells[10] and the specialized conducting tissue of the heart[11] are transmitted to the machine via electric leads attached to the skin of the arms, legs and chest. Special needles on the electrocardiograph trace representations of the impulses on a moving strip of paper. The paper moves at a known speed, which permits calculation of the heart rate and the duration of the various events in the cardiac cycle.[12]

The waves seen on the electrocardiogram represent the stages of the cardiac cycle. The wave that corresponds to the beginning of the heartbeat, that is, the contraction of the atrium, is designated the P wave. The spikes representing the contraction of the ventricles are referred to as the QRS segment. The T wave corresponds to the end of the cardiac cycle, that is, the relaxation phase, when the electric impulses from the heart return to zero. (*See Figure 7–4.*)

The clinician interpreting an electrocardiogram looks for changes from the normal electrocardiogram (e.g., flattening of the waves, lengthening of the intervals between waves and variations in the pattern of the waves) as indicators of the presence of heart disease. The findings of the EKG examination may provide a diagnosis of a patient's heart disease or may indicate a need for further testing by other methods.

[a]   Ambulatory Electrocardiography or Holter Monitoring

This test provides a continuous EKG while the patient goes about his or her daily activities, usually for a period of 24 hours. This technique is used primarily to detect serious arrhythmias that do not show up during a single office visit and to diagnose silent (asymptomatic) cardiac ischemia.[13] It may also be used to determine whether

---

[10] *See* 7.11[3] *supra.*

[11] *See* 7.16 *supra.*

[12] *See* 7.17 *supra.*

[13] *See* 7.44 *infra.*

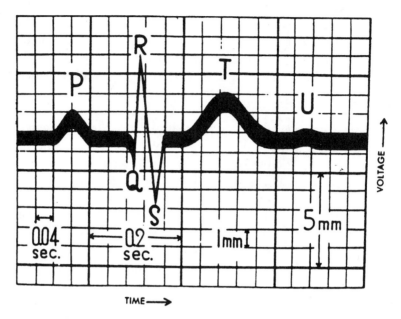

Fig. 7-4. Normal electrocardiographic representation of a single heartbeat.

a heart medication prescribed for the patient is having the desired effect.

The person undergoing ambulatory electrocardiography wears a small cassette recorder on a strap or belt. The recorder is connected to the chest under the clothing by electric leads. After the monitoring period, the information recorded on the cassette tape is played back through a computer, which analyzes the information and allows all or part of it to be printed out as a standard electrocardiogram. Some Holter monitoring devices allow the patient to "mark" the recording at the time symptoms are felt. These marks, together with the information the patient records in a diary about what he or she was doing at the time the symptoms were felt, can provide important diagnostic information.

[b] Signal-averaged Electrocardiography

Signal-averaged electrocardiography is a specialized electrocardiographic method that detects small electric currents, called late potentials, that often are present in the conduction pathways of the heart long after normal activation of the heart muscle.[14] To create a signal-averaged EKG, a conventional EKG is recorded for a longer-than-normal period (usually for about 30 minutes), and a computer superimposes the electrocardiographic impulses (signals) to develop an averaged EKG that is analyzed to detect late potentials. Late potentials generally originate in areas of the heart that have been injured, and patients who have them may have a propensity for cardiac arrhythmia.

[2]   Chest Roentgenography

Another noninvasive technique routinely used in the diagnosis of heart disease is chest roentgenography (also called chest x-ray examination). About 750,000 chest roentgenographic examinations are performed by cardiologists in the United States each year (Zaret, 1992). Other than a minimal exposure to radiation, this diagnostic technique carries no risk for the patient. It also has the advantages of being painless, rapid and relatively inexpensive. The picture produced by chest roentgenography—the roentgenogram or x-ray—provides information on the size and configuration of the heart and the great vessels. In addition, because pulmonary vessel size is proportional to flow, the chest x-ray picture can give information about venous pressures and flows in the pulmonary arteries and veins. The x-ray also may be useful in revealing fluid in the lungs caused by heart failure.

[3]   Echocardiography

Another important technique used in the diagnosis of heart disease is echocardiography. About 970,000 of these examinations are performed in the United States each year (Zaret, 1992). Echocardiography is noninvasive and involves no pain or risk for the patient. For these reasons, and because it exposes the patient to no radiation, it is especially appropriate for use in diagnosing heart problems in children and pregnant women. Good echocardiograms cannot be obtained in 5 to 15 percent of patients, especially in elderly and obese patients and patients with emphysema.

The graphic representation of the heart produced in echocardiography—the echocardiogram—is created by an instrument that transmits a beam of high-frequency sound waves (ultrasound) to the heart and then translates the reflected waves (sound echoes) into images on a

---

[14] *See* 7.16 *supra.*

monitor similar to a television screen. A colorless gel is applied to the patient's chest, and a transducer (a small device that both emits sound waves and receives sound echoes) is held against the chest at various locations to produce different views of the heart.

Echocardiography is widely used to measure the size of the heart and the thickness of the heart muscle, as well as the functioning of the heart. The technique also is suitable for obtaining knowledge about congenital (present at birth) heart disease and valvular heart disease. When it is combined with the Doppler technique, it measures blood flow through the heart chambers and the valves as well as pressure gradients across the valves. When it is coupled with an exercise test, echocardiography can be used to evaluate wall motion of the ventricles and other characteristics of the heart under stress. Echocardiography is the preferred method for identifying masses in the heart, such as tumors and blood clots. It has been found that effective treatment of hypertension (high blood pressure) reduces left ventricular enlargement, and by taking periodic echocardiographic measurements of the size of the left ventricle and the thickness of its wall, it is possible to monitor the effectiveness of therapy for high blood pressure.

The recently developed technique of transesophageal echocardiography, a procedure in which an image is obtained using a probe mounted at the tip of a flexible gastroscope (an instrument used to examine the interior of the stomach) and inserted into the esophagus, is valuable in assessing valvular heart disease and the functioning of artificial (prosthetic) heart valves. The technique also is useful in detecting blood clots in the left atrium, in diagnosing infective endocarditis (inflammation of the endocardium) and in monitoring cardiac function during surgery. Transesophageal echocardiography involves a slight risk for the patient.

Four types of echocardiographic study are performed: M-mode, two-dimensional, contrast and Doppler.

[a] M-mode Echocardiography

In M-mode echocardiography, a single transducer, emitting 1,000 to 2,000 pulses of sound per second along a single line, provides a one-dimensional or "ice-pick" view of the heart with very good temporal resolution. When the direction of the ultrasound beam is changed, the heart can be scanned from the ventricles to the aorta and left atrium.

[b]   Two-dimensional Echocardiography

In two-dimensional echocardiography, an image is produced by an instrument that guides the ultrasound beam through an arc of up to 90 degrees about 30 times per second. This technique provides excellent spatial resolution and permits analysis of the movement of structures of the heart in real time from different positions of the transducer on the chest or abdomen.

[c]   Contrast Echocardiography

In contrast echocardiography, a concentrated mass (bolus) of a liquid contrast medium is injected rapidly into the cardiovascular circulation. Small bubbles that develop in the contrast medium and remain suspended there reflect the beam of ultrasound and produce a "cloud" of echoes within the cardiac chambers. The bubbles formed in the echocardiographic contrast media now in use usually do not pass through the cardiac capillary bed, but agents that have this ability are being developed.

[d]   Doppler Echocardiography

The Doppler technique detects blood flow velocity and turbulence. When sound encounters moving red blood cells, the frequency of the reflected sound is altered. The magnitude of the change, called the Doppler shift, indicates the velocity of blood flow with respect to the sound beam. An upward shift (increased frequency) indicates that the blood is moving toward the transducer, and a downward shift indicates motion away.

Pulsed Doppler echocardiography is used to locate disturbances of blood flow resulting from valvular blockage and regurgitation (backward flow) and intracardiac shunts (a flow of blood from the right to the left or the left to the right side of the heart through a defect in the atrial or ventricular septum).

Continuous-wave Doppler echocardiography allows measurement of flow velocity in the heart. When the velocity of blood flow is known, it is possible to calculate the pressure gradient across a heart valve. Doppler echocardiography combined with imaging echocardiography can be used to determine cardiac output.[15]

---

[15] *See* 7.18 *supra.*

[4] Exercise Stress Testing

An exercise stress test can only be performed by persons whose physical condition allows them to exercise strenuously on a treadmill or stationary bicycle. This test most commonly is performed to evaluate chest pain suspected of being angina pectoris. As the name implies, in an exercise stress test, the patient exercises in order to stress the heart, that is, to cause the heart to work more than it does when the patient is at rest. This stress can reproduce the chest pain that a patient encounters during everyday activities. Exercise stress tests also are used to reveal left ventricular dysfunction and heart rhythm abnormalities, to evaluate cardiac function after a heart attack and to measure the efficacy of treatment over time.

Less frequently, exercise stress testing is included in a physical examination of healthy middle-aged individuals who do not have symptoms of heart disease. The test may be performed to determine a person's fitness for a certain occupation or for beginning a program of vigorous exercise. Stress tests have more false-positive results (indicating that heart disease is present when it is not) in young women without symptoms than in men without symptoms. The false-negative rate is higher in men. An exercise stress test performed as part of a routine physical examination may reveal silent ischemia, that is, ischemia (deficient blood supply) that does not produce chest pain with normal daily activity.

More than a million exercise stress tests are performed each year in the United States. The risk of complications during a stress test is very low, with a nonfatal heart attack occurring during only about 1 in 100,000 tests (Zaret, 1992).

Before the exercise stress test begins, a conventional resting electrocardiogram is recorded. Then the patient walks on a treadmill or pedals an ergometer (stationary bicycle) while his or her heart rate, blood pressure and EKG are monitored on a screen. The exercise is usually sustained until pain occurs, significant changes in the EKG occur or a target heart rate is reached. The goal is to achieve the end point of the test within the first 6 to 15 minutes of physical exertion by gradually increasing the speed and incline of the treadmill or the resistance of the pedals of the ergometer. A test that is too short may not provide enough exercise to cause symptoms, and a longer, less rigorous test may cause the patient to tire before symptoms can occur.

The heart's functional level as revealed by the stress test is expressed in a unit called the metabolic equivalent (MET). One metabolic equivalent is equal to the amount of energy expended by a person standing at rest. A patient's exercise stress test score represents the workload on the heart that was required to provoke symptoms or to reach the target physical state.

[5]   Radionuclide Imaging

Radionuclide imaging (also called scintigraphy) of the heart is an essentially noninvasive method for evaluating heart disease that is easy to perform and exposes patients to less radiation than roentgenographic studies. For adults, this diagnostic method carries a very low risk. Fetuses have a lower tolerance for radiation, however, and therefore radionuclide imaging is not recommended for pregnant women or nursing mothers.

Radionuclide imaging begins with the injection into the bloodstream of a small amount of a radionuclide, that is, a short-lived radioisotope (an atom with an unstable nucleus that emits radiation when it decays). Then a gamma camera (also called a scintillation camera) is used to detect the radiation (gamma rays) emitted by the radioisotope. Finally a computer processes the information supplied by the camera and displays it on a screen as two-dimensional still pictures of the heart. Three-dimensional pictures also can be created by the computer from images obtained from several angles in a single plane.

Radionuclide imaging procedures can be divided into four broad categories:

1. Myocardial perfusion imaging, which shows areas of ischemia and infarcts (groups of cells that have died due to ischemia).

2. Infarct-avid imaging, which is used mainly to detect acute myocardial infarction.

3. Radionuclide ventriculography, which permits evaluation of ventricular function and ventricular wall motion.

4. Shunt scintigraphy, which allows the detection and quantification of left-to-right intracardiac shunts.

[a]   Myocardial Perfusion Imaging

Myocardial perfusion imaging usually is performed with thallium 201 (abbreviated 201-TL) as the radioactive indicator and therefore often is referred to simply as thallium imaging. After intravenous injection, the radioisotope leaves the blood vessels and rapidly enters the cells of the body at a rate proportional to the flow of blood in the region. Healthy myocardial cells take up the radioisotope almost immediately, whereas those that are ischemic (not receiving an adequate supply of blood) take longer to absorb it. Areas of scarring and infarcts usually do not absorb the radioisotope at all and are seen on the image as "cold spots," that is, areas of no radioactivity. Thus by comparing two or three images obtained over time, the examining physician can assess damage to the heart muscle.

Thallium-201 perfusion imaging is most often used to detect exercise-induced ischemia. At peak exercise, the radioisotope is injected intravenously, the patient stops exercising, and images are obtained 5 to 10 minutes later. When a patient is too sick or is physically unable to exercise (because of arthritis, obesity or age, for example), either dipyridamole or adenosine can be injected to simulate the effects of exercise on the heart. Hearts that are healthy show a relatively homogenous distribution of radioactivity, while those with ischemia or infarction show one or more cold spots. Several hours after this initial distribution, a state of equilibrium is reached between the amount of radioisotope in the living cells of the myocardium, including the cells in ischemic areas, and the blood and other structures of the body. Areas of infarction, however, continue to show reduced or no uptake of thallium 201.

Thallium imaging does not distinguish new infarcts from old, but it does provide prognostic information. The presence, size and number of distribution defects correlate with the incidence of future cardiac events. Persons with normal thallium imaging scans have a very low risk of a heart attack in the year following the examination.

[b] Infarct-avid Imaging

Infarct-avid scintigraphy is used primarily in the rare instances in which the traditional methods used to diagnose a heart attack cannot be interpreted or have provided ambiguous results. This method also is used to detect infarction immediately after coronary bypass and other types of heart surgery.

Infarct-avid imaging is based on the principle that certain substances accumulate in irreversibly damaged myocardial cells. Pyrophosphate, for example, a compound that is attracted to bone, collects in myocardial infarcts, presumably because it binds to the calcium that accumulates after the breakdown of the walls of cells that have died. Pyrophosphate labeled with technetium 99m (abbreviated 99mTc) becomes visible to the gamma camera about 12 to 24 hours after a heart attack.

To detect myocardial infarction, technetium 99m-labeled pyrophosphate is injected intravenously, and images of the myocardial region are taken about one hour later. A delay of two to four hours sometimes is necessary to differentiate radioactivity in the myocardium from that in the blood pool. For this reason, diagnosis by this method is more certain when the technetium 99m-labeled pyrophosphate accumulation is focal and intense (greater than or equal to that in the sternum or ribs, for example) rather than faint and diffuse.

Antibodies to cardiac myosin (a constituent of cardiac muscle) that have been labeled with the radioisotope indium 111 have recently been found useful in infarct-avid imaging. These antibodies (called antimyosin) are more specific for acute infarction than are the technetium 99m agents, and they are not taken up by the bone of the ribs or sternum. It is thought that antimyosin will prove to be useful in the assessment of heart transplants by revealing areas of necrosis associated with organ rejection.

[c]   Radionuclide Ventriculography

A number of indicators of ventricular function can be derived from radionuclide ventriculography (RVG), which uses a radioisotope (usually technetium 99m) that generally is attached to red blood cells (called a radiotracer). These studies can be performed by two methods. In the first-pass technique, the radiotracer is injected intravenously, and the gamma camera tracks its progress through the right side of the heart, the lungs and left heart. In the equilibrium or gated method, the radioactivity is recorded from several hundred cardiac cycles after the radiotracer has become uniformly distributed throughout the blood pool. The information for each cycle is divided into 24 or more frames, with the patient's EKG as the timing reference. A computer then generates from these frames a moving picture of the beating heart. Equilibrium scans frequently are made immediately after first-pass scans, because no additional radioisotope is required.

Because the amount of radioactivity detected in radionuclide ventriculography is proportional to blood volume, equilibrium scans permit left and right ventricular ejection fractions (the amount of blood ejected by the ventricle with each heartbeat) and other measures of ventricular performance to be calculated. Since scans can be obtained up to 20 hours after injection, the effects of exercise and medications on ventricular function also can be estimated.

Radionuclide ventriculography also is used to detect chronic ischemia. Scans are made with the patient at rest and at peak exercise level. A failure of the left ventricular ejection fraction to increase by at least 5 percent or the development of one or more regional wall-movement abnormalities indicates significant coronary artery disease. In addition, radionuclide ventriculography can be used to detect mitral valve regurgitation and septal rupture and to assess systolic function in patients with cardiomyopathy.

Equilibrium scans also are useful for monitoring the diastolic functioning of the heart, that is, how well the left ventricle fills between contractions. Elderly cardiac patients, especially, often have a normal ejection fraction but poor filling of the ventricle due to ventricular stiffness. A patient with heart failure caused by poor ventricular filling requires treatment that is altogether different from that of a patient whose heart failure is a result of ventricular weakness.

[d] Shunt Scintigraphy

To detect and evaluate left-to-right intracardiac shunts, first-pass radionuclide ventriculography is modified in such a way that an area of the lung rather than the heart is the area of interest. After the radiotracer has been injected as a bolus into a large vein (usually the external jugular), a curve representing the amount of radioactivity detected by a gamma camera over time is plotted by a computer. If no left-to-right shunt is present, the radiation detected increases sharply as the bolus reaches the lung under the transducer. After this peak, the curve descends smoothly. Later, smaller peaks are seen that represent the normal recirculation of the radiotracer after it has passed through the systemic circulation.[16] A left-to-right shunt causes an interruption in the descent of the curve because of the early reappearance of radioactivity in the lung that is caused by blood passing from the left side of the heart to the right without having to go the normal route through the systemic circulation.

---

[16] *See* 7.10 *supra.*

[6]   Single Photon Emission Computed Tomography

In single photon emission computed tomography (SPECT), a tomogram (three-dimensional picture) is produced by a camera system that rotates around the patient and measures the radioactivity emitted by a radioisotope, usually thallium 201. This technique is somewhat more expensive than the other radionuclide imaging techniques just described, but it may be superior to them in detecting the size and location of defects in the heart caused by coronary artery disease, in identifying the arteries responsible for the defects and in assessing the effectiveness of treatment for ischemic heart disease. Single photon computed tomography also permits determination of the mass of infarcted myocardium—knowledge that is helpful in determining prognosis.

[7]   Positron Emission Tomography

Positron emission tomography (PET) is an imaging technique that measures the metabolic activity of the heart (the way in which the heart uses the energy sources supplied to it) and the flow of blood through the myocardium. The latter information can provide information on the viability of myocardium injured by ischemia and can be useful in predicting the response of injured myocardium to treatment that restores normal blood flow. Knowledge of the metabolic activity of the heart may be helpful in monitoring the response of the heart muscle to treatment. Because the equipment needed for positron emission tomography is very expensive, the technique is used primarily as a research tool and is not employed routinely in the diagnosis of heart disease.

In PET of the heart, a positron emitter (or a combination of emitters) is injected into the patient, and three-dimensional images are produced by a scanner that detects the concentration and position of the emitter. (A positron is a positively charged electron produced during the decay of the nucleus of an atom). Blood flow in the myocardium can be measured with oxygen 15 (15O), rubidium 82 (82Rb) or nitrogen 13 (13N)-labeled ammonia. Metabolic activities, such as glucose utilization, fat utilization and myocardial oxygen consumption, are evaluated by measuring the uptake of fluorine 18 (18F)-labeled deoxyglucose, carbon 11 (11C)-labeled palmitate, and carbon 11-labeled acetate, respectively.

[8] Fast Computed Tomography

Fast computed tomography is capable of providing images of the entire heart that allow highly accurate evaluation of both anatomy and function. In conventional computed tomography, a scanning camera that detects x-rays is rotated around the patient, and a computer processes the electronic information from the scan to produce three-dimensional images or tomograms. In fast computed tomography, the scanner creates a complete tomogram in just 50 milliseconds, which eliminates the interference caused by the motion of the heart. The tomograms produced are connected in a closed-loop cinematic fashion to produce a cine display (hence the other name for fast computed tomography: cine-computed tomography). About 12 to 14 adjacent tomograms are linked to encompass an adult heart. The blood pool can be distinguished from the myocardium by the intravenous injection of a contrast medium (a substance that blocks the passage of x-rays).

Fast computed tomography is used in the detection and evaluation of diseases of the aorta, pericardial diseases, masses (tumors or blood clots) on and in the heart, and complications of myocardial infarction. The technique also is useful in analyzing ventricular function, determining the patency of coronary bypass grafts and evaluating cardiomyopathy.

[9] Magnetic Resonance Imaging (MRI)

Magnetic resonance imaging (MRI) is a noninvasive diagnostic technique that provides highly detailed images of the heart without the use of ionizing radiation or a contrast medium. It is quite expensive, however, and sophisticated MRI equipment is not available everywhere. Presently, therefore, it is used mainly for research.

Magnetic resonance imaging is useful in the diagnosis and assessment of a wide variety of cardiac abnormalities, including aortic and pericardial diseases, tumors, blood clots, myocardial hypertrophy, complications of myocardial infarction and congenital heart disease. It also is helpful in the detection and evaluation of valvular regurgitation.

[10] Diagnostic Cardiac Catheterization and Angiography

Diagnostic cardiac catheterization provides such precise information about the anatomy and physiology of the heart and is so reliable that it is the standard against which all other diagnostic methods are compared. More than 900,000 cardiac catheterizations are performed each year for the evaluation of coronary artery, valvular, congenital and myocardial diseases of the heart (Zaret, 1992). The procedure is used when there is a need to confirm the presence of a heart condition that is suspected on the basis of clinical symptoms and/or the results of another type of diagnostic examination, to determine the severity of a disease and to assess whether other conditions are associated with a disease.

Cardiac catheterization generally is a safe procedure. It is invasive, however, and carries a risk of complications, including myocardial infarction, stroke, perforation of the heart or vessels, local vascular problems and, in rare instances, death. For this reason, cardiac catheterization usually is performed in a hospital so that emergency services are available.

Discomfort associated with cardiac catheterization seems to be unavoidable for some patients, and about 10 percent of patients undergoing the procedure experience nausea and vomiting after the injection of the contrast medium required for angiography. Some patients (generally less than 10 percent) respond to the injection of contrast medium with an allergic reaction, such as headache, sneezing, chills, fever, hives, itching or anaphylactic shock (a violent attack of allergic symptoms that can result in death). Patients with a history of allergic reaction to contrast media may be treated preventively with a glucocorticoid (e.g., prednisone), an antihistamine (e.g., diphenhydramine) and an H_2 blocker (e.g., cimetidine) 18 to 24 hours before cardiac catheterization. It is essential that epinephrine for intravenous injection be readily available during cardiac catheterization for the treatment of anaphylactic shock, should it occur.

The risk factors for death from cardiac catheterization include age (infants and the elderly have a greater risk; elderly women appear to be at a higher risk than elderly men), a high degree of cardiac dysfunction, severe coronary artery obstruction, severe valvular heart disease and severe noncardiac disease (especially renal insufficiency, insulin-dependent diabetes mellitus, severe pulmonary insufficiency and advanced vascular disease) (Grossman, 1991).

Cardiac catheterization has three main uses:

1. Measurement of heart function on the basis of pressure readings taken around the valves and within the ventricles, arteries and veins.

2. Imaging of the ventricles, coronary arteries and other vessels after the injection of a radiopaque contrast medium (a procedure known as cardiac angiography.

3. Biopsy of heart muscle by means of special instruments inserted into the cardiac catheter.

The first two procedures are performed routinely, whereas a biopsy is performed only if there are specific indications for it, such as cardiomyopathy or inflammatory heart disease. A biopsy may also be performed to assess the possibility of transplant rejection. Angiography is particularly useful for diagnosing congenital abnormalities, for assessing the contraction of the ventricles and for identifying narrowed or obstructed coronary arteries.

[a]   The Procedure

To perform cardiac catheterization, the operator inserts a cardiac catheter (a long, thin, flexible tube) through a large needle and a hollow sheath into an artery or vein. (*See Figure 7–5.*) With the aid of a fluoroscope (a machine that shows the shadows of x-rays passed through the body), the operator then threads the catheter through the vein or artery into the heart. The procedure is performed with the patient in a fasting state and sedated but awake.

Right-heart catheterization is usually performed by maneuvering a balloon catheter (a catheter with a sac at its tip that can be distended with gas) from a suitable vein (brachial, femoral, subclavian or internal jugular) into the superior vena cava (one of the two large veins that brings blood to the heart from the body), where blood is withdrawn for the measurement of oxygen content. Then the catheter is advanced to the right atrium, where pressure is measured. The balloon is inflated with air or carbon dioxide and threaded into the right ventricle and pulmonary artery, where pressures are again measured and a blood sample is taken through the catheter tip. With the use of a thermistor (a thermometer than can measure extremely small changes in temperature), it is possible to measure cardiac output after the injection of cold sodium chloride solution.

Comparison of the amount of oxygen in the blood in the vena cava, chambers and pulmonary artery allows the detection of a left-to-right shunt. In addition, careful attention to the course of the catheter as it passes through the chambers of the right heart can reveal the presence of congenital heart disease, such as a defect in the atrial

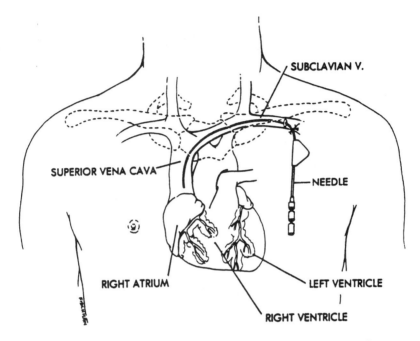

Fig. 7-5. Cardiac catheterization; in this example, the catheter is threaded through the subclavian vein and into the heart.

septum or a patent ductus arteriosus (a fetal blood vessel that normally closes after birth).

Left-side-heart catheterization via the brachial artery begins with a surgical cut in the right or left antecubital fossa (the depression in the anterior region of the elbow) to expose the artery. Then the catheter is advanced to the central aorta, where pressure is measured. Next the catheter is maneuvered across the aortic valve into the left ventricle, where pressure again is measured. If a right-side-heart catheter is in place, the simultaneous measurement of left-heart, right-heart and peripheral arterial pressures for the determination of possible pressure gradients across the cardiac valves is possible. The simultaneous measurement of these pressures and cardiac output provides the information needed to calculate systemic and pulmonary vascular resistance.

When left-heart catheterization is performed via the femoral artery, the artery is punctured with a needle, a guide wire is passed to the abdominal aorta, and a sheath with a side arm is put in place to allow flushing and continuous pressure measurement. Next, a catheter is advanced over the guide wire to the descending aorta, at which time the guide wire is removed and the catheter is threaded to the ascending aorta, where pressure is measured at the same time as peripheral arterial pressure is recorded in the side arm.

[b] Cardiac Angiography

To perform cardiac angiography, the clinician injects a radiopaque contrast medium into a specific chamber or vessel of the heart through the tip of a cardiac catheter using a hand-or power-driven syringe. The flow of the contrast medium is then observed on moving x-ray pictures called angiograms.

The most common type of coronary angiography is coronary arteriography, which is the selective injection of contrast medium into the coronary arteries to allow assessment of the severity of stenosis (blockage), to detect congenital abnormalities of the coronary circulation and to check the patency of coronary bypass grafts. Left ventriculography refers to the injection of roentgenographic contrast medium into the left ventricle to permit calculation of left ventricular chamber volume and ejection fraction, evaluation of regional abnormalities of wall motion, detection of stenosis (narrowing) of the mitral and aortic valves, and the assessment of the thickness of the cusps of the mitral and aortic valves.

A specialized method, known as digital subtraction angiography, uses a computer to digitize high-resolution x-ray images. After the injection of the angiographic contrast medium, an image of the region of interest is subtracted from other images by the computer. The elimination of the images of soft tissue and bone provides good definition of cardiac and vascular structures. Digital subtraction angiography of the heart can be especially valuable in the assessment of ventricular function and the diagnosis of congenital abnormalities.

7.40 CORONARY ARTERY DISEASE

Coronary artery disease is a progressive narrowing of the channels of the coronary arteries due to atherosclerosis that eventually results in myocardial ischemia (an imbalance between the demand of the heart muscle for oxygen and the supply of oxygen reaching the muscle). Atherosclerosis is a condition in which scattered plaques (atheromas) gradually form on the inner wall of an artery, causing the arterial wall to thicken and become less elastic. Atheromas are made of a mixture of cholesterol, fat and fibrous tissue. The major complications of coronary artery disease are angina pectoris, myocardial infarction and sudden cardiac death.

7.41 Angina Pectoris

Angina pectoris (often referred to simply as angina) is a syndrome caused by myocardial ischemia that is characterized by episodes of discomfort and/or pressure felt above the heart. The episodes typically are precipitated by physical exertion and are relieved by rest or the sublingual (under the tongue) administration of nitroglycerin. Stable angina pectoris refers to angina pectoris in which the patient knows fairly well the degree of exertion that will trigger an attack. Unpredictability of the anginal pattern (any increase in the frequency or duration of attacks, decrease in the activity needed to precipitate them or occurrence while the person is at rest) is referred to as unstable angina pectoris.

In some people, angina pectoris most often occurs after a meal. This is because blood pooling in the digestive system increases the work load of the heart, which, in turn, increases the heart's demand for oxygen. Angina also may be more frequent in cold weather, because spasms of the blood vessels caused by cold can increase the work load of the heart and decrease the supply of blood to the heart.

[1] Symptoms and Diagnosis

The discomfort of angina pectoris is usually felt beneath the sternum (breastbone). It may range from a vague ache to an intense crushing sensation. Pain may radiate to the left shoulder and down the inside of the left arm, or it may radiate to the back or into the throat, jaws and teeth. Occasionally pain is felt in the right arm. An episode of angina pectoris usually lasts no more than a few minutes. Attacks vary in frequency from several per day to episodes separated by weeks, months or years. Since the characteristics of a given person's angina are usually constant, the development of unstable angina should be considered serious.

Angina pectoris is diagnosed primarily on the basis of the characteristic complaint of chest discomfort that is brought on by exertion and relieved by rest. The diagnosis can be confirmed by observing characteristic changes in the EKG during an attack that are reversed by the administration of nitroglycerin. An exercise tolerance test or radionuclide imaging during peak exercise stress and after rest can reveal the presence of ischemia, but false-positive and false-negative test results occur (Levinson, et al., 1991). Echocardiography may be useful in the diagnosis of angina pectoris by revealing impaired cardiac function and thickening of the walls of the left ventricle and by helping to rule out other problems, such as valvular heart disease. Coronary angiography will confirm the presence of coronary artery obstruction due to coronary artery disease.[17]

Chest pain caused by other conditions may be mistaken for angina pectoris. Sources of such pain include a pulled muscle in the chest area, a broken rib, reflux of stomach acid into the esophagus (heart-burn), pain due to the obstruction of bile flow (gallbladder disease), inflammation of the cartilage of the chest wall, arthritis of the bones of the neck, infection of the airways (bronchitis) and pericardial disease. Circulatory disorders, such as high blood pressure in the lungs or a blood clot in an artery supplying the lungs, can also result in anginalike symptoms.

[2] Treatment

The first step in treating angina pectoris is the fostering of behavior changes that help halt the progression or reverse the underlying coronary artery disease. As necessary, these measures may be supplemented by drug therapy and surgical procedures such as coronary bypass surgery and balloon angioplasty.

[a] Behavior Modification

Fostering changes in behavior, if necessary through a formal rehabilitation program, is central to the treatment of coronary artery disease, which is the primary cause of angina pectoris (Dennis, 1992). For smokers, quitting is the first and perhaps the most effective behavior change that can be undertaken. Changes in diet also are important. Reducing the intake of saturated fats and cholesterol, while increasing the intake of starches and high-fiber foods, may significantly lower blood cholesterol concentrations.

Also, aerobic exercise has many possible benefits, including weight reduction, lowering of blood cholesterol levels and blood pressure, stress reduction and the creation of a general feeling of well-being.

---

[17] *See* 7.33 *supra* for a discussion of diagnostic methods.

The conditioning effect of exercise also enables the patient to perform more work while requiring less oxygen (Levine and Balady, 1993). Exercise need not be strenuous, but it is essential that it be energetic enough to gradually increase the heart rate. It also is important that exercise be regular, that is, performed at least three to five times a week.

Stress has been shown to be only weakly associated with high blood pressure and coronary artery disease. Changes in behavior that reduce stress may nevertheless be valuable in treating angina pectoris, because reduction in stress benefits the body as a whole. Stress generally is not due so much to having a lot to do but to a sense of being overwhelmed by demands over which one has no control. Regular time set aside to pursue an enjoyable activity may help reduce stress. In some cases, psychological counseling is helpful.

[b]   Drug Therapy

Drug treatment of stable angina pectoris is aimed at reducing ischemia and thereby minimizing symptoms by the administration of compounds belonging to three classes: the nitrates, the beta-adrenergic blocking agents (usually called beta-blockers) and the calcium antagonists (also called calcium-channel blockers). Treatment usually is begun with a beta-blocker and a nitrate. A calcium antagonist may be added later, especially if the patient also has high blood pressure.

Nitrates, which act as vasodilators (drugs that expand the blood vessels), can be used to relieve an attack of angina or can be taken before exertion to prevent an attack. Sublingual nitroglycerin generally is the most effective drug. Amyl nitrate may be effective when severe angina is unresponsive to nitroglycerin and is complicated by hypertension. Tolerance to nitrates develops within 24 hours if blood concentrations are held constant. Therefore, it is recommended that periods without nitrates be provided if symptoms permit. The efficacy of nitroglycerin usually returns after a period of eight hours without use.

The beta-adrenergic blocking agents block stimulation of the heart by the sympathetic nervous system, thereby reducing systolic blood pressure, heart rate and cardiac output. This contributes to a reduction in the demand of the heart muscle for oxygen and increases exercise tolerance. These drugs are very useful in reducing symptoms and are well tolerated by most patients.

Calcium plays an important role in the contraction of the smooth muscle cells of the arteries, and calcium antagonists work by blocking the channels through which calcium normally enters these cells. These drugs help block the muscle contraction that causes coronary artery spasm and thereby improve blood flow to the myocardium.

It currently is thought that unstable angina pectoris is associated with an increase in coronary artery obstruction brought on by the rupture of an atheroma, with subsequent adhesion of blood platelets and the formation of occluding thrombi (blood clots). The anticoagulants heparin and aspirin both have been shown to reduce the incidence of subsequent myocardial infarction in patients with unstable angina pectoris. Nasally administered oxygen, nitrates, beta-adrenergic blockers and calcium antagonists also may be useful in reducing the work load of the heart by slowing the heart rate and lowering blood pressure. Thrombolytic agents (drugs that dissolve clots) have not been found useful in the treatment of unstable angina.

[c] Coronary Bypass Surgery

Coronary bypass surgery provides complete relief of angina pectoris in about 70 percent of patients and partial relief in about 20 percent of patients (Deckelbaum, 1992). This procedure provides new conduits that bypass partially or completely obstructed areas of one or more of the coronary arteries. The new conduits are fashioned from sections of veins removed from the saphenous vein of the leg or from the internal mammary artery of the chest wall. About 320,000 coronary bypass operations are now performed in the United States each year (Deckelbaum, 1992).

The patient selected for coronary bypass surgery ideally should have severe angina, a heart of normal size, no history of myocardial infarction and good ventricular function. In such patients, there is a risk of about 5 percent that myocardial infarction will occur during surgery, and the mortality rate is about 1.5 percent. After one year, about 85 percent of bypass grafts are patent (open). Mortality during a second bypass operation is three to five times that during the first operation (Berkow and Fletcher, 1992).

[d] Balloon Angioplasty

In this procedure (also called percutaneous transluminal coronary angioplasty), a balloon catheter is inserted into an artery and maneuvered to the site of an obstructing atherosclerotic plaque. Inflation of the balloon flattens and/or breaks the plaque and simultaneously dilates the vessel by disrupting its lining and wall. In the United States, more than 200,000 balloon angioplasty procedures are performed each year (Deckelbaum, 1992).

Care must be exercised in the selection of patients to undergo this operation. Ideally the patient will have only one or two obstructed coronary arteries, and the obstructions must be in areas that can be reached by the catheter. Improvements in technique and devices have made balloon angioplasty an increasingly effective method for treating angina pectoris that does not respond to drug treatment (Lange, 1991; Tenaglia and Stack, 1993), but about 30 percent of blockages recur within six months (Meier, 1991). Mortality and myocardial infarction rates during the procedure are about 1 to 3 percent and 3 to 5 percent, respectively (Berkow and Fletcher, 1992).

7.42   Acute Myocardial Infarction

Acute myocardial infarction (often referred to simply as myocardial infarction or heart attack) is due to myocardial necrosis (death of tissue) resulting from an abrupt reduction in coronary artery blood flow to a segment of the myocardium. An infarct that affects as little as 10 percent of the myocardium can cause death if it involves a critical area or if it causes arrhythmia (irregular heartbeat) or perforation of the heart wall. On the other hand, infarcts that affect up to 40 percent of the myocardium,can be survived if a less critical area is involved (Deckelbaum, 1992).

In the United States, about 1.5 million people have heart attacks each year, and about 25 percent of the stricken individuals die. About half of all heart attack sufferers die before they can reach a hospital. Of those who survive a myocardial infarction, 5 to 10 percent die within the first year after the attack (Pasternak and Braunwald, 1991).

The vast majority of heart attacks are a direct result of coronary artery disease. In more than 90 percent of cases of acute myocardial infarction, a thrombus (clot), usually forming on a ruptured atheroma, occludes the coronary artery (previously partially obstructed by the atheroma) that supplies the necrotic area of the myocardium (Forrester, et al., 1991). Acute myocardial infarction also may be caused by an embolus (a clot that has traveled from a distant site in the body), especially in persons with aortic valve stenosis or infective endocarditis, or by a coronary artery spasm, but the latter two causes are rare.

[1] Symptoms

Deep visceral pain is the most common symptom in patients experiencing acute myocardial infarction. The pain may be excruciating and commonly is described as heavy, squeezing or crushing. The pain of myocardial infarction is similar to that of angina pectoris but is usually more severe and lasts much longer. Typically, it is felt in the center of the chest and, in about 30 percent of cases, it radiates to the arms. Less common sites of pain are the abdomen, back, lower jaw and neck.

The pain of a heart attack is often accompanied by weakness, nausea, vomiting, sweating, dizziness and anxiety. In about two thirds of cases, the pain starts when the patient is at rest, and the most common time of occurrence is the early morning. When the pain of acute myocardial infarction is brought on by exertion, it does not subside with rest. About half of the patients who suffer acute myocardial infarction have previously experienced unstable angina pectoris.[18]

In about 15 to 20 percent of cases of myocardial infarction, there is no pain, especially in patients with diabetes mellitus and in the elderly (Pasternak and Braunwald, 1991). In the elderly, myocardial infarction may be manifested by sudden breathlessness. Other, less common symptoms of heart attack, which may or may not be accompanied by pain, include sudden loss of consciousness, arrhythmia, confusion and an unexplained drop in arterial blood pressure.

[2] Diagnosis

Acute myocardial infarction is often suspected from the patient's history and should be considered in all men over the age of 35 and all women over the age of 50 when the major symptom is chest pain. The diagnosis is confirmed on the basis of the results of the physical examination and the laboratory test findings.

[a] Physical Examination

The patient experiencing acute myocardial infarction is usually restless, apprehensive, pale, sweating and in severe pain. Blood pressure is variable, but many patients show some degree of hypertension. Arrhythmia is common, and of the patients who die during acute myocardial infarction, at least half succumb to ventricular fibrillation

---

[18] *See* 7.41 *supra.*

(an arrhythmia characterized by rapid contractions of the ventricular muscle due to repetitive excitation of myocardial fibers without coordinated contraction of the muscle) [19] before reaching the hospital (Berkow and Fletcher, 1992). The heart sounds are usually somewhat distant, and third and fourth heart sounds often are present. Other possible abnormalities include a systolic murmur (a reflection of dysfunction of the papillary muscle) and a friction rub (a scraping or grating sound created by the rubbing together of the inflamed surfaces of the pericardium).

[b] Laboratory Test Findings

Routine laboratory blood tests reveal nonspecific abnormalities typical of tissue necrosis, including an increase in white blood cell count and in erythrocyte sedimentation rate that appears within a few hours of the onset of pain and persists for several days.

Enzymes are released into the blood from necrotic heart muscle after myocardial infarction, and the rate of release of specific enzymes is diagnostic. The level of creatine kinase in the blood increases within 8 to 24 hours of myocardial necrosis and usually returns to normal within 48 to 72 hours. The lactate dehydrogenase level rises later, within 24 to 48 hours, and remains elevated for 7 to 14 days. The MB enzyme of creatine kinase (CK-MB) is especially useful in the diagnosis of myocardial infarction because it is not present in significant concentrations in tissue outside the heart.

The most important step in the diagnosis of acute myocardial infarction is analysis of the electrocardiogram, which shows striking abnormalities recognizable to the trained observer. Radionuclide imaging with thallium 201 or technetium 99m pyrophosphate may be used to identify infarction and to measure the area affected. These evaluations are time consuming and expensive, however, and the information gained from them often is of little benefit in the diagnosis or treatment of myocardial infarction. Information on intracardiac blood pressures and cardiac output gained by cardiac catheterization may be valuable in the management of certain complications of myocardial infarction. such as severe heart failure, hypoxia (inadequate supply of oxygen) or hypertension.

---

[19] See 7.52[2] infra.

[3] Treatment

The four principle objectives in treating the heart attack victim are relief of distress, limiting the size of the infarct, reduction of heart activity and prevention of death from complications.

[a] Prehospital Treatment

The immediate threat to life from acute myocardial infarction is ventricular fibrillation, with consequent low blood pressure that leads to cardiac arrest (absence or inadequacy of ventricular contraction, with immediate systemic circulatory failure). Optimal early treatment by an emergency medical team includes alleviation of pain and apprehension, stabilization of heart rhythm and blood pressure, and administration of a thrombolytic agent (e.g., streptokinase or recombinant tissue plasminogen activator [rtPA], agents that dissolve blood clots), if one is available. Thrombolytic therapy, if it is applied before damage to the myocardium is irreversible, may allow the return of blood flow to the infarcted area, thereby limiting infarct size and ventricular dysfunction.

Intravenous (IV) morphine is highly effective in alleviating the pain of myocardial infarction, but it depresses the respiration. Continued pain may be relieved in some patients by the sublingual or intravenous administration of nitroglycerin.

An extremely low heart rate and hypotension may respond to treatment with atropine sulfate. Severe hypotension may be treated with a vasopressor, a drug that stimulates contraction of the muscle of the capillaries and arteries (e.g., isoproterenol, norepinephrine, dopamine or amirone). Ventricular arrhythmia may be treated with an intravenous antiarrhythmic drug, such as procainamide or lidocaine. In patients who do no have hypotension or another contraindication, the administration of a beta-blocker may reduce the likelihood of ventricular fibrillation.

[b] Hospital Treatment

Patients suspected of having acute myocardial infarction should be admitted as soon as possible to a hospital with an emergency room equipped to treat acute heart problems and a cardiac care unit. If the diagnosis is unmistakable, an aspirin tablet should be chewed immediately, and a thrombolytic agent should be administered. Some authorities recommend the intravenous administration of a beta-blocker (atenolol or metoprolol, for example). Heart rate and rhythm should be continuously monitored by EKG.

The quality of heart function after recovery from a heart attack depends on the amount of functioning myocardium that remains. If more than 50 percent of the heart muscle has been damaged, survival is unusual. Using a vasodilator (nitroglycerin) to effect reduction of cardiac work and consumption of oxygen by the heart muscle, and using a a beta-blocker to effect reduction of heart rate and contractility, may help minimize the area of infarction.

Anxiety, mood changes, denial and depression are common in patients who have experienced acute myocardial infarction. The administration of a mild tranquilizer (diazepam, for example) may be helpful in alleviating distress.

[c]   Treatment of Complications

Cardiac arrest due to ventricular fibrillation is treated by immediate defibrillation (also called cardioversion), which involves the administration of a brief electric shock to the heart through paddles applied to the chest. The shock temporarily halts all electric activity in the heart, allowing the heart to reestablish its normal rhythm. Antiarrhythmic drugs are usually administered preventively after the patient has been resuscitated.

Heart failure, usually with a predominance of left ventricular dysfunction, occurs in about two thirds of hospitalized patients with acute myocardial infarction. Treatment in this circumstance depends on the severity of the heart failure. The administration of a loop diuretic drug, such as furosemide, to reduce ventricular filling pressure may be all that is necessary. Treatment of heart failure caused by acute myocardial infarction is similar to that of heart failure due to other diseases. The major difference is that cardiac glycosides, such as digitalis, have not been found to be particularly effective in patients with myocardial infarction.

Hypoxemia (low blood level of oxygen) is common in patients with acute myocardial infarction. The administration of oxygen through a nasal cannula may be effective in maintaining an adequate level of oxygen in the blood, which, in turn, may limit the extent of infarction or ischemia.

Cardiogenic shock, a condition characterized by hypotension, rapid heart rate, reduced urine output, confusion, profuse sweating and cold extremities, carries a mortality rate of 65 percent or greater. This complication of acute myocardial infarction is usually associated with massive infarction and loss of left ventricular function. Treatment with dopamine, dobutamine or both may be temporarily effective. Injection into the coronary artery of a thrombolytic agent or emergency balloon angioplasty to break up the occluding clot may be effective in patients who do not respond to drug treatment.

Myocardial rupture is a complication of myocardial infarction that is marked by sudden disappearance of the pulse and blood pressure and loss of consciousness, even though the EKG continues to show normal sinoatrial heart rhythm. The myocardium continues to contract, but blood flow to the arteries ceases as blood escapes into the pericardium. The result is cardiac tamponade (compression of the heart) and, in the vast majority of cases, death. In rare instances, emergency heart surgery has been successful in preventing death.

Rupture of the interventricular septum is recognized by the sudden appearance of a characteristic systolic murmur accompanied by hypotension, with or without left ventricular failure. The diagnosis may be confirmed by the insertion of a balloon catheter and comparison of the oxygen levels in the right atrium, right ventricle and pulmonary artery, or by Doppler echocardiography.[20] Mortality is high with this complication, too, but surgical repair may be possible.

Ventricular aneurysm is a common complication of myocardial infarction in which an outpocketing is formed by a dilation of the wall of the ventricle. Ventricular aneurysms, which may not develop until weeks or months after acute infarction, are composed of scar tissue and do not predispose the patient to cardiac rupture. They may be associated with heart failure and ventricular arrhythmia. The EKG shows characteristic changes in the ST segment; the chest x-ray may show a characteristic bulge in the heart, and two-dimensional echocardiography may reveal a thrombus in the aneurysm. Surgical repair may be necessary if persistent heart failure or arrhythmia is present.

7.43 Sudden Cardiac Death

The term sudden cardiac death, which literally implies a swift and unexpected death due to a cardiac cause, is used by different clinicians to mean different things. It may be used to refer to death occurring within moments of the onset of symptoms (the victim may be said

---

[20] *See* 7.33[3][d] *supra.*

to have "dropped dead"). More commonly, however, it is used to designate death that occurs within one to several hours—or even 24 hours—after the appearance of symptoms. Some practitioners use "sudden cardiac death" to refer to one that occurs before the patient reaches the hospital, and some restrict their use of the term to the death of persons thought to be free of heart disease or to persons with mild heart disease and no acute symptoms.

The vast majority of sudden cardiac deaths are due to coronary artery disease, and in about 20 percent of cases, it is the first manifestation of the disease. The more severe the coronary artery disease (severity is manifested by acute heart failure and arrhythmia), the more likely is sudden cardiac death. Another important risk factor for sudden cardiac death is a history of myocardial infarction. Other diseases that can lead to sudden cardiac death are cardiomyopathy,[21] congenital heart disease, rheumatic heart disease,[22] cor pulmonale[23] and bacterial endocarditis.

Obstruction due to a thrombus or a ruptured atheroma is found in only a minority of patients who have experienced rapid sudden cardiac death but in most patients with later sudden death. The tissue changes typical of acute myocardial infarction are found in only a small fraction of victims of sudden cardiac death, because the changes do not have time to develop before death ensues. Ventricular fibrillation is the most common arrhythmia observed immediately after collapse. Cardiac standstill (cessation of contraction of the myocardium) usually occurs later after collapse.

[1] Symptoms

Questioning of the family and associates of the person who has succumbed to sudden cardiac death often reveals new or progressive symptoms of heart disease that occurred for several days—or for only a few hours or minutes—before death. Such symptoms include chest discomfort, palpitations, increased angina pectoris, dyspnea (difficulty breathing), overwhelming fatigue and depression. The symptoms may not seem particularly noteworthy to the victim and may not be recognized as warning signs.

---

[21] *See* 7.70 *infra.*

[22] *See* 7.90 *infra.*

[23] *See* 7.80 *infra.*

[2] Diagnosis

Sudden cardiac death is diagnosed on the basis of the clinical symptoms that preceded death and the autopsy finding of coronary artery disease or other heart disease. Causes of death that must be excluded include pulmonary embolism, the action of prescribed or illegally obtained drugs, stroke, infection and gastrointestinal bleeding or perforation.

[3] Prevention

The prevention of sudden cardiac death includes prompt attention to acute symptoms and the cardiac resuscitation (re-establishment of heart and lung action by artificial respiration and heart massage) of persons who develop cardiac arrest. The most effective prevention against sudden cardiac death, however, is the prevention of coronary artery disease, which includes the avoidance of smoking, obesity and a sedentary life-style, and the control of high blood levels of cholesterol and hypertension.

7.44 Asymptomatic ("Silent") Ischemia

The increasing use of exercise-tolerance tests during routine physical examinations has revealed that a large number of people have severe coronary artery disease—and may even have experienced acute myocardial infarction—but show no symptoms (Valle, 1990). Ambulatory EKG performed in these people may reveal frequent episodes of asymptomatic or "silent" ischemia during daily activities. Studies have shown an increased incidence of sudden cardiac death, myocardial infarction and angina pectoris in these patients.

The decision of whether and how to treat patients with asymptomatic ischemia is based on a number of factors, including:

- the stage of exercise at which the EKG signs of ischemia appear;

- the number and size of the areas of poor cardiac blood flow revealed by thallium imaging;[24]

- the change in left ventricular ejection fraction, as shown by radionuclide ventriculography, that occurs during exercise; and

---

[24] *See* 7.33[5][a] *supra.*

● the patient's age, occupation and general health. Patients with evidence of severe ischemia revealed by noninvasive testing should undergo coronary arteriography.

The incidence of episodes of asymptomatic ischemia may be reduced by treatment with beta-blockers, calcium antagonists and nitrates, but there is no consensus on whether such treatment is desirable in patients who have not experienced a myocardial infarction. Asymptomatic patients with severe coronary artery disease and impaired left ventricular function may be considered candidates for coronary artery bypass surgery.

7.50   CARDIAC ARRHYTHMIA

A disturbance of heart rhythm, referred to as a cardiac arrhythmia, represents a medical paradox. Nearly everyone has experienced the extra or skipped heartbeats or the fluttering, racing or thumping of the heart known medically as palpitations. These symptoms of arrhythmia may be merely annoying occurrences in an otherwise healthy heart, or they may indicate the presence of a serious or even life-threatening heart condition. Some people with cardiac arrhythmia experience more distressing symptoms, such as dizziness, fainting, chest pain and dyspnea (shortness of breath). The seriousness of the symptoms, however, does not necessarily indicate the seriousness of the disorder underlying the arrhythmia, and many people with arrhythmia have no symptoms.

The physician confronted with a patient with arrhythmia has the difficult task of assessing the risks posed by the disturbance and deciding whether to attempt to suppress the arrhythmias with drugs. Antiarrhythmic drug treatment carries the potential for adverse effects that in themselves may be life threatening. In addition, there is considerable evidence that the suppression of some types of arrhythmia does not improve the patient's prognosis (McPherson and Rosenfeld, 1992; Berkow and Fletcher, 1992).

Although a number of heart ailments may underlie abnormal heart rhythm, the immediate cause is a malfunction of the heart's conduction system.[25] There are two general types of arrhythmia: bradyarrhythmia (or bradycardia), which is an excessively slow heart rate, and tachyarrhythmia (tachycardia), which is an overly rapid heart rate.

---

[25] *See* 7.16 *supra.*

7.51 Bradyarrhythmia

The three types of bradyarrhythmias are sinus bradyarrhythmia, sick sinus syndrome and heart block.

[1] Sinus Bradyarrhythmia

Sinus bradyarrhythmia is defined as a heart rate lower than 60 beats per minute that has its origin in a normal sinoatrial node. A slow heart rate is considered abnormal when it reduces cardiac output to the point of reducing the flow of blood to the body enough to cause symptoms such as fatigue, dyspnea and fainting (syncope). Exercise may trigger these symptoms when the heart rate fails to increase enough to meet the body's need for an increased blood supply.

[2] Sick Sinus Syndrome

A bradyarrhythmic condition known as sick sinus syndrome occurs when the sinoatrial node (the "pacemaker" of the heart) fails to generate or conduct impulses as it should. The cause may be a disease that has damaged the sinoatrial node, the accumulation of fibrous or scar tissue in the node or a failure of the autonomic nervous system to properly regulate the activity of the node. In addition, certain antiarrhythmic, antihypertensive and other drugs can adversely affect the sinoatrial node. Children and adolescents who have had surgery to repair a congenital heart disease may develop sick sinus syndrome later in life as a result of scarring from the disease itself or from the surgery.

[3] Heart Block

A bradyarrhythmia known as heart block may be caused by a defect in the transmission of electric impulses through the atrioventricular node or another part of the heart's conduction system (e.g., the bundle of His or the Purkinje fibers), even when the sinoatrial node is generating the impulses properly.

Heart block usually is caused by inflammation and scarring of the conducting tissue of the heart, which often are due to coronary artery disease or high blood pressure but may also be caused by the aging process. Certain drugs can also cause heart block.

First-degree heart block is a result of slow conduction of impulses through the atrioventricular node. Second-degree heart block occurs when some of the impulses from the atria intermittently fail to reach and activate the ventricles, resulting in "skipped" or "dropped" beats. Third-degree heart block (or complete atrioventricular block) results when no impulses from the atria reach the ventricles. If an independent ventricular pacemaker takes over (myocardial cells outside the nodes are capable of generating impulses on their own), the ventricles will continue to contract. If there is a lag between the atrial contraction and the impulse from the ventricular pacemaker, however, the lack of ventricular contraction may cause fainting in what is called an Adam-Stokes attack. Patients with third-degree heart block also may develop heart failure.

7.52 Tachyarrhythmia

Two general types of tachyarrhythmia are recognized: supraventricular tachyarrhythmia (arising above the ventricle, that is, in the atria or the atrioventricular node), and ventricular tachyarrhythmia (arising in the ventricle). Both types may be triggered by an extra or early beat called an ectopic beat, which occurs when islands of cells in the heart outside the normal pacemaker express their latent ability to produce impulses. This can occur when conduction to some part of the myocardium is blocked or when the heart is overstimulated. Extra or early beats arising in the atria are called premature atrial contractions, atrial premature beats, atrial ectopic beats or atrial extrasystoles. These beats often occur in normal hearts and are usually benign and easily treated. They can precipitate supraventricular tachycardia, however.

[1] Supraventricular Tachyarrhythmia

A type of supraventricular tachyarrhythmia known as atrial flutter occurs when an extra or early beat triggers an electric impulse that travels in regular cycles around the atrium, causing the atrium to contract 250 to 350 times per minute. If the atrioventricular node blocks one of every two of these beats, the ventricle will contract only 125 to 175 times per minute. At this rate, a normal heart can effectively function for hours or even days, but a patient with structural heart disease may experience chest pain, faintness or heart failure.

Atrial fibrillation results when the impulse does not travel in regular cycles around the atrium but divides and follows many pathways, creating a confusion of beats that occurs at a rate of 350 or more per minute. The ventricular beat also becomes uncoordinated, and a rapid, irregular pulse is felt. Although atrial fibrillation can cause the heart to lose 20 to 30 percent of its pumping ability, the volume of blood pumped usually remains adequate. Fibrillation often occurs when the atrium is enlarged, but it can also occur in the absence of structural heart disease.

Sleep deprivation, excessive consumption of caffeine or alcohol and drugs such as amphetamines and cocaine can increase a person's susceptibility to atrial flutter or fibrillation. Underlying diseases include heart valve disease, hyperactivity of the thyroid gland, pulmonary disease and pericarditis (inflammation of the pericardium, the membranous sac surrounding the heart).

Paroxysmal supraventricular tachycardia, a condition characterized by heart rates ranging from 140 to 250 beats per minute, often occurs in persons born with an extra conduction pathway between the atria and the ventricles. These extra circuits usually are located in the sinoatrial node, but in some individuals, accessory pathways (or bypass tracts, as they sometimes are called) are situated outside the node. When the EKG of a patient with atrial fibrillation is found to have an accessory pathway, the patient is said to have Wolff-Parkinson-White syndrome. If it is properly treated, this syndrome may pose no serious threat. Rarely, however, persons with Wolff-Parkinson-White syndrome develop ventricular fibrillation that may result in death.

[2] Ventricular Tachyarrhythmia

Ventricular tachyarrhythmia is potentially more dangerous than supraventricular tachyarrhythmia, and it is more often associated with structural heart disease. Like supraventricular tachyarrhythmia, ventricular tachyarrhythmia may have no symptoms. The most common ventricular tachyarrhythmia is premature ventricular contraction. Such early or extra beats are common and benign in persons with a healthy heart. In rare circumstances, however, premature ventricular contractions can cause the ventricles to lapse into fibrillation, in which case, death usually occurs in a matter of minutes.[26]

7.53 Diagnosis

Patients often are able to describe their arrhythmias reliably enough to establish a working diagnosis. If the patient is examined during an arrhythmia, palpation of the peripheral pulse (which reflects ventricular activation) and the jugular venous pulse (reflecting both atrial and

---

[26] See 7.43 supra.

ventricular activation) may aid in differentiating a ventricular arrhythmia from a supraventricular arrhythmia and from second-and third-degree heart block.

The primary approach to the diagnosis of arrhythmia is the electrocardiogram (EKG), which is most useful if it is recorded when symptoms are occurring. Because exertion often provokes arrhythmia, an exercise test with electrocardiographic monitoring may be helpful. Signal-averaged EKGs are a means of predicting the risk that a person will experience potentially dangerous ventricular arrhythmia. Transesophageal EKG may be useful in the diagnosis of atrial arrhythmia, because the esophagus lies directly behind the atria. Ambulatory (Holter) monitoring that provides a record of the patient's heartbeat during regular activities for 24 or 48 hours may be especially beneficial in detecting the more serious types of premature ventricular contraction that are associated with the risk of ventricular fibrillation.

Invasive electrophysiology studies can be very useful in determining the best means of preventing a recurrence of sudden cardiac arrest and in evaluating patients at high risk of sudden cardiac death and those with paroxysmal supraventricular tachyarrhythmia. In these studies, electrodes are threaded through a venous catheter into the heart to make detailed recordings of the heart's electric activity. The electrodes can also be used to simulate extra beats to determine whether the beats trigger arrhythmia and to assess the effectiveness of therapy.

7.54   Treatment

The treatment approaches to cardiac arrhythmias include antiarrhythmic drugs, pacemakers, implantable defibrillators and surgery.

[1]   Antiarrhythmic Drugs

Antiarrhythmic drugs are the mainstay treatment for most potentially dangerous types of arrhythmia. No one drug is universally effective, all have limiting adverse side effects and all can aggravate or even promote arrhythmia. The selection of the right drug is difficult and often involves trial and error.

When employed as an antiarrhythmic agent, digitalis (digoxin) is used to treat atrial fibrillation and other supraventricular tachyarrhythmia because it slows the conduction of the electric impulse through the atrioventricular node, thereby reducing the ventricular contraction rate. Digitalis is contraindicated in the treatment of patients with conduction via accessory pathways. [27]

Beta-blockers are used to inhibit the effects of hormones that increase the heart rate and to enhance the effects of other antiarrhythmics. Propranolol is an often-used beta-blocker. The calcium antagonists slow the heart rate generated by the sinoatrial node and slow conduction through the atrioventricular node by changing the electric properties of heart tissue. They do this by inhibiting the flow of calcium in and out of cells. The calcium antagonists most commonly used to treat arrhythmia are diltiazem and verapamil. Beta-blockers and calcium antagonists may be useful in treating atrial fibrillation and paroxysmal supraventricular tachyarrhythmia.

Quinidine, procainamide, disopyramide, lidocaine, tocainide, mexiletine, flecainide, propafenone and moricizine are antiarrhythmics that stabilize irregular heart rhythm by blocking sodium channels and thereby slowing conduction. These drugs are very effective in suppressing ectopic beats, but they also depress left ventricular performance. Amiodarone is the most potent antiarrhythmic drug in use. It suppresses virtually all types of arrhythmia and also acts as a beta-blocker and a calcium antagonist. Because of its many side effects, however, it is approved only for the treatment of serious arrhythmia that does not respond to other drugs.

[2] Pacemakers

Some patients require an artificial pacemaker to correct their arrhythmia. These small, surgically implanted devices use batteries to produce electric impulses that stimulate the cardiac chambers to contract in much the same way as the heart's natural pacemaker, the sinoatrial node. The pacemaker is programmed to suit the needs of the individual. After implantation, minor surgery is occasionally required to allow replacement of the batteries. New interference-resistant circuitry has greatly reduced the risk that automobile distributors, radar antennae, microwave devices and metal detectors will interfere with pacemakers. Magnetic resonance imaging (MRI) examinations, however, may interfere with pacemaker function and should be avoided.

---

[27] See 7.52 supra.

[3]   Implantable Defibrillators

Implantable defibrillators deliver relatively low energy shocks to the heart to stop ventricular fibrillation. They currently are used to treat patients who have been resuscitated from sudden death and patients with life-threatening ventricular tachyarrhythmia that does not respond to drug treatment (Kutalek and Dreifus, 1993). Implantable defibrillators do not prevent arrhythmia, and it therefore is essential that they be used in conjunction with suppressive antiarrhythmic therapy.

[4]   Surgery

In patients with Wolff-Parkinson-White syndrome,[28] it may be possible to destroy the accessory pathway by surgery or with an intracardiac catheter (Prystowsky, et al., 1990). Surgical success rates are high, and the mortality rate is low. Surgery may be particularly beneficial for young people who might face a lifetime of antiarrhythmic therapy without it.

7.60   VALVULAR HEART DISEASE

Because the left side of the heart has a greater workload than the right, the mitral and aortic valves are more susceptible to disease than the tricuspid and pulmonary valves.[29] The narrowing of a valve opening is referred to as valvular stenosis. Stenosis occurs when the cusps of a valve become rigid, thickened or fused, and results in obstruction of the flow of blood through the affected valve. When a valve fails to close properly, the condition is known as valvular insufficiency or valvular incompetence, and a result is regurgitation (backward flow of a portion of the blood that has been ejected from a heart chamber). When the cusps of a valve shrink, the valve can become fixed in a partially open position, resulting in both stenosis and insufficiency.

Valvular stenosis and insufficiency cause the myocardium to dilate and thicken gradually as the heart attempts to compensate for the extra work it must do to pump an adequate amount of blood. Eventually, however, the enlarged heart may become weak, and heart failure may

---

[28] See 7.52[1] supra.

[29] See 7.12 supra for a complete discussion of the anatomy and physiology of the valves of the heart.

occur. Heart failure is responsible for the breathlessness and swelling of the ankles that are major symptoms of valvular heart disease. Heart valve disease can also lead to cardiomyopathy (disease of the myocardium) and arrhythmia.

Another serious complication of valvular heart disease is the formation of blood clots, which may then detach and travel through the bloodstream as emboli. An embolus that lodges in the brain may cause stroke, and one that blocks an artery in the leg may cause pain, discoloration and even gangrene. Such clots form when the rough surface of a damaged valve creates an area of blood stagnation.

Diseases of the heart valves may take decades to develop, and they may be in an advanced stage before they are detected. Many damaged valves cause no problems, however, and require no treatment other than the use of antibiotics before certain dental or surgical procedures to reduce the risk of endocarditis from microorganisms that may enter the bloodstream during the operation.

7.61 Mitral Valve Disease

Included among the conditions that can affect the mitral valve are prolapse, regurgitation and stenosis.

[1] Mitral Valve Prolapse

Mitral valve prolapse (also called systolic click murmur syndrome, Barlow's syndrome, billowing mitral valve syndrome and ballooned valve syndrome) is a bulging of one or both mitral cusps into the left atrium during systole, with the result that the valve fails to close properly. A crisp systolic sound (click) and late systolic regurgitation murmur may be audible. This condition may be inherited, and it usually is associated with myxomatous degeneration—a series of metabolic changes of unknown etiology that cause the tissue of the valve to lose its elasticity and become covered with starch deposits. Breakage of the chords that connect the valve to the ventricular walls may result. Mitral valve prolapse, which usually is very mild, occurs at a rate of about 5 to 10 percent in the otherwise normal population (Bender, 1992). Women are affected much more often than men.

[a] Symptoms and Diagnosis

Most patients with mitral valve prolapse have no symptoms. Those who do may experience fatigue, migraine, dizziness, dyspnea or palpitations. When a click and a murmur are present, the degree of regurgitation is usually mild to moderate. A cardiac angiogram will show contraction abnormalities, and an echocardiogram often reveals a prolongation and reduction in the velocity of the shortening of the circumferential muscle fibers in the inflow tract.

A click without a murmur is usually associated with prolapse of only the anterior mitral cusp. Patients who experience severe pain or arrhythmia frequently have left ventricular dysfunction that is apparent with myocardial perfusion imaging[30] and on the EKG. Cerebral emboli occur but are rare. The incidence of sudden death due to ventricular fibrillation in patients with mitral valve prolapse is less than 1 percent (Berkow and Fletcher, 1992).

[b] Treatment

When there are no symptoms or the symptoms are mild, mitral valve prolapse generally requires no treatment. Patients who have mitral regurgitation may be advised to refrain from strenuous activities, such as competitive sports. Arrhythmia and dizziness may be relieved by the administration of a beta-blocker. The use of a beta-blocker may also reduce the risk of fibrillation in patients with dangerous ventricular tachyarrhythmia.

[2] Mitral Regurgitation

Mitral regurgitation (also called mitral incompetence or mitral insufficiency) is defined as the backward flow of blood from the left ventricle into the left atrium through an incompetent mitral valve. In adults, the most common causes are mitral valve prolapse, papillary muscle dysfunction, valve damage due to rheumatic fever and ruptured chordae tendineae. Myocardial infarction may cause mitral insufficiency if the portion of the heart that supports the valve is damaged. Severe mitral regurgitation may cause heart failure.

[a] Symptoms and Diagnosis

The patient with mitral regurgitation may experience palpitations due to atrial fibrillation or dyspnea long before heart failure develops. In moderate to severe mitral regurgitation, the physical examination reveals a rapid pulse, a characteristic heart movement caused by enlargement of the left atrium and splitting of the second heart sound.

---

[30] *See* 7.33[5][a] *supra.*

If the condition is caused by mitral valve prolapse, papillary muscle dysfunction or ruptured chords, murmurs characteristic of these defects may be heard. The chest x-ray of patients with moderate to severe mitral regurgitation shows an enlarged left atrium and left ventricle, and the EKG exhibits signs of left atrial and left ventricular overload. Doppler echocardiography and left ventriculography may be useful in assessing the degree of regurgitation.

[b] Treatment

A patient with extreme heart failure or atrial fibrillation should receive anticoagulant therapy to prevent the formation of emboli. If the patient experiences symptoms of heart failure with less than ordinary exertion while receiving maximum drug treatment for heart failure, surgery to repair or replace the valve is advisable (Grunkemeier and Rahimtoola, 1990; McKay and Ross, 1993).

[3] Mitral Stenosis

Mitral stenosis is obstruction of the flow of blood from the left atrium into the left ventricle due to a narrowing of the mitral orifice. In the adult, this stenosis is nearly always a sequela of rheumatic fever, which can cause valvular fibrosis (overgrowth of fibrous tissue) and fusion and calcification accompanied by shortening and thickening of the chordae tendineae.

A left atrial myxoma (a benign gelatinous tumor whose cells resemble endothelium) may also obstruct the mitral orifice. The symptoms of this valvular heart disease usually do not appear until 10 to 20 years after the patient has had rheumatic fever. Once symptoms appear, they tend to progress. Because of the relative rarity of rheumatic fever in the United States, the incidence of mitral stenosis also is low.

[a] Symptoms and Diagnosis

Many patients with mitral stenosis, even when it is relatively severe, have no symptoms. The first symptoms are usually fatigue and dyspnea on exertion. Heart failure may occur, and emboli associated with atrial fibrillation are produced in as many as 15 percent of patients with the disorder.

The physical examination may reveal diagnostic snaps, murmurs and heart movements. The EKG shows signs of left atrial overload and may reveal right ventricular hypertrophy and atrial fibrillation. The chest x-ray shows straightening of the left border of the heart due to a dilated left atrial appendage; the pulmonary artery may be prominent and the right cardiac border may show signs of an enlarged left atrium. An echocardiogram may be useful in indicating the extent of calcification of the valve and the size of the left atrium. A two-dimensional echocardiogram may reveal the exact size of the mitral opening.

[b] Treatment

Drug treatment of mitral stenosis consists of the use of beta-blockers or calcium antagonists to slow the heart rate and the use of anticoagulants to prevent emboli. If atrial fibrillation is present, digitalis may be used together with a beta-blocker and a calcium antagonist.

Surgery to correct mitral stenosis is considered if the patient shows symptoms of heart failure with less-than-ordinary exertion despite the best medical treatment. If the valve is not heavily calcified, valvotomy or balloon valvuloplasty may be performed; otherwise valve replacement is necessary.

7.62 Aortic Valve Disease

The aortic valve may be subject to regurgitation and stenosis.

[1] Aortic Regurgitation

Aortic regurgitation (also called aortic incompetence or aortic insufficiency) is the backward flow of blood from the aorta into the left ventricle through an incompetent aortic valve. The most common causes of severe aortic regurgitation in adults are degeneration of the aortic valve, rheumatic heart disease, infective endocarditis and trauma. Severe regurgitation may be accompanied by valvular calcification.

The most common causes of mild adult aortic regurgitation are bicuspid aortic valve (the presence of two cusps rather than three) and severe hypertension. In patients with aortic regurgitation, the left ventricle dilates and the stroke volume increases, because the left ventricle must receive blood regurgitated during diastole as well as the blood flowing into it normally from the pulmonary veins. Hypertrophy of the left ventricle develops in response to the dilation to allow the maintenance of adequate blood pressure.

[a] Symptoms and Diagnosis

Even if their aortic regurgitation is severe, most patients tolerate effort well for many years. Eventually, however, dyspnea on exertion, orthopnea (difficulty breathing except when in an upright position) and paroxysmal nocturnal dyspnea (a form of respiratory distress that occurs while the patient is reclining at night that is thought to be related to heart failure) develop. About 5 percent of patients experience angina pectoris, primarily at night. Physical examination reveals a "slapping" pulse (a rapid rise of the pulse with a large volume). The second heart sound is usually slightly sharp or slapping and loud. If aortic regurgitation is severe, however, the second heart sound may be missing. Characteristic murmurs are heard, depending on the cause of the regurgitation. An EKG may show left ventricular hypertrophy. Echocardiography may show reduced ejection fraction (the amount of blood ejected with each heartbeat). Coronary angiography should be performed before surgery to replace a diseased aortic valve, because some patients with severe aortic regurgitation also have significant coronary artery disease.

[b] Treatment

Replacement of the aortic valve is considered the treatment of choice for patients with heart failure or a dangerously low ejection fraction. The usual drug treatment for heart failure includes both digitalis and a vasodilator. Antibiotic treatment to prevent endocarditis is administered before and after valve replacement.

[2] Aortic Stenosis

Aortic stenosis is defined as a narrowing of the aortic outflow tract causing obstruction of the flow of blood from the left ventricle into the aorta and resulting in a pressure gradient across the obstruction of 10 mmHg or greater. The narrowing may be located at the aortic valve or above or below it. Even in adults, aortic stenosis is considered a congenital heart disease, unless there is accompanying mitral valve disease or the patient is 70 years of age or older. In the elderly, a previously normal aortic valve may become so hardened and calcified that significant narrowing is produced. Severe calcification of the cusps of the valve may also occur in persons with congenital aortic valve stenosis.

The first response of the heart to aortic stenosis is ventricular hypertrophy due to inward growth and a resultant reduction in the size of the ventricular cavity (as opposed to the ventricular dilation that occurs in aortic regurgitation). The ventricle becomes enlarged only when extreme obstruction causes heart failure or damages the myocardium.

[a]   Symptoms and Diagnosis

The classic symptoms of aortic stenosis are syncope (fainting), angina pectoris (chest pain) and dyspnea (shortness of breath) on exertion. Syncope on exertion usually is a sign of severe aortic stenosis, but syncope also may be due to arrhythmias that are unrelated to exertion. The angina pectoris of patients with this type of valvular disease may be due to coronary artery disease. In at least half of these patients, however, angina is caused by an insufficient supply of blood to a thickened left ventricle, despite normal coronary arteries. The mean survival time of patients after the appearance of any of the symptoms just described ranges from three to five years.

Physical examination reveals a carotid pulse that is slow in rising. When aortic regurgitation also is present, the pulse may show a notch or dip in midsystole. In cases of severe aortic stenosis, the blood pressure and the pulse pressure are low. In mild or moderate cases, the systolic pressure may be high. A characteristic ejection murmur may be heard. The chest x-ray and the echocardiogram may show calcification of the valvular cusps and hypertrophy of the septum and chamber walls. An EKG reveals various degrees of left ventricular hypertrophy. Doppler echocardiography and/or cardiac catheterization may be used to determine the pressure gradients across the valve and detect the presence of coronary artery disease. Considered significant are gradients during cardiac catheterization of 50 mmHg.

[b]   Treatment

Patients with the gradients just described should restrict their activity to avoid sudden cardiac death. Treatment with a beta-blocker may slow the heart rate and improve coronary artery flow. If syncope, angina pectoris and dyspnea on exertion are present, valve replacement surgery should be considered. The prophylactic administration of antibiotics is necessary to prevent endocarditis, and continuous anticoagulant therapy is required if the replacement valve is artificial. In adults with low cardiac output, balloon valvuloplasty may produce a large decrease in the pressure gradient without necessarily greatly increasing the size of the valvular orifice.

7.63 Tricuspid Valve Disease

Diseases of the tricuspid valve account for less than 5 percent of valvular heart disease, and they usually accompany valve problems of other types.

[1] Tricuspid Regurgitation

Tricuspid regurgitation (also called tricuspid incompetence or tricuspid insufficiency) is the backward flow of blood from the right ventricle to the right atrium, due to an inadequate juxtaposition of the cusps of the tricuspid valve. This type of valvular heart disease is usually due to a combination of right ventricular dilation and high blood pressure due to severe pulmonary hypertension or obstruction of right ventricular outflow. Less commonly, tricuspid regurgitation is caused by infective endocarditis or by dysfunction of the papillary muscles after right ventricular infarction. Tricuspid regurgitation may be diagnosed shortly after valvotomy to correct mitral stenosis. This phenomenon probably is due to the unmasking of latent tricuspid regurgitation as blood flow increases.

[a] Symptoms and Diagnosis

The only specific symptom of severe tricuspid regurgitation is the sensation of pulsations in the neck due to waves in the jugular veins that result from the regurgitation. Atrial fibrillation or flutter, which usually occurs when the right atrium is enlarged, may precipitate sudden, severe heart failure. A characteristic murmur may be heard during systole.

The EKG may reveal right ventricular overload, depending on the severity of the regurgitation. A chest x-ray shows enlargement of the superior vena cava, the right atrium and the right ventricle. These findings can be confirmed by echocardiography. Cardiac catheterization and angiography can be used to demonstrate the regurgitation directly and to measure pressure in the right ventricle.

[b] Treatment

Patients often tolerate even severe tricuspid regurgitation for years (in fact, the tricuspid valve has been removed entirely to eliminate infective endocarditis). If severe heart failure is present, tricuspid regurgitation may be corrected by valvuloplasty (the surgical fashioning of an artificial valve). In patients in whom tricuspid regurgitation and mitral valve disease occur together, tricuspid valve repair frequently is performed at the same time as mitral valve surgery to prevent death from low cardiac output.

[2]   Tricuspid Stenosis

Tricuspid stenosis is defined as a narrowing of the tricuspid orifice that obstructs blood flow from the right atrium to the right ventricle. This type of valvular disease is usually due to rheumatic fever and nearly always occurs together with mitral stenosis. Usually the mitral stenosis is dominant, but occasionally the tricuspid stenosis dominates. Tricuspid stenosis produces distension and hypertrophy of the right atrium, while the right ventricle remains underfilled and small.

[a]   Symptoms and Diagnosis

The symptoms of severe tricuspid stenosis are a fluttering discomfort in the neck caused by giant waves in the jugular veins, and fatigue due to low cardiac output. A presystolic murmur may be heard. The EKG shows signs of right atrial overload, and the chest x-ray and echocardiogram reveal dilation of the superior vena cava and the right atrium. Cardiac catheterization shows a diastolic pressure gradient across the tricuspid valve.

[b]   Treatment

In rare instances, tricuspid stenosis is severe enough to require valvotomy (surgical repair of the valve).

7.70   CARDIOMYOPATHY

A cardiomyopathy is a structural or functional abnormality of the myocardium (membrane surrounding the heart) that is not due to ischemic, hypertensive, valvular or pericardial disease or a congenital developmental defect. A variety of systems have been proposed for the classification of the different types of cardiomyopathy. Because cardiomyopathy can be due to any of a large number of diseases or can occur without an identifiable cause, the classification most useful to the clinician (and the one used here) is based on the pathophysiology of the disease (Wynne and Braunwald, 1992). Once the pathophysiologic type has been identified, a cause can be sought. If none is found, the cardiomyopathy is referred to as primary or idiopathic.

The three basic types of cardiomyopathy are dilated, hypertrophic and restrictive.

7.71 Dilated Congestive Cardiomyopathy

Dilated cardiomyopathy (also called congestive cardiomyopathy) is a disorder of myocardial function accompanied by symptoms of heart failure in which ventricular dilation is the dominant characteristic. The pathophysiology includes acute inflammation of the myocardium, chronic fibrosis and diffuse loss of muscle cells that probably is due to an autoimmune reaction. The dilation of the ventricles leads to secondary mitral or tricuspid regurgitation and atrial dilation. The functional consequence of these abnormalities is a depression of ventricular systolic function such that cardiac output is maintained only by sinoatrial tachycardia (overly rapid heart rate)[31] and diastolic filling that is greater than normal.

The prognosis of patients with dilated cardiomyopathy is poor. Seventy percent die within 5 years of diagnosis. Poor prognosis is related to poor ventricular function or the finding of frequent ventricular arrhythmia on a 24-hour ambulatory EKG. Half of the deaths due to dilated cardiomyopathy are sudden, suggesting that ventricular fibrillation is the terminal event (Berkow and Fletcher, 1992).

[1] Symptoms and Diagnosis

Most patients with dilated cardiomyopathy experience dyspnea on exertion and fatigability as their first symptoms. If an infective agent is responsible for the disease, fever may be the first symptom. The inflammation of the myocardium caused by infection is referred to as myocarditis. Infection with the Coxsackie B virus is the most common cause of dilated cardiomyopathy in temperate North America, whereas Chagas' disease (infection with the parasite *Trypanosoma cruzi*) is the most prevalent infection in Central and South America.

A diagnosis of dilated cardiomyopathy relies primarily on the exclusion of other causes of ventricular failure (e.g., systemic hypertension, primary valvular disease and previous myocardial infarction), the patient's medical history and the physical examination. In about a fourth of patients, differentiation from myocardial infarction may be complicated by the presence of chest pain that mimics angina pectoris.

The physical examination reveals a normal or low blood pressure, distension of the neck veins and peripheral edema (swelling due to

---

[31] *See* 7.51[2] *supra.*

accumulation of fluid). In severe cases, an enlarged liver, ascites (accumulation of fluid in the abdominal cavity) and wasting of the skeletal muscles are found. Murmurs due to mitral and/or tricuspid regurgitation may be heard. The EKG may show sinoatrial tachycardia, left bundle-branch block (heart block due to the absence of conduction in the left branch of the bundle of His) and other characteristic signs. The chest x-ray reveals enlargement of the heart that usually involves all four chambers.

M-mode and two-dimensional echocardiography show dilated chambers with reduced shortening on contraction and help rule out primary valvular disease and myocardial infarction. Echocardiography may reveal a thrombus on the wall of a chamber, a complication that often accompanies dilated cardiomyopathy. Magnetic resonance imaging shows an abnormal texture of the myocardial tissue. A diagnosis of dilated cardiomyopathy may be confirmed by the examination of a myocardial biopsy sample obtained by cardiac catheterization.

[2]   Treatment

Usually no primary cause of dilated cardiomyopathy can be found, but unless one is present, there is no treatment for dilated cardiomyopathy that will prolong life. Treatable causes include alcoholism, exposure to certain psychotherapeutic drugs and environmental toxins, electrolyte disorders and infection by microorganisms. Palliative measures include therapy for low cardiac output and heart failure, and specific treatment for complications. Adequate rest, sleep and stress avoidance are important, but prolonged bed rest should be prescribed only if symptoms require it.

Because of the high mortality associated with dilated cardiomyopathy, more patients with this condition receive heart transplants than any other group.

7.72   Hypertrophic Cardiomyopathy

Hypertrophic cardiomyopathy is an inherited or acquired disorder characterized by marked ventricular hypertrophy in the absence of a condition (aortic stenosis or systemic hypertension, for example) that creates an increased afterload (pressure on the wall of the ventricles during systolic ejection) demand on the heart. The contractility of the myocardium in patients with hypertrophic cardiomyopathy usually is normal or even enhanced. The primary functional results of ventricular hypertrophy are stiffness of the chamber and resistance to diastolic filling, which ultimately increases pulmonary venous pressure.

Because the hypertrophied myocardium requires more oxygen than it can receive via the coronary arteries, the patient experiences angina pectoris. Light-headedness and fainting on exertion are caused by an increase in the pressure gradient across the left ventricular outflow tract (caused by a combination of arrhythmia and poor diastolic filling of the ventricle) that results in a decrease in cardiac output. The distal left ventricle sometimes thins and dilates in an aneurysmlike manner. Infective endocarditis and heart block sometimes occur as complications of hypertrophic cardiomyopathy, and sudden death from ventricular tachyarrhythmia may occur.

[1]   Symptoms and Diagnosis

The symptoms of hypertrophic cardiomyopathy are chest pain, syncope, palpitations, dyspnea on exertion and sudden death, which may occur alone or in combination. In patients in the terminal phase of the disease, the physical examination reveals signs of elevated venous pressure (e.g., distension of the jugular vein, ascites and swelling of the ankles). A conventional or 24-hour ambulatory EKG may reveal arrhythmia. Cardiac catheterization may be used to confirm the presence of outflow obstruction.

[2]   Treatment

Treatment for hypertrophic cardiomyopathy consists mainly of the use of beta-blockers, calcium antagonists or both to decrease myocardial contractility and thereby dilate the heart and decrease the obstruction of outflow. The ultimate result is an improvement in diastolic ventricular function. Verapamil is currently the calcium antagonist of choice. Nitrates and diuretics are not recommended for these patients, because they decrease the size of the chambers and worsen the symptoms of the disease. Antiarrhythmic drugs may be used to suppress arrhythmia, but it has not been shown that this helps prevent sudden death. Amiodarone seems to be the most effective antiarrhythmic (Hopf and Kaltenbach, 1990), but it has severe side effects, some of which are irreversible. Antibiotics to prevent infective endocarditis are recommended. Extreme exertion should be avoided as a means of preventing sudden death.

Septal myectomy (excision of part of the septal myocardium) is recommended only for patients with confirmed outflow tract obstruction and incapacitating symptoms that do not respond to drug therapy. This procedure usually ameliorates the symptoms of hypertrophic cardiomyopathy but has not been shown to reduce mortality.

7.73   Restrictive Cardiomyopathy

Restrictive cardiomyopathy is a disorder characterized by rigid, noncompliant (not yielding to pressure) ventricular walls. The noncompliance causes one or both of the ventricles (usually the left) to resist diastolic filling. The resultant high diastolic pressure leads to pulmonary venous hypertension. Restrictive cardiomyopathy is the least prevalent of the three types of cardiomyopathy.

The cause of restrictive cardiomyopathy usually cannot be found. Identifiable causes include hypereosinophilic syndrome (a massive increase in the number of eosinophils, a type of white blood cell, with infiltration by eosinophils of the heart), Loffler's disease (an illness characterized by arteritis with eosinophilia, the formation of thrombi on the endocardium and atrioventricular valves) and endocardial fibrosis. Sarcoidosis (a progressive granulomatous condition), Fabry's disease (a rare hereditary disease in which glycolipids are deposited in the tissues) and amyloidosis (the accumulation of amyloid, an abnormal material that superficially resembles starch) also may involve the myocardium and lead to restrictive cardiomyopathy.

[1]   Symptoms and Diagnosis

The symptoms of restrictive cardiomyopathy include dyspnea on exertion and orthopnea (discomfort on breathing that is relieved by sitting or standing), which are due to a fixed cardiac output that is caused by resistance to ventricular filling. When the right ventricle is involved, peripheral edema is also seen. Angina pectoris and syncope occur rarely, but both atrial and ventricular arrhythmia and heart block are common. The EKG usually shows abnormalities, but they are not specific to restrictive cardiomyopathy. A chest x-ray often shows the heart to be of normal size or small, but in late-stage amyloidosis, the heart can be enlarged. Echocardiography shows normal systolic function and often reveals dilation of the atria and myocardial hypertrophy.

Cardiac catheterization and myocardial biopsy are usually necessary to confirm a diagnosis of restrictive cardiomyopathy. Constrictive cardiomyopathy also leads to a noncompliant heart but is due to a diseased pericardial encasement of the heart, as opposed to a problem of the cardiac muscle proper. Differentiating these two entities may be quite difficult clinically.

[2]   Treatment

There is no therapy for patients with restrictive cardiomyopathy unless an underlying disease can be identified and treated. The prognosis of patients with the disease is poor.

7.80   COR PULMONALE

Cor pulmonale is an enlargement of the right ventricle, accompanied by right ventricular failure, that is due to the increase in right ventricular afterload that occurs in diseases of the thorax, lung and pulmonary circulation. Enlargement of the right ventricle caused by left ventricular failure, congenital heart disease or acquired valvular heart disease are not classified as cor pulmonale. The disease is usually chronic but may be acute and reversible.

The most common cause of chronic cor pulmonale is chronic obstructive pulmonary disease (chronic bronchitis and/or emphysema, often referred to simply as COPD). Other causes are extensive loss of lung tissue due to surgery or trauma, pulmonary emboli, primary pulmonary hypertension, scleroderma (chronic hardening and shrinking of the connective tissue), interstitial fibrosis, kyphoscoliosis (curvature of the spinal column), obesity with alveolar hypoventilation (a state in which a reduced amount of air enters the alveoli of the lungs), idiopathic hypoventilation and diseases that involve the respiratory muscles. Acute cor pulmonale usually is due to massive pulmonary embolism (the closure of the pulmonary artery or one of its branches by an embolus, sometimes associated with pulmonary infarction), but exacerbations of chronic cor pulmonale often occur in patients with COPD, usually during bouts of respiratory infection.

The prognosis of patients with cor pulmonale depends on the degree of pulmonary hypertension. In patients with obstructive airflow disease, however, it is difficult to separate the distress, morbidity and mortality of cor pulmonale from those of the primary disease. Death due to right ventricular failure per se probably is very rare (Butler, 1991).

7.81   Diagnosis

Dyspnea (shortness of breath) on exertion is the most common symptom of patients with pulmonary hypertension, and some patients suffer syncope and substernal pain on exertion. Cough, cyanosis and wheezing may be present in patients with a primary pulmonary vascular disease. Murmurs due to insufficiency of the tricuspid and pulmonary valves and a characteristic loud pulmonary sound may be heard. The chest x-ray may reveal enlargement of the right ventricle and the proximal pulmonary artery, but this examination may be insensitive to right ventricular enlargement because hyperinflation of the lungs may realign the heart. The EKG may show evidence of right ventricular hypertrophy that correlates with the degree of pulmonary hypertension. Blood gas analysis may reveal hypoxemia, hypercapnia (excessive amount of carbon dioxide in the blood) and acidosis.

In patients in whom cor pulmonale is due to a disease of the lung tissue, the symptoms of the primary disease may eclipse those of cor pulmonale. The symptoms of left heart failure, furthermore, can be similar to those of cor pulmonale, and it may be difficult to distinguish between the two diseases. Evaluation of left ventricular function by echocardiography or radionuclide imaging may be helpful in the latter situation.

7.82   Treatment

The primary lung diseases seen in cor pulmonale have their own treatment regimens. Digitalis is not effective in patients with hypoxia (reduction of the supply of oxygen to the tissues, despite adequate blood flow) due to cor pulmonale, and those who respond to the drug may actually have left ventricular dysfunction. Diuretics, however, may improve pulmonary gas exchange in hypoxic cor pulmonale by relieving accumulation of fluid in the lungs. Continuous use of oxygen decreases pulmonary hypertension, prevents polycythemia (abnormally high level of red blood cells) and may reduce the risk of death. If venous thromboembolism occurs, long-term anticoagulant therapy is essential.

7.90   RHEUMATIC HEART DISEASE

Rheumatic fever is an inflammatory disease that occurs as a delayed sequela of infection of the throat by group A streptococci (a group of spherical bacteria that occur primarily in chains; the infection is referred to colloquially as strep throat). The inflammation of rheumatic fever can involve the joints, central nervous system, skin and subcutaneous tissues, but the primary importance of the disease is its effect on the heart. The inflammation of the heart, or carditis, that occurs in acute rheumatic fever can be fatal or lead to rheumatic heart disease, a chronic condition characterized by scarring and deformity of the heart valves.

7.91 Diagnosis

The vast majority of patients with rheumatic carditis do not have symptoms referable to the heart. For this reason, unless noncardiac manifestations are present (e.g., chorea [ceaseless rapid, jerky involuntary movements] or polyarthritis [inflammation of several joints occurring at the same time]), patients frequently are not diagnosed as having rheumatic fever but later in life may be found to have rheumatic heart disease without a history of rheumatic fever.

Acute rheumatic carditis, if it has symptoms at all, is first manifested by the appearance of heart murmurs caused by either mitral or aortic regurgitation. In severe cases, symptoms of pericarditis and heart failure may be noted. Death may result from heart failure during the acute stage of the disease, or permanent valvular damage that results in serious disability may occur. Tachycardia (rapid heart rate) usually is present, and the EKG may show varying degrees of heart block. Involvement of the pericardium may cause pain over the heart, and a pericardial friction rub[32] may be audible. The chest x-ray shows an increase in the size of the heart. There are no specific laboratory tests that indicate the presence of rheumatic fever.

7.92 Treatment

There is no specific treatment for rheumatic fever, and no measures are known that can change the course of an attack. In patients with carditis, the goal of treatment is to suppress inflammation while avoiding a recurrence of the inflammation after therapy is discontinued (post-therapeutic rebound). The administration of a salicylate (a salt of salicylic acid, of which aspirin is one) is the treatment of first choice, but a program of corticosteroid administration may be necessary when the carditis is severe, especially when heart failure is present.

---

[32] *See* 7.42[2][a] *supra.*

A course of antibiotics also is recommended to eradicate persistent streptococci. Preventive antistreptococcal therapy should be maintained continuously after an attack of rheumatic fever to prevent recurrent attacks. Some physicians recommend preventive therapy for life; others favor prophylaxis for only a few years after an attack and for life only if there has been severe damage to the heart. In patients with known or suspected rheumatic valvular disease, therapy to prevent bacterial endocarditis should be administered before dental procedures that are likely to cause bleeding of the gums and before surgery on the upper respiratory tract, the genitourinary tract or the gastrointestinal tract.

7.100   ENDOCARDITIS

Endocarditis is an inflammation of the endocardium that most often involves a heart valve but may also affect the lining of the chambers of the heart. It may occur as a primary disease or in association with another disease.

7.110   CARDIAC TUMORS

Tumors may occur on the outside of the heart or within the myocardium or endocardium. Cardiac tumors frequently mimic other types of heart disease and therefore are often diagnosed by chance or because cancer outside the heart suggests that metastasis to the heart has occurred. Secondary (metastatic) cardiac tumors are much more common than primary tumors.

7.111   Primary Cardiac Tumors

Primary cardiac tumors can be malignant or benign.

[1]   Malignant Cardiac Tumors

Malignant cardiac tumors occur mostly in children. The most common are sarcomas (e.g., hemangiosarcoma, fibrosarcoma, rhabdomyosarcoma and liposarcoma). Malignant tumors may be associated with the sudden appearance of heart failure, rapid development of pericardial effusion and tamponade, and various forms of arrhythmia or heart block. Malignant cardiac tumors may spread to the spine, neighboring soft tissues and major organs. The prognosis of patients with malignant cardiac tumors is poor, and treatment is limited to radiation therapy, chemotherapy and the management of complications.

[2] Benign Cardiac Tumors

Benign cardiac tumors, which include myxomas, rhabdomyomas, fibromas, lipomas and teratomas (tumors made up of a number of types of tissue), may threaten life if they are not treated.

Myxomas account for about half of all primary heart tumors. Seventy-five percent of myxomas occur in the left atrium, with most of the rest occurring in the right atrium. Myxomas appear either as semitransparent or gelatinous growths with a lobular or shaggy surface, or as firm, round masses. The cells of myxomas resemble endothelial cells. Atrial myxomas, especially those of the right atrium, may contain calcium deposits.

Myxomas result in three major clinical syndromes: (1) embolic phenomena, (2) obstruction of blood flow, and (3) systemic symptoms that include fever, weight loss, anemia, clubbing of the fingers, increased white blood cell count, decreased blood platelet count and abnormal serum protein levels. Calcification may be visible on a chest x-ray. A diagnosis of myxoma made on the basis of symptoms usually can be confirmed by echocardiography. Cardiac catheterization and biopsy may also be useful in diagnosis. Radionuclide imaging, CT or MRI are useful as preparations for surgery.[33] Myxoma usually can be cured by surgical removal.

Fibromas and rhabdomyomas occur as multiple nodules within the myocardium or endocardium and are most often found in children or infants. Rhabdomyomas, which account for about 20 percent of primary cardiac tumors, are the most common of the two. Most cases are associated with tuberous sclerosis (a congenital, inherited disease characterized by sclerotic patches on the surface of the brain) and adenoma sebaceum (tumors of the oil glands) of the skin, kidney tumors and arrhythmia.

The symptoms of cardiac fibroma and rhabdomyoma include heart block, paroxysmal supraventricular and ventricular tachyarrhythmia, enlargement of the heart and obstruction of ventricular outflow. The latter may result in heart failure and murmurs due to pulmonary or aortic stenosis. Association of these symptoms with the signs of

---

[33] *See* 7.30 *supra* for a discussion of diagnostic methods.

tuberous sclerosis suggests a diagnosis of cardiac fibroma or rhabdomyoma. The diagnosis can be confirmed by echocardiography or
cardiac angiography.

Surgical treatment of these tumors is usually ineffective, and most
infants with cardiac fibroma or rhabdomyoma do not live longer than
one year.

Lipomas (benign tumors composed of fat cells) are more common
than teratomas, and the latter are seen most frequently in infants. These
tumors generally are asymptomatic and are often discovered on routine
chest x-rays. Surgery is performed only to rule out a more serious
tumor.

7.112   Secondary Cardiac Tumors

A number of types of malignant tumor, including carcinomas (a
tumor made up of endothelial cells), sarcomas, leukemias and reticulo-
endothelial tumors, can metastasize to the tissues of the heart.
Carcinomas of the lung and breast have the highest incidence of
metastasis to the heart. Metastatic involvement of the heart may be
seen on the chest x-ray as a sudden enlargement of the heart or bizarre
changes in its contour. Other possible manifestations include tamponade, arrhythmia and unexplained heart failure. As with primary
malignant tumors, treatment for secondary cardiac tumors is limited
to palliation (treatment of symptoms).

7.120   DRUG AND CHEMICAL EFFECTS ON THE HEART

Numerous drugs (both illicit and therapeutic) and chemicals (including animal venoms) may act on and injure the heart. In some cases,
the damage is acute and transient and associated with myocardial
necrosis. In others, an acute hypersensitivity (allergic) reaction occurs,
with no evidence of necrosis but with allergic myocarditis characterized by infiltration of the myocardium by eosinophils, giant cells and
leukocytes (types of white blood cells).

Allergic myocarditis is rarely recognized clinically and therefore
is often discovered only during autopsy. Some agents cause chronic
changes that result in fibrosis and dilated cardiomyopathy, and others
are associated with both acute and chronic phases.[34] A cardiac

---

[34] *See also* ch. 16 for a full discussion of drug treatment in the elderly.

response to a drug or chemical often is related to the size of the dose and the frequency of exposure. The adverse effects of a number of agents are presented in this section[35] (Wynne and Braunwald, 1992).

Acetaminophen: The frequently used analgesic acetaminophen (brand name Tylenol®) is best known for its potential to produce massive liver damage. Overdoses occasionally also cause fatty degeneration and focal necrosis of the myocardium.

Antimony: Various compounds containing antimony, such as stibophen and tartar emetic, are used in the treatment of schistoso-miasis (infection with flukes belonging to the genus *Schisto-soma*). Almost all patients treated with these compounds show EKG changes, but the majority show no cardiac symptoms. However, chest pain, bradycardia (slow heartbeat), hypotension (low blood pressure), ventricular arrhythmia (irregular heartbeat) and sudden death have been reported.

Arsenic: Adverse effects on the myocardium may be seen in persons exposed to arsenic, a chemical used in pesticides. The heart may become dilated, and fluid may accumulate in the pericardium. Hemorrhage beneath the endocardium is characteristic. The myocardium usually is abnormal, with evidence of infiltration by white cells. Electrocardiographic abnormalities usually resolve within two to four weeks after exposure.

Carbon monoxide: Carbon monoxide poisoning occasionally results in fatal heart abnormalities. Carbon monoxide has a greater affinity for hemoglobin (the carrier of oxygen in the blood) than oxygen does, which results in the delivery of reduced amounts of oxygen to the tissues. It is thought that the adverse effects of the gas on the heart may be due to myocardial hypoxia. A direct toxic effect on the heart also may play a role. Postmortem examination of heart tissue sometimes reveals areas of necrosis.

Catecholamines: Catecholamines (dopamine, epinephrine and norepinephrine) may produce cardiomyopathy, acute myocarditis with focal myocardial necrosis, tachycardia and arrhythmia. The toxic effect may be due to direct toxicity or to hypoxia due to increased metabolic demands on the myocardium.

Chloroquine: Chloroquine, a compound used in the prevention and treatment of parasitic and other diseases, can be very toxic

---

[35] *See* 7.28 *supra* for a discussion of the effects of alcohol on the heart.

to the heart. Electrocardiographic changes may be seen with routine doses, and large doses may result in a reduction in cardiac output, bradycardia, arrhythmia, heart block and death.

Cocaine: The illicit use of cocaine is often associated with chest pain, profuse sweating and palpitations. In some cases, there is evidence of myocardial ischemia or infarction resulting from an increase in blood pressure and heart rate that leads to an increase in myocardial oxygen demand. Myocarditis and accelerated atherosclerotic occlusion of the coronary arteries sometimes are found on examination of cardiac tissue samples from cocaine abusers. Spasm of the coronary arteries may lead to acute myocardial infarction. Ventricular arrhythmia and sudden cardiac death may occur (Isner and Chokshi, 1991).

Cyclophosphamide: High doses of cyclophosphamide (a chemo-therapeutic cancer drug) may be associated with EKG changes, heart failure and death from hemorrhagic myocarditis. The myocardial injury appears to be caused by direct damage to the endothelium and the resultant formation of fibrin thrombi in the capillaries.

Emetine: Cardiovascular changes are common in patients who use emetine (a drug used for the treatment of parasitic diseases), but fatalities have been reported only rarely. Myocardial lesions have been found at autopsy, but clinical symptoms of cardiomyo-pathy usually are lacking. The EKG may show abnormalities, but they usually resolve within weeks or months after emetine treatment has been discontinued.

Hydrocarbons: The ingestion of hydrocarbons, which are used extensively as propellants and solvents, may cause fragmentation of the muscle fibers of the heart, with resultant EKG changes, arrhythmia and enlargement of the heart.

Interferon: Interferon, a protein derived from white blood cells, is used in the treatment of cancer and other diseases, including infection with the human immunodeficiency virus (HIV). This agent has been found to cause cardiotoxicity manifested by hypotension, arrhythmia, dilated cardiomyopathy and symptoms of ischemic heart disease, including myocardial infarction and sudden cardiac death (Sonnenblick and Rosin, 1991).

Interleukin-2: Interleukin-2, a protein released by lymphocytes that is used in the treatment of cancer, has significant toxic effects on the capillaries that result in hypotension and oliguria (diminished excretion of urine in relation to fluid intake). Cardiotoxicity consisting of myocardial ischemia, myocardial infraction, arrhythmia and myocarditis, is seen in a small percentage of patients treated with interleukin-2.

Lead: Lead is known primarily for its effects on the gastrointestinal tract and the central nervous system. In some fatal cases of lead poisoning, however, effects on the myocardium may contribute to or be the principal cause of death. Electrocardiographic changes, atrioventricular conduction defects and heart failure may occur.

Lithium carbonate: Lithium, used in the treatment of manic-depressive (bipolar) disorders, is associated with EKG changes in about a fourth of the patients who use it. Overdose may be manifested by ventricular arrhythmia, conduction disturbances, heart failure and, rarely, death.

Methyldopa: Sudden cardiac death has been reported in a number of patients taking methyldopa, an antihypertensive agent. On autopsy, these patients have been found to have allergic myocarditis characterized by inflammatory reactions, vasculitis and focal myocardial necrosis. The EKG findings indicate sinoatrial node bradycardia and first-and second-degree atrioventricular block.

Methysergide: The long-term use of methysergide (a drug used to treat migraine) results in widespread fibrotic reactions that can involve the heart. Lesions of the valves of the left side of the heart that lead to stenosis and regurgitation occur in up to 1 percent of long-term methysergide users. Fibrotic endocardial lesions occasionally produce the clinical symptoms of restrictive cardiomyopathy.

Penicillin: Allergic reactions to penicillin are fairly common, but allergic myocarditis. due to its use is rare. Myocardial necrosis may occur and cause EKG abnormalities.

Phenothiazines: The phenothiazines (drugs used in the treatment of psychiatric disorders) have been reported to cause a variety of cardiac disturbances, including atrial and ventricular arrhythmia and sudden death. Cardiomyopathic changes have been observed in biopsy specimens from patients who have died suddenly, but whether there is a direct relationship between phenothiazine use and cardiomyopathy is not known.

Scorpion venom: Scorpion venom has mainly neurotoxic effects, but its effects on the heart may be significant and even fatal. The EKG is altered, and arrhythmia, tachycardia and hypertension may occur. The arrhythmia is thought to be the cause of sudden death in some victims of scorpion sting. Examination of tissue samples from the myocardium may reveal degeneration and necrosis of the muscle fibers.

Snake venom: Occasionally snake venom has adverse effects on the myocardium, and the effects may contribute to morbidity and death. Electrocardiographic changes attributable to myocardial damage may be seen, and death may be caused by circulatory collapse or myocardial infarction brought on by hypotension and coronary artery thrombosis or coronary artery spasm.

Sulfonamides: Sulfonamides may result in allergic vasculitis and myocarditis, which, in turn, can cause myocardial damage. Even though the damage usually is asymptomatic, severe and even fatal heart failure can occur.

Tetracycline: Antibiotics of the tetracycline class can produce fever, tachycardia and first-degree atrioventricular block. Autopsy findings include cardiac dilation, degeneration of the cardiac muscle cells and infiltration by inflammatory cells.

Tricyclic antidepressants: Exacerbation of postural hypotension, arrhythmia, heart block and sudden cardiac death have been observed in conjunction with the use of tricyclic antidepressants, especially when taken in overdose.

Wasp venom: Wasp stings may lead to hypotension, cyanosis, symptoms of anaphylactic shock and circulatory collapse. Occasionally victims have chest pain and symptoms of acute myocardial infarction. The mechanism of damage to the heart is not known, but a direct toxic effect on the myocardium or coronary arteries may be involved.

7.130   HEART TRANSPLANTATION

The transplantation of hearts from cadavers as a treatment for heart disease began in 1967, and by 1991, over 12,000 transplants had been performed (Hunt and Billingham, 1991). Today about 1,500 per year are being performed worldwide, and certainly there would be a further increase if more donors were available. The current one- and five-year survival rates of heart transplant recipients are 90 percent and 70 percent, respectively, which indicates that the procedure is the treatment of choice for end-stage heart disease (Schroeder, 1991).

7.131   Selection of Candidates

It is estimated that there are at least 20,000 candidates for only 2,000 potential donors each year in the United States (Schroeder, 1991). The limited number of donors and the high cost of cardiac transplantation restrict its use to those patients who are most likely to survive and resume a functional life. It is generally accepted that this requires a mentally vigorous, medically compliant person who has not suffered extensive organ damage from heart failure and does not have chronic systemic diseases such as diabetes mellitus or collagen vascular disease.

A recommendation for heart transplantation requires difficult assessments of the patient's present disability, the stability of the course of his or her disease and the likelihood of survival without the operation. Generally a left ventricular ejection fraction of less than 20 percent and the presence of serious ventricular arrhythmia indicate a one-year survival rate without transplantation of about 50 percent.

Usually no attempt is made to "match" the tissues of the heart donor and the recipient, because it is difficult to obtain good matches and because a good correlation between match and outcome has not been found.

7.132   Procedure

In the heart transplant operation, the surgeon removes most of the diseased heart but leaves the posterior wall of the right atrium, together with the superior and inferior vena cavae, in place. Also left in place are the posterior wall of the left atrium and the pulmonary veins. The donor heart is then removed completely, and cuts are made in the posterior walls of the right and left atria. The rims of the two atria of the donor heart are then sutured to the corresponding recipient rims, and the aorta and the pulmonary artery are attached to the donor heart.

7.133   Controlling Transplant Rejection

Crucial to the success of a heart transplantation operation is control of the tissue-rejection process of the recipient with immunosuppressive agents. Because early rejection may produce no symptoms, repeated biopsy samples of the right ventricular endocardium are taken via a catheter introduced through the skin and the right internal jugular vein to determine the state of immunosuppression and rejection.

Immunosuppressive regimens vary but usually include cyclosporine, azathioprine and prednisone. It is crucial that the side effects of these agents, which include nephrotoxicity, suppression of bone marrow activity and opportunistic infections, be carefully monitored.

7.134   Physiology and Function

Transplanted hearts are denervated (without a nervous system), and their function therefore differs from that of native hearts during both rest and exercise. The EKG shows two P waves as a reflection of the residual sinoatrial node activity of the recipient's native heart (although it does not control the donor heart rate, the recipient's sinoatrial node remains innervated and is under the influence of the autonomic nervous system). The donor sinoatrial node maintains the rate of the transplanted heart at about 100 to 110 beats per minute, and increases in rate in response to activity depend on the arrival via the bloodstream of catecholamines. A cardiac transplant recipient usually can achieve about 70 percent of the maximum cardiac output expected for his or her age.

7.200   BIBLIOGRAPHY

Text References

Bender, J. R.: Heart Valve Disease. In: Zaret, B. L., et al. (Eds.): Yale University School of Medicine Heart Book. New York: Hearst Books, 1992.

Berkow, R. and Fletcher, A. J. (Eds.): The Merck Manual of Diagnosis and Therapy, 16th ed. Rahway, N.J.: Merck, 1992.

Bisno, A. L.: The Resurgence of Acute Rheumatic Fever in the United States. Annu. Rev. Med. 41:319-329, 1990.

Braunwald, E.: Approach to the Patient with Heart Disease. In: Wilson, J. D., et al. (Eds.): Harrison's Principles of Internal Medicine, 12th ed. New York: McGraw-Hill, 1991.

Butler, J.: Cor Pulmonale. In: Wilson, J. D., et al. (Eds.): Harrison's Principles of Internal Medicine, 12th ed. New York: McGraw-Hill, 1991.

Cohen, L. S.: What Can Go Wrong. In: Zaret, B. L., et al. (Eds.): Yale University School of Medicine Heart Book. New York: Hearst Books, 1992.

Deckelbaum, L.: Heart Attacks and Coronary Artery Disease. In: Zaret, B. L., et al. (Eds.): Yale University School of Medicine Heart Book. New York: Hearst Books, 1992.

Dennis, C. A.: Rehabilitation of Patients with Coronary Artery Disease. In: Braunwald, E. (Ed.): Heart Disease. A Textbook of Cardiovascular Medicine, 4th ed. Philadelphia: Saunders, 1992.

Farmer, J. A., and Gotto, A. M., Jr.: Risk Factors for Coronary Artery Disease. In: Braunwald, E. (Ed.): Heart Disease. A Textbook of Cardiovascular Medicine, 4th ed. Philadelphia: Saunders, 1992.

Forrester, J. S., et al.: Initiating Events of Acute Coronary Arterial Occlusion. Annu. Rev. Med. 42:35-45, 1991.

Friedman, W. F. and Child, J. S.: Congenital Heart Disease. In: Wilson, J. D., et al. (Eds.): Harrison's Principles of Internal Medicine, 12th ed. New York: McGraw-Hill, 1991.

Friedewald, W. T.: Epidemiology of Cardiovascular Disease. In: Wyngaarden, J. B., et al. (Eds.): Cecil Textbook of Medicine, 19th ed. Philadelphia: Saunders, 1992.

Glantz, S. A., et al.: Passive Smoking and Heart Disease. Epidemiology, Physiology, and Biochemistry. Circulation 83:1-12, 1991.

Grossman, W.: Diagnostic Cardiac Catheterization and Angiography. In: Wilson, J. D., et al. (Eds.): Harrison's Principles of Internal Medicine, 12th ed. New York: McGraw-Hill, 1991.

Grunkemeier, G. L. and Rahimtoola, S. H.: Artificial Heart Valves. Annu. Rev. Med. 41:251-263, 1990.

Gunby, P. H.: Two New Reports Help Put Nation's No. 1 Killer Disease Challenges into Perspective for 1993. J.A.M.A. 269:449-450, 1993.

Hopf, R., and Kaltenbach, M.: Management of Hypertrophic Cardiomyopathy. Annu. Rev. Med. 41:75-83, 1990.

Hunt, S., and Billingham, M.: Long-Term Results of Cardiac Transplantation. Annu. Rev. Med. 42:437-447, 1991.

Isner, J. M. and Chokshi, S. K.: Cardiac Complications of Cocaine Abuse. Annu. Rev. Med. 42:133-138, 1991.

Kutalek, S. P. and Dreifus, L. S.: Implantable Cardioverter-Defibrillators. Adv. Intern. Med. 38:421-438, 1993.

Lange, R. A., et al.: Restenosis after Coronary Balloon Angioplasty. Annu. Rev. Med. 42:127-132, 1991.

Levine, G. N. and Balady, G. L.: The Benefits and Risks of Exercise Training: The Exercise Prescription. Adv. Intern. Med. 38:57-99, 1993.

Levinson, J. R., et al.: Functional Tests for Myocardial Ischemia. Annu. Rev. Med. 42:119-126, 1991.

McKay, R. and Ross, D. N.: Primary Repair and Autotransplantation of Cardiac Valves. Annu. Rev. Med. 44:181-188, 1993.

McPherson, C. A. and Rosenfeld, L. E.: Heart Rhythm Disorders. In: Zaret, B. L., et al. (Eds.): Yale University School of Medicine Heart Book. New York: Hearst Books, 1992.

Meier, B.: Long-Term Results of Coronary Balloon Angioplasty. Annu. Rev. Med. 42:47-59, 1991.

Pasternak, R. C. and Braunwald, E.: Acute Myocardial Infarction. In: Wilson, J. D., et al. (Eds.): Harrison's Principles of Internal Medicine, 12th ed. New York: McGraw-Hill, 1991.

Prystowsky, E. N., et al.: Nonpharmacologic Treatment of the Wolff-Parkinson-White Syndrome and Other Supraventricular Tachycardias. Annu. Rev. Med. 41:239-250, 1990.

Ross, J., Jr.: Cardiac Function and Circulatory Control. In: Wyngaarden, J. B., et al. (Eds.): Cecil Textbook of Medicine, 19th ed. Philadelphia: Saunders, 1992.

Schroeder, J. S.: Cardiac Transplantation. In: Wilson, J. D., et al. (Eds.): Harrison's Principles of Internal Medicine, 12th ed. New York: McGraw-Hill, 1991.

Sonnenblick, M. and Rosin, A.: Cardiotoxicity of Interferon. A Review of 44 Cases. Chest 99:557-561, 1991.

Steenland, K.: Passive Smoking and the Risk of Heart Disease. J.A.M.A. 267:94-99, 1992.

Tenaglia, A. N. and Stack, R. S.: Angioplasty for Acute Coronary Syndromes. Annu. Rev. Med. 44:465-479, 1993.

Tribble, D. L., and Krauss, R. M.: HDL and Coronary Artery Disease. Adv. Intern. Med. 38:1-29, 1993.

Valle, G. A.: Silent Ischemia: A Clinical Update. Chest 97:186-191, 1990.

Wynne, J., and Braunwald, E.: The Cardiomyopathies and Myocarditis: Toxic, Chemical, and Physical Damage to the Heart. In: Braunwald, E. (Ed.): Heart Disease. A Textbook of Cardiovascular Medicine, 4th ed. Philadelphia: Saunders, 1992.

Zaret, B. L.: Diagnosis of Heart Disease. In: Zaret, B. L., et al. (Eds.): Yale University School of Medicine Heart Book. New York: Hearst Books, 1992.

CHAPTER 8

CEREBROVASCULAR INJURIES (STROKE)

SCOPE

Cerebrovascular injuries may result from trauma to the head or as a result of cerebrovascular disease. Intracranial vascular injury can be caused by penetrating or closed head trauma, resulting in compressive hematomas (accumulations of blood) within the brain or its enveloping meningeal tissues. The manifestations of cerebrovascular disease are commonly referred to as stroke or cerebrovascular accident (CVA). Cerebrovascular disease can lead to intracranial hemorrhage, most commonly from a ruptured aneurysm. More often, cerebrovascular disease results in brain ischemia and infarction from thrombosis or occlusion of an artery by an embolus. Cerebrovascular injury can have a devastating effect on all body systems and ultimately be fatal. Many systemic diseases cause problems in the cerebral vasculature similar to those of stroke. CT scan, MRI and arteriography are the mainstays of diagnosis. Treatment includes the administration of antihypertensive, anticoagulant and thrombolytic medications, and surgical procedures, such as carotid endarterectomy, to correct problems in the arteries. Treatment is determined by the nature of the lesion, its size and site.

SYNOPSIS

317

8.00   THE CEREBROVASCULAR SYSTEM

The vascular system is composed of arteries, veins and capillaries. Arteries transport blood away from the heart to peripheral organs. Veins return blood to the heart. Thin-walled capillaries interposed between arteries and veins connect arterioles (small arteries) and venules (small veins continuous with capillaries) in organs and allow for the exchange of substances between tissues and the bloodstream. (*See Figure 8-1.*)

This network of vessels is referred to as the *peripheral vasculature.* Arteries transport oxygen and metabolic substrates (substances that are affected by enzymes) in the blood to peripheral organs, and veins return blood saturated with waste products to be eliminated.

Blood is circulated throughout the body as arterial pressure is generated by contraction of the heart, facilitated by contraction and relaxation of muscle fibers in arterial walls. Tension in these muscle fibers is controlled by an intricate system of nerves called the vasomotor nerves. The vasomotor system is part of the autonomic (involuntary) nervous system and regulates the supply of varying amounts of blood to different organs, according to their metabolic

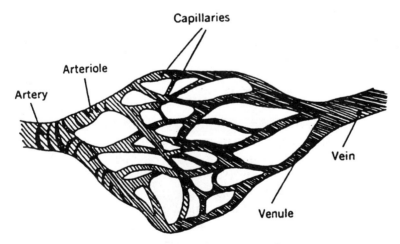

Fig. 8-1. The peripheral vascular system is composed of arteries, veins and capillaries. Capillaries connect arterioles and venules in organs and allow for the exchange of substances between tissues and the bloodstream.

requirements. The autoregulation of the intracranial arteries (the arteries that supply the brain) is very intricate, allowing for maintenance of critical amounts of blood flow and blood pressure in various parts of the brain.

8.01   Structure of Blood Vessel Walls

Each blood vessel is a hollow tube with walls composed of three tissue layers: the intima, the media and the adventitia. (*See Figure 8-2.*) The intima is a smooth inner lining of endothelial cells, which are important for metabolism and for maintaining a barrier to the cellular components of blood. The media, or middle layer, consists of connective tissue and smooth muscle and is important for regulating tissue tension in the vessel wall. Muscle fibers of the media form oblique concentric bands that can regulate vessel diameter and thus blood flow and perfusion pressure. Muscle contraction increases perfusion pressure but decreases blood flow. Muscular relaxation results in dilation (expansion), which decreases perfusion pressure and increases blood flow. Autoregulation of muscle tension in the media of cerebral arterioles is particularly well developed and allows for meticulous regulation of the distribution of regional blood flow in the brain. The adventitia—the outermost vessel wall layer—consists of elastic connective tissue that provides for vessel distension and structural maintenance.

Arterial walls must be relatively strong to withstand the force of blood being pumped under pressure, but this three-ply composition permits flexibility and resilience. Veins have a larger diameter than arteries, and thus venous blood is under lower pressure than arterial blood. Vein walls are thinner and more fibrous than artery walls, and they have less smooth muscle.

8.02   Brain Anatomy and Circulation

The brain and the spinal cord comprise the central nervous system. (*See Figure 8-3.*) The brain is divided into the cortical and subcortical cerebral lobes, the cerebellum and the various parts of the brain stem. (*See Figure 8-4.*) The brain and spinal cord are covered by three layers of meninges (connective tissue): the dura mater, arachnoid membrane and pia mater. Cerebrospinal fluid (CSF) circulates through the ventricles (cavities within the brain) and is also found in the subarachnoid space (the space separating the arachnoid from the pia mater). (*See Figure 8-5.*)

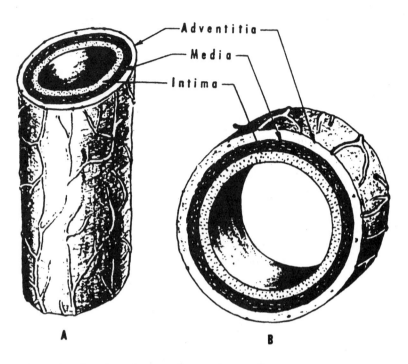

Fig. 8-2. The three layers of an artery wall.

The brain is supplied with blood by the two internal carotid arteries and the two vertebral arteries. The two internal carotid arteries enter the skull anterior to (in front of) the foramen magnum at the skull base and branch to form the anterior and middle cerebral arteries. The two vertebral arteries enter the skull through the foramen magnum at the skull base and converge to form the basilar artery, which divides into the posterior cerebral arteries after supplying branches to the brain stem and cerebellum. (*See Figure 8-6.*) The internal carotid arteries and the posterior cerebral arteries are connected at the base of the brain by the posterior communicating arteries, forming the circle of Willis, an anastomotic (connected) vascular ring. (*See Figure 8-7.*) The basilar and cerebral arteries and their branches are positioned beneath the thin arachnoid membrane in the subarachnoid space.

Blood is returned from brain tissue by a system of veins that tend to parallel the major arteries. These veins empty into venous sinuses (of no relation to the paranasal sinuses) that are formed between the two layers of the dura mater (the thickest of the brain meninges). The venous sinuses drain into the internal jugular veins, and thus blood is returned to the heart (Carpenter, 1991).

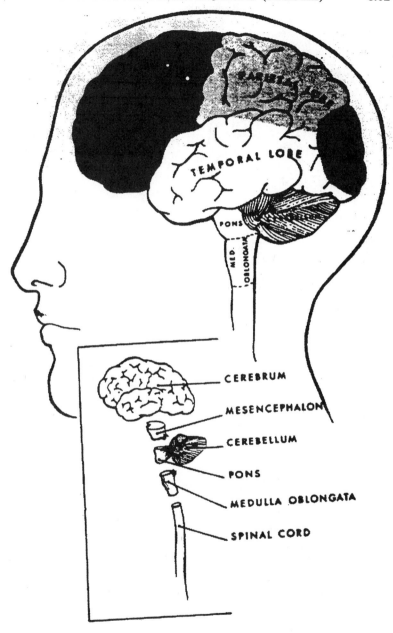

Fig. 8-3. The brain and spinal cord.

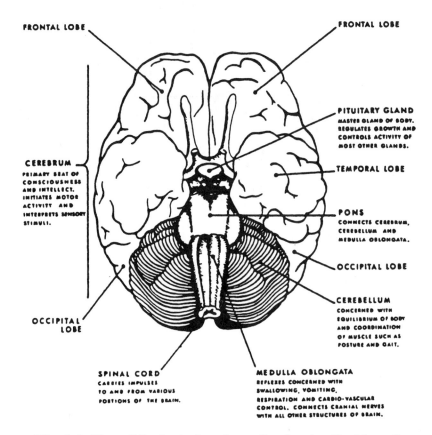

FRONTAL LOBE

FRONTAL LOBE

PITUITARY GLAND
MASTER GLAND OF BODY.
REGULATES GROWTH AND
CONTROLS ACTIVITY OF
MOST OTHER GLANDS.

CEREBRUM
PRIMARY SEAT OF
CONSCIOUSNESS
AND INTELLECT.
INITIATES MOTOR
ACTIVITY AND
INTERPRETS SENSORY
STIMULI.

TEMPORAL LOBE

PONS
CONNECTS CEREBRUM,
CEREBELLUM AND
MEDULLA OBLONGATA.

OCCIPITAL LOBE

CEREBELLUM
CONCERNED WITH
EQUILIBRIUM OF BODY
AND COORDINATION
OF MUSCLE SUCH AS
POSTURE AND GAIT.

OCCIPITAL
LOBE

SPINAL CORD
CARRIES IMPULSES
TO AND FROM VARIOUS
PORTIONS OF THE BRAIN.

MEDULLA OBLONGATA
REFLEXES CONCERNED WITH
SWALLOWING, VOMITING,
RESPIRATION AND CARDIO-VASCULAR
CONTROL. CONNECTS CRANIAL NERVES
WITH ALL OTHER STRUCTURES OF BRAIN.

Fig. 8-4. View of the brain from beneath, showing the lobes, the cerebellum and various parts of the brain stem.

8.03 Diagnostic Techniques in Cerebrovascular Trauma and Disease

Neuroimaging and neurophysiologic diagnostic tests help locate the site of a central nervous system lesion and determine the cause and extent of injury. Computed tomography (CT), an x-ray procedure that generates cross-sectional "slice" views through the body, is noninvasive, rapidly provides good quality images of the brain and is widely available. Magnetic resonance imaging (MRI) utilizes radio waves and is completely noninvasive. CT is generally superior to MRI for the evaluation of acute trauma and acute hemorrhage, although MRI typically provides superior brain images in most other situations. Single photon emission computerized tomography (SPECT) is used to track a radioisotope that is administered intravenously and provides information about blood flow.

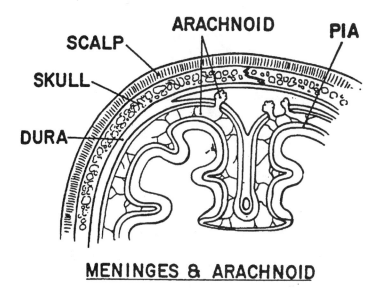

MENINGES & ARACHNOID

Fig. 8-5. The meningeal tissues and their relation to the brain.

With the development of carotid duplex Doppler ultrasound and transcranial Doppler ultrasound, vascular imaging is becoming increasingly sophisticated. The resolution of magnetic resonance angiography (MRA) is also rapidly improving. Definitive vascular imaging still calls for arteriography (x-ray study of arteries that have been injected with a contrast medium), although this invasive procedure may become obsolete as the resolution of noninvasive neuroimaging techniques improves. Electroencephalography (EEG, which measures electrical activity in the brain) has a limited role in the evaluation of cerebrovascular injury, although it does provide functional information and is useful for identifying epileptiform (related to epilepsy) activity.

8.10 TRAUMATIC INTRACRANIAL VASCULAR INJURIES

Trauma to the intracranial vasculature most commonly produces symptoms that manifest acutely, within minutes or hours of the trauma. However, symptoms may develop in a more chronic manner and not become apparent for days or weeks. The two major causes of acute and chronic symptoms that represent abnormal function of various brain structures and pathways are *ischemia* and *mass effect*.

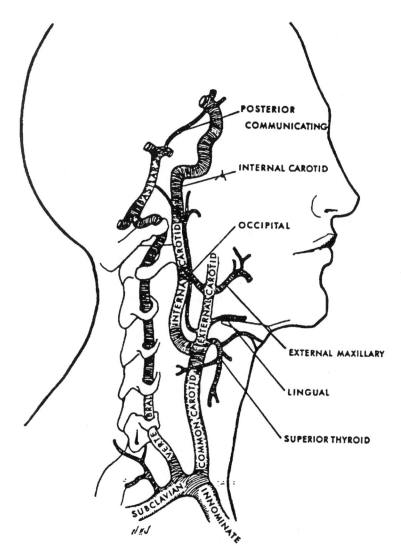

Fig. 8-6. The arteries that supply the head and neck. The carotid and vertebral arteries are the main blood source for the brain.

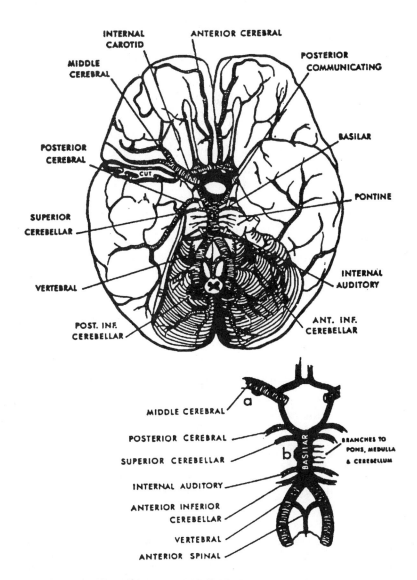

Fig. 8-7. The vascular system of the brain as seen from its underside. The centrally located Circle of Willis lies at the juncture of the cerebral and basilar arteries.

When trauma interrupts blood flow through an artery, tissues distal to (beyond) the injury may not be adequately perfused, and thus they will be deprived of oxygen and nutrients. *Ischemia* is the term used to describe the state of such tissue. The brain is particularly sensitive to ischemia. If ischemia persists, the ischemic brain tissue is irreversibly damaged, and infarction (permanent destruction) of the tissue occurs, accompanied by edema (swelling due to accumulation of fluid) of the infarcted tissue. Infarcted brain tissue cannot regenerate.

The brain is contained in a fixed and limited space by the skull. Normal brain tissue can be displaced (herniated) and functionally damaged or destroyed by any type of mass that compresses it. This mass effect can occur after intracranial vascular trauma by formation of a hematoma (accumulation of blood), edema, infarction or contusion (bruising) of tissue, or accumulation of an abnormal volume of CSF if the normal outflow route of the fluid is blocked (Poirier, 1990; Plum and Posner, 1980).

8.11 Mechanisms of Injury

A variety of traumatic mechanisms that affect blood flow to the brain or the integrity of the cerebral vasculature can contribute to cerebrovascular disorders.

[1] Ischemia

Ischemia, which refers to diminution or cessation of blood flow, can result from functional impedance or obstruction of arterial blood flow. When ischemia is sufficient, the supply of oxygen to tissue is inadequate, and the tissue is said to be hypoxic. This results in acidosis (intracellular accumulation of metabolic acids), edema (swelling of the cells due to fluid accumulation) and an influx of calcium ions into the neurons (nerve cells). If this process is prolonged, infarction (cellular death) of the ischemic tissue occurs.

The brain is the organ most vulnerable to ischemia, with permanent damage occurring within a few minutes. As the duration of ischemia continues, it becomes increasingly difficult to restore perfusion of blood to the tissue, and the likelihood of infarction rises.

Ischemic damage to the brain can be global (widespread) or regional (limited to a particular area). A common cause of global brain ischemia is hypoperfusion (low perfusion) resulting from a cardiac arrhythmia (irregular heartbeat) or myocardial infarction (heart attack), with inadequate cardiac output of blood to perfuse the brain. Another common cause is asphyxiation from strangling or choking. Regional ischemia can result from occlusion, laceration or spasm of an artery, or from compression of arteries by regional brain edema or hematoma (Poirier, 1990; Schochet, 1983; Adams, 1995; Yatsu, 1995a).

[2]   Arterial and Venous Laceration and Transection

Laceration (tearing) and transection of arteries occurs commonly, usually as a result of penetrating head injury. Traumatic intracranial arterial laceration can range in severity from a simple puncture to a ragged tear of the vessel wall or complete arterial transection. It is usually caused by a penetrating missile, such as a bullet, or a bone fragment after a skull fracture. Closed (nonpenetrating) head trauma can result in venous and, less commonly, arterial intracranial laceration.

Hemorrhage may be more severe after arterial laceration than after complete arterial transection. When a blood vessel is completely transected, the severed ends retract and constrict, facilitating thrombus (blood clot) formation. This does not occur after incomplete laceration, and the edges of the wound tend to gape and continue to bleed (Poirier, 1990; Schochet, 1983).

[3]   Arterial Contusion and Thrombosis

Contusion (bruising) of blood vessels usually results from blunt trauma that disrupts the intima of the vessel but does not lacerate the arterial wall.[1] The media and adventitia may also be contused. This can occur even after minor head trauma. Contusion tends to disrupt the arterial intima, causing an effusion of blood and the formation of a hematoma (an accumulation of semi-clotted blood) within the adventitia of the vessel.[2] A large tear of the intima may result in a thrombus in the vessel wall that blocks blood flow through the artery. The thrombus may slowly enlarge and extend along the vessel wall. This is commonly referred to as arterial dissection.

Pieces of intravascular thrombi may break off and be carried in the blood vessel to distal sites (at which point the clots are called emboli), where they lodge in small blood vessels and promote further thrombus formation, tissue ischemia and infarction. This process is referred to

---

[1] *See* 8.01 *supra* for further discussion of the structure of blood vessel walls.

[2] *See* 8.12 *infra* for further discussion of intracranial hematoma.

as embolization (Poirier, 1990; Schochet, 1983; Adams and Victor, 1993).

[4]   Traumatic Vascular Spasm

Traumatic intracranial arterial spasm, or vasospasm, results from autoregulated contraction of the involuntary muscle of the media layer of the arterial wall. It may occur independently or in association with other vascular lesions, such as contusion or laceration. Spasm can result from blunt trauma and also from the force generated by the shock wave of a penetrating missile, such as a bullet. High-velocity missiles generate the greatest force. Severe spasm can completely obstruct distal blood supply, causing ischemia and infarction of brain tissue supplied by the artery in spasm (Poirier, 1990; Schochet, 1983; Mayberg, et al., 1994).

[5]   Traumatic Aneurysm

An aneurysm is an expansion in an artery caused by damage to the vessel wall. The pressure of blood within the artery creates a saclike enlargement at the weakened area.

Rupture, the most serious complication of an aneurysm, can occur if the weakened adventitia suddenly breaks down. This results in hemorrhage under arterial pressure into and around the brain, under the arachnoid membrane (subarachnoid hemorrhage).

Thrombi can form within aneurysms. Although this reduces the risk of rupture, thrombi can impede blood flow in the artery. Thrombi of this type also can embolize to distal arterial sites.

Aneurysms are usually caused by a congenital (present from birth) defect of the arterial wall. The role of arteriosclerosis (hardening of blood vessels, most commonly due to the deposition of fatty plaques in vessel walls) in aneurysm formation is uncertain. Infection of a blood vessel can also result in aneurysm formation. Venous aneurysms are rare (Poirier, 1990; Schochet, 1983; Mayberg, et al., 1994).

[6]   False Aneurysm

False aneurysm (pseudonaneurysm) usually occurs after laceration of all layers of an arterial wall from penetrating trauma, with the hemorrhage contained in the surrounding tissue. A fibrous membrane forms around the hematoma; the hematoma's interior liquefies, and the mass pulsates with arterial blood flow. (*See Figure 8-8.*) Arterial pressure progressively enlarges the false aneurysm, and rupture can occur. Although false aneurysms are common in the peripheral vasculature, they do not tend to occur intracranially. This is because brain tissue is too soft to contain a hematoma adjacent to an artery adequately for a false aneurysm to develop (Poirier, 1990; Schochet, 1983).

[7]   Traumatic Arteriovenous Fistula

An arteriovenous fistula is an abnormal direct communication between an artery and a vein. Arteriovenous fistulas may develop acutely following simultaneous perforation of an artery and an adjacent vein. In such cases, arterial blood is diverted from the injured artery into the adjacent vein immediately after the trauma. Sometimes a hematoma forms around the damaged artery and the fistula does not develop until the clot liquefies, days or weeks after the trauma.

The fistula diverts arterial blood flow directly into the venous system, because arterial pressure is greater than venous pressure. (*See Figure 8-9.*) This diversion of blood flow into the venous system can result in a relative decrease in arterial blood flow to areas distal to (farther from the point of origin) the fistula that are normally supplied by the artery. The pathologic significance of the diverted blood depends on the size of the fistula, the sizes of the involved vessels and the duration of the fistula. With time, collateral blood vessels can develop around the fistula to enhance arterial circulation to tissue distal to the fistula.

Although extracranial arteriovenous fistulas develop commonly after penetrating trauma and procedures, traumatic intracranial arteriovenous fistulas are not common. Carotid artery to cavernous venous

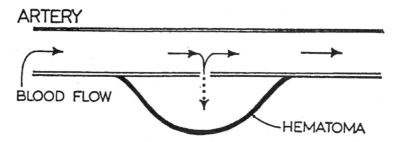

Fig. 8-8. A false aneurysm, in which hemorrhage through an artery wall is held in place by surrounding tissues.

sinus fistulas are most often seen. The carotid artery passes directly through the cavernous venous sinus behind the orbit (eye socket). Penetrating or blunt trauma to the intracavernous portion of the carotid artery can produce a fistula. Patients with this type of fistula tend to develop exophthalmos (bulging of the eyeball) with ocular pulsation synchronous with the heartbeat. Congenital arteriovenous fistulas are usually referred to as arteriovenous malformations (Poirier, 1990; Schochet, 1983; Adams and Victor, 1993).

8.12 Traumatic Intracranial Hematoma

Traumatic intracranial hematomas may be epidural, subdural, subarachnoid or intraparenchymal in location. (*See Figure 8-10.*)

[1] Epidural Hematoma

Epidural (extradural; outside the dura mater) hemorrhage most commonly occurs acutely from head trauma resulting in a linear fracture of the temporal bone (on the side of the head), with subsequent laceration of the underlying middle meningeal artery. The hematoma accumulates in the space between the skull and the dura mater. (*See Figure 8-11.*)

It is common for patients with an extradural hematoma to experience a brief loss of consciousness at the time of injury, due to cerebral concussion, and then to regain consciousness. They often have a characteristic "lucid interval," followed in a few hours by increased intracranial pressure and compression of brain structures as the hematoma enlarges. Compression of the third cranial nerve by herniated brain tissue results in a dilated pupil that does not respond to

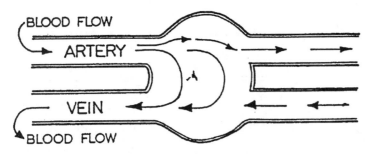

Fig. 8-9. An arteriovenous fistula diverts blood directly into the venous bed, owing to the higher pressure of arterial blood.

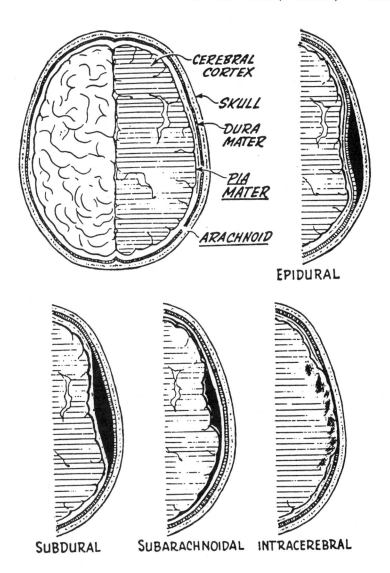

Fig. 8-10. The cerebral cortex (outer layer) and surrounding meninges, with different types of intracranial hematoma that may occur.

bright light. There may be weakness of the contralateral (opposite) side of the body.

Epidural hematomas are often fatal if not rapidly diagnosed and surgically evacuated. Diagnosis is usually accomplished by computed tomography (Poirier, 1990; Schochet, 1983; Rowland, 1995a; Adams and Victor, 1993).

[2] Subdural Hematoma

Subdural (between the dura mater and the arachnoid) hematomas result from arterial or venous bleeding in the subdural space, usually over the convexity of the cerebral hemisphere, and may be unilateral or bilateral (on one or both sides). (*See Figure 8-12.*) Symptoms result from painful stretching of the dura, increased intracranial pressure and displacement of brain structures as the hematoma enlarges.

Acute subdural hematoma typically follows acute trauma, as a result of arterial bleeding, and may combine with epidural hemorrhage, cerebral contusion and cerebral laceration. The clinical presentation

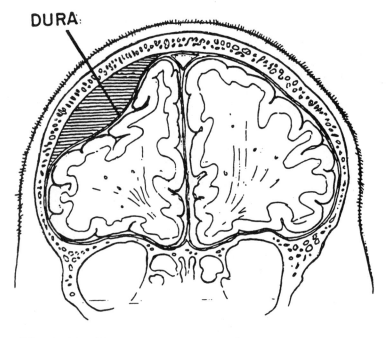

Fig. 8-11. Classic presentation of an epidural (extradural) hematoma.

is similar to that of epidural hematoma. CT is diagnostic, and prompt surgical evacuation is necessary if the hematoma causes mass effect.[3]

Chronic subdural hematoma results from venous bleeding and may not cause symptoms for weeks to months after head trauma. The trauma that precipitated the bleeding may have been so minor that the patient has no recollection of it. Stretching of the dura may cause headache, and compression of brain tissue from the enlarging hematoma may produce contralateral weakness. Increased intracranial pressure and displacement of brain structures may eventually occur, with potentially fatal herniation of brain tissue if a critical degree of brain displacement occurs.

CT is usually diagnostic, although it can fail to diagnose hematomas of a certain age that have the same density as brain tissue as seen on radiography. Magnetic resonance imaging (MRI) may be necessary for diagnosis in such cases.

Treatment consists of surgical evacuation if the hematoma results in significant mass effect. However, small chronic subdural hematomas that result in only minimal mass effect may be treated

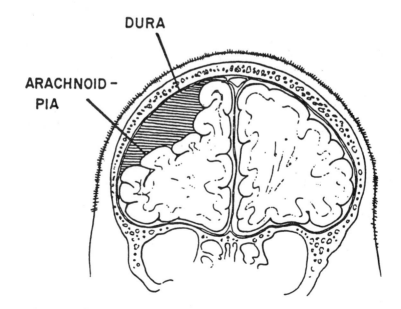

Fig. 8-12. Classic presentation of a subdural hematoma.

---

[3] *See* 8.10 *supra.*

conservatively with corticosteroid drugs and their course followed with serial CT (Poirier, 1990; Schochet, 1983; Rowland, 1995a; Adams and Victor, 1993).

[3] Traumatic Intraparenchymal Hemorrhage

Acute intraparenchymal (within the functional tissue) hemorrhage may result from penetrating or closed head injuries that cause laceration of intraparenchymal intracranial blood vessels. This can cause a rapid rise in intracranial pressure, with compression and displacement of normal brain structures. Such injuries are very often fatal, especially following penetrating injuries. Diagnosis is by computed tomography. Medical management of increased intracranial pressure and surgical hematoma evacuation are of limited value (Poirier, 1990; Schochet, 1983; Rowland, 1995a; Adams and Victor, 1993).

8.20 NONTRAUMATIC CEREBROVASCULAR DISEASE

Stroke and *cerebrovascular accident* (CVA) are terms used to refer to manifestations of nontraumatic cerebrovascular disease. A minority of strokes are caused by hemorrhage, usually either spontaneous subarachnoid hemorrhage or intraparenchymal brain hemorrhage. Most strokes consist of brain infarctions (tissue death) that are either thrombotic or embolic in origin.

8.21 Spontaneous Subarachnoid Hemorrhage

Primary subarachnoid hemorrhage accounts for 3 to 11 percent of strokes in the United States (Sacco, 1995). Approximately 26,000 nontraumatic subarachnoid hemorrhages occur in the United States each year, accounting for about 10 percent of all stroke deaths. Half of those who sustain spontaneous subarachnoid hemorrhage are over the age of 45.

[1] Etiology

An aneurysm is a sac in the wall of an artery whose underlying pathology involves a defect in the muscular coat and the internal elastic layers of the vessel wall. The weak area allows the arterial wall to bulge outward under pressure in the artery.

Aneurysms typically develop at areas of bifurcation (branching) of arteries. By far the majority of intracranial aneurysms are located in carotid artery territory, and 10 percent are in vertebrobasilar artery territory. Common sites are:

- the vicinity of the anterior communicating artery;
- the origin of the posterior communicating artery from the internal carotid artery;
- the first major bifurcation of the middle cerebral artery;
- the bifurcation of the internal carotid artery into the anterior and middle cerebral arteries;
- the origin of the ophthalmic artery (the first intracranial branch of the internal carotid artery, which supplies the eye with blood);
- the junction of the posterior communicating artery with the posterior cerebral artery;
- the bifurcations of the three pairs of cerebellar arteries; and
- the top of the basilar artery.

The most common type of aneurysm is a "saccular" or "berry" aneurysm. It is commonly accepted that these aneurysms are a result of a congenital defect of the arterial wall. This produces a localized area of arterial dilation, with the aneurysm sac usually connected to the arterial wall by a narrow neck. The wall of the sac consists of elastic tissue that often is very thin.

Saccular aneurysms are rarely seen before puberty, but it is estimated that 5 percent of persons age 20 and older have one or more, and that 25 percent of these people have multiple aneurysms. Saccular aneurysms are slightly more prevalent in women than men. They range in size from 2 mm to several cm, with the average size being 7 to 10 mm. Aneurysms greater than 3 cm in diameter are referred to as *giant aneurysms,* and these are at lower risk than smaller aneurysms (7 to 12 mm) of producing massive hemorrhage.

Mycotic aneurysms result from the inflammation of infected arterial walls, most commonly as a result of septic (infected) emboli in people with infective endocarditis (inflammation of the lining of the heart).[4] They usually occur in peripheral branches of the intracranial arteries.

Arteriosclerotic aneurysms are relatively uncommon; when they occur, they are usually cylindrical or fusiform (spindle-shaped;

---

[4] *See* 8.37 *infra* for further discussion of endocarditis.

tapering at both ends) in shape. They most commonly involve the proximal (closer to the point of origin) intracranial internal carotid arteries and the basilar artery, and they are often very large. Rupture is uncommon; more often, these aneurysms partially or completely thrombose (clot closed).

Angiomas are congenital malformations of vessels. There are four major types: venous, cavernous and capillary angiomas, and arteriovenous malformations. Venous angiomas are the most common and consist of anomalous veins. Rupture of this type of angioma is uncommon. Cavernous angiomas are composed of a mass of sinusoidal vessels. Capillary angiomas (telangiectases) are composed of small, capillarylike vessels. Arteriovenous malformations consist of masses of arteries and veins with abnormal direct connections. They vary greatly in size and location, although they most commonly occur in the cerebral hemispheres and are the type of angioma most likely to be symptomatic (Mayberg, et al., 1994; Schochet, 1983).

[2]   Pathogenesis

Theories for the pathogenesis of saccular aneurysms include congenital defects of the arterial media, vestigial remnants of embryonic vessels and arteriosclerosis. None of these explanations is completely satisfactory. Hypertension (high blood pressure) is considered by some to have etiologic significance, but hypertension is less common in patients with aneurysms.

There is also no satisfactory explanation for the cause of rupture of saccular aneurysms. The relationship of physical activity to rupture is not at all clear. The role of trauma in precipitating the rupture of an intracranial aneurysm has long been a matter of controversy. Trauma can only be implicated as a cause by a temporal relationship between the trauma and evidence of aneurysm rupture. It is likely that in many cases, loss of consciousness from a vehicular accident occurred at the time of aneurysm rupture, and that the accident did not cause the rupture. About a third of aneurysmal ruptures occur during sleep.

Angiomas are congenital malformations. Arteriovenous and cavernous angiomas occasionally grow, although most are smaller than 3 cm in size and tend to remain so. Only a minority—perhaps 10 percent—rupture with massive bleeding. No definite cause of angioma rupture has been identified A close association between head trauma and rupture is difficult or impossible to prove (Mayberg, et al., 1994; Schochet, 1983).

[3] Clinical Presentation

Most aneurysms are asymptomatic until they rupture. Giant aneurysms can compress normal brain structures and have a mass effect on the function of these structures.[5] Occasionally smaller aneurysms enlarge and produce mass effect by compression of normal intracranial structures. The most common example of this phenomenon is compression of the oculomotor nerve by an enlarging posterior communicating artery aneurysm, resulting in ptosis (drooping eyelid), pupillary dilation and impaired extraocular movement (dysfunction of the extraocular muscle, which contributes to excursion of the eye). Retroorbital pain may result from compression of the ophthalmic division of the trigeminal nerve (the fifth cranial nerve).

About 30 percent of patients with acute aneurysmal rupture report suspicious symptoms a few hours, days or weeks prior to rupture. Symptoms include "sentinel headache," stiff neck, nausea, dizziness, syncope (fainting) and disturbances of vision. These symptoms are often minor or absent but, in retrospect, their presence may signal initial aneurysmal leak (Brust, 1995c).

Arteriovenous malformations more commonly cause symptoms without rupture, including seizures and chronic recurrent headache that is clinically indistinguishable from migraine. A minority of arteriovenous malformations result in subarachnoid hemorrhages, most often in pregnant women.

Subarachnoid hemorrhage is the hallmark of aneurysmal rupture, owing to the arterial saccular aneurysm's rupture into the subarachnoid space. If the aneurysm tip is pointed toward the parenchyma of the brain, blood may rupture into the brain tissue or the ventricular system of the brain. If the arachnoid membrane ruptures, blood can enter the subdural space and form a subdural hematoma.

The first symptom of rupture is usually very sudden onset of excruciating headache, typically described as the worst headache a person has ever experienced. This may be accompanied by neck pain, loss of consciousness and seizure activity. Confusion may be present if consciousness is preserved or regained. There is often moderate

---

[5] *See* 8.10 *supra* for further discussion of mass effect.

fever (102° to 103° F) and elevation of the peripheral white blood cell count (leukocytosis). Many cases have a more subtle presentation (Mayberg, et al., 1994; Adams and Victor, 1993).

[4]   Neurologic Complications

Because the cranium is a rigidly enclosed space, any increase in its contents can raise pressure within the head. With subarachnoid hemorrhage due to aneurysmal rupture, the sudden rush of blood into the subarachnoid space under arterial pressure can cause a sudden, tremendous increase in intracranial pressure. This results in compression and dysfunction of normal brain structures, often with coma and rapidly ensuing death (Plum and Posner, 1980).

Pressure on the hypothalamus can cause impaired body temperature regulation and the inappropriate secretion of antidiuretic hormone (ADH), resulting in excessive fluid retention and hyponatremia (low sodium content in circulating blood). This can cause confusion, stupor and seizures.

[a]   Rebleeding

Without surgical intervention, about 30 percent of patients who survive an initial aneurysmal rupture will rebleed (experience recurrent hemorrhage) within a month. This occurs most commonly between the fifth and ninth day after the initial hemorrhage. Rebleeding has been the cause of death in almost 40 percent of fatal subarachnoid hemorrhages (Sahs, et al., 1981). The use of epsilon aminocaproic acid to reduce rebleeding has been abandoned, owing to complications, its lack of proven effect on outcome and the increasing acceptance of early surgical intervention. After six months, the rate of rebleeding drops to about 3 percent a year (Jane, et al., 1985).

[b]   Vasospasm

Vasospasm is a more common cause of clinical deterioration than rebleeding. The severity of spasm of arteries in the subarachnoid space correlates with the amount of blood that is present. Although the pathogenesis is not entirely clear, there is some evidence that chemical mediators such as histamine, serotonin and angiotensin may be involved. Vasospasm occurs 3 to 21 days after subarachnoid hemorrhage, resulting in ischemia and infarction of brain tissue in the distribution of the arteries in spasm. Brain infarctions can produce a variety of focal neurologic symptoms and signs, including aphasia (difficulty speaking), hemiparesis (paralysis on one side of the body), sensory and visual abnormalities and disturbances of consciousness.

[c] Hydrocephalus

The presence of clotted blood in the subarachnoid space or the ventricles of the brain can impede the resorption of CSF, resulting in hydrocephalus (ventricular enlargement due to fluid accumulation). This type of hydrocephalus is seen in 5 to 10 percent of persons who sustain nontraumatic subarachnoid hemorrhage. Fibrin (a blood component that is essential to clotting) from the hemorrhage can obstruct the foramina of Luschka and Magendie (openings in the brain stem that connect the fourth ventricle of the brain with the subarachnoid space), or adhesions can develop between the pia mater and arachnoid membrane, blocking the resorption of CSF. This increases intracranial pressure, resulting in generalized brain compression and dysfunction, usually with headache, confusion and a decline in consciousness. Hydrocephalus usually appears two to four weeks after hemorrhage but may present more insidiously (Mayberg, et al., 1994; Adams and Victor, 1993).

[5] Diagnosis

Definitive diagnosis of an aneurysm or arteriovenous malformation is currently made by conventional cerebral arteriography. Unruptured giant aneurysms and many arteriovenous malformations can be visualized with brain MRI or CT. The technology of intracranial magnetic resonance angiography (MRA) is rapidly evolving. The resolution of intracranial MRA is already adequate for visualizing most saccular aneurysms and arteriovenous malformations, and MRA may eventually replace conventional radiographic arteriography. Some small, asymptomatic aneurysms are identified by MRI, MRA or CT performed for an unrelated indication (Mayberg, et al., 1994; Greenberg, 1995).

Diagnosis of subarachnoid hemorrhage can be difficult and is frequently delayed or missed. Diagnosis begins with a high index of clinical suspicion, especially when patients present to an emergency department with acute headache or other subtle symptoms. The patient may abruptly lose consciousness, remain conscious but confused or remain alert and oriented. Nausea, vomiting, hypertension (high blood pressure) and altered level of consciousness are commonly observed. Seizures and fever are sometimes seen. Neck stiffness is often a prominent complaint, with nuchal (nape) rigidity present on examination. This is due to irritation of the meninges as blood circulates through the CSF into the spinal subarachnoid space. Focal neurologic findings are often absent, unless the aneurysm has ruptured into the parenchyma (functional tissue) of the brain or there is occlusion of an artery distal to the aneurysm, in which case hemiparesis or other focal deficits may be present. Cranial nerve palsies (paralyses), particularly involving the oculomotor (third cranial) nerve, may develop due to sudden compression. Hemorrhage into the retina of the eye may occur; subhyaloid retinal hemorrhage (hemorrhage between the retina of the eye and the hyaloid membrane separating it from the vitreous humor) is virtually diagnostic of subarachnoid hemorrhage (Adams and Victor, 1993; Yatsu, 1995a).

[a]   CT Scan

Diagnosis of subarachnoid hemorrhage can usually be confirmed by cranial CT, which is generally superior to MRI for this purpose. CT also allows for the diagnosis of intraparenchymal hemorrhage, subdural hemorrhage and acute obstructive hydrocephalus. If subarachnoid blood is identified on CT, lumbar puncture is usually unnecessary. However, CT will miss a small percentage of cases of subarachnoid hemorrhage. If the CT is nondiagnostic and subarachnoid hemorrhage is still suspected, a lumbar puncture (spinal tap; withdrawal of cerebrospinal fluid through a needle inserted into the low back) should be performed.

[b]   CSF Studies

CSF drawn from a person with subarachnoid hemorrhage is uniformly bloody. Any bloody CSF should be centrifuged. The supernatant (top) layer of the fluid after centrifuging is xanthochromic (yellow), indicating that blood has been present for at least six hours. This differentiates between subarachnoid hemorrhage and the presence of blood from a traumatic lumbar puncture. Spinal fluid pressure is usually elevated, ranging from 200 to 500 mm of water. In addition to red blood cells, excessive white blood cells may be present in the CSF, owing to inflammation of the meninges (chemical meningitis). CSF glucose concentration is often modestly reduced, and CSF protein concentration may be slightly increased (Brust, 1995c; Yatsu, 1995a).

[c] Arteriography

Following confirmation of subarachnoid hemorrhage by CT or lumbar puncture, complete arteriography of the intracranial vessels is necessary to identify one or more aneurysms. This should typically be done in a timely fashion (within 12 to 48 hours). Arteriography should be complete, because many patients have multiple aneurysms.

The presence of multiple aneurysms can present a challenge regarding diagnosing which aneurysm has ruptured, since clinical symptoms may not accurately reflect the location of the hemorrhage. However, when CT is combined with complete arteriography, the correct site of bleeding can be identified in most cases. If an aneurysm or arteriovenous malformation is not identified, arteriography is commonly repeated after 10 to 14 days.

Arteriography also allows for the identification of vasospasm[6] in cases of subarachnoid hemorrhage (Yatsu, 1995a; Greenberg, 1995; Mayberg, et al., 1994; Brust, 1995c). Vasospasm can also be diagnosed and monitored by transcranial Doppler ultrasonography (Babikian and Wechsler, 1993). Skull radiographs, electroencephalography (which measures the brain's electrical activity) and radionuclide brain scanning (which measures the uptake of radioactive isotopes in the bloodstream as a gauge of pathology) have very limited utility in the diagnosis and evaluation of subarachnoid hemorrhage (Mayberg, et al., 1994).

[6] Treatment

Diagnosis should be made in a timely fashion, and patients should generally be placed in a quiet, dark room. Fluid and electrolyte abnormalities should be corrected, blood sugar levels should be controlled, excessive hypertension should be treated and seizures should be managed with anticonvulsant medications. The administration of oral nimodipine has been demonstrated to reduce the incidence of vasospasm (Pickard, et al., 1989).

Surgery is considered the definitive treatment for saccular aneurysm. In the past, surgery was typically delayed for one or two weeks, due to increased morbidity and mortality associated with vasospasm. However, this introduced a significant risk of rebleeding. Recent technical advances allow neurosurgeons to surgically clip or obliterate

---

[6] *See* 8.11[4] *supra* for a discussion of vascular spasm.

most aneurysms soon after rupture (within 24 to 72 hours) and to flush blood from the subarachnoid cisterns (Miyaoka, et al., 1993). Surgery is sometimes still delayed in medically unstable or neurologically devastated patients, in patients with demonstrated severe vasospasm and in patients in whom the source of bleeding cannot be identified.

Three types of surgical failure may necessitate reoperation. During exploration, the surgeon may abandon clipping as dangerous or impractical and choose to wrap the aneurysm with fat or muscle tissue, or to ligate (tie off) the carotid artery. Imperfect placement of a clip can result in slipping. Carotid artery ligation, which is now uncommon, may fail to terminate blood flow to the aneurysm (Drake, et al., 1984).

Surgical evacuation of an intraparenchymal or a subdural hematoma may be necessary to eliminate mass effect. If acute hydrocephalus develops, ventricular drainage by ventriculostomy (surgical opening of the ventricle) may be required (Mayberg, et al., 1994; Adams and Victor, 1993).

Interventional neuroradiology involves the obliteration of some aneurysms, especially giant aneurysms, with balloons, wires and coils introduced via an arterial catheter. These techniques, along with interventional embolization with plastic spheres, are more commonly used to obliterate arteriovenous malformations. Sometimes the obliteration is partial, prior to surgical excision or noninvasive radiosurgical obliteration using a "gamma knife." These treatment modalities are not widely available and are currently experimental (Mayberg, et al., 1994).

[7]   Prognosis

Age and condition of the patient; size, location and configuration of the aneurysm; presence of multiple aneurysms; time interval between rupture and surgery; quality of the medical facility; and skill of the surgeon are all important variables that influence survival and quality of life following rupture and repair of a saccular aneurysm.

A commonly applied grading system is based on the preoperative neurologic status of the patient:

Grade 1: alert, oriented, with or without headache, with no motor or sensory deficit.

Grade 2: moderate alteration in sensorium or focal deficit; severe headache and meningeal signs.

Grade 3: obtunded (sensorium blunted) and/or major focal deficit.

Grade 4: stuporous or comatose, with or without major lateralizing findings.

The rate of mortality increases progressively with increase in preoperative clinical grade. There is also a close correlation between clinical grade and quality of survival. Patients with grade 3 or 4 clinical status have a much poorer postoperative outcome. Surgery for such patients is sometimes delayed, although this introduces the risk of rebleeding. About 40 percent of patients with ruptured aneurysms die of the initial bleed. At least 40 to 50 percent of patients who rebleed die, and morbidity for survivors of rebleeding is increased (Nishioka, et al., 1984; Ingall, and Wiebers, 1993). Intraventricular hemorrhage is usually fatal.

The results of surgical treatment of saccular aneurysms have improved dramatically over the years. The experience and skill of the surgeon are very important: Operative results tend to be better for neurosurgeons who perform such procedures relatively regularly and frequently (Adams and Victor, 1993).

Restoration of function depends on age of the patient, severity of neurologic damage and absence of rebleeding. With mild to moderate neurologic deficit, full recovery often takes place, especially in the absence of focal neurologic signs indicating intracerebral hemorrhage or infarction from vasospasm. If patients with intraparenchymal bleeding or infarction survive, they often exhibit permanent neurologic sequela, including mental changes, paralysis, aphasia (difficulty speaking), visual field defects and epilepsy.

8.22 Spontaneous Intraparenchymal Brain Hemorrhage

Primary intracerebral hemorrhage accounts for 5 to 10 percent of strokes in the United States (Sacco, 1995).

[1] Etiology

Trauma is the most common cause of intraparenchymal (intracerebral) brain hemorrhage. Acute intraparenchymal hemorrhage may result from penetrating or closed head injuries that cause laceration of intraparenchymal intracranial blood vessels.

Arteriovenous malformation, which can be a source of subarachnoid hemorrhage, usually results in intraparenchymal brain hemorrhage when it ruptures.[7] It is commonly believed that spontaneous intra-parenchymal brain hemorrhage with no identifiable cause may be due to a small, "cryptic" arteriovenous malformation that occludes or destroys itself when it ruptures (Schochet, 1983).

Hypertension (high blood pressure) is a common cause of intra-parenchymal brain hemorrhage. Hypertensive hemorrhages may be massive, small or petechial (pinpoint size). The most common locations, in descending frequency, are the basal ganglia (a cluster of gray matter at the base of the brain; 50 percent), the cerebral lobes ("lobar hemorrhage"), the thalamus, the cerebellum and the pons of the brain stem (Adams and Victor, 1993; Sacco, 1995; Schochet, 1983). A small number of intraparenchymal hemorrhages arise from a degenerative disorder affecting the media of smaller arteries in elderly people that is referred to as congophilic amyloid angiopathy (Yatsu, 1995b).

Brain tumors typically present subacutely or chronically as they grow, but they may present acutely due to hemorrhage into the tumor. This is especially prevalent with metastatic (traveling from the site of origin to more distant areas) melanoma (a type of skin cancer), renal (kidney) cell carcinoma, choriocarcinoma (a highly malignant tumor with common metastases to the brain) and bronchogenic (related to the lungs) carcinoma (Mohr, 1995b; Schochet, 1983).

Illicit drug use must be considered in the etiology of intraparenchymal brain hemorrhage in a person with drug-induced vasculitis. The two substances most commonly implicated are methamphetamine and crack cocaine.

Mycotic (septic) aneurysms typically result from endocarditis. These present as intraparenchymal brain hemorrhage more commonly than as subarachnoid hemorrhage (Schochet, 1983).

[2] Pathogenesis

Trauma and arteriovenous malformations both can precipitate intraparenchymal hemorrhage. Hypertensive hemorrhages are believed to result from the rupture of microaneurysms on small intracerebral arteries, and subsequent mechanical distension by arterial hypertension. Referred to as microaneurysms of Charcot and Brouchard, these result in the total replacement of the normal endothelial, muscular and elastic elements of the vessel by a thin layer of connective tissue. This

---

[7] *See* 8.21 *supra* for further discussion of arteriovenous malformations.

destruction of the normal vascular architecture results in the deposition of lipid (fat) and fibrin (fibrous clotting elements) products (lipohyalinosis), predisposing to fragility of the vessel wall and potentiating rupture and hemorrhage (Poirier, et al., 1990). With congophilic amyloid angiopathy, vascular fragility results from the deposition of amyloid protein in the vessel walls. Drug use can contribute to the development of arteritis (inflammation of the arterial walls), with subsequent vascular fragility.

[3]   Clinical Presentation

Neurologic symptoms and signs vary with the site and size of the hemorrhage.The neurologic deficit resulting from intraparenchymal hemorrhage typically begins abruptly, depends on the site of hemorrhage, is usually accompanied by hypertension and may be accompanied by headache, nausea, vomiting and loss of consciousness. Headache may be absent in as much as 50 percent of cases. Seizures occur in about 10 percent of cases of intracerebral hemorrhage. With the advent of CT, many small hemorrhages are now identified that would previously have been clinically diagnosed as cerebral infarctions.

Basal ganglionic hemorrhages tend to involve the internal capsule and result in hemiplegia, with large hemorrhages (greater than 2 to 3 cm in diameter) producing stupor and coma. Similar symptoms are seen with lobar and thalamic hemorrhages. Lobar hemorrhages also commonly produce visual field defects and aphasia. Pontine (referring to the pons; part of the brain stem) hemorrhages are usually devastating, with oculomotor (referring to eye movement) disturbances and deep coma typically developing within minutes. Cerebellar hemorrhage may develop over several hours, with vomiting, headache, vertigo and ataxia (incoordination). Prompt diagnosis of cerebellar hemorrhage is very important if fatal, progressive brain stem compression is to be prevented. Surgical decompression can be lifesaving in such cases (Adams and Victor, 1993; Patten, 1996; Plum and Posner, 1980).

[4]   Neurologic Complications

Focal neurologic symptoms and signs vary with the site and size of the hematoma. A zone of edema (swelling due to accumulation of fluid) develops around the hematoma, contributing to the size of the mass. Within the rigidly enclosed space of the cranium, any increase in contents can raise intracranial pressure. This results in compression, brain tissue herniation (protrusion through the foramen magnum, or opening at the base of the skull), ischemia and dysfunction of normal brain structures, often with coma and rapid death. Brain stem hemorrhages have a particularly high mortality. Cerebellar hemorrhages are also extremely dangerous, due to the risk of progressive brain stem compression, which can be rapid and fatal (Plum and Posner, 1980).

[5] Diagnosis

Intraparenchymal and intraventricular intracranial bleeding is very easy to diagnose by CT, which is typically superior to MRI in this situation. The primary purpose of emergent neuroimaging with CT of patients presenting to an emergency department with coma or focal neurologic signs is to diagnose intracranial bleeding (Caplan, et al., 1995; Plum and Posner, 1980; Schochet, 1983).

[6] Treatment

Fluid and electrolyte abnormalities should be corrected; blood sugar levels should be controlled; excessive hypertension (high blood pressure) should be treated and seizures should be treated with anticonvulsants. Ventilatory (respiratory) support may be necessary, as may hyperventilation, which lowers intracranial pressure. A corticosteroid (usually dexamethasone) may be administered to reduce edema, especially in patients with large hemorrhages and poor neurologic condition. However, the value of corticosteroid therapy for improving neurologic deficits is unproved. With acute, massive intracranial pressure and herniation, the administration of mannitol (a hyperosmotic agent) may lower intracranial pressure and be lifesaving (Adams and Victor, 1993).

The goal for treating arterial hypertension after intracerebral hemorrhage is a subject of controversy. Proponents of aggressive treatment favor lowering arterial blood pressure to prevent further bleeding. However, there is evidence that bleeding stops spontaneously within 30 minutes and that excessive lowering of arterial blood pressure can worsen the patient's neurologic status by reducing cerebral blood flow, aggravating ischemia and promoting infarction (Adams and Victor, 1993; Mohr, 1995a).

Cerebellar hemorrhages resulting in brain stem compression and a decline in consciousness should be surgically evacuated. Most other intraparenchymal brain hemorrhages are treated medically, unless there is significant decline in neurologic status resulting from increased intracranial pressure and herniation of brain tissue. Some advocate surgical evacuation of the hematoma at this point, although there is wide variation in the degree of enthusiasm with which neurosurgeons evacuate intracerebral hemorrhages. The outcome is often poor with this type of surgical intervention, because patients for whom it is reserved have typically suffered acute, massive brain injury.

[7] Prognosis

The overall mortality rate is high for patients with intraparenchymal brain hemorrhage, with 30 to 35 percent of patients dying within 30 days (Adams and Victor, 1993). The mortality rate is extremely high for pontine hemorrhages and basal ganglionic hemorrhages that rupture into the ventricular system, regardless of the type of treatment that is rendered. The mortality rate following basal ganglionic, thalamic and lobar hemorrhages depends on the size of the hemorrhage and ranges from 13 percent to 40 percent. With cerebellar hemorrhage, mortality relates to the size of the hemorrhage. Neurosurgical evacuation of the hematoma can be lifesaving in cases of brain stem compression, if it is performed in a timely fashion (Mohr, 1995a; Adams and Victor, 1993; Plum and Posner, 1980; Lampl, et al., 1995).

8.23 Thrombotic Ischemic Brain Infarction

Ischemic infarction accounts for 70 to 80 percent of strokes in the United States.

[1] Etiology

Thrombotic ischemic brain infarction (death of brain tissue caused by a blood clot that blocks a cerebral artery) is the most common type of stroke. Cardioembolism (a blood clot from the heart that travels through the bloodstream) accounts for 15 to 30 percent of strokes,[8] and thrombotic ischemic cerebrovascular infarction makes up the majority of the remainder. Atherosclerosis (deposition of fatty plaques in the arterial wall) is by far the most important underlying pathophysiologic factor for thrombosis of a cerebral artery.

Risk factors for noncardiac cerebral infarction include age, hypertension, diabetes mellitus, cigarette smoking, coronary artery disease,

---

[8] *See* 8.24 *infra* for further discussion of cardioembolic ischemic brain infarction.

lipid abnormalities and a family history of atherosclerotic disease. Excessive alcohol consumption is a recognized risk factor for stroke. However, there is evidence that light alcohol use may be protective against the development of atherosclerosis (Sacco, 1995; Adams and Victor, 1993; Hachinski, et al., 1996; Whisnant, 1996). Migraine may be an independent risk factor for cerebral infarction (Buring, et al., 1995).

[2] Pathogenesis

The common denominator in the pathogenesis of the most common type of stroke is atherosclerosis, which results from the deposition of lipids, fibrin and platelets on the arterial endothelium and the formation of plaques. Atherosclerosis most commonly affects large arteries, such as the internal carotid, vertebral and basilar, and has a predilection for sites of arterial bifurcation (division). Calcification (hardening due to calcium deposition), intramural hemorrhage (bleeding in the blood vessel wall) and mural thrombosis (clotting in the blood vessel wall) lead to an increase in plaque size.

Atherosclerotic plaque predisposes to cerebral ischemia, thrombosis and infarction by three mechanisms: ischemia, arterial thrombosis and microembolization. Small vessel occlusion and trauma can also play a role.

[a] Ischemia

Ischemia distal to the site of an atherosclerotic plaque can occur if the lumen of the vessel is sufficiently stenotic (narrowed) to compromise blood flow in the artery. Arterial stenosis is typically not hemodynamically significant unless the arterial lumen is at least 70 to 80 percent stenotic. In such cases, superimposed arterial hypotension (low blood pressure) can lead to ischemia and infarction without thrombosis.

[b] Arterial Thrombosis

Arterial thrombosis tends to occur at areas of atherosclerotic plaque. Platelet and fibrin deposition on a plaque results in mural (pertaining to a vessel wall) thrombus formation, with occlusion of the artery. The ensuing ischemia results in infarction of the brain tissue that is supplied by the occluded artery.

[c] Microembolization

Microembolization probably plays a major role in the pathogenesis of ischemic cerebrovascular symptoms associated with atherosclerosis. Platelet and fibrin deposition on a large-vessel atherosclerotic plaque may result in nonocclusive mural thrombus formation. Small parts of this thrombus (microemboli) may then break off and flow to more distal arterial branches, resulting in transient or permanent occlusion, with transient or permanent focal neurologic symptoms.

[d] Small Vessel Occlusion

Noncardiac cerebral infarction may also result from small vessel occlusion. This is most commonly due to lipohyalinosis (degeneration of smooth tissue and replacement with fatty tissue) of small arteries associated with arterial hypertension (sometimes referred to as arteriosclerosis). It may also be related to microembolism from atherosclerotic plaques in larger vessels. Small vessel disease is also common in diabetic individuals (Poirier, et al., 1990; Schochet, 1983; Sacco, 1995).

[e] Trauma

Trauma can play a role in thrombotic infarction. This applies primarily to dissection of the carotid and vertebral arteries (enlargement and extension of a thrombus along the vessel wall) during manipulation of the neck, as well as during other activities associated with sudden neck movement.[9]

[3] Clinical Presentation

Ischemic cerebrovascular disease manifests clinically as one or more focal neurologic symptoms and signs. Subjective symptoms can include having trouble speaking, visual problems, difficulty swallowing, dizziness, imbalance, weakness and numbness. Objective signs can include aphasia (difficulty speaking), visual field defects, loss of ocular motility, ataxia (incoordination), dysarthria (slurred speech), inattention, loss of spatial organization, sensory loss, paresis (partial paralysis) and paralysis. (*See Figure 8-13.*)

Symptoms of ischemic cerebrovascular disease typically begin acutely. They may be transient, evolve and progress, or remain stable. The combination of symptoms and signs depends on the location and

---

[9] *See* 8.11[3] *supra* for further discussion of arterial dissection.

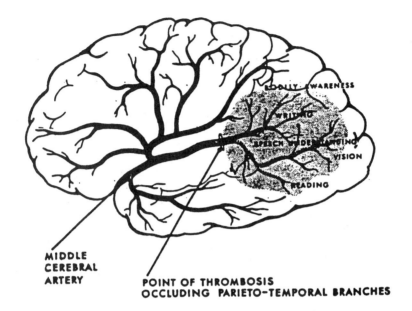

Fig. 8-13. Thrombotic occlusion of a cerebral artery that produces visual field defects, among other problems.

size of the ischemic area of the brain. (*See Figure 8-14.*) Cerebral cortical (in the lobes) ischemic lesions produce symptoms experienced on the contralateral (opposite) side of the body and may rarely be accompanied by seizures. Cerebellar ischemic lesions are accompanied by symptoms on the ipsilateral (same) side of the body. Cranial nerve involvement is the hallmark of brain stem ischemic lesions.

A number of common stroke syndromes have been described (Patten, 1996; Poirier, et al., 1990; Adams and Victor, 1993; Brust, 1995b; Kistler, et al., 1994). Stupor and coma may be present with brain stem lesions, bilateral cerebral lesions and large unilateral cerebral lesions with mass effect and increased intracranial pressure (Plum and Posner, 1980).

[a]   Lacunar Strokes

Lacunar strokes (characterized by the development of lacunae, or empty spaces in brain tissue) are caused by occlusion of small penetrating arterioles in the subcortical cerebrum and brain stem, resulting in small infarctions that can be clinically silent or devastating,

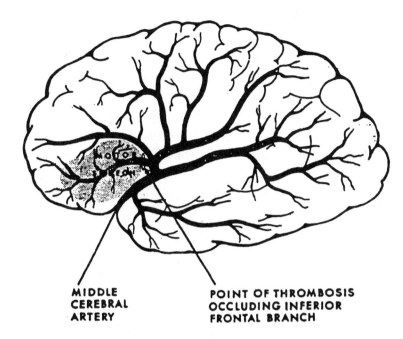

MIDDLE
CEREBRAL
ARTERY

POINT OF THROMBOSIS
OCCLUDING INFERIOR
FRONTAL BRANCH

Fig. 8-14. Thrombotic obstruction of a cerebral artery, leading to weakness of the lower part of the right side of the face and tongue that causes disabilities of speech.

depending on the location. They are most commonly a result of long-standing, untreated hypertension (high blood pressure) that causes arteriosclerosis. As many as 35 percent of lacunar infarctions may be asymptomatic, but most are symptomatic as transient ischemic attacks (TIAs) or sudden, focal neurologic deficit, with a stepwise pattern of deterioration over time as more lacunae develop. Discrete clinical syndromes that have been described include pure motor hemiplegia (motor paralysis on one side of the body), pure hemisensory (loss of sensation on side of the body) stroke, sensorimotor pseudobulbar palsy (paralysis of nerves in the rhombencephalon, or hindbrain, which is comprised of the pons, cerebellum and medulla oblongata), ipsilateral ataxia (incoordination on the same side as the stroke), hemiparesis and dysarthria. Multiple lacunae tend to occur bilaterally in the basal ganglia and brain stem, with dementia, rigidity and gait disturbances developing (Yatsu, 1995b; Adams and Victor, 1993; Critchley, 1983).

[b]   Transient Ischemic Attacks (TIAs)

Transient ischemic attacks (TIAs) are groupings of focal neurologic symptoms resulting from ischemia to the eye (*amaurosis fugax,* a form of temporary blindness) or a part of the brain supplied by the carotid or vertebro-basilar arteries. By definition, such symptoms last less than 24 hours and clinically resolve completely. They typically last a few minutes to a few hours before complete clinical resolution.

Most TIAs probably result from platelet-fibrin microemboli that arise from a more proximal atherosclerotic plaque, although they can result from cardiogenic emboli. Patients who experience TIAs are at increased risk of stroke and myocardial infarction. Improved diagnosis of TIAs in recent years may be partially responsible for an observed reduction of the incidence of strokes. Although clinical resolution is complete within 24 hours, CT and MRI have demonstrated that many patients with clinical TIAs actually experience a small brain infarction. Transient symptoms that resolve after more than 24 hours have often been referred to as reversible ischemic neurologic deficits (rinds), although this is a term with little meaning (Yatsu, 1995b; Brust, 1995a; Adams and Victor, 1993; Kistler, et al., 1994; Waxman, et al., 1983; Hachinski, 1984).

[c]   Ischemic Penumbra

Many patients who have symptoms of brain dysfunction due to ischemic cerebrovascular disease undergo progressive evolution of the neurologic deficit due to complications. However, the concept of the "ischemic penumbra" is of paramount importance. The ischemic penumbra is a zone of viable brain tissue with critically reduced blood flow surrounding an area of ischemic infarction. Factors that further reduce blood flow to this ischemic zone can result in extension of a brain infarction, with evolution of clinical symptoms (Yatsu, 1995a; Adams, 1994; Adams and Victor, 1993).

[d]   Completed Stroke

Many patients with focal neurologic deficits due to ischemic cerebrovascular disease do not experience resolution of their symptoms; neither do they undergo clinical evolution (progression). Such patients, as well as those whose condition has evolved, are said to have a "completed stroke" (Yatsu, 1995a).

[4] Neurologic Complications

Neurologic deterioration after ischemic brain infarction can occur by several mechanisms, among them evolution of infarction due to loss of viability of the ischemic penumbra. This process is promoted by ischemia-induced collection of neural excitotoxins (products toxic to nerve cells) and calcium in the ischemic, but still viable, neurons of the ischemic penumbra.

Ischemic and infarcted neurons become edematous (swollen due to an influx of water), contributing to the size of the mass. With brain infarctions, maximum edema typically occurs on the third or fourth day after infarction. Brain infarctions can undergo hemorrhagic transformation due to bleeding into the infarcted area of brain tissue. This is more common with infarctions caused by cardiogenic emboli and venous occlusion. Any increase in contents within the rigidly enclosed space of the cranium can raise intracranial pressure. This results in compression, brain tissue herniation, ischemia and dysfunction of normal brain structures, often with coma and rapid death. Distortion of penetrating pontine arteries due to downward herniation of brain tissue can lead to brain stem hemorrhages known as Duret's hemorrhages, which usually lead to death.

There is no convincing evidence that corticosteroid therapy benefits the cerebral edema associated with cerebral infarction. Seizures can occur with acute ischemic brain infarction (Yatsu, 1995a; Adams and Victor, 1993; Plum and Posner, 1980; Poirier, et al., 1990; Schochet, 1983; Kilpatrick, et al., 1990).

[5] Diagnosis

The initial step in the proper management of patients with cerebral infarction is correct diagnosis in a timely fashion. Diagnosis of brain infarction can usually be made correctly on clinical grounds, although it is important to exclude a diagnosis of intraparenchymal brain hemorrhage, subdural hematoma, neoplasm (tumor) and other causes of focal neurologic deficits. It is also impossible to absolutely differentiate between cardiogenic embolic and thrombotic ischemic infarctions on clinical grounds.

Patients who present with a focal neurologic deficit should undergo a complete medical history and physical examination, as well as an urgent CT scan, primarily to exclude hemorrhage and other pathologic processes.

Acute infarctions may not be visualized initially on early CT. Other routine emergent tests include electrocardiogram (EKG, a measure of the electrical activity of the heart), complete blood count (CBC), platelet count, serum electrolyte levels (measures of substances that facilitate electrical activity in the tissues), blood sugar levels, renal (kidney) function testing, prothrombin time (a measure of the blood's clotting ability), partial thromboplastin time (another measure of the blood's clotting ability) and pulse oximetry or arterial blood gases. These tests should allow for differentiation of most TIAs and brain infarctions from other causes of acute focal neurologic deficits, often by exclusion, although they do not always allow for the differentiation between cardiogenic embolic and thrombotic ischemic infarctions. In addition, the severity of illness and clinical stability of the patient are simultaneously observed.

If the CT scan is not diagnostic and subarachnoid hemorrhage or meningoencephalitis (inflammation of the brain and meninges) is suspected, a lumbar puncture (spinal tap) should be performed. Additional laboratory tests in selected situations can include blood ethanol (alcohol) level, drug screen and liver function tests. Serum calcium and magnesium levels should be checked if seizures have occurred (Adams, 1994; Adams, 1995; Feinberg, et al., 1994; Mohr, 1995b; Adams and Victor, 1993).

The diagnosis of cardiogenic embolic causes of stroke is sometimes indefinite, but important. The decision that a patient has had a cardiogenic embolus is usually made based on circumstantial evidence provided by the clinical history, physical examination, electrocardiogram, carotid Doppler ultrasound, arteriography and echocardiography.[10]

All patients with TIAs or acute ischemic cerebral infarction should be evaluated for the presence of significant carotid artery stenosis (narrowing). Technologic advances in carotid Doppler ultrasonography now allow for screening of patients, with high-quality studies eliminating the need for conventional arteriography for many patients. Patients with greater than 50 percent carotid artery stenosis by Doppler should probably undergo conventional arteriography. Technologic advances in the resolution of magnetic resonance angiography may eliminate the need for conventional arteriography (Adams, 1995; von Reutern and von Büdingen, 1993; Greenberg, 1995).

---

[10] *See* 8.24[5][c] *infra* for further discussion of echocardiography.

[6] Medical Treatment

Optimally, patients with acute ischemic neurologic events should be admitted to the hospital and undergo continuous cardiac monitoring. There is significant cardiac co-morbidity with ischemic cerebrovascular disease, and as many as 40 percent of patients with symptomatic carotid artery disease have asymptomatic severe coronary artery disease. Cardiac deaths are the major cause of mortality with cerebrovascular disease (Adams, 1995).

Fluid and electrolyte abnormalities should be corrected, hyperglycemia (high blood sugar level) and hypoxemia (low blood oxygen level) managed, and seizures treated with anticonvulsant medications. Airway and ventilatory support should be provided to patients with depressed levels of consciousness.

[a] Antihypertensives

There is general agreement that hypertension (high blood pressure) should not be treated aggressively in the patient with acute focal brain ischemia. This is because aggressive treatment of hypertension can decrease cerebral blood flow to the ischemic penumbra, resulting in extension of infarction with subsequent clinical worsening.[11] It is acceptable to withhold antihypertensive treatment for systolic (while the heart is contracting end ejecting blood) blood pressures lower than 200 to 220 mm Hg and diastolic (while the heart is filling with blood) blood pressures less than 120 to 130 mm Hg (Adams, 1995; Adams, et al., 1994). Some experts advocate aggressive hydration (fluid infusion) and volume expansion in order to enhance cerebral blood flow and decrease blood viscosity.

[b] Anticoagulants

Heparin (an anticoagulating agent) binds with intrinsic antithrombin III to inactivate thrombin and the propagation of blood clots. The treatment approach of acute anticoagulation with heparin after TIA and noncardiogenic cerebral infarction is somewhat controversial. Heparin has been recommended and used extensively as an anticoagulant in patients with "crescendo" TIAs and with evolving cerebral infarction (Adams, 1995; Kistler, et al., 1994; Adams and Victor, 1993). However, American Heart Association guidelines conclude that there is no evidence to recommend the routine administration of

---

[11] See 8.23[3][c] supra for further discussion of the ischemic penumbra.

anticoagulants to patients with TIAs (Feinberg, et al., 1994). These guidelines further conclude that data about the safety and efficacy of using heparin in acute ischemic stroke is insufficient and conflicting. Hemorrhage can be a serious complication of heparin therapy. The use of heparin in this clinical setting remains a matter of preference for the treating physician (Adams, et al., 1994).

[c]   Thrombolytic Therapy

There is currently great interest in the application of acute thrombolytic (clot-dissolving) therapy to ischemic stroke victims. The thrombolytic agents streptokinase and urokinase have not yet been demonstrated to be of definite benefit. Intravenous tissue plasminogen activator (tPA) has recently been shown to improve patient outcome following acute ischemic stroke, and it is currently being used at times. However, it has significant limitations, not the least of which is that it must be administered within three hours of the onset of symptoms. In addition, CT of the brain must be obtained prior to administration of tPA to exclude the presence of hemorrhage.

Although the overall outcome is improved, an increased percentage of patients who receive tPA hemorrhage into an ischemic brain infarction, a complication that can be very critical. In addition, use of tPA for acute thrombolytic therapy of stroke has not currently been approved by the FDA; currently stroke is listed as a contraindication to the administration of tPA. Until FDA approval, the use of tPA for acute thrombolytic therapy of stroke is not likely to be widespread (The National Institute of Neurological Disorders and Stroke rt-PA Stroke Study Group, 1995; Adams, et al.,1994).

[d]   Cytoprotective Therapy

There is also currently great interest in the application of cytoprotective therapy to acute ischemic stroke victims. The most commonly used drugs include corticosteroids, barbiturates and calcium channel blockers. However, none of these has been demonstrated to be effective. Current experimental trials are mainly centered around calcium channel blockers, excitatory amino acid inhibitors, 21-aminosteroids (lazaroids), free radical scavengers and antioxidants (Adams, et al., 1994; Yatsu, 1995a).

[e]   Chronic Platelet Antiaggregant Therapy

Additional medical therapy for prevention of recurrent TIA and noncardiogenic ischemic brain infarction involves acute and chronic platelet antiaggregant therapy.

American Heart Association guidelines conclude that there is no evidence to recommend the routine administration of anticoagulants (heparin or warfarin) to patients with TIAs or acute noncardiogenic ischemic brain infarction (Feinberg, et al., 1994; Adams, et al., 1994). Although oral anticoagulants (warfarin) have been used for decades to prevent stroke in TIA patients, there is no conclusive data supporting this use (Feinberg, et al., 1994). The situation is quite different for chronic platelet antiaggregant therapy. There is convincing evidence that aspirin and ticlopidine reduce the risk of primary and recurrent cerebral thrombosis in patients with TIAs or acute noncardiogenic ischemic brain infarction. Aspirin doses ranging from 75 mg to 1,500 mg per day have been shown to be efficacious, although the optimal dosage has not been determined. In the acute phase, a loading dose of 160 mg to 325 mg of aspirin is recommended. In clinical practice, doses of 325 mg to 1500 mg daily are most commonly used for chronic stroke prophylactic therapy (Fuster, et al., 1983; Antiplatelet Trialists' Collaboration, 1994; Antiplatelet Trialists' Collaboration, 1988).

Ticlopidine is a relatively new antiplatelet agent approved in the United States for stroke prevention. It is at least as effective as aspirin, and it may be more effective in certain groups of patients, including women, diabetics and patients with small vessel disease (Feinberg, et al., 1994; Gent, et al., 1989; Hass, et al., 1989).

For patients with TIAs or noncardiogenic ischemic brain infarction, the current recommendation is for the chronic administration of aspirin or ticlopidine. Aspirin should probably be used for most patients, and ticlopidine for selected patients, due to the increased cost and side effects of the latter. Chronic warfarin treatment, although it is unproven, may be used for patients who are allergic or refractory to aspirin or ticlopidine. Persantine and sulfinpyrazone are of unproven value for these patients (Feinberg, et al., 1994; Fuster, et al., 1983; Grotta, et al., 1992; Raps and Galetta, 1995; Kistler, et al., 1994; Adams and Victor, 1993).

[f]   Lowering Risk Factors for Atherosclerosis

After the acute phase, risk factors for atherosclerosis should be modified. Hypertension (high blood pressure) is the most important treatable risk factor for stroke, and it should be treated aggressively on a chronic basis (Whisnant, 1996). Diabetes mellitus should be treated with optimal control of blood sugar levels. Cigarette smoking should be discontinued, and hyperlipidemia (increased blood fat levels) should be treated (Sacco, 1995; Feinberg, 1994). Recent guidelines recommend more aggressive treatment of patients with atherosclerotic disease and hyperlipidemia, as well as of individuals with multiple atherosclerotic risk factors and hyperlipidemia (Hachinski, et al., 1996; Expert Panel, 1993; LaRosa, 1993).

[7]   Surgical Treatment

Atherosclerotic plaque can lead to stenosis (narrowing) of arteries prior to occlusion (blockage). Surgical methods have been devised to open stenosed arteries that supply the brain.

[a]   Carotid Endarterectomy

The carotid arteries are surgically accessible in the neck. Carotid endarterectomy, a surgical technique to re-establish blood flow through the carotid arteries, involves excision of the tunica intima (the innermost layer of the artery) that is thickened with plaque. Carotid endarterectomy with plaque removal has been performed since the 1950s, with minimal evidence of efficacy. However, recent landmark investigations have demonstrated the efficacy of the procedure and clarified acceptable surgical risk for various subgroups of patients.

Carotid endarterectomy definitely reduces the risk of recurrent TIA and noncardiogenic ischemic cerebral infarction in patients with symptomatic carotid artery stenosis greater than 70 percent, and possibly in selected patients with symptomatic carotid artery stenosis greater than 50 percent. Acceptable risk of surgical morbidity and mortality is 3 to 5 percent. For patients with asymptomatic carotid artery stenosis greater than 70 percent, carotid endarterectomy reduces the risk of noncardiogenic ischemic cerebral infarction, and acceptable risk of surgical morbidity and mortality is 3 percent.

Risk of surgical morbidity and mortality up to 10 percent is acceptable for certain patients with symptomatic carotid artery disease. There remains some controversy regarding the appropriate management of patients with asymptomatic carotid artery stenosis (Moore, et al., 1995; Goldstein, et al., 1995; North American Symptomatic Carotid Endarterectomy Trial Collaborators, 1991; European Carotid

Surgery Trialists' Collaborative Group, 1991; Mayberg, et al., 1991; The Asymptomatic Carotid Atherosclerosis Study Group, 1989; Clinical Advisory, 1995; National Institute of Neurological Disorders and Stroke, 1995; Barnett, et al., 1996; Barnett, et al., 1995; Brott and Toole, 1995).

Complications of endarterectomy can include stroke, infection, wound hematoma, nerve transection and other general surgical complications.

[b] Bypass Surgery

Extracranial to intracranial (EC-IC) bypass surgery was transiently popular for the treatment of patients with TIAs or acute ischemic cerebral infarction due to surgically inaccessible carotid disease. However, an international randomized trial found EC-IC bypass to be no more efficacious than medical therapy, and the procedure has largely been abandoned (EC-IC Bypass Study Group, 1985). Controversy persists about the possibility that certain groups of patients might benefit from EC-IC bypass, but this remains unproven (Feinberg, et al., 1994).

[8] Prognosis

The 30-day stroke mortality rate after acute ischemic or embolic cerebral infarction is 8 to 15 percent. Mortality after 30 days is more likely to be due to co-morbid disease, particularly cardiovascular disease. Patients with major hemispheric or brain stem infarctions have a cumulative mortality rate of 90 percent at five years. The risk of stroke recurrence is 3 to 8 percent in the first 30 days, with a five-year cumulative recurrence risk of 25 to 40 percent (Sacco, 1995; Sacco, 1982).

8.24 Cardiac Embolic Ischemic Brain Infarction

Ischemic infarction accounts for 70 to 80 percent of strokes in the United States, and cardioembolism results in 15 to 30 percent of these infarctions (Sacco, 1995).

[1] Etiology

Emboli can originate from thrombi in the heart associated with atrial fibrillation (irregular contraction of the atria, or upper chamber of the heart), myocardial infarction (heart attack) and dilated cardiomyopathy (disorder of the heart muscle), infected heart valves (valves that prevent backflow of blood into the chambers of the heart), thrombus on noninfected but diseased heart valves and prosthetic heart valves. Embolism can also occur as a complication of open heart surgery. Intracardiac tumors are rarely a source of cardioembolism (Kistler, et al., 1994; Adams and Victor, 1993; Yatsu, 1995b).

[2] Pathogenesis

Cardioembolism can result from infectious material, tumor or thrombus resident on a heart valve or adherent to the endocardium (inner lining of the heart) breaking loose and migrating through the circulation.

Septic emboli from infected heart valves in persons with bacterial endocarditis is a systemic disease that can present as stroke.[12] In rare instances, tumors called myxomas develop in the heart (most commonly in the left atrium, or upper left chamber of the heart) and embolize to the brain, presenting initially as stroke (Kistler, et al., 1994).

Congenital heart disease, including valvular and septal (referring to the septum, which separates the right and left sides of the heart) defects, can result in an embolic stroke, even in the absence of infection. Mild valvular deformities, in the absence of cardiac arrhythmias, probably do not carry a significant risk of stroke. However, more serious valvular deformities can predispose an individual to an embolic stroke, especially in the presence of significant cardiac arrhythmias, such as atrial fibrillation (Gold, 1995; Yatsu, 1995b; Adams and Victor, 1993).

The role of nonvalvular atrial fibrillation in embolic strokes was not clearly defined until recently. It has now been established that persistent or paroxysmal nonvalvular atrial fibrillation is the most important cause of cerebral embolisms from the heart. Another common source of cerebral embolism from the heart is a left ventricular thrombus forming within the first few weeks after a myocardial infarction. This probably also occurs more commonly than is recognized with dilated cardiomyopathy (Kistler, et al., 1994).

A TIA or embolic stroke is uncommon after cardiac catheterization (threading of a catheter through a blood vessel into the heart for

---

[12] *See* 8.37 *infra.*

diagnostic purposes). It occurs in fewer than 1 percent of procedures and usually involves the vertebrobasilar circulation. A clinically detectable neurologic deficit is present in as many as 12 percent of people after cardiac bypass surgery. This is most likely a result of microembolization (Heyer and Rowland, 1995). Mitral and aortic valve (the valve between the aorta, or central artery of the body, and the left ventricle) prostheses are associated with embolisms in up to 70 percent of cases (Adams and Victor, 1993). Embolism is more common in persons with metal than with porcine valves.

[3] Clinical Presentation

In general, the clinical presentation of cardioembolic infarction is similar to that of thrombotic infarction or small intraparenchymal hemorrhage. Cardioembolic cerebrovascular disease manifests clinically as one or more focal neurologic symptoms and signs. Subjective symptoms can include trouble speaking, visual problems, difficulty swallowing, dizziness, imbalance, weakness and numbness. Objective signs can include aphasia (difficulty speaking), visual field defects, loss of ocular motility, ataxia (incoordination), dysarthria (slurred speech), inattention, loss of spatial organization, sensory losses, paresis (partial paralysis) and paralysis.

The combination of symptoms and signs depends on the location and size of the ischemic area of the brain. Cerebral cortical embolic lesions are accompanied by symptoms on the contralateral side of the body, and seizures are probably more common than with thrombotic ischemic infarctions.[13] Cerebellar embolic lesions are accompanied by symptoms on the ipsilateral (same) side of the body. Cranial nerve involvement indicates brain stem ischemic lesions.

A number of common stroke syndromes (constellation of findings) have been described (Patten, 1996; Poirier, et al., 1990; Adams, and Victor, 1993; Brust, 1995b; Kistler, et al., 1994). Stupor and coma can be present with brain stem lesions, bilateral cerebral lesions and large unilateral cerebral lesions with mass effect and increased intracranial pressure (Plum and Posner, 1980). Symptoms of embolic cerebrovascular disease typically begin acutely. They may be transient, evolve and progress, or they may remain stable.

---

[13] *See* 8.23[3] *supra.*

Concepts regarding transient ischemic attacks, the ischemic penumbra and completed stroke with regard to thrombotic ischemic brain infarction also pertain to cardioembolic brain infarction.[14]

[4]   Neurologic Complications

Neurologic complications following cardiogenic embolic ischemic brain infarction occur through the same mechanisms as those for thrombotic ischemic brain infarction.[15]

[5]   Diagnosis

The initial step in the proper management of patients with any type of cerebral infarction is correct and timely diagnosis. Diagnosis of brain infarction can usually be made correctly on clinical grounds, although it is important to exclude a diagnosis of intraparenchymal brain hemorrhage, subdural hematoma, neoplasm and other causes of focal neurologic deficits. It is impossible to absolutely differentiate between cardiogenic embolic and thrombotic ischemic infarctions on clinical grounds.

Indications for CT scan and additional laboratory tests in the diagnosis of persons with cardiogenic embolic ischemic brain infarction are the same as those for persons with thrombotic ischemic brain infarction.[16]

The diagnosis of cardiogenic embolic causes of stroke is sometimes indefinite, but important. The decision that a patient has had a cardiogenic embolism is usually made on circumstantial evidence provided by the clinical history, physical examination, electrocardiogram, carotid Doppler ultrasonography, arteriography and echocardiography. Cardiogenic embolic infarction should be suspected in patients with atrial fibrillation, heart valve prostheses or evidence on examination of valvular heart disease, myocardial infarction or endocarditis. Such patients should undergo echocardiography (the use of ultrasound to create an image of the heart on an oscilloscope for diagnostic viewing).

Echocardiography is a low-yield procedure for other patients. However, it is definitely indicated for those at significant risk of

---

[14] *See* 8.23 *supra.*

[15] *See* 8.23[4] *supra.*

[16] *See* 8.23[5] *supra.*

cardiogenic embolic brain infarction. Transesophageal echocardiography (in which the ultrasound transducer is inserted into the opening of the throat to place it nearer the heart) is more sensitive than transthoracic (through the chest wall) echocardiography, although both have a significant false-negative rate (incorrectly indicate that pathology is not present) (Yatsu, 1995a; Kistler, et al., 1994; Adams and Victor, 1993).

[6] Treatment

Patients with acute thrombotic or embolic ischemic neurologic events should be admitted to the hospital and undergo continuous cardiac monitoring. There is significant cardiac co-morbidity with ischemic cerebrovascular disease, with as many as 40 percent of patients who have symptomatic carotid artery disease also having asymptomatic severe coronary artery disease. Cardiac deaths are the major cause of mortality with cerebrovascular disease (Adams, 1995).

Fluid and electrolyte abnormalities should be corrected, hyperglycemia and hypoxemia should be treated, and seizures should be treated with anticonvulsants. Airway and ventilatory support should be provided to patients with depressed levels of consciousness.

[a] Antihypertensives

There is general agreement that hypertension should not be treated aggressively in the patient with acute focal brain ischemia. This is because aggressive treatment of hypertension can decrease cerebral blood flow to the ischemic penumbra, resulting in extension of infarction with subsequent clinical worsening. It is acceptable to withhold antihypertensive treatment for systolic blood pressures less than 200 to 220 mm Hg and diastolic blood pressures less than 120 to 130 mm Hg (Adams, 1995; Adams, et al., 1994). Some advocate aggressive hydration and volume expansion in order to enhance cerebral blood flow and decrease blood viscosity.

[b] Anticoagulants

Heparin binds with intrinsic antithrombin III to inactivate thrombin and the propagation of blood clots. Acute anticoagulation with heparin after noninfective cardiogenic TIA and cerebral infarction is somewhat controversial, but accepted by most authorities. After three to five days, patients are generally switched to warfarin (Sherman, et al., 1995; Adams, 1995; Kistler, et al., 1994; Adams and Victor, 1993).

One controversy surrounding anticoagulation of such patients involves the timing of anticoagulation. Because emboli migrate and lyse (dissolve), revascularization (reopening a vessel) is more likely to cause hemorrhagic transformation of an embolic infarction than a thrombotic infarction. Thus, some authorities advocate a delay of three to five days before giving anticoagulants to patients with embolic infarction. However, because there is also a significant risk of re-embolization in this waiting period, with up to 20 percent of patients experiencing recurrent emboli within ten days after the initial embolus, some experts advocate immediate anticoagulation. Whether anti-coagulation is immediate or delayed, brain CT should always be obtained first, to ensure that patients with intracerebral hemorrhage are not anticoagulated (Kistler, et al., 1994; Adams and Victor, 1993). Hemorrhage is the most common complication of anticoagulation. It can involve any part of the body and be very serious if it occurs.

A major recent advance in prevention of cardioembolic stroke has been the recognition that anticoagulation reduces the risk of stroke in patients with nonvalvular atrial fibrillation. Strokes occur in 4.5 percent of untreated atrial fibrillation patients per year. Independent risk factors for stroke in patients with nonrheumatic atrial fibrillation include advanced age, history of prior embolism, hypertension, diabetes mellitus and echocardiographic evidence of left atrial enlargement or left ventricular dysfunction. Warfarin decreases stroke by two thirds and aspirin by one third in these patients. Recommended treatment of patients with nonrheumatic atrial fibrillation at the present time is with warfarin, especially for patients with any of the risk factors noted and patients over the age of 70. For persons at risk of falling and persons with significant risk of bleeding, treatment with aspirin is acceptable. The value of persantine and sulfinpyrazone has not been proved for these patients (Laupacis, et al., 1995; Streifler and Katz, 1995; Blackshear, et al., 1996; Ezekowitz, et al., 1992; Connolly, et al., 1991). There is some controversy regarding the optimal level of anticoagulation with nonvalvular atrial fibrillation (The European Atrial Fibrillation Trial Study Group, 1995).

[7]   Prognosis

The 30-day stroke mortality rate after acute ischemic or embolic cerebral infarction is 8 to 15 percent. Mortality after 30 days is most likely due to co-morbid disease, particularly cardiovascular disease. Patients with major hemispheric or brain stem infarctions have a cumulative mortality rate of 90 percent at five years. The risk of stroke recurrence is 3 to 8 percent in the first 30 days, with a five-year cumulative recurrence risk of 25 to 40 percent (Sacco, 1995; Sacco, 1982).

8.30 SYSTEMIC DISEASES THAT CAN PRESENT AS STROKE

A variety of systemic diseases can affect the cerebral vasculature and produce symptoms similar to those of stroke.

8.31 Sickle Cell Anemia

Sickle cell disease is an inherited abnormality of hemoglobin (the oxygen-carrying component of blood) that is seen primarily in people of African heritage, but also in Greek and Latin American ethnic groups. Abnormal hemoglobin leads to distortion of the shape of red blood cells, hemolysis (breakdown of the blood cell) and occlusion of vessels in kidney, bone, lung, liver, heart, spleen and brain. Occlusion of vessels in the brain results in ischemic brain infarction.

Brain infarctions are more common in the vicinity of large vessels than small vessels. The clinical presentation does not differ from that of infarction or intraparenchymal hemorrhage resulting from other causes.[17] Diagnosis is made on the basis of clinical suspicion for a victim of appropriate ethnic background, and confirmation by cranial CT or MRI and hemoglobin electrophoresis. Transfusion reduces the risk of recurrent strokes. Within three years of stroke, there is a 67 percent recurrence rate in patients who are not transfused and a 10 percent recurrence in patients who are transfused (Weksler, 1995; Menkes, et al., 1995; Balmaceda and Fetell, 1995; Schochet, 1983).

8.32 Arteritis

Brain infarctions can result from infective or noninfective inflammatory arteritis of the cerebral arteries. Noninfective inflammatory arteritis of the cerebral arteries is most commonly associated with autoimmune diseases (in which the body mistakenly launches an immune response against its own tissues), especially systemic lupus erythematosus (an autoimmune disease with characteristic skin lesions). It can also be seen with giant cell arteritis, polyarteritis nodosa,

---

[17] See 8.20 supra.

Churg-Straus disease and Wegener's granulomatosis, and as an isolated intracranial arteritis. Intracranial arteritis with infarction also occurs with abuse of illicit drugs, most notably heroin.

Diagnosis can usually be made with arteriography and appropriate blood studies, although a biopsy is sometimes necessary. Treatment is with corticosteroids and other immunosuppressant drugs (Futrell, 1995; Rowland, 1995b; Moore and Cupps, 1983; Futrell and Millikan, 1989; Harris and Hughes, 1985).

8.33 Polycythemia Vera

Polycythemia vera is characterized by excessive production of red blood cells. This is believed to increase the viscosity of the blood, resulting in tissue hypoxia (low blood level of oxygen) and ischemia. Alternatively, there is evidence that polycythemia results in infarction as a physiologic response to elevated arterial level of oxygen. Whatever the pathophysiology, brain infarction and, less commonly, hemorrhage can occur with polycythemia. An emergency phlebotomy (cutting into a vein) is indicated in cases with a hematocrit (the volume of blood composed of cells) greater than 60 percent. The presence of hypoglycemia (low blood sugar level) increases the risk of cerebral thrombosis in polycythemic neonates (Weksler, 1995; Menkes, et al., 1995; Balmaceda and Fetell, 1995).

8.34 Hypercoagulable States

Thrombotic thrombocytopenic purpura manifests as thrombocytopenia (low platelet count), purpura (bruising), fever and fluctuating neurologic symptoms due to brain infarction. Diagnosis can be difficult but is crucial, because this is a treatable entity, with recovery in as many of 70 percent of patients.

Protein C deficiency, protein S deficiency and antithrombin III deficiency are rarely recognized entities that can cause a hypercoagulable state and stroke.

Primary antiphospholipid antibody syndrome, an autoimmune disease in which individuals produce autoantibodies to the phospholipid compounds that are embedded in blood vessel walls, is an entity that has been increasingly associated with stroke. Antiphospholipid antibodies are referred to as the lupus anticoagulant and anticardiolipin antibodies (immunoglobulin G and M). They are most commonly associated with spontaneous abortion and venous thrombosis, but they can result in intracranial arterial or venous occlusion. There is some evidence that drug-induced antiphospholipid antibodies may be of little consequence. These entities should be considered in unusual presentations of cerebral thrombosis. They account for about 20 percent of all strokes (Adams and Victor, 1993; Antiphospholipid Antibody Stroke Study Group, 1993; Yatsu, 1995b; Balmaceda and Fetell, 1995).

8.35 Hemophilia

Intracranial hemorrhage can occur with any type of hemophilia, including deficiency of factor VII, factor VIII, factor IX and von Willebrand's disease. Intracranial hemorrhage is the leading cause of death in factor VIII deficiency, with as many as 10 percent of afflicted individuals experiencing intracerebral hemorrhage. Epidural or subdural hematomas develop in about half, often after minor head trauma but sometimes spontaneously. Any hemophiliac who experiences head trauma should undergo cranial CT. The missing factor should be replaced immediately, and surgical evacuation of the clot may be necessary (Weksler, 1995; Menkes, et al., 1995; Balmaceda and Fetell, 1995; Kistler, et al., 1994).

8.36 Polycystic Kidney Disease

Polycystic kidney disease is an inherited renal disorder that can cause flank pain, hematuria (blood in the urine), hypertension (high blood pressure) and chronic renal failure. The incidence rates of intracranial saccular aneurysms and subarachnoid hemorrhages are increased in people with polycystic kidney disease, with reports of subarachnoid hemorrhage in as many as 10 percent of afflicted individuals.[18] Routine screening with cerebral arteriography has not generally been recommended, although this position is being modified with the evolving resolution of noninvasive magnetic resonance angiography (Coe and Kathpalia, 1994; Brust, 1995c; Schochet, 1983).

8.37 Infection

Intracranial mycotic aneurysms develop from septic emboli originating in infected heart valves in persons with bacterial endocarditis (infection of the membranous sac surrounding the heart). These

---

[18] *See* 8.21 *supra* for further discussion of saccular aneurysms and their relation to subarachnoid hemorrhage.

aneurysms are seen most often in people with valvular heart disease and in intravenous drug abusers.[19]

Mycotic aneurysms occur in about 10 percent of individuals with infective endocarditis, and a stroke may be the initial manifestation. They result from dilation and destruction of inflamed and infected intracranial peripheral arterial walls. Rupture and hemorrhage are common. Diagnosis is by CT, MRI, MRA and arteriography. Treatment is with antibiotics. Anticoagulation is relatively contraindicated, because septic brain emboli are commonly hemorrhagic. Surgical replacement of the infected cardiac valve with a prosthetic valve is sometimes necessary (Schochet, 1983; Kaye, 1994; Kistler, et al., 1994).

Cerebral infarction can also occur with any type of infectious meningitis, most commonly with bacterial meningitis caused by tuberculosis, syphilis and *Haemophilus*. Brain infarction of this kind results from infective inflammatory arteritis of the cerebral arteries, a condition known as Heubner's arteritis. Any part of the brain can be involved. Individuals with acquired immunodeficiency syndrome (AIDS) resulting from human immunodeficiency virus (HIV) infection are at particular risk for tuberculous meningitis and neurosyphilis (Schochet, 1983; Menkes, 1995; Scheld, 1994; Igarashi, et al., 1984).

8.38   Neoplasm

Stroke can occur as a complication of all forms of leukemia (a disease characterized by excessive production of white blood cells), primarily the acute forms. Three mechanisms may be involved (Weksler, 1995; Balmaceda and Fetell, 1995; Menkes, et al., 1995):

1. With markedly elevated white blood cell counts (greater than 150,000/mm^3), leukostasis (stagnation of white blood cells) can lead to thrombosis of cerebral vessels, with subsequent brain infarction.

2. Leukemic nodules in the brain can predispose to intracerebral hemorrhage.

3. Hemorrhage may also result from thrombocytopenia (low platelet count) caused by chemotherapy.

Brain tumors, both primary and metastatic (spreading from an origin at a distant site), can manifest acutely as stroke. The mechanism is

---

[19] *See* 8.21 *supra.*

intratumoral hemorrhage, and the clinical presentation is the same as that of any other intracerebral hemorrhage, usually lobar or cerebellar in location. Among primary brain tumors, this is seen most commonly in glioblastoma multiforme. Among metastatic brain tumors, intratumoral hemorrhage is particularly common with melanoma (skin cancer), renal (kidney) cell carcinoma, choriocarcinoma (a highly malignant tumor with common metastases to the brain) and bronchogenic carcinoma (a type of lung cancer). Diagnosis can be difficult at times but is greatly facilitated by MRI (Balmaceda and Fetell, 1995; Kistler, et al., 1994; Adams and Victor, 1993; Schochet, 1983).

Some patients with systemic malignancy develop nonbacterial thrombotic endocarditis, with sterile platelet–fibrin heart valve vegetations resulting in embolization and subsequent brain infarction. Emboli to other organs may also occur (Balmaceda and Fetell, 1995).

8.40 SYSTEMIC COMPLICATIONS OF CEREBROVASCULAR INJURY

A number of systemic complications can occur after any type of stroke. These complications can also occur after traumatic cerebrovascular injury.

8.41 Respiratory Complications

Aspiration pneumonia (inflammation of the lungs caused by the inhalation of food or other substances) is very common in stroke victims with impaired swallowing or cough mechanisms. Many patients should not receive anything by mouth initially. Assessment of the ability to swallow is critical if there is clinical suspicion of impairment. Pneumonia is an important cause of death after strokes, and fever should prompt evaluation by chest x-ray. Pneumonia should be appropriately treated with antibiotics (Adams, et al., 1994; Horner, et al., 1988; Adams, 1993).

Pulmonary embolism (migration of a blood clot to the pulmonary circulation) resulting from deep vein thrombophlebitis (DVT) of the lower extremities accounts for about 10 percent of strokes. Proximal DVT can be identified in up to a third of patients with moderately severe stroke. Prevention includes early mobilization, alternating pressure stockings and anticoagulation if it is not contraindicated (Adams, et al., 1994; Adams, 1993).

Respiratory failure can occur in stroke victims, especially those with pre-existing cardiopulmonary disease, large infarction or hemorrhage and brain stem infarction or hemorrhage. Patients with a predisposing condition have a worse prognosis than those without, and they may require ventilatory support (Adams, 1995).

8.42   Cardiovascular Complications

Cardiac death is the major cause of mortality in patients with cerebrovascular disease. Concurrent brain infarction and myocardial infarction are not uncommon. However, a minority of cerebrovascular disease patients have clear symptoms of coronary artery disease. Forty percent of patients with symptomatic carotid artery disease have asymptomatic coronary artery disease.

Cardiac arrhythmias due to atrial fibrillation and ventricular arrhythmias (uneven, irregular rhythms) are also common among stroke victims.

Minimum cardiovascular evaluation of patients with cerebrovascular disease should include an electrocardiogram (EKG, which measures the heart's electrical activity) and a chest x-ray. Optimally, all patients should undergo continuous cardiac monitoring for the first few days. Hospital stroke units should be utilized when they are available, and patients suspected of having myocardial infarction (heart attack) should be admitted to a coronary care unit. Echocardiography (ultrasonography of the heart) and anticoagulation therapy should be used when indicated, and cardiac arrhythmias (irregular heartbeats) should be treated appropriately. The cardiac evaluation of ischemic stroke patients with severe atherosclerotic disease should probably include stress thallium testing or treadmill stress testing, with coronary arteriography when indicated (Adams, 1995; Adams, et al., 1994).

8.43   Gastrointestinal Complications

Impairment of swallowing ability is a common complication of stroke. Other common gastrointestinal complications include loss of intestinal motility (ileus), constipation and fecal impaction (inability to pass feces). Gastrointestinal bleeding can also occur, particularly in patients who are anticoagulated and have pre-existing peptic ulcer disease (Adams, 1993).

8.44   Genitourinary Complications

In-dwelling urinary catheters are often necessary after a stroke, but their use increases the risk of urinary tract infections, which are common in stroke patients. Secondary septicemia (systemic disease caused by proliferation of microorganisms in the blood) can develop and be fatal. Fever should prompt evaluation of the urine, and infection should be appropriately treated with antibiotics (Adams, et al., 1994; Adams, 1993).

8.45   Endocrine System Complications

Diabetes mellitus is a risk factor for atherosclerosis, and ischemic strokes are common among diabetic individuals. Hyperglycemia (elevated blood sugar level) is common in diabetic stroke victims, and there is suggestive evidence that it may worsen ischemic infarction. Hypoglycemia and hyperglycemia should be controlled after a stroke (Adams, et al., 1994).

Hyponatremia (low blood sodium levels) occurs in up to 34 percent of patients after subarachnoid hemorrhage, usually due to intravascular volume contraction caused by diabetes insipidus (chronic excretion of large amounts of pale urine and excessive thirst). Intravascular volume status may need to be closely monitored. Hyponatremia due to volume contraction should be treated with intravenous isotonic fluids (Mayberg, et al., 1994).

8.46   Dermatologic Complications

Meticulous nursing care, with frequent turning, attention to skin care and early mobilization, is necessary for the prevention of decubitus ulcers (pressure sores). Once they develop, decubitus ulcers can contribute significantly to the morbidity involved in stroke. Treatment is time consuming, expensive and not always effective (Bergstrom, et al., 1994; Adams, 1993).

8.47   Psychiatric Complications

Depression after a stroke is common, occurring in 23 to 63 percent of patients. It is more common with left cerebral lesions than right cerebral lesions. It should be recognized and treated (Kelly-Hayes and Paige, 1995; Adams, 1995; Adams, 1993).

Dementia after multiple large or lacunar strokes is common. Deficiencies are common in orientation, attention, memory, calculation and spatial organization. There is no satisfactory treatment, other than attempts at preventing more strokes.

8.50   REHABILITATION AFTER CEREBROVASCULAR INJURY

A large percentage of survivors of cerebrovascular injury have substantial motor impairment, sensory impairment, difficulty swallowing, cognitive deficit, language deficit, depression and incontinence. Many of these patients will benefit from multidisciplinary rehabilitation if their neurologic deficit is not too severe. Assessment of each patient's individual social support system is important in the decision regarding a patient's potential to achieve the ultimate goal of rehabilitation: to return to the community and be able to perform instrumental activities of daily living. Most patients realize maximal functional recovery in three to six months, but the rehabilitation period is usually much shorter than this. Expectations should be realistic (Agency for Health Care Policy and Research, 1995; Jeffery and Good, 1995; Kelly-Hayes and Paige, 1995; Jorgensen, et al., 1995; Granger, et al., 1992).

8.100   BIBLIOGRAPHY

Text References

Adams, H. P. (Ed.): Handbook of Cerebrovascular Disease. New York: Marcel Dekker, 1993.

Adams, H. P., et al.: Guidelines for the Management of Patients with Acute Ischemic Stroke—A Statement for Healthcare Professionals From a Special Writing Group of the Stroke Council, American Heart Association. Circulation 90(3):1588-1601, Sept. 1994.

Adams, R. D. and Victor, M.: Principles of Neurology, 5th ed. New York: McGraw-Hill, 1993.

Adams, R.J.: Management Issues for Patients with Ischemic Stroke. In: Dobkin, B. (Ed.): Management of the Patient with Stroke. Neurology 45(2, Suppl.1):S15-S18, Feb. 1995.

Agency for Health Care Policy and Research: Post-Stroke Rehabilitation: Assessment, Referral, and Patient Management. Rockville, Md.: U.S. Department of Health and Human Services, 1995.

Antiphospholipid Antibody Stroke Study Group: Anticardiolipin Antibodies are an Independent Risk Factor for First Ischemic Stroke. The Antiphospholipid Antibodies in Stroke Study (APASS). Neurology 43(10):2069-2073, Oct. 1993.

Antiplatelet Trialists' Collaboration: Collaborative Overview of Randomised Trials of Antiplatelet Therapy, I: Prevention of Death, Myocardial Infarction, and Stroke by Prolonged Antiplatelet Therapy in Various Categories of Patients. Br. Med. J. 308(6921):81-106, Jan. 1994.

Antiplatelet Trialists' Collaboration: Secondary Prevention of Vascular Disease by Prolonged Antiplatelet Treatment. Br. Med. J. 296(6618):320-331, Jan. 1988.

The Asymptomatic Carotid Atherosclerosis Study Group: Study Design for Randomized Prospective Trial of Carotid Endarterectomy for Asymptomatic Atherosclerosis. Stroke 20(7):844-849, July 1989.

Babikian, V. L. and Wechsler, L. R. (Eds.): Transcranial Doppler Ultrasonography. St. Louis: Mosby, 1993.

Balmaceda, C. M. and Fetell, M. R.: Hematologic and Related Disorders. In: Rowland, L. P. (Ed.): Merritt's Textbook of Neurology, 9th ed. Baltimore: Williams & Wilkins, 1995.

Barnett, H. J. M., et al.: Do the Facts and Figures Warrant a 10-Fold Increase in the Performance of Carotid Endarterectomy on Asymptomatic Patients? Neurology 46(3):603-608, Mar. 1996.

Barnett, H. J. M., et al.: The Dilemma of Surgical Treatment for Patients with Asymptomatic Carotid Disease. Ann. Intern. Med. 123(9):723-725, Nov. 1995.

Bergstrom, N., et al.: Agency for Health Care Policy and Research: Clinical Practice Guideline Number 15: Treatment of Pressure Ulcers. Rockville Md.: U.S. Dept. of Health and Human Services, Dec. 1994.

Blackshear, J. L., et al.: Management of Atrial Fibrillation in Adults: Prevention of Thromboembolism and Symptomatic Treatment. Mayo Clin. Proc. 71(2):150-160, Feb. 1996.

Brott, T. and Toole, J. F.: Medical Compared with Surgical Treatment of Asymptomatic Carotid Artery Stenosis. Ann. Intern. Med. 123(9):720-722, Nov. 1995.

Brust, J. C. M.: Transient Ischemic Attacks. In: Rowland, L. P. (Ed.): Merritt's Textbook of Neurology, 9th ed. Baltimore: Williams & Wilkins, 1995a.

Brust, J. C. M.: Cerebral Infarction. In: Rowland, L. P. (Ed.): Merritt's Textbook of Neurology, 9th ed. Baltimore: Williams & Wilkins, 1995b.

Brust, J. C. M.: Subarachnoid Hemorrhage. In: Rowland, L. P. (Ed.): Merritt's Textbook of Neurology, 9th ed. Baltimore: Williams & Wilkins, 1995c.

Buring, J. E., et al.: Migraine and Subsequent Risk of Stroke in the Physicians' Health Study. Arch. Neurol. 52(2):129-134, Feb. 1995.

Caplan, L. R., et al.: Neuroimaging in Patients with Cerebrovascular Disease: In: Greenberg, J. O. (Ed.): Neuroimaging. New York: McGraw-Hill, 1995.

Carpenter, M. B.: Core Text of Neuroanatomy, 4th ed. Baltimore: Williams & Wilkins, 1991.

Clinical Advisory: Carotid Endarterectomy for Patients with Asymptomatic Internal Carotid Artery Stenosis. Stroke 25(12):2523-2524, Dec. 1994.

Coe, F. L. and Kathpalia, S.: Polycystic Renal Disease in Adults. In: Isselbacher, K. J., et al. (Eds.): Harrison's Principles of Internal Medicine, 13th ed. New York: McGraw-Hill, 1994.

Connolly, S. J., et al.: Canadian Atrial Fibrillation Anticoagulation (CAFA) Study. J. Am. Coll. Cardiol. 18(2):349-355, Aug. 1991.

Critchley, E. M.: Recognition and Management of Lacunar Strokes [Editorial]. Br. Med. J. [Clin. Res.] 287(6395):777-778, Sept. 1983.

Drake, C. G., et al.: Failed Aneurysm Surgery. Reoperation in 115 Cases. J. Neurosurg. 61(5):848-856, Nov. 1984.

EC/IC Bypass Study Group: Failure of Extracranial-Intracranial Arterial Bypass to Reduce the Risk of Ischemic Stroke: Results of International Randomized Trial. N. Engl. J. Med. 313(19):1191-1200, Nov. 1985.

The European Atrial Fibrillation Trial Study Group: Optimal Oral Anticoagulant Therapy in Patients with Nonrheumatic Atrial Fibrillation and Recent Cerebral Ischemia. N. Engl. J. Med. 333(1):5-10, July 1995.

European Carotid Surgery Trialists' Collaborative Group: MRC European Carotid Surgery Trial: Interim Results for Symptomatic Patients with Severe (70-99%) or with Mild (0-29%) Carotid Stenosis. Lancet 337(8752):1235-1243, May 1991.

Expert Panel: Summary of the Second Report of the National Cholesterol Education Program (NCEP) Expert Panel on Detection, Evaluation, and Treatment of High Blood Cholesterol in Adults (Adult Treatment Panel II). J.A.M.A. 269(23):3015-3023, June 1993.

Ezekowitz, M. D., et al.: Warfarin in the Prevention of Stroke Associated with Nonrheumatic Atrial Fibrillation. N. Engl. J. Med. 327(20):1406-1412, Nov. 1992.

Feinberg, W. M., et al.: Guidelines for the Management of Transient Ischemic Attacks—From the Ad Hoc Committee for the Management of Transient Ischemic Attacks of the Stroke Council of the American Heart Association. Stroke 25(6):1320-1335, June 1994.

Fuster, V., et al.: Aspirin As a Therapeutic Agent in Cardiovascular Disease. Circulation 87(2):659-675, Feb. 1993.

Futrell, N.: Inflammatory Vascular Disorders: Diagnosis and Treatment in Ischemic Stroke. Curr. Opin. Neurol. 8(1):55-61, Feb. 1995.

Futrell, N. and Millikan, C.: Frequency, Etiology, and Prevention of Stroke in Patients with Systemic Lupus Erythematosus. Stroke 20(5):584-591, July 1989.

Gent, M., et al.: The Canadian American Ticlopidine Study (CATS) in Thromboembolic Stroke. Lancet 1(8649):1215-1220, June 5, 1989.

Gold, A. P.: Stroke in Children. In: Rowland, L. P. (Ed.): Merritt's Textbook of Neurology, 9th ed. Baltimore: Williams & Wilkins, 1995.

Goldstein, L. B., et al.: Comparison and Meta-Analysis of Randomized Trials of Endarterectomy for Symptomatic Carotid Artery Stenosis. Neurology 45(11):1965-1970, Nov. 1995.

Granger, C. V., et al.: Discharge Outcome after Stroke Rehabilitation. Stroke 23(7):978-982, July 1992.

Greenberg, J. O. (Ed.): Neuroimaging. New York: McGraw-Hill, 1995.

Grotta, J. C., et al.: Prevention of Stroke with Ticlopidine: Who Benefits the Most? Neurology. 42(1):111-115, Jan. 1992.

Hachinski, V.: Hypertension in Acute Ischemic Strokes. Arch. Neurol. 42(10):1002, Oct. 1985.

Hachinski, V.: Decreased Incidence and Mortality of Stroke. Stroke 15(2):376-378, Mar.-Apr. 1984.

Hachinski,V., et al.: Lipids and Stroke. Arch. Neurol. 53(4):303-308, Apr. 1996.

Harris, E. N. and Hughes, G. R. V.: Cerebral Disease in Systemic Lupus Erythematosus. Springer Semin. Immunopathol. 8(3):251-266, 1985.

Hass, W. K., et al.: A Randomized Trial Comparing Ticlopidine Hydrochloride with Aspirin for the Prevention of Stroke in High-Risk Patients. N. Engl. J. Med. 321(8):501-507, Aug. 1989.

Heyer, E. J. and Rowland, L. P.: Cerebral Complications of Cardiac Surgery. In: Rowland, L. P. (Ed.): Merritt's Textbook of Neurology, 9th ed. Baltimore: Williams & Wilkins, 1995.

Horner, J., et al.: Aspiration following Stroke. Clinical Correlation and Outcome. Neurology 38(9):1359-1362, Sept. 1988.

Igarashi, M., et al.: Cerebral Arteritis and Bacterial Meningitis. Arch. Neurol. 41(5):531-535, May 1984.

Ingall, T. J. and Wiebers, D. O.: Natural History of Subarachnoid Hemorrhage. In: Whisnant, J. P. (Ed.): Stroke: Populations, Cohorts, and Clinical Trials. Boston: Butterworth-Heinemann, 1993.

Jane, J. A., et al.: The Natural History of Aneurysms and Arteriovenous Malformations. J. Neurosurg. 62(3):321-323, Mar. 1985.

Jeffery, D. R. and Good, D. C.: Rehabilitation of the Stroke Patient. Curr. Opin. Neurol. 8(1):62-68, Feb. 1995.

Jorgensen H. S., et al.: Outcome and Time Course of Recovery in Stroke. Part II: Time Course of Recovery. The Copenhagen Stroke Study. Arch. Phys. Med. Rehabil. 76(5):406-412, May 1995.

Kaye, D.: Infective Endocarditis. In: Isselbacher, K. J., et al. (Eds.): Harrison's Principles of Internal Medicine, 13th ed. New York: McGraw-Hill, 1994.

Kelly-Hayes, M. and Paige, C.: Assessment and Psychologic Factors in Stroke Rehabilitation. In: Dobkin, B. (Ed.): Management of the Patient with Stroke. Neurology 45(2,Suppl.1):S15-S18, Feb. 1995.

Kilpatrick, C. J., et al.: Epileptic Seizures in Acute Stroke. Arch. Neurol. 47(2):157-160, Feb. 1990.

Kistler, J. P., et al.: Cerebrovascular Disease. In: Isselbacher, K. J., et al. (Eds.): Harrison's Principles of Internal Medicine, 13th ed. New York: McGraw-Hill, 1994.

Lampl, Y., et al.: Neurological and Functional Outcome in Patients with Supratentorial Hemorrhages. Stroke 26(12):2249-2253, Dec. 1995.

LaRosa, J.C.: Cholesterol Lowering, Low Cholesterol, and Mortality. Am. J. Cardiol. 72(11):776-786, Oct. 1993.

Laupacis, A., et al.: Antithrombotic Therapy in Atrial Fibrillation. Chest 108(4,Suppl.):352S-359S, Oct. 1995.

Mayberg, M. R., et al.: Guidelines for the Management of Aneurysmal Subarachnoid Hemorrhage—A Statement for Healthcare Professionals From a Special Writing Group of the Stroke Council, American Heart Association. Circulation 90(5):2592-2605, Nov. 1994.

Mayberg, M. R., et al.: Carotid Endarterectomy and Prevention of Cerebral Ischemia in Symptomatic Carotid Stenosis: Veterans Affairs Cooperative Studies 309 Trialist Group. J.A.M.A. 266(23):3289-3294, Dec. 1991.

Menkes, J. H., et al.: Neurologic Manifestations of Systemic Disease. In: Menkes, J. H.(Ed.): Textbook of Child Neurology, 5th ed. Baltimore: Williams & Wilkins, 1995.

Miyaoka, M., et al.: A Clinical Study of the Relationship of Timing to Outcome of Surgery for Ruptured Cerebral Aneurysm—A Retrospective Analysis of 1622 Cases. J. Neurosurg. 79(3):373-378, Sept. 1993.

Mohr, J. P.: Cerebral and Cerebellar Hemorrhage. In: Rowland, L. P. (Ed.): Merritt's Textbook of Neurology, 9th ed. Baltimore: Williams & Wilkins, 1995a.

Mohr, J. P.: Differential Diagnosis of Stroke. In: Rowland, L. P. (Ed.): Merritt's Textbook of Neurology, 9th ed. Baltimore: Williams & Wilkins, 1995b.

Moore, P. M. and Cupps, T. R.: Neurological Complications of Vasculitis. Ann. Neurol. 14(2):155-167, Aug. 1983.

Moore, W. S., et al.: Guidelines for Carotid Endarterectomy—A Multidisciplinary Consensus Statement From the Ad Hoc

Committee, American Heart Association. Circulation 91(2):566-579, Jan. 1995.

National Institute of Neurological Disorders and Stroke: Carotid Endarterectomy for Patients with Asymptomatic Internal Carotid Artery Stenosis. J. Neurol. Sci. 129(1):76-77, Mar. 1995.

The National Institute of Neurological Disorders and Stroke rt-PA Stroke Study Group.: Tissue Plasminogen Activator for Acute Ischemic Stroke. N. Engl. J. Med. 333(24):1581-1587, Dec. 1995.

North American Symptomatic Carotid Endarterectomy Trial Collaborators: Beneficial Effect of Carotid Endarterectomy in Symptomatic Patients with High-Grade Carotid Stenosis. N. Engl. J. Med. 325(7):445-453, Aug. 1991.

Nishioka, H., et al.: Cooperative Study of Intracranial Aneurysms and Subarachnoid Hemorrhage: A Long-Term Prognostic Study, II. Ruptured Intracranial Aneurysms Managed Conservatively, III. Subarachnoid Hemorrhage of Undetermined Etiology. Arch. Neurol. 41(11):1142-1146, Nov. 1984.

Patten, J.: Neurological Differential Diagnosis, 2nd ed. London: Springer-Verlag, 1996.

Pickard, J. D., et al.: Effect of Oral Nimodipine on Cerebral Infarction and Outcome after Subarachnoid Hemorrhage. Br. Med. J. 298(3):636-642, Mar. 1989.

Plum, F. and Posner, J. B.: The Diagnosis of Stupor and Coma, 3rd ed. Philadelphia: Davis, 1980.

Poirier, J., et al.: In: Rubenstein, L. J. (Trans.): Manual of Basic Neuropathology, 3rd ed. Philadelphia: Saunders, 1990.

Raps, E. C. and Galetta, S. L.: Stroke Prevention Therapies and Management of Patient Subgroups. In: Dobkin, B. (Ed.): Management of the Patient with Stroke. Neurology 45(2,Suppl.1):S15-S18, Feb. 1995.

Rowland, L. P.: Head Injury. In: Rowland, L. P. (Ed.): Merritt's Textbook of Neurology, 9th ed. Baltimore: Williams & Wilkins, 1995a.

Rowland, L. P.: Vasculitis Syndromes. In: Rowland, L.P. (Ed.): Merritt's Textbook of Neurology, 9th ed. Baltimore: Williams & Wilkins, 1995b.

Sacco, R. L.: Risk Factors and Outcomes for Ischemic Stroke. In: Dobkin, B. (Ed.): Management of the Patient with Stroke. Neurology 45(2,Suppl.1):S10-S14, Feb. 1995.

Sacco, R. L., et al.: Survival and Recurrence Following Stroke: The Framingham Study. Stroke 13(3):290-295, May-June 1982.

Sahs, A. L., et al.: Aneurysmal Subarachnoid Hemorrhage: Report of the Cooperative Study. Baltimore: Urban & Schwartzenberg, 1981.

Scheld, W. M.: Bacterial Meningitis and Brain Abscess. In: Isselbacher, K. J., et al. (Eds.): Harrison's Principles of Internal Medicine, 13th ed. New York: McGraw-Hill. 1994.

Sherman, D. G., et al.: Antithrombotic Therapy for Cerebrovascular Disorders: An Update. Chest 108(4,Suppl.):444S-456S, Oct. 1995.

Schochet, S. S. (Ed.): Neuropathology: In: Rosenberg, R.N. (Ed.): The Clinical Neurosciences. New York: Churchill Livingstone, 1983.

Streifler, J. Y. and Katz, M.: Cardiogenic Cerebral Emboli: Diagnosis and Treatment. Curr. Opin. Neurol.8(1):45-54, Feb. 1995.

von Reutern, G-M. and von Büdingen, H. J.: Ultrasound Diagnosis of Cerebrovascular Disease. New York: Thieme Medical Publishers, 1993.

Waxman, S. G., et al.: Temporal Profile Resembling TIA in the Setting of Cerebral Infarction. Stroke 14(3):433, May-June 1983.

Weksler, B. B.: Hematologic Disorders and Ischemic Stroke. Curr. Opin. Neurol. 8(1):38-44, Feb. 1995.

Whisnant, J. P.: Effectiveness Versus Efficacy of Treatment of Hypertension for Stroke Prevention. Neurology 46(2):301-307, Feb. 1996.

Yatsu, F.: Treatment and Prevention of Stroke. In: Rowland, L. P. (Ed.): Merritt's Textbook of Neurology, 9th ed. Baltimore: Williams & Wilkins, 1995a.

Yatsu, F.: Other Cerebrovascular Syndromes. In: Rowland, L. P. (Ed.): Merritt's Textbook of Neurology, 9th ed. Baltimore: Williams & Wilkins, 1995b.

Additional References

Chimowitz, M. I., et al.: The Warfarin-Aspirin Symptomatic Intracranial Disease Study. Neurology 45(8):1488-1493, Aug. 1995.

Fisher, M., et al. (Eds.): Current Review of Cerebrovascular Disease, 2nd ed. New York: Churchill Livingstone, 1995.

Gorelick, P. B. (Ed.): Atlas of Cerebrovascular Disease. New York: Churchill Livingstone, 1996.

Hirsh, J., et al.: Oral Anticoagulants: Mechanism of Action, Clinical Effectiveness, and Optimal Therapeutic Range. Chest 108(4):231S-246S, Oct. 1995.

Kalra, L. and Eade, J.: Role of Stroke Rehabilitation Units in Managing Severe Disability After Stroke. Stroke 26(11):2031-2034, Nov. 1995.

Lincoln, N. B., et al.: Comparison of Rehabilitation Practice on Hospital Wards for Stroke Patients. Stroke 27(1):18-23, Jan. 1996.

Mohr, J. P. and Prohovkik, I.: Neurovascular Imaging. In: Rowland, L. P. (Ed.): Merritt's Textbook of Neurology, 9th ed. Baltimore: Williams & Wilkins, 1995.

Pollock, B. E., et al.: Factors that Predict the Bleeding Risk of Cerebral Arteriovenous Malformations. Stroke 27(1):1-6, Jan. 1996.

Solomon, R. A., et al.: Relationship Between the Volume of Craniotomies for Cerebral Aneurysm Performed at New York State Hospitals and In-Hospital Mortality. Stroke 27(1):13-17, Jan. 1996.

Sturzenegger, M.: Spontaneous Internal Carotid Artery Dissection: Early Diagnosis and Management in 44 Patients. J. Neurol. 242(4):231-238, Mar. 1995.

Yatsu, F.: Stroke. St. Louis: Mosby, 1995.

CHAPTER 9

DIABETES MELLITUS

SCOPE

Patients with NIDDM are likely to be older than those with IDDM and therefore to be taking medications for other medical problems. For such patients, possible adverse drug interactions and side effects are important considerations when developing a therapeutic regimen. For example, beta-blockers impair glucose tolerance and also mask physiologic responses to hypoglycemia. Hyperosmolar coma occurs most frequently in middle-aged and elderly patients who have severe illnesses, and therefore it has a mortality rate more than ten times higher than that of diabetic ketoacidosis. Frequently the patient has not consumed adequate fluid, often because of gastrointestinal distress or because of being elderly or bedridden with no way of obtaining water. Hypoglycemic reactions can also occur in type II diabetics who take oral hypoglycemic drugs, especially those who are elderly or have renal or hepatic impairment. A deep hypoglycemic coma can result in permanent neurologic impairment or even death. Diabetic amyotrophy is a motor neuropathy that involves bilateral pain and weakness of thigh muscles, with wasting and weight loss. It occurs mostly in elderly men.

SYNOPSIS

9.00   DEFINITION AND CLASSIFICATION

Diabetes mellitus may be defined as a chronic disease in which an absolute or a relative lack of insulin results in abnormal fat, carbohydrate and protein metabolism. Diabetes is characterized by hyperglycemia (increase of blood glucose beyond the normal concentration), resulting either from inadequate secretion of insulin by the pancreas or because the insulin that is secreted cannot be utilized by the cells. Strictly speaking, diabetes is not a single disease but rather a group of diseases with similar symptoms but different etiologies and pathologies, all of which have in common an abnormal blood glucose level.

If it remains untreated, a complete lack of insulin will result in metabolic changes that develop into ketoacidosis, a toxic condition that leads to coma and death. By contrast, some people with diabetes, who suffer only a minimal lack of insulin, are asymptomatic. However, in most cases, diabetes is associated with a variety of vascular, neurologic, renal and other complications that result in serious morbidity and mortality (Guthrie and Guthrie, 1991; Lee, 1991).

In the past, diabetes was classified as juvenile-onset or adult-onset, depending on the patient's age when symptoms began. However, in 1979, the Diabetes Data Group of the National Institutes of Health (NIH) recommended classifying diabetes mellitus into two types according to whether the patient is dependent on exogenous (from an outside source) insulin. The etiology, course and nature of treatment needed are different for each type (Guthrie and Guthrie, 1991; Karam, et al., 1991).

9.01   Type I: Insulin-Dependent Diabetes Mellitus

Patients with type I diabetes are those who require insulin injections in order to survive. They have an absolute lack of insulin, and their blood glucose levels are elevated when fasting and after eating. Lack of insulin also causes depletion of stored fat and protein in the body. Insulin-dependent diabetes mellitus (IDDM), previously referred to as juvenile-onset diabetes, brittle diabetes, ketosis-prone diabetes and unstable diabetes, is most frequent in young people but also occurs in nonobese adults (Guthrie and Guthrie, 1991; Karam, et al., 1991). Type I accounts for 20 to 30 percent of diabetes in Europe and North America (Karam, et al. 1991; Lee, 1991).

9.02   Type II: Non-Insulin-Dependent Diabetes Mellitus

Type II consists of a group of different forms of less severe diabetes; it occurs mostly in adults over 30. Non-insulin-dependent diabetes mellitus (NIDDM) was previously called adult- or maturity-onset diabetes. In NIDDM, both insulin secretion and the body's ability to use insulin are impaired. NIDDM is further divided into two subgroups (Guthrie and Guthrie, 1991; Lee, 1991).

[1]   Obese NIDDM

About 60 to 65 percent of people with diabetes are in the obese NIDDM subgroup; this group accounts for 85 percent of all adults with diabetes. These individuals produce their own insulin and usually do not need exogenous insulin, except when they are under stress. Often their disease can be managed simply by losing weight (Guthrie and Guthrie, 1991).

[2]   Nonobese NIDDM

People with nonobese NIDDM constitute about 15 percent of type II diabetics (Karam, et al., 1991). They generally have normal or slightly decreased levels of insulin and may require insulin to control their hyperglycemia (Guthrie and Guthrie, 1991).

[3]   Maturity-Onset Diabetes of the Young

Maturity-onset diabetes of the young (MODY) is a recently recognized subgroup of NIDDM. Patients have mild hyperglycemia, which manifests during late childhood or young adulthood. MODY appears to have an autosomal dominant genetic transmission (Karam, et al., 1991; Guthrie and Guthrie, 1991).

9.03   Gestational Diabetes

Gestational diabetes is that which appears in pregnant women who have no previous history of diabetes. Usually it is mild and it may be asymptomatic, but there is a greater risk of complications for both mother and fetus. After birth, the mother's disease must be reclassified (Guthrie and Guthrie, 1991).

9.04   Impaired Glucose Tolerance

This term is used to describe people who have had an abnormal glucose tolerance test,[1] but who have a fasting blood glucose level that is either normal or only slightly elevated. Previously this condition was referred to as asymptomatic diabetes, chemical diabetes, borderline diabetes or latent diabetes. The use of the word "diabetes" to classify it was discarded because employers and insurance companies did not distinguish between this condition and full-blown diabetes, even though many people with impaired glucose tolerance revert to normal and most do not develop the disabling complications of diabetes mellitus (Guthrie and Guthrie, 1991).

9.10   EPIDEMIOLOGY

It has been difficult to acquire precise epidemiologic data for diabetes mellitus for several reasons. In the past, criteria for diagnosis varied considerably among different investigators. Another difficulty is that many people who are surveyed will not admit to having diabetes.

---

[1] *See* 9.43[2][b] *infra.*

There are over 7 million known cases of diabetes in the United States. The prevalence is increasing because the population is aging, even though half the patients are under 65 and three quarters of newly diagnosed patients are under 65. Both prevalence and incidence increase with age; whereas about 1 of every 700 people under 17 have diabetes, 1 out of every 12.5 people 65 and over have the disease. In addition to the known cases, statistical projections indicate that there are between 4 and 7 million undiagnosed cases of diabetes in the United States, bringing the total number of cases to 11 to 14 million.

Worldwide, diabetes is slightly more common in women than in men and more common in nonwhites than in whites. The incidence of IDDM is lowest in Asians and highest in Scandinavians. In the United States, the incidence and prevalence are highest in the Pima Indians of Arizona, somewhat lower in other Native Americans and still lower, in descending order, in Mexican-Americans, blacks and whites (Guthrie and Guthrie, 1991).

Precise mortality rates are also difficult to determine, because diabetes is usually not recorded as the cause of death even for people who are known to have it. Estimates of the number of deaths from cardiovascular, cerebrovascular and renal (kidney) disease in which diabetes is the underlying cause suggest that about 365,000 deaths per year are caused by diabetes and its complications (Guthrie and Guthrie, 1991).

9.20 PATHOPHYSIOLOGY

The basis of diabetes mellitus is the failure of the pancreas to produce enough insulin, or the inability of the body to use the insulin that is available. Describing the different pathologies of IDDM and NIDDM requires an explanation of normal glucose metabolism.

9.21 Glucose Metabolism

Glucose is the body's primary fuel, and half of the body's supply of glucose is used by the brain. Adequate brain function requires that the level of glucose in the blood be maintained at between 60 and 120 mg/dL (milligrams per deciliter).

Insulin regulates the level of blood glucose. It is a hormone produced by clusters of cells called the islets of Langerhans, which are located in the pancreas. Insulin controls the rate at which glucose is taken up by fat, muscle and liver cells. Each of these three types of cells has a different enzyme system that controls how the cell uses glucose. In fat cells, glucose is converted to triglycerides, and triglycerides are broken down into fatty acids, to be released as required and converted by the liver into ketones (acidic by-products of fat metabolism). These processes are regulated by insulin. When insulin levels are low, uptake of glucose into fat cells is poor, which means that more triglycerides are broken down than are formed, and stored fat is lost.

Similarly, insulin stimulates glucose uptake into muscle cells, which convert the glucose either into energy for contraction or into glycogen (a storage form of glucose). The liver also stores glycogen and, in addition, can covert amino acids (protein) to glucose when required, in a process called gluconeogenesis (the use of protein to make glucose). Insulin promotes glucose uptake by the liver, increases the synthesis of glycogen and decreases gluconeogenesis.

Insulin is secreted by the beta cells of the islets of Langerhans according to a feedback system whereby the beta cells release an amount of insulin that corresponds to the blood glucose level. A higher level of blood glucose stimulates a greater release of insulin. More precisely, glucose metabolism stimulates the synthesis of proinsulin, the precursor of insulin, which is converted into insulin in the beta cells. Increased insulin secretion stimulates the liver to synthesize glycogen, decrease the release of glycogen and reduce gluconeogenesis. The tissue cells take up more glucose.

When the blood sugar level is low, insulin release is diminished, and the necessary glucose is fed into the blood by means of glycogenolysis (release of glycogen) and gluconeogenesis (Lee, 1991).

Uptake of insulin by tissue cells depends on insulin receptors on the surface of each cell that bind insulin to the cell. The insulin then stimulates the cell to take up glucose. Without insulin, glucose cannot be used by the tissue cells, even when there is adequate glucose in the blood. Defective receptor functioning is a factor in NIDDM (Lee, 1991).

9.22   Effects of Insulin Deficiency

The initial effect of insulin deficiency is that fat and muscle cells do not take up glucose, which means that the body is not receiving the fuel it requires and that the blood glucose level increases. In response to this condition, which resembles starvation, the body tries to use glycogen, protein and fat from its stores. Muscle cells break down glycogen, liver cells convert amino acids into glucose, and fat cells convert triglycerides into free fatty acids, which in turn are converted into ketones. However, without insulin, the body cannot use these substances for fuel either, and the blood glucose level continues to rise.

At a level of about 180 mg/dL, the kidneys are no longer able to reabsorb glucose from the blood (this level is called the renal threshold), and the sugar is excreted in the urine (glycosuria). The glucose in the urine functions as a diuretic, and large quantities of water and salts are also excreted, resulting in cellular dehydration and electrolyte imbalance. This is the mechanism underlying the typical excessive urination (polyuria) and thirst (polydipsia) of diabetics. Excessive hunger (polyphagia) and fatigue are other typical symptoms that result from the lack of glucose uptake.

As the acidic ketones (also known as ketone bodies) accumulate in the blood, the condition known as diabetic ketoacidosis (a pathologic condition of excess acidity) develops. The body tries to compensate by a typical deep, labored breathing known as Kussmaul's respiration. If all these changes go untreated, brain function is impaired and coma results, followed by death.

Type II diabetes progresses mores slowly than type I; patients often have no symptoms and are unlikely to develop ketoacidosis except under stressful conditions (Lipsky, 1994). However, they still often develop the chronic complications of the disease, such as neuropathy, vascular disease, recurrent infection and ocular problems (Lee, 1991). The pathophysiology of type II involves long-term insulin resistance or inability of the cells to use insulin.[2] Initially the pancreas compensates by secreting extra insulin, but over time it is unable to continue to do so. An additional factor is increased production of glucose by the liver, despite the presence of hyperglycemia and insulin (Fore, 1995).

9.30 ETIOLOGY

The etiology of diabetes involves a genetic predisposition acted upon by environmental factors that cause the disease to manifest.

---

[2] See 9.32 infra.

However, the underlying causes for insufficient delivery of insulin to the tissues are different for type I and type II diabetes. Genetic influences are less strong in type I than in type II, and the derangements in metabolism develop differently in the two types.

9.31   Type I

Type I diabetes mellitus is caused by a genetic defect of the immune system that leaves a person susceptible to an autoimmune process that gradually destroys the beta cells. This defect is carried in the genes responsible for the human leukocyte antigens (HLAs). These histocompatibility antigens are proteins located on cell surfaces that enable the immune system to differentiate a person's own body cells from foreign cells such as viruses (Gearhart and Forbes, 1995; Karam, et al., 1991).

HLA antigens have been divided into several groups, each of which has multiple variations. Certain HLA antigens—in particular, types DR3 and DR4—have been strongly associated with type I diabetes, although the specific antigens involved vary among different racial groups. Recently another HLA system, the DQ group, has been shown to be an even more specific genetic marker for type I diabetes. One variety of this group, HLA-DQw3.2, is always found in HLA-DR4 patients who have type I diabetes.

Although the precise mechanism is not known, it appears that the genetic defect produces an immune deficiency, leaving the person susceptible to an infection or an environmental insult that results in the production of cytotoxic lymphocytes (white cells) and autoantibodies that cause beta cell destruction (Karam, et al., 1991). These genetic factors, however, only determine susceptibility; most people with these genes do not develop type I diabetes. The finding that the incidence of diabetes changes in populations that migrate indicates the importance of nongenetic, environmental factors in inducing the disease in susceptible individuals. The specific environmental factors that play this role are unknown, although possibilities include viruses, dietary factors and toxic chemicals. Whatever the factor is, it is probably widespread and affects children at an early age. It has been found, for example, that breast-feeding children for three months protects them from IDDM, possibly because breast milk provides immune factors that protect against infection.

Further, the incidence of IDDM decreases after puberty, suggesting that the environmental factor operates only during childhood, although the disease would then take a variable number of years to manifest clinically (Leslie and Elliot, 1994).

9.32 Type II

Although it is not linked to HLA antigens, NIDDM is a genetic disease. The gene for it is present worldwide, but type II diabetes generally appears only when societies become industrialized, which means that more calories are consumed while fewer are expended in physical labor (Guthrie and Guthrie, 1991).

Twin studies have found that whereas only half of identical twins of type I diabetics will develop IDDM, nearly all identical twins of type II diabetics will develop NIDDM within a year of the first twin's developing it. The genetic factor in MODY (maturity-onset diabetes of the young) is stronger; when a parent has a mild diabetes, MODY will occur in half that individual's children. Among individuals who develop NIDDM between 25 and 40 years of age, there is also a high family prevalence. If each of two parents has inherited a gene for diabetes from one of their parents (that is, they are heterozygous), they may or may not develop diabetes after 40, but up to 75 percent of their children have a high risk for diabetes, and up to 25 percent of these children will develop the disease before age 40 (Karam, et al., 1991).

Although it is clear that there is a strong genetic factor determining inheritance of NIDDM, its actual cause in most patients is presently not clearly understood. Generally there is both beta cell dysfunction, resulting in a defect in insulin secretion, and insulin resistance. Insulin resistance is a metabolic abnormality that involves insensitivity of tissues to insulin, for which several possible mechanisms have been suggested. These include factors that inhibit insulin receptors, such as autoantibodies, and postreceptor influences promoting poor responsiveness to insulin, such as excessive amounts of certain hormones (Karam, et al., 1991). Recent evidence suggests that deficient insulin secretion by the beta cells actually is secondary to insulin resistance, which appears first (Bogardus, 1995).

While the cause of insulin resistance has not been defined, it is clearly related to obesity. Insensitivity to endogenous insulin is associated with the presence of fat in the abdominal area. Resistance to insulin in obese patients appears to be related to saturation of storage areas in liver, muscle and fat cells. Failure to absorb insulin results in hyperinsulinism, which may down-regulate insulin receptors, increasing insulin resistance. When the patient goes on a diet so that storage areas are no longer saturated, insulin sensitivity improves (Karam, et al., 1991).

9.40 DIAGNOSIS

Adults should undergo testing for diabetes when they have hyperglycemia (high amount of glucose in the blood), glycosuria (glucose in the urine), obesity, a history of past diabetes, a strong family history of the disease, a history of babies weighing over 9 pounds at birth or of loss of a fetus, lipid abnormalities, early coronary artery disease or peripheral atherosclerosis,[3] or symptoms of hypoglycemia (low blood level of glucose),[4] neuropathy or retinopathy. The physician should have a high index of suspicion for older people, Native Americans, African-Americans and Mexican-Americans.

In the past, criteria varied for diagnosing diabetes mellitus. Since 1979, with the publication of clinical criteria by the National Diabetes Study Group, there has been a consensus that a fasting blood glucose level equal to or above 140 mg/dL present on two occasions, or a random glucose level equal to or above 200 mg/dL associated with polyuria and polydipsia, establishes the diagnosis (Fore, 1995).

9.41 Clinical Features

Diabetes mellitus can be either quite easy or very difficult to diagnose. Type I often has a rapid onset, and patients may present for treatment in a state of ketoacidosis, while type II patients may be symptomless.

[1] Type I

Many characteristic symptoms of IDDM are related to fluid loss. Increased urination is typical. Loss of water in the urine results in thirst and also in blurred vision due to the hyperosmolarity (abnormally increased concentration of osmotically active particles) of the body fluids. Decreased fluid volume leads to dizziness, weakness and postural hypotension (dizziness upon standing upright), since the brain is not receiving adequate circulation. The patient may be alert if the

---

[3] *See also* ch. 7.

[4] *See* 9.74 *infra*.

disease has developed slowly enough that water intake can be maintained. However, when there is vomiting due to ketoacidosis, osmolarity increases and the patient may become stuporous or comatose.

Weight loss when the appetite is normal or increased is another common symptom when IDDM develops subacutely, over a number of weeks. The patient may also experience paresthesias (abnormal sensations) due to dysfunction of sensory nerves (Karam, et al., 1991).

[2]   Type II

Like type I patients, those with NIDDM experience thirst, increased urination, paresthesias, blurred vision and weakness. However, in these patients, especially those who are obese, the onset of symptoms may be insidious and remain unnoticed for years, during which time complications affecting other body systems may begin to develop. A common symptom is a chronic skin infection. For women, the initial symptom is often a vaginal yeast infection.

In obese patients, diabetes appears to be most frequently associated with fat deposits in the abdomen, chest, face and neck, as opposed to the arms and legs. CT scans have documented an association between insulin resistance and fat deposits deep inside the abdomen, as opposed to fat in subcutaneous abdominal tissues (Karam, et al., 1991).

9.42   History and Physical Examination

A complete assessment should be carried out in order to classify the patient's disease and detect any co-existing or complicating disease. Diabetics often have a variety of other diseases, including hypertension, obesity and dyslipidemia (abnormal levels of cholesterol and other lipids), which also need to be evaluated and treated.

The history should document the patient's symptoms—especially those of hypoglycemia and complications involving the kidneys, eyes or peripheral or autonomic nerves—acute complications (such as coma), eating habits, gestational history and history of cardiovascular risk factors, such as smoking, use of oral contraceptives or hypertension. It should include the presence and age at onset of diabetes in other family members, whether these individuals are obese and whether they need insulin.

The physical examination should include evaluation of peripheral arterial pulses, neurologic and ophthalmic examinations, and skin examination. If the patient is obese, fat distribution should be described (Karam, et al., 1991; Fore, 1995).

9.43   Laboratory Tests

A number of tests are available for diagnosing diabetes. They include techniques for screening urine for the presence of glucose and ketone bodies, and tests of the glucose level of whole blood or plasma. The purpose of laboratory studies is to document the presence of hyperglycemia either when the patient is fasting or after ingesting glucose (postprandial). Certain other studies are also useful, either for initial assessment or to evaluate treatment.

[1]   Urine Tests

Urine testing is not used for initial diagnosis but may be helpful for ongoing evaluation during treatment.

[a]   Testing for Glucose

Urine testing for glucosuria is inexpensive and simple but not particularly sensitive. The most common form is the dipstick method, in which a paper strip dipped in the sample turns a color that corresponds to the concentration of glucose in the urine.

[b]   Testing for Ketones and Protein

Various products such as dipsticks are available to test for the presence of ketone bodies in the urine. However, such products may not measure all three major types of ketones, and they become ineffective soon after they are opened, which means they may result in false-negatives.

Albuminuria (excess albumin, or serum protein, in the urine) can be detected by the dipstick method and may be an early sign of renal complications. It can also be detected in smaller concentrations by a radioimmunoassay technique (Karam, et al., 1991).

[2]   Blood Tests

Random blood sampling (done at any time that is convenient) is widely used for mass screening, but because there is no standard value with which to compare the result, this type of test is hard to interpret. Blood glucose levels fluctuate depending on when food is eaten and on time of day. Blood tests are therefore more accurate if performed at specific times related to when food has been consumed.

Laboratory testing usually measures the level of glucose in plasma, while whole blood glucose is measured in patient self-testing.[5] Normal whole-blood levels range from 60 to 110 mg/dL, while for plasma glucose, the range is 70 to 120 mg/dL. Since glucose tolerance changes with age, in people over 60, the range must be corrected upward by 1 mg/dL for each year (Guthrie and Guthrie, 1991; Karam, et al., 1991).

[a]   Fasting Blood Glucose Test

This is probably the laboratory test most frequently used to diagnose diabetes. The blood sample is drawn in the morning, after the patient has fasted overnight. In symptomatic individuals, this test can confirm the diagnosis when the value is above 140 mg/dL on more than one occasion (Karam, et al., 1991; Guthrie and Guthrie, 1991).

[b]   Oral Glucose Tolerance Test

The oral glucose tolerance test is the most sensitive technique for detecting diabetes mellitus, but it is difficult to administer and interpret accurately (Guthrie and Guthrie, 1991). In most cases, this test is not necessary. It should generally be given only to patients who have complications associated with diabetes but whose fasting plasma glucose levels are under 140 mg/dL (Fore, 1995).

Patients must be on a high-carbohydrate diet for three days prior to the test, eating nothing after midnight the day before it is administered. Adult patients are given 7.5 g of glucose in 300 mL of water. The dose should be drunk within 5 minutes. Blood and urine samples are taken before the test and then at 30-, 60-, 90- and 120-minute intervals. Two hours is the length called for by the NIH criteria; some examiners extend the test to three to six hours.

In the past, the test was interpreted according to various criteria. According to the stricter NIH criteria, fasting venous plasma glucose levels greater than 140 mg/dL or any value during the test above 200 mg/dL is diagnostic of diabetes. A fasting level above 110 mg/dL but below 140 mg/dL or a value above 200 mg/dL during the test is diagnostic of impaired glucose tolerance. A fasting level less than 140 mg/dL plus two or more values of 200 mg/dL or greater also constitute diabetes (Guthrie and Guthrie, 1991).

---

[5] *See 9.52 infra.*

Certain drugs can produce false-positives, including diuretics, oral contraceptives, glucocorticoids, excess thyroxine, nicotinic acid, phenytoin and some psychoactive agents. Patients who are malnourished, under severe emotional stress, bedridden or have an infection may also have false-positive results (Karam, et al., 1991).

[c]   Glycosylated Hemoglobin Test

Glycosylated hemoglobin is also known as glycohemoglobin; its major form is hemoglobin A_{1c}. It is produced by a chemical reaction between glucose and the hemoglobin molecule such that the glucose attaches to the red blood cell. The amount of glycosylation is an indication of the concentration of blood glucose over the preceding 8 to 12 weeks. Thus, an assay (test) of glycosylated hemoglobin can demonstrate the effectiveness of diabetic control over the preceding 2 to 3 months. The test is therefore useful for evaluating the effectiveness of treatment as well as the reliability of the patient's self-monitoring (Karam, et al., 1991).

[d]   Serum Insulin Values

Insulin levels can be measured during the glucose tolerance test by separating serum or plasma and performing a radioimmunoassay. Some experts claim this information is generally not clinically useful; others say it improves the reliability of the oral glucose tolerance test (Karam, et al., 1991; Guthrie and Guthrie, 1991).

[3]   Other Tests

The intravenous glucose tolerance test is usually given to patients who have gastrointestinal problems that interfere with normal absorption of glucose. It is not as sensitive as the oral glucose tolerance test and requires care in interpretation (Karam, et al., 1991).

New tests under development involve HLA gene typing and screening for anti-beta-cell and anti-insulin antibodies. These tests identify individuals at risk for diabetes before the disease develops. However, at the present time, use of these procedures is generally limited to research (Guthrie and Guthrie, 1991).

9.50   TREATMENT

Treatment of diabetes must be individualized according to each patient's characteristics. In general, however, the goal is to normalize the patient's physiology by administering insulin in such a way as to maintain a continuous basal blood glucose level, with an eight- to tenfold rise with each meal. The hope is that this treatment will delay or prevent the development of microvascular disease.

There is controversy over what is the best method to achieve this goal. In any case, treatment requires that the patient cooperate in adjusting his or her diet, exercise and use of drugs (Karam, et al., 1991).

9.51 Principles of Dietary Control

Appropriate diet is a fundamental component of treatment for all diabetics. Currently recommended diabetic diets do not involve undue restrictions; they are similar to general guidelines for healthy eating. Nevertheless, over half of patients do not stick to their diet (Karam, et al., 1991).

Maintaining a normal blood glucose level requires a proper balance between insulin, exercise and food. The basis for managing diabetes successfully is developing a routine incorporating the same insulin dose, the same amount of activity and the same number of calories at the same time each day (Quinn, 1993). Varying the regimen requires that the patient understand the relationships among all three components, in order to make the necessary adjustments. Strenuous exercise uses up glucose and requires consuming more food, and may precipitate hypoglycemia. Insulin also lowers plasma glucose level. Both food consumption and stress caused by illness or emotional disturbance raise the plasma glucose level. Achieving an appropriate balance between the size and frequency of meals and regular, moderate exercise can stabilize the amount of insulin needed by diabetics who have difficulty maintaining glycemic control (Karam, et al., 1991).

[1] Components of Diet

In the past, diabetics were told that eating sugar could raise blood glucose to dangerous levels. Traditionally the American Diabetes Association (ADA) recommended that diabetics eat starches rather than sugars, and also recommended specific percentages of protein, carbohydrate and fat intake. In May 1994, however, the ADA issued new nutrition guidelines based on the discovery that it is the total amount of carbohydrates in the diet, regardless of whether they are from starch or sugar, that determines blood sugar levels.

The new recommendations give diabetics more flexibility in food choices. Diabetics do not have to avoid sugars and fruit completely, but they should count these foods as part of their total carbohydrate consumption. Further, instead of recommending specific proportions of protein, carbohydrate and fat in the diet, the ADA now advises that these be individualized according to the metabolic outcome desired in a given case (Dinsmoor, 1994; Gearhart and Forbes, 1995).

Weight control is a critical component of the diabetic diet. Weight-loss programs that include behavior modification techniques appear to be most successful. Fasts or extremely low calorie regimens should only be undertaken by very obese patients and then only with medical monitoring. Diabetics who are prone to ketosis or who have liver disease, renal impairment or recent myocardial infarction should not undertake such diets. Exercise is more useful for maintaining weight than for losing it, and the most effective type of exercise is of moderate intensity but long duration (Quinn, 1993).

To facilitate meal planning, the ADA has developed a so-called exchange system, which categorizes all foods into six groups and lists foods in each group in specific serving amounts, in such a manner that each item is equal in protein, carbohydrate and fat content, as well as in calories, to all other items on the same list. Thus if a patient's diet includes five servings of carbohydrate, any type of starch on the list can be "exchanged" for any other.

It has been established that once kidney disease exists, restricting protein intake can prevent or retard the associated decrease in creatinine clearance. It is also possible that protein restriction may help prevent renal complications from developing. However, restricting protein intake may require that the patient take amino acid supplements (Quinn, 1993).

[2] Type I Diabetes

The total calories in the diet for the patient with IDDM are calculated to maintain ideal body weight. The diet must also be adjusted according to the insulin regimen the patient is on. The timing and size of meals depends on the timing and type of insulin being taken. Most patients take insulin at least twice a day, frequently combining intermediate-acting with short-acting types. They should eat breakfast within a half-hour to an hour of the first dose, a carbohydrate snack three hours later, lunch within five hours after the morning dose and an afternoon snack within seven to eight hours. Dinner should be eaten one-half to one and a half hours after the second insulin dose, and a bedtime snack should be consumed three hours later. The more frequent the insulin doses in a day, the more flexibility the patient has in timing meals (Karam, et al., 1991).

[3] Type II Diabetes

Since most type II diabetics are obese, standard treatment for NIDDM involves caloric restriction and exercise in order to induce weight loss and thereby improve insulin resistance. Successful weight reduction requires close supervision of the diet and of an exercise program. A team approach in which patients can meet individually with a nutritionist or in a group session is most effective. The actual number of calories in the diet should depend on the patient's activity level and life-style (Quinn, 1993; Karam, et al., 1991; Gearhart and Forbes, 1995).

9.52 Self-Monitoring

Patients whose diabetes is hard to control are taught to monitor their own blood glucose levels so they can make corrections in insulin dosage and adjust exercise and food intake in order to maximize glycemic control and prevent episodes of hyperglycemia and hypoglycemia. Self-monitoring also enables them to be more flexible in their life-style habits (Karam, et al., 1991).

[1] Blood Glucose Monitoring

Home kits are available for self-monitoring of blood glucose. The diabetic pricks the finger using a specially designed lancet to obtain a drop of blood, which is then applied to an enzyme-impregnated test strip. The strip changes color corresponding to the blood glucose level. The result can be read using either a color chart or a more complicated meter that gives a digital readout.

Type I patients usually need to check their blood glucose at least four times a day initially. After treatment has brought some improvement, levels are checked at least twice a day and also if the patient experiences symptoms of hypoglycemia. Logs of the results should be kept (Karam, et al., 1991).

[2] Urine Self-monitoring

Patients who cannot or do not want to perform finger-sticks to draw blood can check for glucose in the urine by the dipstick method, although this method is not as accurate as blood testing. Self-monitoring for ketones may also be useful (Gearhart and Forbes, 1995).

9.53 Insulin

Patients with IDDM and those with NIDDM whose hyperglycemia cannot be controlled by diet or hypoglycemic drugs[6] must take insulin, which is usually administered by subcutaneous injection but sometimes by use of a portable infusion pump. Various types of commercial insulin preparations are available.

[1] Types of Insulin

Over 40 different insulin formulations are available. They differ with respect to the animal source from which they are made, their concentration, purity and solubility, and the length of time they remain active (Karam, et al., 1991). The three basic types are short acting (regular), intermediate acting (NPH or lente) and long acting (ultralente). The longer-acting types are modified to make them less soluble, thus delaying their time of onset, time of peak action and overall duration of action (Hollander, 1994).

[a] Sources of Insulin

Commercial insulin is derived from beef or pork pancreas or is a synthesized human insulin. Beef insulin differs from human insulin by three amino acids and therefore is more antigenic than pork insulin, which differs by only one amino acid. These types are available either as mixed beef and pork or as pure pork. Synthetic human insulin is produced by recombinant DNA techniques or by an enzymatic conversion process in which pork insulin is converted to human insulin by replacing the single different amino acid with the human one (Arslanian and Drash, 1994; Karam, et al., 1991).

[b] Purification and Concentration of Insulin

Recent purification techniques have reduced or eliminated impurities—specifically proinsulin—in commercial insulin that induced formation of anti-insulin antibodies. Insulin labeled "new improved single peak insulin" contains less than 25 ppm (parts per million) of proinsulin but more than 10 ppm. Insulin labeled "purified" contains

---

6 *See* 9.54 *infra.*

less than 10 ppm of proinsulin. "Highly purified" insulin has the additional advantage that it can maintain its potency for long periods without refrigeration. Most insulin comes in a concentration of 100 units/mL (also referred to as U100) (Karam, et al., 1991).

[c]   Regular Insulin

Regular or short-acting insulin starts acting within 15 minutes of injection, reaches its peak at between 1 and 3 hours, and lasts for between 5 and 7 hours. It is used to control glucose levels after meals and is thus injected 15 to 30 minutes before eating. Semilente is a form of regular insulin with a slightly longer onset of between 30 and 60 minutes. It peaks at around 6 hours and lasts 12 to 16 hours. When it is used in a pump, regular insulin is buffered to improve stability (Karam, et al., 1991; Hollander, 1994).

[d]   NPH or Lente Insulin

NPH and lente are intermediate-acting preparations composed of mixtures of different insulins to produce an onset of action at between 2 and 4 hours, and a peak response at 8 to 10 hours. The duration of action is between 18 and 24 hours. Intermediate-acting insulins are used to provide basal levels of insulin but may also be adequate to cover lunch. The standard insulin regime of two injections a day combines regular with NPH insulins. Premixed preparations are available (Karam, et al., 1991; Hollander, 1994).

[e]   Ultralente Insulin

Ultralente is generally made from beef insulin, which is less soluble than pork, providing a longer duration of action of 28 to 36 hours. Because of this slow action, ultralente is used as a basal insulin, along with injections of regular insulin before meals. Ultralente made from human insulin has a somewhat shorter duration of 24 to 28 hours (Karam, et al., 1991; Hollander, 1994).

[2]   Methods of Administration

Various delivery systems are available for administering insulin.

[a]   Syringes

Most diabetics self-administer their insulin by subcutaneous injection. Plastic syringes have been developed to make this process as painless as possible. Low-dose syringes with calibrations make it possible to measure each dose and to mix intermediate and regular insulins together in one injection. A variation on the syringe is the pen injector, which is useful for diabetics who need several before-meal injections of regular insulin during the day. The pen contains a cartridge of insulin and has a retractable needle (Karam, et al., 1991).

Injections are commonly given in the upper arm, thigh, abdomen, flank and buttock. Physicians advise rotating sites to avoid delayed absorption resulting from fibrosis or lipohypertrophy (excess accumulation of fatty tissue), which can develop at sites that are used repeatedly. Patients must be aware, however, that rates of absorption of insulin vary at different sites, with regular insulin being more rapidly absorbed from sites in the upper body. Exercise also facilitates absorption when the injection site is next to the muscle being contracted. To avoid possible fluctuation in glycemic control, many experts recommend that diabetics use just one body area for injections but rotate sites within that area. For most patients, this is the abdomen.

[b] Pumps

Use of pumps is based on the idea that continuous subcutaneous infusion of insulin can imitate the continuous insulin production of the normal pancreas. "Closed-loop" infusion systems utilize a glucose sensor that controls the amount of insulin or glucose to be infused. Such systems are useful in emergencies such as ketoacidosis but are too cumbersome for constant use (Karam, et al., 1991).

"Open loop" systems are small, ambulatory infusion pumps that can be programmed to deliver a basal dose of regular insulin at a specified rate and to change this rate for certain time periods, as before meals or just before dawn, when some patients' blood glucose level starts to rise (the "dawn phenomenon").[7] This device requires self-monitoring and adjustment by the patient. This type of pump can be useful when insulin absorption is erratic and it is difficult to establish a stable basal level (Hollander, 1994). However, complications are associated with pump use, including infection at the infusion site and ketoacidosis resulting from the flow of insulin being cut off because of a kink in the tube (Karam, et al., 1991). Also, pumps have not been effective for children or adolescents (Arslanian and Drash, 1994).

---

[7] *See* 9.55[3] *infra.*

[3]   Complications of Insulin Therapy

The most serious complication of insulin use is the development of hypoglycemia.[8] A number of less severe side effects of insulin therapy are due to the immunogenicity of insulin. Reactions are more common among diabetics who use preparations containing some beef insulin.

[a]   Allergic Reactions

Antibodies to insulin develop after two to three weeks of taking it. Rarely, a patient develops a generalized hypersensitivity reaction that manifests as urticaria (hives) after an injection. This problem can often be resolved by switching to pure pork or human insulin, although treatment with antihistamines and corticosteroids has sometimes been required. Severe reactions can also be treated by a desensitization procedure in which the patient stops taking insulin for 12 to 24 hours, then is given small amounts that gradually increase to a full dose over a 6-hour period (Karam, et al., 1991).

[b]   Insulin Resistance

All diabetics except those who take highly purified pork or human insulin develop a low concentration of IgG antibodies, which neutralize to some extent the action of insulin. Some patients who have used insulin intermittently develop a high concentration of these antibodies, especially if they are obese NIDDM patients who already have some degree of insensitivity to insulin. Such individuals may need 200 units or more of insulin a day. Often this resistance is temporary and resolves spontaneously. Switching to pork or human insulin may reduce the resistance or shorten its duration. If it does not, the patient may be given prednisone, which improves the response to insulin (Karam, et al., 1991).

[c]   Lipodystrophy

Lipodystrophy is a loss (atrophy) of subcutaneous fatty tissue at the site of an insulin injection, which is thought to be an immune reaction. It occurs mostly in females; since it can be a cosmetic problem, patients are advised to inject into the abdominal wall. This problem is less common since highly purified insulin has come into

---

[8] *See* 9.74 *infra.*

widespread use. It can often be reversed by injecting purified insulin directly into the atrophied area.

Lipohypertrophy is an excess of subcutaneous fatty tissue, creating a puffy effect. It is not caused by an immune response but appears to be a result of repeatedly injecting insulin into a single site. Lipohypertrophy can be avoided by rotating sites. If necessary, the excess tissue can be removed by liposuction (Karam, et al., 1991).

9.54   Oral Hypoglycemic Drugs

Type II diabetics who are unable to achieve glycemic control with diet and exercise alone are given an oral hypoglycemic drug. This type of drug is believed to lower blood glucose levels by increasing the functioning of insulin receptors and stimulating secretion of endogenous insulin by the beta cells. The two types of oral hypoglycemic drugs, sulfonylureas and biguanides, have different modes of action. Patients with type I diabetes should not take these drugs (Gearhart and Forbes, 1995).

[1]   Sulfonylureas

Sulfonylureas appear to work by binding to receptors on the surface of the beta cells. This depolarizes the cell, allowing calcium to enter and promote release of insulin. Thus these agents require functioning beta cells to be effective. They are most effective in NIDDM patients who develop diabetes after the age of 40, have had the disease for under five years, are obese or of normal weight, and have never taken insulin or have been able to control diabetes while taking less than 40 U/d (Gearhart and Forbes, 1994; Karam, et al., 1991).

Six types of sulfonylureas are available in the United States. Tolbutamide has a short duration (6 to 10 hours) and rarely causes acute toxic reactions; it therefore seems safest for elderly patients who are at particular risk for hypoglycemia. Chlorpropamide may last up to 60 hours and should not be taken by patients with renal impairment. It is a potent drug that often controls hyperglycemia when other agents have failed, but it poses a greater risk of prolonged hypoglycemia and may be inappropriate for people over 65.

The potency of tolazamide resembles that of chlorpropamide, but this drug is more slowly absorbed. Its action lasts up to 20 hours. Acetohexamide has a duration of action of 10 to 16 hours. Because acetohexamide is metabolized into a compound that remains hypoglycemically active and is excreted in the urine, it should not be given to patients with renal impairment.

Glyburide and glipizide are highly potent sulfonylureas that should not be given to patients with renal or hepatic impairment because of the risk of hypoglycemia. Caution should be used when prescribing them for elderly patients or those with cardiovascular disease (Gearhart and Forbes, 1994; Karam, et al., 1991).

[2] Biguanides

Biguanides are thought to act by increasing the function of insulin receptors, delaying absorption of nutrients from the intestine and decreasing gluconeogenesis. These drugs do not require functioning beta cells to be effective. In the past, phenformin was the only biguanide available in this country, but its use was discontinued because it was reported to be associated with lactic acidosis (accumulation of excess lactic acid in the blood)[9] in patients who also had kidney or liver disease. In 1994, the Food and Drug Administration (FDA) approved another biguanide, metformin, which is less likely to cause hypoglycemia than other drugs. Many experts prefer it for obese patients who are newly diagnosed with NIDDM (Gearhart and Forbes, 1994; Karam, et al., 1991).

[3] Safety of Oral Hypoglycemic Drugs

The University Group Diabetes Program reported that diabetics treated with tolbutamide or phenformin had an excess number of deaths from cardiovascular disease, compared to patients given insulin or placebo. However, methodologic criticisms of this study generated controversy about its validity. Currently the ADA does not restrict use of sulfonylureas, although a label warning of cardiovascular risk is included with each pack (Karam, et al., 1991).

9.55 Management of Type I Diabetes

The theoretic objective of IDDM management is to restore and maintain metabolic normality. Unfortunately, achieving this goal is more or less impossible, since attempts to do so are likely to lead to hypoglycemia or ketoacidosis. Therefore, patient and physician need to determine together a set of compromise goals that are achievable.

---

9 *See 9.75 infra.*

These goals include (Gearhart and Forbes, 1995; Arslanian and Drash, 1994):

- eliminating symptomatic hyperglycemia;
- restoring fluid and electrolyte balance;
- preventing hypoglycemia, obesity and dyslipidemia;
- maintaining physical fitness;
- keeping blood glucose levels close to normal to prevent diabetic complications; and
- maintaining a normal life-style.

[1]   Insulin Therapy

To attain these objectives, it is necessary to move toward target glucose levels gradually. The need for insulin varies considerably from one patient to another, as well as over time in the same patient. Newly diagnosed patients, who may still be secreting some insulin, need a relatively low dose unless they present with ketoacidosis. The initial dose for an adult within 20 percent of ideal body weight ranges from 0.25 to 1.0 U/kg/day.

During the first few weeks, beta cell function often recovers temporarily. During this "honeymoon period," patients need less exogenous insulin than they did right after the diagnosis. After this remission, however, most patients lose all or nearly all beta cell function and must begin a regimen of insulin therapy (Gearhart and Forbes, 1995; Arslanian and Drash, 1994).

The choice of an insulin regimen is based on the patient's self-discipline, physiologic needs and schedule, and on how much the patient is willing to do. The fundamental principle is to use the simplest regimen that can achieve the agreed-on objectives. With three different types of insulin available, many different regimens have been developed. Any regimen must provide both a basal level of insulin that is continuously present in order to suppress glucose production by the liver, and bolus (concentrated doses) insulin, which is given before meals to prevent a rise in blood glucose level after eating (Hollander, 1994). Insulin requirements increase during infections with fever and during severe illness (Karam, et al., 1991).

[a]   Conventional Insulin Therapy

A conventional insulin regimen consists of a split dose of regular- and intermediate-acting insulin, of which 50 to 70 percent is injected in the morning before breakfast and the remainder in the evening. This is the most frequently used regimen in the United States. Its disadvantages are that it does not always cover the midday meal, hypoglycemia frequently occurs at night and the regimen does not provide for supplemental doses. A variation of this regimen moves the second injection to bedtime to avoid nighttime hypoglycemia (Gearhart and Forbes, 1995; Hollander, 1994).

Patients must be educated to monitor their blood glucose levels initially before breakfast and again before dinner. The next phase is to monitor postprandial (after-meal) and middle-of-the-night blood glucose values to make glucose control tighter. Morning glucose values reflect the effectiveness of the previous evening's NPH dose; 5 p.m. values reflect the effects of the morning NPH; and 9 p.m. values, the effect of the evening regular insulin.

The regimen can be individualized for each patient's meal and exercise schedule and life-style. Gradually, as the patient learns to adjust diet, activity level and insulin dose to correct for a specific blood glucose value, the target blood glucose level decreases (that is, approaches closer to normal). In making adjustments, the patient must be aware that absorption of insulin varies considerably even when the dose is injected into the same area (Gearhart and Forbes, 1995; Karam, et al., 1991).

[b]   Intensive Insulin Therapy

A conventional regimen frequently does not result in adequate control of glucose values during the day and may also produce hypoglycemia at night. Thus other regimens have been developed that involve multiple daily injections. These involve varying combinations of regular, NPH and ultralente administered in the morning, at noon, in the evening and at bedtime. A regimen that uses multiple injections or an insulin pump is referred to as intensive insulin therapy. Its purpose is to move more aggressively toward normal levels of blood glucose (Hollander, 1994).

The question of how important it is to maintain what is known as tight control of blood glucose levels, which had been a subject of controversy, was answered in 1993 with the publication of the *Diabetes Control and Complications Trial* (DCCT), which investigated the effect of blood glucose levels on the development of microvascular complications. The results clearly demonstrated that both the incidence and the progression of microvascular disease are related to blood glucose level. The study compared patients on standard and intensive insulin regimens and found that whether or not diabetic complications are already present, early intensive insulin therapy prevents complications and lengthens remissions. However, patients on the intensive regimen had more episodes of hypoglycemia and gained more weight.

The question, then, is whether all type I diabetics should be on an intensive regimen. One answer is that if the goals of therapy can be met with two injections a day, there is no reason to prescribe more. A candidate for intensive therapy is healthy except for the diabetes, is motivated enough to perform extra self-monitoring and learn to adjust doses, and has no signs of diabetic complications. Intensive therapy is generally contraindicated for patients who are unable to recognize the symptoms of hypoglycemia or who have angina or poor counter-regulatory responses to hypoglycemia. The risk of hypoglycemia is also a contraindication for some people who live alone, since severe hypoglycemia can impair brain development (Gearhart and Forbes, 1995; Hollander, 1994).

An intensive insulin regimen has several components. The first is setting goals for blood glucose levels. Ultimately the level should be within 1 to 1.5 percent of normal for most patients. Second, to best adjust the dose, self-monitoring four to seven times a day may be required, and the patient's Hb A_{1c} should be tested every three to four months by the physician. This measurement also serves to reveal falsification of self-monitoring glucose data, which all patients are at least tempted to engage in.

A third component is self-adjustment of the insulin dose by the patient according to a set of guides or algorithms supplied by the physician. Usually the patient changes the amount of regular insulin, but sometimes intermediate or long-acting doses are also adjusted. The fourth component is patient education[10] (Hollander, 1994).

One example of an intensive regimen starts out with four doses of regular insulin: 35 percent of the total before breakfast, 20 percent before lunch, 30 percent before dinner and 15 percent at bedtime or midnight. As the patient's need for insulin stabilizes, two thirds of the total is injected before breakfast and a third before supper. A more

---

[10] *See* 9.57 *infra.*

complicated regimen allows for flexible mealtimes. In this regimen, of the total daily dose, about a third is taken as NPH at night. The remaining two thirds is divided into fifths. Two fifths is taken in the morning, one fifth at lunch and two fifths with dinner (Gearhart and Forbes, 1995).

This is an example of a basic regimen combining basal and bolus insulin. Most patients need an additional active insulin regimen, which includes supplemental doses of regular insulin. These supplements are either added to or subtracted from the basic regimen, based on measured glucose levels or the expectation of extra food consumption or additional exercise. The goal of supplementation is to make the next glucose level measurement conform to the target value. The patient is given schedules for different times of day, listing the amounts of supplements that may be needed at each time, corresponding to the measured blood glucose level. Extra insulin may be needed to compensate for a large meal; by contrast, insulin must be subtracted when particular physical activities are contemplated. The patient eventually learns how much regular insulin must be added to cover a specific food and how much subtracted for a given activity (Hollander, 1994).

[2] Diet

In most cases, diet is the greatest obstacle to glycemic control. The patients with the best results in the DCCT (Diabetes Control and Complications Trial) were those who adhered most closely to their diet. Although an intensive regimen allows greater flexibility in eating, in order to consume additional food safely, the patient must learn how much insulin she or he requires for different quantities of food. With carbohydrates, for example, 1 U of regular insulin covers 15 g of carbohydrate. Patients must also learn to treat a hypoglycemic reaction with a limited amount of carbohydrate instead of a large amount.

Weight gain resulting from an intensive regimen frequently occurs when glycosuria is controlled, since calories are no longer being lost in the urine. Unless consumption of calories is reduced, the patient will gain weight (Hollander, 1994).

[3] Early Morning Hyperglycemia

Many patients experience high blood glucose levels in the early morning. This phenomenon may result from the Somogyi effect, in which nighttime hypoglycemia triggers a hormonal reaction that causes blood glucose levels to rise by 7 a.m. More often, early morning hyperglycemia is caused by a decrease in the level of insulin and thus must be corrected by increasing the evening dose. These two reactions can also co-exist, resulting in higher levels of blood glucose than either alone might produce.

Another cause of early morning hyperglycemia is the "dawn phenomenon," which affects most diabetics with NIDDM, up to 75 percent of those with IDDM and normal individuals as well. These people experience a decreased sensitivity to insulin between 5 and 8 a.m., which seems to be due to growth hormone that was secreted earlier, when they fell asleep (growth hormone, which is secreted by the pituitary gland, counteracts the effects of insulin). By itself, the dawn phenomenon may cause only mild hyperglycemia, but it can occur along with the previous two causes, making the hyperglycemia more severe. In order to diagnose the cause of early morning hypoglycemia, the patient may have to monitor glucose at 3 a.m.

The Somogyi effect can be treated by decreasing the evening dose of intermediate-acting insulin, giving some of it at bedtime or eating more food at bedtime. Decreasing insulin levels are treated by increasing the evening dose or shifting it to bedtime, or both. The dawn phenomenon can be treated by giving part of the patient's intermediate-acting insulin at bedtime instead of dinnertime or, if the patient is using a pump, the pump can be set to increase the infusion rate after 6 a.m. (Karam, et al., 1991).

[4]   Other Drug Therapies

Various other drug treatments for diabetes have been investigated.

[a]   Immunotherapy

Since IDDM is caused by a genetic immune system defect, drug treatment with cyclosporine, an immunosuppressive agent, has been tried at the onset of the disease in an attempt to halt the autoimmune process and save the remaining functioning beta cells. Although some patients experience a partial remission, they do not achieve permanent remission. Because immunotherapy has serious side effects, including renal toxicity, the benefits are not sufficient to justify clinical use of cyclosporine (Gearhart and Forbes, 1995; Karam, et al., 1991).

[b] Nonimmunosuppressive Therapies

Nicotinamide, which inhibits an enzyme whose action depletes a coenzyme vital to cell function, has also been studied as a possible way to preserve beta cells, but it has not produced permanent remission (Karam, et al., 1991; Gearhart and Forbes, 1995). Another possible therapeutic agent is insulinlike growth factor-1, which has been found to stimulate glucose uptake. Patients with severe insulin resistance have experienced improved metabolic control after using it, and type II patients have experienced improved glucose tolerance and decreased hyperinsulinemia and hypertriglyceridemia (increased level of triglycerides in the blood). However, possible complications of this drug are unknown (Kolaczynski and Caro, 1994).

[5] Transplantation Procedures

Even using tight control, it is impossible to achieve the level of glucose metabolism that is possible with an endogenous source of insulin provided in response to constant variations in blood glucose levels. Pancreas transplantation procedures were developed in an attempt to provide such a source of insulin. This is now the only treatment that can achieve a normal level of blood glucose without insulin injections. Currently, the one-year survival rate for pancreas transplantation is 91 percent, with 72 percent of patients needing no exogenous insulin (Larsen, et al., 1994). At three years, 59 percent of pancreases transplanted between 1987 and 1992 were still functioning (Remuzzi, et al., 1994). Whether the benefits of this procedure outweigh its risks is still being investigated.

[a] Indications

Pancreas transplantation is performed only for patients with IDDM, since a new organ will not improve the body's inability to use insulin, the condition that characterizes NIDDM. When patients have IDDM and severe nephropathy, combined pancreas-kidney transplantation should be considered. Candidates for a pancreas transplantation alone should have either complications such as neuropathy that would be improved by better blood glucose control or such poor glucose control that the risks of hypoglycemia and/or ketoacidosis outweigh those of the immunosuppression required to prevent graft rejection after transplantation (Larsen, et al., 1994).

[b]   Pancreas Transplant Alone

Patients who have a pancreas transplant alone must consider that although they become free of the need to take insulin, they become dependent on immunosuppressive drugs, which carry an increased risk of infections and neoplasms (tumors), as well as other side effects. In addition, increased morbidity from complications of surgery may offset the improvement in quality of life provided by freedom from exogenous insulin and dietary control. Thus some experts have concluded that solitary pancreas transplantation is not justified except for diabetics whose metabolic control is so fragile that their disease is life threatening or their quality of life intolerable (Remuzzi, et al., 1994).

Others would also perform this procedure for patients with clear early signs of diabetic complications, in the expectation that improved glucose control would either prevent or reverse these complications. Solitary pancreas transplantation is currently being performed in only a few centers in this country as an experimental procedure (Larsen, et al., 1994).

[c]   Combined Pancreas-Kidney Transplant

When diabetics have renal failure and are dependent on dialysis as well as insulin injections, combined pancreas-kidney transplantation can relieve them of both dependencies. The toxic effects of immunosuppression are not an issue, since a kidney transplant will require them anyway. Further, for unknown reasons, pancreas survival is better in patients who have a combined transplant. Thus, in properly selected patients, this procedure has a better outcome and considerably improves quality of life. However, this operation involves greater morbidity and mortality than kidney transplants alone. There is also insufficient information to determine whether the combined operation prevents diabetic complications, although one study has reported an improvement in peripheral neuropathy (Remuzzi, et al., 1994).

[d]   Islet Transplantation

A number of attempts have been made to transplant islets of Langerhans alone. However, the transplants were mostly rejected, despite immunosuppressive therapy. Efforts to encapsulate islets in various types of membranes to protect them from immune attack have been successful in animals, but these procedures are as yet far from being applied to humans (Remuzzi, et al., 1994).

[6] Gene Transfer Techniques

Another approach to treating diabetes uses molecular strategies to replace the normal mechanism of insulin delivery. Gene transfer techniques are being used to insert genetically engineered insulin-secreting cells into the islets of Langerhans. Engineered cells can be grown at a relatively low cost in large numbers, and since they are cloned, their function should be highly reproducible. Several methods for transferring genes for such cells into the islets are being investigated. One uses a recombinant adenovirus that contains the genes for certain components of the insulin-secreting process. It is possible that engineered cell lines that imitate the insulin-secreting response of normal beta cells stimulated by glucose can be developed. Their value as treatment for diabetes will depend on whether their makeup remains stable over time and whether they cause an autoimmune response (Newgard, 1994).

9.56 Management of Type II Diabetes

Treatment of NIDDM begins with diet and exercise to improve insulin sensitivity and the response of beta cells to glucose stimulation. If necessary, the patient also receives an oral hypoglycemic drug. If these measures do not control the disease, the patient may need insulin. Insulin may additionally be needed during periods of emotional stress, surgery, traumatic injury or infection (Gearhart and Forbes, 1995).

In obese patients, weight reduction alone can normalize blood glucose values and restore insulin sensitivity to the tissues. Unfortunately, very obese diabetics rarely lose a significant amount of weight. Less obese diabetics can lose more, if they are sufficiently motivated. Obese patients with mild diabetes generally should not be given hypoglycemic drugs or insulin. Not only does insulin tend to lead to weight gain, but such a patient may already have high circulating levels of insulin, so that adding more will only exacerbate insulin insensitivity.

Patients with moderately severe diabetes who are symptomatic are candidates for oral hypoglycemic drugs. If these do not prevent symptoms of hyperglycemia, insulin may be indicated to control the symptoms. Use of drugs in these patients should be temporary, for the purpose of improving symptoms until weight loss eliminates them (Karam, et al., 1991). Oral hypoglycemic medications are contraindicated in cases of ketoacidosis, serious infection, liver or kidney impairment, chronic debilitating disease and when the patient is allergic to them (Gearhart and Forbes, 1995).

In nonobese type II diabetics, beta cells that do not produce insulin in response to glucose in the blood are more significant in the disease process than is insulin resistance. If hyperglycemia is mild, normal blood glucose levels can sometimes be achieved through a diet that avoids simple sugars and contains only enough calories to maintain ideal body weight. If diet is not effective, hypoglycemic drugs may be added. The goal is to maintain plasma glucose levels below 200 mg/dL to protect the patient from vascular or retinal complications.

According to some experts, insulin is indicated if the highest recommended dosage of oral hypoglycemic drug does not maintain this level. For these nonobese type II patients, a single dose of intermediate-acting insulin may be sufficient (Karam, et al., 1991). Other authorities, however, suggest that early use of insulin may avoid the cycle by which glucotoxicity injures beta cells, which secrete less insulin, which results in increased hyperglycemia and consequently further beta cell destruction (Gearhart and Forbes, 1995).

There is no consensus regarding the combining of insulin with hypoglycemic drugs, and various regimens have been proposed. There is agreement, however, that when a type II patient needs extremely large amounts of insulin, it is preferable to add oral hypoglycemics rather than give the high insulin dose (Karam, et al., 1991).

Patients with NIDDM are likely to be older than those with IDDM and therefore to be taking medications for other medical problems. For such patients, the physician needs to consider possible adverse drug interactions and side effects when developing a therapeutic regimen. For example, beta-blockers impair glucose tolerance and also mask physiologic responses to hypoglycemia (Gearhart and Forbes, 1995).

A new drug has recently been recommended for approval by a team of advisers to the FDA. The drug, called Rezulin®, is the first to attack an underlying cause of type II diabetes. Rezulin®, known chemically as troglitazone, acts to resensitize the body to insulin. Researchers believe it stimulates a gene to produce more insulin-controlled proteins. This, in turn, removes glucose from the bloodstream, thus giving insulin more opportunity to do its job. Studies have shown that patients taking Rezulin® regularly for six months were able to reduce their daily insulin dose by approximately 58 percent.

9.57   Team Management Approach

A diagnosis of diabetes is likely to have a strong emotional impact on the patient and family, leading to denial. At the same time, the patient needs to absorb a great deal of information and adapt to life-style changes. For these reasons, optimal management requires a team approach. The team generally includes a nurse-educator, a dietitian and a social worker or psychologist, as well as the patient's family (Gearhart and Forbes, 1995; Arslanian and Drash, 1994).

Patients require individual instruction in diet, the effects of exercise, self-monitoring, the action and self-administering of insulin, hypogly-cemic drugs, the need for good hygiene of the skin, feet and teeth, how to adjust insulin dosage in the presence of infection and the need to avoid psychological stress (Karam, et al., 1991).

9.60   SURGERY FOR DIABETIC PATIENTS

Surgery involves stress, with concomitant secretion of substances, such as corticosteroids and catecholamines, that function as insulin antagonists. Thus diabetics who undergo surgery must be managed so as to avoid hyperglycemia or ketoacidosis brought on by inadequate insulin. The specifics depend on how the individual's diabetes is controlled and on the type of surgery (Karam, et al., 1991).

9.61   Diabetics Not Taking Insulin

Diabetics who control their disease by diet require no specialized management unless the surgery significantly affects blood glucose levels, in which case control can usually be re-established by taking two small doses of insulin a day. Diabetics taking oral hypoglycemics continue to take them in their usual doses and should be given carbohydrates orally or intravenously while their blood glucose is monitored. There is some risk of hypoglycemia, and if necessary, medication may be omitted before the surgery. If patients develop symptoms of hyperglycemia or ketosis, they can be given insulin (Karam, et al., 1991; Barash, et al., 1993).

9.62   Diabetics Taking Insulin

Management is more complicated for insulin-dependent diabetics. Patients undergoing minor surgery requiring only a local or regional anesthetic or a short-acting intravenous anesthetic should be given half their usual dose of insulin in the morning. Such patients should be operated on as early in the day as possible, and if there is a delay, should be given an infusion of glucose and water, with regular determinations of blood glucose levels.

For major surgery, the patient should have a snack at 9 p.m. the evening before and consume nothing orally thereafter. The next morning, instead of an injection, the patient should have an infusion of glucose in water with regular insulin added to it. This infusion may continue for several days, with blood glucose values monitored every two to four hours and the insulin dose adjusted if required. The infusion is stopped once the patient starts eating by mouth, and two hours later, the first insulin injection can be given. Rising and falling insulin needs in the first few days after surgery may necessitate multiple doses, the sizes of which are determined by blood glucose checks (Karam, et al., 1991).

9.70 ACUTE COMPLICATIONS OF DIABETES

The most common acute complications of diabetes in patients with IDDM are hypoglycemic reactions, the most severe form of which is coma. Diabetes and its treatment causes four forms of coma. In addition to hypoglycemic coma, these include two types of hyperglycemic coma (diabetic ketoacidosis and hyperosmolar, nonketotic coma) and coma due to lactic acidosis. These different types must be considered in the differential diagnosis before treatment is instituted (Arslanian and Drash, 1994; Karam, et al., 1991).

9.71 Emergency Management and Diagnosis

For any comatose patient, the first step is to establish an airway. The second is to establish intravenous access and draw a blood sample for analysis. The third is to administer a glucose solution unless monitoring reveals significant hyperglycemia. Giving glucose will reverse hypoglycemic coma but will not have a significant effect on a patient with only mild hyperglycemia. The fourth step is to administer naloxone and thiamine intravenously.

It is then possible to determine—based on the history, physical examination and laboratory studies—the cause of the coma (Karam, et al., 1991).

9.72 Diabetic Ketoacidosis

Diabetic ketoacidosis is a common complication of IDDM. Before insulin was discovered in the 1920s, diabetics usually died from it;

and even today, the mortality rate is between 5 and 10 percent. Those with IDDM are most at risk, although diabetics with NIDDM may also develop the condition under stress, as, for example during a heart attack (Lipsky, 1994).

[1] Causes

Infection is the precipitating factor in 25 to 50 percent of cases. Another important cause is failure to take insulin, either because of poor compliance or because the patient believed that she or he should not take insulin while eating little during an illness. Other causes include alcohol abuse, renal failure, trauma and certain medications, such as beta-blockers, calcium channel blockers and steroids. In 15 to 30 percent of cases, no cause can be determined (Lipsky, 1994).

[2] Clinical Features and Diagnosis

Signs and symptoms range from mild nausea to a patient being in coma. Often the condition develops over several days, with the diabetic experiencing polyuria (increased urination) and thirst, nausea and vomiting, and weakness. Severe abdominal pain is present in about a third of cases. Signs include tachycardia (rapid heart rate), dehydration, mental stupor, a fruity breath odor indicating the presence of ketones and typical rapid, deep Kussmaul respirations (Lipsky, 1994).

Urinalysis showing glycosuria and ketonuria should lead to measuring of the blood glucose level. The diagnosis is confirmed by the finding of a blood glucose level over 250 mg/dL, strong ketonuria, a low arterial blood pH (below 7.3) and a low level of plasma bicarbonate (Lipsky, 1994).

[3] Treatment

Immediate fluid and electrolyte replacement is crucial, since patients with diabetic ketoacidosis have a considerable fluid deficit. Usually therapy involves giving 1 liter of normal saline in the first hour, followed by 1 liter over the next two hours. Often, in order to avoid triggering congestive heart failure[11] or cerebral edema, especially in older patients, physicians do not give sufficient fluids. However, evidence indicates that rapid rehydration does not lead to these complications.

---

[11] *See also* ch. 8.

A second component of therapy is intravenous administration of regular human insulin, in a low dose in order to avoid hypoglycemia and hypokalemia (abnormally low level of potassium in the blood, which can occur as potassium flows back into the cells once acidosis is corrected). After the first hour, the insulin dose is adjusted according to blood glucose determinations. Insulin administration should be continued until the ketosis resolves, even if the blood glucose level drops first. To avoid hypoglycemia, some glucose is added to the infused fluid. Once the patient can eat, the serum ketones have disappeared and the glucose level is below 250 mg/dL, the infusion can be stopped and subcutaneous insulin injections resumed.

Patients recovering from diabetic ketoacidosis also require potassium replacement. Although diabetic ketoacidosis also causes phosphate deficiency, there is no evidence confirming that giving phosphate improves the outcome. However, most clinicians do administer phosphate replacement if the level is below 1.5 mg/dL. Administration of potassium phosphate can replace both potassium and phosphate at the same time.

Use of sodium bicarbonate to normalize the pH is recommended by some, although certain risks are associated with this therapy, including hypokalemia, tissue anoxia and cerebral edema. It should be stopped once the pH is above 7.1.

Additional supportive measures include antibiotic treatment for infection and supplemental oxygen (Lipsky, 1994).

9.73 Nonketotic Hyperosmolar State

Hyperosmolar coma occurs in diabetics with NIDDM when high blood glucose levels are combined with dehydration and hyperosmolarity (abnormally increased concentration of osmotically active particles). Ketosis is not present. Because hyperosmolar coma occurs most frequently in middle-aged and elderly patients who have severe illnesses, it has a mortality rate more than ten times higher than that of diabetic ketoacidosis (Karam, et al., 1991).

[1] Causes

Hyperosmolar coma is most likely to occur when the diabetic's fluid intake is insufficient because of illness or when he or she has lost large amounts of fluid. Decreased fluid volume leads to renal insufficiency, which further increases both the blood glucose level (since less glucose is being excreted in the urine) and osmolarity. Hyperosmolarity causes altered mental state and, if it is severe enough, coma (Karam, et al., 1991).

[2]   Clinical Features and Diagnosis

The onset of the hyperosmolar state may occur after several days of thirst, frequent urination and weakness. Frequently the patient has not consumed adequate fluid, often because of gastrointestinal distress or because of being elderly or bedridden with no way of obtaining water. Dry mucous membranes, orthostatic hypotension and other signs of dehydration are present, and the patient may be mentally confused.

Laboratory tests show severe hyperglycemia and high serum sodium levels. Since signs of ketoacidosis are not present, there may be a delay in diagnosis, so the patient's condition may be more severe than in diabetic ketoacidosis (Karam, et al., 1991).

[3]   Treatment

The most important treatment measure is fluid replacement. The patient may need 4 to 7 liters of fluid over eight to ten hours. Blood pressure, urine output and pulse should be monitored. Hypotonic saline (which causes a flow of water into the tissue cells) is given initially unless the patient is suffering circulatory collapse, although as plasma glucose and serum osmolarity decrease, it may be necessary to switch to isotonic saline (which causes no flow of water into the cells) in order to maintain the blood pressure. Potassium and sometimes phosphate replacement are also required.

Fluid replacement reduces blood glucose levels significantly in these patients, but some regular insulin is also needed. Patients who have severe co-existing medical problems may need continuous intravenous infusion of insulin.

Finally, it is important to determine what event triggered the condition, if this has not already been established. Unrecognized myocardial infarction [12] and occult infection are two possibilities. The patient should also be taught how to recognize circumstances, such as infection, that make recurrences likely and how to prevent dehydration from becoming severe (Karam, et al., 1991).

---

[12] *See also* ch. 7.

9.74   Hypoglycemia

Hypoglycemia is a common, important complication of IDDM. An insulin-dependent diabetic taking two injections a day for 30 years can expect to have about 1,482 hypoglycemic episodes that are amenable to self-treatment and 6 serious episodes that cause a seizure or coma or require treatment with intravenous glucose or glucagon (Santiago, et al., 1994). Hypoglycemic reactions can also occur in type II diabetics who take oral hypoglycemic drugs, especially those who are elderly or have renal or hepatic impairment. A deep hypoglycemic coma can result in permanent neurologic impairment or even death (Karam, et al., 1991).

[1]   Causes

There are four common causes of hypoglycemia. The first is excess insulin. Even when the diabetic adheres to his or her insulin regimen, the rate of insulin absorption from the skin is subject to unpredictable increases that alter the balance between blood glucose and insulin. A diabetic who takes the same amount of insulin every day can expect to experience a peak effect comparable to that of a higher dose about twice a month. Other causes of insulin excess are lowered insulin resistance occurring after an infection and greater insulin sensitivity, which can occur after exercise. Differences in commercial insulin formulas can also affect absorption.

The second common cause of hypoglycemia is a delayed, missed or irregularly absorbed meal that leaves the body without adequate glucose to balance the high level of insulin that the patient's regimen creates after mealtimes. The third cause is exercise, which increases glucose utilization. Patients need to know how much and what type of carbohydrate they require to balance a given type and amount of exercise. This requirement can also vary according to the time of day.

Fourth, alcohol consumption causes hypoglycemia, in two ways. It interferes with gluconeogenesis,[13] which is important for maintaining blood glucose levels when no food has been eaten, and it can mask awareness of early hypoglycemic symptoms (Santiago, et al., 1994).

[2]   Risk Factors

There are also a number of risk factors for hypoglycemia. A major one is failure by the patient to follow his or her treatment plan and

---

[13] *See* 9.21 *supra.*

to make appropriate daily adjustments, either from carelessness or due to lack of training. It must be noted, however, that even highly motivated diabetics who follow their treatment plan rigorously are subject to unexpected, uncontrollable factors that cause severe hypoglycemic episodes. As one group of investigators comments, "The main reason for increased hypoglycemia during intensive treatment of IDDM is not . . . problems with patient adherence but limitations of current forms of treatment" (Santiago, et al., 1994).

Another risk factor is the attempt by a patient or health care practitioner to maintain tight control to an unrealistic degree. Many patients are unable, even with multiple injections and frequent monitoring, to maintain normal blood glucose levels without risking hypoglycemia.

A third risk factor is longer duration of diabetes, which makes hypoglycemia more likely in several ways. Over time, the body loses its ability to secrete endogenous insulin and becomes more dependent on injected insulin. The body also loses its ability to release glucagon when there is hypoglycemia. What is more, the body becomes unable to secrete epinephrine, which compensates for the lack of glucagon in responding to hypoglycemia. Finally, patients who over a long period have not had severe hypoglycemic episodes develop false confidence and begin to take risks.

A fourth risk factor is what is called hypoglycemia unawareness. Some patients lose the ability to recognize the warning symptoms of hypoglycemia before it becomes so severe that they are unable to treat themselves or get assistance. More often, the symptoms of hypoglycemia change over time or become less noticeable.

Fifth, the risk of hypoglycemia is greater at night. More than half of episodes of severe hypoglycemia occur at night or in the early morning. One reason for this is that 20 to 30 percent less insulin is needed to maintain a normal level of blood glucose during the predawn period than at dawn. Further, patients are generally not awakened by nocturnal hypoglycemia, which means they cannot take measures to treat it. Also, attempts to decrease early morning hyperglycemia (the dawn phenomenon[14]) by adjusting the evening dose of insulin may cause hypoglycemia.

---

[14] *See* 9.53[2][b] *supra.*

Finally, one episode of severe hypoglycemia increases the risk of another, since it diminishes the hormonal response to hypoglycemia and adds to hypoglycemic unawareness (Santiago, et al., 1994).

[3]   Clinical Features

Hypoglycemia can be defined as a blood glucose level below 50 mg/dL or, clinically, in terms of signs and symptoms. In mild hypoglycemia, the diabetic has symptoms of autonomic nervous system hyperactivity: perspiration, tachycardia (rapid heartbeat), shakiness and palpitations. Moderate hypoglycemia involves symptoms due to insufficient glucose supply to the central nervous system, such as confusion, blurred vision, impaired concentration and poor coordination. Patients in these two categories can treat themselves for the condition. In severe hypoglycemia, function is so impaired that the patient requires assistance, manifesting seizure, profound disorientation, bizarre behavior, stupor and possibly loss of consciousness (Santiago, et al., 1994).

[4]   Treatment

Hypoglycemia is relieved by administration of glucose. Patients who are conscious can treat themselves by consuming candy, orange juice or some other sugar-containing food. Glucose tablets are also available. Diabetic patients should always carry some such food with them. Unconscious patients must be treated by others. The family and friends of diabetics should have access to a glucagon emergency kit containing the materials necessary to give an injection of glucagon. If no glucagon is available, glucose gel, honey or syrup can be rubbed into the mucous membranes between the cheek and gums. Once the patient is conscious, she or he consumes some type of sugar orally (Karam, et al., 1991).

Patients whose hypoglycemia was due to taking an oral hypoglycemic drug need to be hospitalized and given intravenous glucose with monitoring of blood glucose levels (Karam, et al., 1991).

9.75   Lactic Acidosis

Lactic acid is the final product of anaerobic (without oxygen) metabolism of glucose. Lactic acidosis occurs when the body either produces too much lactic acid due to tissue hypoxia (insufficient oxygen) or is unable to excrete it due to liver failure. In cases involving circulatory collapse, both causes operate together. Patients who develop lactic acidosis usually have serious illnesses, such as pulmonary or liver disease and myocardial infarction.

Most often, the patient with lactic acidosis hyperventilates and manifests confusion that may develop into coma. Management involves first establishing an adequate airway and sufficient oxygenation of the tissues, then treatment of the underlying cause (Karam, et al., 1991).

9.80 CHRONIC COMPLICATIONS

Diabetic patients develop a number of chronic illnesses over the course of the disease. Most of these involve the vascular system, but the kidneys, nerves, skin and lens of the eye are also affected. Although type I and type II patients can have the same complications, microvascular complications are less prevalent and less severe in type II patients. For them, macrovascular disease is the most prevalent complication, possibly because of the later onset of diabetes in this group (Fore, 1995).

9.81 Results of the Diabetes Control and Complications Trial (DCCT)

The Diabetes Control and Complications Trial (DCCT) showed that intensive management delayed or prevented the microvascular complications of diabetes—neuropathy, nephropathy and retinopathy—but made no significant change in macrovascular complications. Although the DCCT studied only IDDM patients, the American Diabetes Association and the American Association of Clinical Endocrinologists have recommended that the same level of tight control be applied to the management of NIDDM. This involves maintaining an average glucose level of 150 mg/dL or a hemoglobin A_{1c} level of 7 to 8 percent. In type II patients, macrovascular and microvascular disease can exist before diabetes is diagnosed and thereby go untreated for a considerable period, eventually resulting in a poor outcome (Fore, 1995).

9.82 Diabetic Vascular Disease

Vascular complications of diabetes are categorized as microvascular and macrovascular.

[1]   Microvascular Disease

Disease of the capillaries and precapillary arterioles manifests primarily as thickening of the capillary basement membrane (single-layered connective-tissue membrane). In the eye, microvascular disease results in diabetic retinopathy;[15] in the kidney, it causes diabetic nephropathy.[16] Microvascular disease has also been found in the heart in some diabetics whose coronary arteries were not blocked (Karam, et al., 1991).

[2]   Macrovascular Disease

More common (and the most frequent complication of NIDDM) is large-vessel atherosclerosis (hardening of vessel walls, with formation of fatty plaques) involving the coronary, cerebral and large peripheral arteries of the legs. Atherosclerosis of the coronary arteries (which supply blood to the heart muscle) causes myocardial infarction, the major cause of death in patients with NIDDM. In diabetics, atherosclerosis tends to appear earlier and progress more rapidly than in the general population. The result is reduction of blood flow to the organs supplied by the affected vessels. In addition to heart attack, this leads to stroke and, in the legs and feet, lower resistance to infection and delayed wound healing, which may cause gangrene.

Often, macrovascular disease manifests clinically as delayed wound healing or gangrene before the patient has been diagnosed as diabetic, since the narrowed vessels may be able to provide sufficient circulation until an infection or injury increases the requirement for blood. What is more, diabetics may have atherosclerosis even when laboratory tests for lipids in the blood are normal. Consequently it is essential to detect the earliest indications of complications and to treat diabetes aggressively.

The results of the DCCT suggested that keeping the glucose level below 150 mg/dL may reduce macrovascular disease in type I diabetics. Levels of hemoglobin A_{1c} are used to indicate the tightness of glucose control needed to prevent complications; thus a patient whose hemoglobin A_{1c} is 10 percent or above requires more intensive control.

Currently there is no evidence that insulin or oral hypoglycemic drugs can decrease the prevalence or the progression of atherosclerosis

---

[15]   *See* 9.86 *infra.*

[16]   *See* 9.83 *infra.*

in type II patients. Nevertheless, it is prudent to implement a prevention strategy of controlling hypertension and lowering blood cholesterol through diet, exercise and blood glucose control. If these measures are unsuccessful, the patient is given cholesterol-lowering drugs such as gemfibrozil, lovastatin, pravastatin and simvastatin (Fore, 1995).

9.83 Renal Complications

Kidney failure caused by capillary basement membrane thickening in the renal glomeruli (microscopic clusters of vessels in the kidney that produce urine) is the major cause of death among diabetics with IDDM (Karam, et al., 1991). The vascular pathology results in intercapillary glomerulosclerosis, a fibrosis (overgrowth) of the glomeruli that reduces the filtration rate. Diabetics are at high risk for hypertension, which, by increasing pressure on vessel walls, can exacerbate renal disease.

The initial manifestation of diabetic renal disease is proteinuria, which over about five years generally progresses to uremia (presence in the blood of waste products normally excreted by the kidneys) and renal failure (Karam, et al., 1991). Between 25 and 30 percent of patients receiving some form of kidney replacement therapy are diabetics; half of these have NIDDM, half IDDM (Fore, 1995).

The DCCT demonstrated that tight control of blood glucose levels can decrease the onset and progression of proteinuria in type I patients. Studies of patients with NIDDM have been unable to confirm a relationship between glycemic control and proteinuria. The presence of microalbuminuria has not reliably predicted renal failure. However, for the sake of prevention, microalbumin in the urine should be assessed in both groups of patients. If it is elevated over 30 mg per day or 20 (some say 30) grams per minute (g/min), the patient requires tight control plus a low-protein diet. Antihypertensive drugs, particularly angiotensin converting enzyme (ACE) inhibitors, also decrease proteinuria. However, beta-blockers and thiazide diuretics should be avoided, since these drugs increase blood lipid levels. Patients should be educated about the importance of discontinuing tobacco use in order to reduce hypertension (Fore, 1995).

Diabetic kidney disease may also be caused by renal artery atherosclerosis and by infection. Due to diabetic neuropathy that impairs bladder emptying, diabetics are more susceptible to bladder infections that can ascend to the kidneys.

Hemodialysis has not been particularly successful in treating diabetic kidney failure, since macrovascular disease is likely to progress to stroke, myocardial infarction and death. Ambulatory dialysis may be more useful. For some patients, renal transplantation[17] is the best solution (Karam, et al., 1991).

9.84 Neurologic Complications

Another common complication of diabetes is neuropathy, which may involve peripheral and autonomic nerves. The etiology is poorly understood, but is thought to involve both abnormal metabolism in the nerves and ischemia (lack of oxygen supply) due to microvascular disease (Fore, 1995).

[1] Peripheral Neuropathy

About half of diabetics are affected by peripheral neuropathy 25 to 30 years following diagnosis. This complication causes some of the most distressing disabilities associated with diabetes. Peripheral neuropathies are classified as symmetric and asymmetric (Swenson, 1994).

[a] Symmetric Syndromes

Symmetric neuropathies affecting several sensory nerves on both sides of the body are the most common type of nerve disorder. The diabetic individual experiences sensory loss, with variable degrees of pain in the extremities. Paresthesias (abnormal sensations) such as tingling or itching precede a diminished sense of touch, temperature and vibration, absent reflexes and severe burning pain, mostly in the feet but also in the hands. Symptoms are made worse by hypertension and smoking (Fore, 1995; Swenson, 1994).

Diabetic amyotrophy is a motor neuropathy that involves bilateral pain and weakness of the thigh muscles, with wasting and weight loss. It occurs mostly in elderly men. Motor function returns in a period ranging from weeks to months (Karam, et al., 1991).

[b] Asymmetric Syndromes

Asymmetric neuropathies affecting one or more isolated peripheral nerves in the trunk or extremities are also common. The cranial nerves most often develop isolated dysfunction, resulting in palsies such as

---

[17] *See* 9.55[5] *supra.*

lid droop or facial paralysis. Diabetics are more susceptible to entrapment syndromes, such as carpal tunnel syndrome. Also commonly affected are the femoral nerve, radial nerve (causing wrist drop) and peroneal nerve (causing foot drop). These asymmetric neuropathies usually recover in a few weeks to a year and a half or more (Swenson, 1994; Fore, 1995; Karam 1991).

[c] Treatment of Peripheral Neuropathy

Better blood glucose control serves as both prevention and cure for diabetic neuropathy. Pain is reduced and clinical signs improve if blood glucose level remains close to normal over a number of months. Clinical trials are underway of drugs that show promise of restoring function by manipulating nerve metabolism. In the meantime, patients with peripheral nerve disease are generally advised to take vitamin supplements, although there is no conclusive evidence that they are effective.

Symptomatic treatment of pain from symmetric syndromes may include aspirin and other nonsteroidal anti-inflammatory drugs, tricyclics, carbamazepine, phenothiazines and infusion of lidocaine. Carbamazepine use is limited by its side effects and must be administered with caution. Phenytoin interferes with insulin secretion but has been used for intractable pain. Transcutaneous electrical nerve stimulation (TENS), acupuncture and biofeedback may also be of benefit.

Asymmetric neuropathies are treated by splinting or bracing, physical therapy and sometimes surgical release of an entrapped nerve, although since diabetics are susceptible to delayed wound healing and infection, such a procedure requires a specially trained neurosurgeon (Swenson, 1994).

[2] Autonomic Neuropathy

Neuropathy affecting the autonomic system is usually associated with peripheral neuropathy. Autonomic neuropathy can affect a wide variety of functions, resulting in postural hypotension with fainting; heart rate abnormalities; gastrointestinal disorders including diarrhea, constipation and gastroparesis (stomach paralysis) with nausea, vomiting and bloating; urologic disorders including impotence, urinary incontinence and incomplete bladder emptying; hypoglycemic unawareness due to absence of response to adrenaline; and dysfunction of the sweat glands.

Treatment depends on the symptoms. Thus postural hypotension is treated with elastic stockings and leg elevation; gastroparesis with metoclopramide, an antiemetic, or bethanechol, which has anticholinergic effects; diarrhea with bulking agents or tetracycline; and impotence with penile implants (Swenson, 1994).

9.85   Foot Problems

Foot problems, a potentially serious complication of diabetes, affect 15 percent of diabetics, who have a 15 to 40 times greater risk of amputation than nondiabetics. Diabetics also have an increased risk of surgical complications and mortality: Half die within three years of amputation (Shenaq, et al., 1994). Since foot ulcers can progress to gangrene with a need to amputate, it is imperative to prevent and treat foot injury.

[1]   Etiology

Foot ulcers are caused by a combination of atherosclerosis of the peripheral arteries (which results in insufficient blood supply to the lower extremities), microvascular disease, peripheral neuropathy causing loss of sensation in the feet, and diminished cellular immune response. Together, these factors make the diabetic more susceptible to infection (Shenaq, et al., 1994). Further, because of diminished sensation, the diabetic may not notice blisters or small sores and may continue to walk on them, preventing them from healing and leading to infection that does not heal because of inadequate blood supply to the feet.

[2]   Prevention

Prevention of foot ulcers requires both avoiding injury and early detection of any injury that does occur. The patient must be educated in standard measures to prevent and avoid exacerbation of foot ulcers. These involve, first, preventing infection through tight blood glucose control, frequent examination of the feet and daily hygiene. Patients are given detailed instructions regarding inspection, washing in lukewarm water, using moisturizers and avoiding applying chemical products to the feet.

A second group of measures is intended to avoid pressure that can cause sores. These involve choosing shoes properly, using insoles that distribute pressure evenly, managing nail growth and not walking barefoot. Third are measures to reduce arterial insufficiency: reducing lipid levels,[18] controlling hypertension with drugs, life-style changes such as quitting smoking, and relieving claudication (leg pain causing lameness) with pentoxifylline, a drug that also enhances microcirculation. Sometimes vascular bypass surgery is indicated.

Another important measure is evaluation of the feet by the physician, who should examine each foot in detail. Ischemia is indicated by chalky-white skin color with red-purple mottling in areas of sluggish circulation and by atrophy of the skin, which becomes thin, shiny and hairless. Neuropathy is manifested by loss of sensation, claw toe due to motor nerve degeneration, and diminished or absent reflexes. Most foot lesions are mixed, caused by both ischemia and neuropathy (Shenaq, et al., 1994).

[3] Treatment

Skin ulcers that extend only into the tendon and/or joint capsule can be treated on an outpatient basis. The ulcer is debrided, calluses are trimmed, and the wound is irrigated and dressed. If there are signs of infection, the patient is given oral antibiotics. The patient needs to use crutches or a walker, along with periods of bed rest, to allow the ulcers to heal.

Ulcers that penetrate bone or are moderately or severely infected are treated in the hospital with intravenous antibiotics. High doses are necessary because of poor circulation in the foot. At the same time, an attempt is made to regain tight blood glucose control by switching to regular insulin. Thorough debridement is required, sometimes repeatedly. Special dressing systems have been developed to accelerate wound healing. Other adjunctive measures to facilitate healing include treatment with growth factors, electrical nerve stimulation and collagen, and various surgical techniques such as grafting and surgical flaps.

When deep ulcers fail to heal, revascularization by bypass surgery or angioplasty can effectively promote healing. If all measures fail, amputation is necessary. If possible, a below-knee procedure is performed, since the patient will have an easier time walking with a prosthesis. Forty percent of these patients need a second amputation within five years (Shenaq, et al., 1994).

---

[18] See 9.82[2] supra.

9.86   Ocular Complications

Diabetics are at greater risk of both retinal pathology and cataracts.

[1]   Diabetic Retinopathy

Diabetes is the major cause of new blindness in people between the ages of 20 and 74 in the United States (Fore, 1995). The first stage is nonproliferative (also called "background") retinopathy, involving weakness of the walls of the retinal capillaries, which develop microaneurysms, hemorrhages and edema. Leakage of proteins, lipids or red cells into the retina results in vision loss when the macula (point of clearest vision in the center of the retina) is affected.

In the next stage, proliferative retinopathy, occlusion of capillaries results in retinal hypoxia (deficient oxygenation), which leads to growth of new capillaries and fibrous tissue into the retina and vitreous. Blindness results from retinal detachment or vitreous hemorrhage (Karam, et al., 1991). Neovascularization, by interfering with the drainage of aqueous humor, can also lead to glaucoma.[19]

Among IDDM patients, 90 percent have nonproliferative retinopathy and 40 percent have proliferative retinopathy. By contrast, 80 percent of NIDDM patients develop nonproliferative retinopathy after 30 years and only about 25 percent have proliferative retinopathy. NIDDM patients also have a lower risk of blindness (Fore, 1995).

The DCCT[20] showed that good glucose control as reflected in a reduction in glycosylated hemoglobin levels is associated with decreased risk of diabetic retinopathy. Patients should have annual examinations by an ophthalmologist to detect abnormalities as early as possible. Since high blood pressure is associated with more severe retinopathy, control of hypertension is important.

Loss of vision is not inevitable in diabetic patients. Those whose blood glucose is maintained at a mean level of 150 mg/dL, with early diagnosis and treatment, can reduce the risk of blindness from proliferative diabetic retinopathy to under 5 percent in five years (Fore, 1995).

---

[19] *See also* ch. 10 for a discussion of glaucoma.

[20] *See* 9.81 *supra.*

[2]   Cataracts

Diabetics are susceptible to two types of cataracts.[21] Subcapsular cataract appears mostly in patients with IDDM. It develops just underneath the capsule as flocculated (flaking) opacities. This type can develop rapidly and is clearly related to hyperglycemia when diabetes is uncontrolled.

The second type, senile cataract, is also common in nondiabetic adults but is likely to appear in diabetics at a younger age. In this type, the opacification begins at the center of the lens and gradually extends toward the periphery (Karam, et al., 1991).

9.87   Skin Problems

Poor circulation and the resulting inadequate flow of nutrients to the skin result in skin changes. Atrophy of the skin manifests as brown patches, usually on the fronts of the legs, known as shin spots. Also appearing on the shins are the lesions of necrobiosis lipoidica diabeticorum, a rare condition characterized by shiny plaques with yellow centers and red borders.

When diabetes is poorly controlled and triglyceride levels in the blood are high, eruptive xanthomas may develop. These are clusters of small yellow papules that appear all over the body (Karam, et al., 1991).

The skin of diabetics may be dry and itchy, and individuals are particularly susceptible to various infections (boils, carbuncles, fungal and yeast infections).

9.88   Joint Complications

Patients who have had diabetes for many years are subject to complications affecting the joints. Cheirarthropathy, or joint disease affecting the hand, is a syndrome that may manifest five to six years after the onset of IDDM. It is thought to be caused by glycosylation of collagen and possibly other connective tissue proteins. The hand becomes progressively stiffer as a result of contracture and tightening of the skin over the joints, and the affected person cannot flatten the hand on a flat surface.

Diabetics have an increased incidence of bursitis, especially of the hips and shoulders, and of gout (Karam, et al., 1991).

---

[21] *See also* ch. 11 for a discussion of cataracts.

9.90 PROGNOSIS

Patients who pass the 20-year mark of diabetes without severe microvascular complications have a good chance of continuing in relatively good health. Current methods of preventing or delaying the progression of complications have improved the outlook. A good outcome, however, continues to depend heavily on the patient's own motivation, cooperation in treatment and life-style changes (Karam, et al., 1991).

9.100 AMA EVALUATION OF PERMANENT IMPAIRMENT

Much of the impairment caused by diabetes is related to the complications of the disease. Thus the clinician must both determine whether neuropathy, retinopathy and other complications are present and assess the other body systems affected by the complications. In the American Medical Association scheme for evaluating permanent impairment due to diabetes mellitus, the degree of impairment of these other systems is expressed as a percentage of impairment of the whole person and then combined with a percentage of impairment caused by poor glucose control.

The criteria for evaluating impairment due to diabetes are categorized into four classes of impairment of the whole person (American Medical Association, 1993).

9.101 Class 1: 0 to 5 Percent Impairment

A person with NIDDM controlled by diet, and who may or may not have microvascular disease as indicated by retinopathy or microalbuminuria over 30 mg/dL, is deemed to have class 1 impairment. For example, an obese woman of 45 had an elevated fasting plasma glucose level on a first examination and signs of retinopathy 14 months later, but no visual impairment. She was judged to have 5 percent total impairment.

9.102 Class 2: 5 to 10 Percent Impairment

Patients with a diagnosis of NIDDM who require both a restricted diet and either an oral hypoglycemic drug or insulin to control blood glucose values are deemed to be in Class 2. They may or may not have retinopathy or albuminuria indicating microvascular disease.

A 55-year-old man who had indications of NIDDM for several years had no signs of retinopathy or albuminuria. He lost weight on a diet but required an oral hypoglycemic, which controlled his blood glucose level reasonably well. He was considered to have 5 percent impairment.

9.103   Class 3: 10 to 20 Percent Impairment

Patients who have IDDM with or without signs of microvascular disease are deemed to be in Class 3.

A 45-year-old man who had had IDDM for 25 years had proliferative retinopathy as well as signs of renal impairment. His blood glucose level was satisfactorily controlled by diet and two daily insulin injections, but he had visual loss in both eyes that combined for a 55 percent visual impairment. His impairment from diabetes was 20 percent. His total impairment would be a combination of these totals with an estimate of urinary system impairment.

9.104   Class 4: 20 to 40 Percent Impairment

Patients with IDDM who experience hypoglycemia or hyperglycemia frequently despite ongoing attempts by them and their physicians to control blood glucose levels are considered to be in Class 4.

9.200   BIBLIOGRAPHY

Text References

American Medical Association: Guides to the Evaluation of Permanent Impairment, 4th ed. Chicago: American Medical Association, 1993.

Arslanian, S. and Drash, A. L.: Insulin-Dependent Diabetes Mellitus in Children and Adolescents. In: Bardin, C.W. (Ed.): Current Therapy in Endocrinology and Metabolism, 5th ed. St. Louis: Mosby, 1994.

Barash, P. G., et al.: Handbook of Clinical Anesthesia, 2d ed. Philadelphia: Lippincott, 1993.

Bogardus, C.: Agonist: The Case for Insulin Resistance as a Necessary and Sufficient Cause of Type II Diabetes Mellitus. J. Lab. Clin. Med. 125(5):556-558, May 1995.

Dinsmoor, R. S.: Lifting the Sugar Embargo. Harvard Health Letter 19(12):7-8, Oct.. 1994.

Fore, W. W.: Noninsulin-Dependent Diabetes Mellitus: The Prevention of Complications. Med. Clin. North Am. 79(2):287-298, Mar. 1995.

Gearhart, J. G. and Forbes, R. C.: Initial Management of the Patient with Newly Diagnosed Diabetes. Am. Fam. Physician 51(8):1953, June 1995.

Guthrie, D. W. and Guthrie, R. A.: Nursing Management of Diabetes Mellitus, 3d ed. New York: Springer Publishing, 1991.

Hollander, P.: Intensified Insulin Regimens. Should They Be Used in All Patients with Type I Diabetes? Postgrad. Med. 96(3):63, Sept. 1, 1994.

Karam, J. H., et al.: Pancreatic Hormones and Diabetes Mellitus. In: Greenspan, F. S. (Ed.): Basic and Clinical Endocrinology, 3d. ed. Norwalk, Conn.: Appleton & Lange, 1991.

Kitzmiller, J. L.: Diabetes Mellitus and Pregnancy. In: Greenspan, F.S. (Ed.): Basic and Clinical Endocrinology, 3d. ed. Norwalk, Conn.: Appleton & Lange, 1991.

Kolaczynski, J. W. and Caro, J. F.: Insulin-Like Growth Factor-1 Therapy in Diabetes: Physiologic Basis, Clinical Benefits, and Risks. Ann. Intern. Med. 120(1):47-55, Jan. 1, 1994.

Larsen, J. L., et al.: Pancreas Transplantation for Type I Diabetes Mellitus. Do the Benefits Offset the Risks and Cost? Postgrad. Med. 96(3):105-111, Sept. 1, 1994.

Lee, C. A. B.: Physiology of Glucose Metabolism. In: Guthrie, D.W., and Guthrie, R.A.: Nursing Management of Diabetes Mellitus, 3d ed. New York: Springer Publishing, 1991.

Leslie, R. D. and Elliot, R. B.: Early Environmental Events as a Cause of IDDM: Evidence and Implications. Diabetes 43(7):843-850, July 1994.

Lipsky, M. S.: Management of Diabetic Ketoacidosis. Am. Fam. Physician 49(7):1607-1612, May 15, 1994.

Newgard, C. B.: Cellular Engineering and Gene Therapy Strategies for Insulin Replacement in Diabetes. Diabetes 43(3):341-350, Mar. 1994.

Quinn, S.: Diabetes and Diet: We Are Still Learning. Med. Clin. North Am. 77(4):773-782, July 1993.

Remuzzi, G., et al.: Pancreas and Kidney/Pancreas Transplants: Experimental Medicine or Real Improvement? Lancet 343(8888):27-31, Jan. 1, 1994.

Santiago, J. V., et al.: Definitions, Causes, and Risk Factors for Hypoglycemia in Insulin-Dependent Diabetes. In: Bardin, C. W. (Ed.): Current Therapy in Endocrinology and Metabolism, 5th ed. St. Louis: Mosby, 1994.

Shenaq, S. M., et al.: How to Help Diabetic Patients Avoid Amputation: Prevention and Management of Foot Ulcers. Postgrad. Med. 96(5):177, Oct. 1994.

Swenson, M. S.: Diabetic Peripheral Neuropathy. In: Bardin, C. W. (Ed.): Current Therapy in Endocrinology and Metabolism, 5th ed. St. Louis: Mosby, 1994.

CHAPTER 10

GLAUCOMA

<table>
<tr><td>

SCOPE

Glaucoma is a syndrome including different forms of illness with different causes, treatments and outcomes. It is best detected by examination of the optic disk. Primary open-angle glaucoma is the most common form. Secondary open-angle glaucoma may arise from causes such as trauma, hemorrhage within the eye, uveitis, exfoliation syndrome, pigment dispersion syndrome and use of corticosteroids. Open-angle glaucoma is often not detected until the disease is advanced, while angle-closure glaucoma has a sudden onset with alarming rises in intraocular pressure. Important diagnostic tests include ophthalmoscopy, tonometry, gonioscopy and perimetry.

</td></tr>
</table>

SYNOPSIS

10.00   INTRODUCTION

Glaucoma is not one disease but many. It is a syndrome including different forms of illness with different causes, treatments and outcomes. What all these conditions have in common is increased pressure within the eyeball that causes optic nerve damage and defects in the field of vision.

The eye with glaucoma can be compared to an overinflated basketball, in which the air in the ball exerts equal pressure on its entire interior surface. Similarly, elevated pressure in the eye strains every structure within the globe. If the condition is left untreated, the excessive pressure can exert enough force on the retina and optic nerve and on their blood supply to destroy both the neural pathways to the optic nerve and the nerve itself.

Although ophthalmologists treat active cases of glaucoma, primary care physicians play an important role in controlling the disease through early diagnosis and referral. The effects of glaucoma cannot be reversed, but the progress of the disease can be stopped; if glaucoma is detected early in its course, medication, surgery or a combination of treatments usually keep the disease under control and save the patient's sight.

Glaucoma is best detected by examination of the optic disk, since intraocular pressure is not always elevated in patients with the condition. Changes in the optic disk can easily be observed with an ophthalmoscope; therefore, ophthalmoscopy should be part of every patient's regular eye examination (Pederson, 1991).

10.01   Epidemiology

Primary open-angle glaucoma is the most common form and as such is a leading cause of blindness in the United States (Ghezzi and Renner, 1992). Glaucoma is particularly common among blacks and is the foremost cause of blindness for that group: in those between ages 45 and 65, glaucoma is 15 times more prevalent than in whites of the same age. Other groups with high rates of glaucoma include those from Southeast Asia, Europe and Java. Heredity plays a large role in the disease, since it occurs more frequently in patients with a family history of glaucoma. Individuals with diabetes are also at high risk for glaucoma.

10.02   Anatomy

The eye is composed of three primary layers, called tunics. The outer coat, the tunica fibrosa, is the protective layer of the eye. The middle layer, the tunica vasculosa, also called the uvea, is blood-rich and highly pigmented. The inner layer, the tunica nervosa, is composed of the sensory retina and the optic nerve. *(See Figure 10-1.)*

The outer, protective layer is composed of elastic, collagen-rich connective tissue. The cornea forms the front sixth of this layer, and the sclera, the rear five sixths. *(See Figure 10-2.)* The tissues in the cornea are arranged in a parallel pattern that gives it a geometrically regular appearance and renders the cornea transparent to incoming light. The fibers of the sclera are more random and irregular, an arrangement that renders it white and opaque to incoming light.

The middle layer lies just inside the sclera and consists of three parts: the iris, the ciliary body and the choroid. An important function of this layer is to transport blood to the eye, particularly to the outer portion of the sensory retina. The muscles of the ciliary body serve to focus the lens of the eye. Of special interest to a discussion of glaucoma, the epithelium (lining) of the ciliary body secretes aqueous humor, the fluid that fills the chambers between the lens and the cornea. Aqueous primarily drains via the canal of Schlemm. When the flow of aqueous is impaired or stopped, pressure builds up within the eye, and glaucoma results.

The inner layer of the eye is composed of the sensory retina, pigment epithelium and optic nerve. The front part of the inner lining forms the two-layered epithelia (linings) of the iris and the ciliary body. Aqueous humor is a liquid produced and discharged by the ciliary body

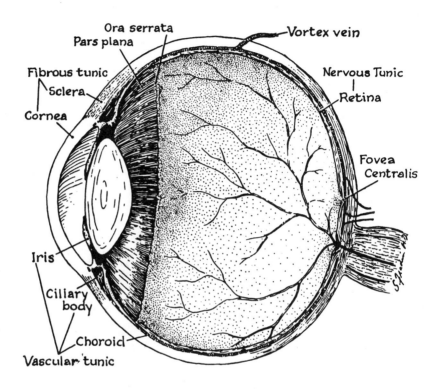

Fig. 10-1. A side view of the structures of the eyeball.

into the anterior space; the aqueous flows outward through the canal of Schlemm. The optic disk is a circular, light-colored area at the back of the retina where the optic nerve joins the eye. The center part of the globe is filled with vitreous humor.

10.03   Classification of Glaucoma

The various forms of glaucoma may be divided into three major categories: *angle-closure, open-angle* and *congenital glaucoma.* Angle-closure and open-angle glaucoma may be further subdivided as *primary* and *secondary.* Primary glaucoma is thought to develop independent of any other disorder and without a known cause, while secondary glaucoma may be traumatic, postsurgical or an aftermath of local or systemic infection, ocular tumors or a systemic disease such as diabetes.

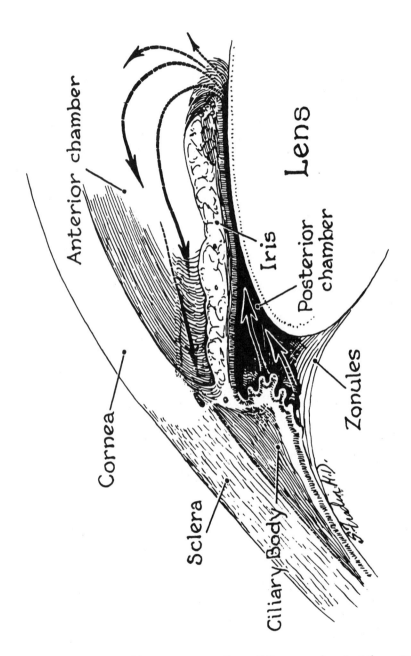

Fig. 10-2. An oblique cross section of the eye, showing the origin (in the ciliary body) and direction of flow of the aqueous humor.

10.10 PATHOPHYSIOLOGY

Glaucoma arises from an increase in intraocular pressure caused by the excessive accumulation of aqueous humor within the eye. Aqueous humor, or more simply, aqueous, is a fluid produced by the lining of the ciliary body that nourishes the cornea and the lens, and stabilizes intraocular pressure. It flows through the posterior chamber, the narrow area between the lens and the iris, and passes through the pupil into the anterior, or front, chamber. *(See Figure 10-3.)* Drainage from the anterior chamber is through the trabecular meshwork, a sievelike structure located in the anterior chamber angle recess, an area bounded by the root of the iris, the front fourth of the ciliary body and the junction of the cornea and the sclera. After passing though the spongelike tissue of the anterior chamber angle recess, aqueous then passes into the canal of Schlemm, a drainage duct located within the sclera. Intraocular pressure depends on the balance between aqueous formation and outflow. When adequate outflow of aqueous is not maintained, intraocular pressure increases, and glaucoma is the result (Apple and Rabb, 1991).

Disorders of the trabecular meshwork can inhibit or block the outflow of aqueous, as can certain eye injuries. When the iris is stripped from its roots but not completely torn, it damages the

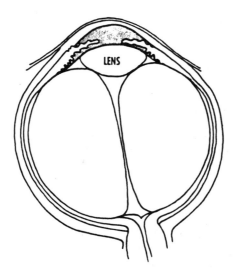

Fig. 10-3. The aqueous humor as it appears in front of the lens of the eye.

meshwork and causes angle recession, thus squeezing the meshwork into a tighter space and making normal outflow difficult or impossible. Traumatic iritis (inflammation of the iris) is a common, but difficult to diagnose, injury that results in the release of protein and inflammatory cells into the anterior angle recess. Traumatic hyphema (bleeding into the anterior chamber following blunt injury) is potentially serious and may be followed by glaucoma. Lens debris and other ocular debris can block the trabecular meshwork. Adhesions (fibrous growths) between the iris and the vitreous body when the lens is absent can also block outflow of aqueous.

10.11   Intraocular Pressure

Excessive intraocular pressure can affect eyesight by constricting the ocular nerves or by interfering with their blood supply. Intraocular pressure is measured in terms of millimeters of mercury (mm Hg) over and above the atmospheric pressure. The "normal" range of pressure is quite large—10 mm Hg to 21 mm Hg (Pederson, 1991)—with the majority of subjects testing in the mid-range of 16 to 18 mm Hg. However, the eye is far more capable of withstanding pressure on the low end of normal. When intraocular pressure is high, there is a significant risk of constricted blood vessels within the eye, a condition that can lead to damage resulting from inadequate blood circulation. Thus any intraocular pressure higher than 22 mm Hg is cause for concern and should alert the clinician to the need for further tests for the diagnosis of glaucoma.

10.12   The Cupped Disk

The normal optic disk is a light-colored area at the back of the retina where the optic nerve enters the eyeball. It is rounded in shape and slightly oval vertically. The central area may contain a shallow depression—the cup—that appears lighter than the surrounding area, which is usually a pink color. The cup-disk ratio compares the diameter of the cup to the diameter of the entire optic nerve head. A cup-disk ratio of 0.2 to 0.4 is considered normal; 0.5 to 0.6, borderline; and 0.7 or greater, abnormal (Pederson, 1991).

Optic nerve cupping in glaucoma is a result of loss of nerve fibers, which causes an increase in the size of the cup (Newell, 1992). This loss of nerve fibers takes place when blood flow to the head of the optic nerve is impaired, which usually occurs when intraocular pressure is elevated. Intraocular pressure often produces precise areas of infarction (death) of the optic nerve head, resulting in vision loss in some parts of the visual spectrum but not in others.

In glaucoma, the first areas most commonly interrupted lie in the peripheral visual field. This may eventually lead to a classic symptom of glaucoma, tunnel vision, in which a patient's straight-ahead vision is apparently normal, but peripheral vision gradually diminishes. The progress of glaucoma is often slow, and the gradual narrowing of a patient's field of vision may be almost unnoticeable until the disease has substantially destroyed the visual field. For screening purposes, the best early indicator of the presence of glaucoma is optic nerve cupping, the detection of which requires no special equipment other than an ophthalmoscope (Pederson, 1991).

10.20 DIAGNOSIS OF GLAUCOMA

The signs and symptoms of glaucoma depend upon its etiology. Open-angle glaucoma, the most common form of the disorder, is often not detected until the disease is advanced, while angle-closure glaucoma has a sudden onset with alarming rises in intraocular pressure. Diagnosis of all the glaucomas rests on a careful history followed by a combination of examination methods and laboratory tests.

Several tests are of particular importance in the diagnosis of glaucoma: (1) ophthalmoscopy—evaluation of the optic cup and the rim of the optic disk; (2) tonometry—measurement of ocular tension; (3) gonioscopy—observation of the anterior chamber angle; and (4) perimetry—measurement of visual function in the central field of vision.

Visual field defects may be caused by a number of conditions other than glaucoma that must be considered in the differential diagnosis of glaucoma. Furthermore, the following variations on the diagnostic procedure must be taken into account: constriction of the pupil, which may exaggerate visual defects; refractive errors during perimetric examination, which must be corrected for an accurate reading; aging in the patient, as well as the patient's alertness and cooperation; and, very importantly, the skill of the examiner. All these factors influence the accuracy of glaucoma testing.

10.21 Ophthalmoscopy

Ophthalmoscopy is the examination of the interior of the eye with an instrument, which may be done either with a direct ophthalmoscope—a biomicroscope combined with a contact lens—or with a +90 diopter field lens (Newell, 1992). The ophthalmoscope consists of three parts: a concave mirror with a hole in the middle through which the observer examines the eye, a source of light that is reflected into the eye by the mirror, and lenses that can be manipulated to make clear the image of the fundus (the part of the eye opposite the pupil). *(See Figure 10-4.)*

The nerve fiber of the retina may be seen with a direct ophthalmoscope using a bright illumination and a red-free (green) filter to enhance its appearance. The nerve fiber becomes progressively more difficult to see with aging and lighter pigmentation. Progressive changes in the optic disk caused by glaucoma are difficult to evaluate, since they may be very subtle. Color stereophotographs taken over a period of time permit serial evaluation and take some of the guesswork out of the diagnosis of optic disk cupping.

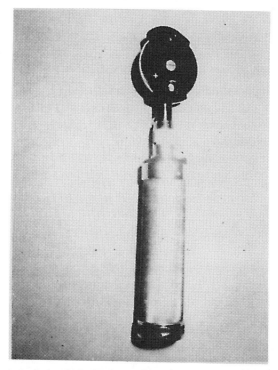

Fig. 10-4. The ophthalmoscope contains rotating lenses to facilitate examination of the patient's eye.

10.22   Tonometry

Tonometry is the measurement of intraocular pressure, in which a tonometer is pressed directly on the eye to measure its degree of resistance. The intraocular pressure is then estimated by measuring the force required either to flatten a standard area (3.6 mm in diameter) of the cornea or to indent the cornea.

The international standard instrument is the Goldmann applanation tonometer, which measures the force required to flatten a standard circle in the cornea. In applanation tonometry, the patient's cornea is anesthetized and injected with a fluorescent dye. The corneal circle is observed through a biomicroscope to which the tonometer is attached. This test is generally accurate, but it is difficult to use in patients with scarred corneas.

The Schiotz tonometer measures the ease with which the cornea may be indented by the plunger of the instrument. *(See Figure 10-5.)* A soft eye is easily indented, indicating low pressure. A hard eye is less easily indented, indicating high pressure. Indentation tonometry is adversely affected by more factors than is the method of applanation tonometry, but it is easier to use and less expensive than the Goldmann applanation tonometer. The Schiotz tonometer is sometimes given to patients for home use.

A third type of tonometer has been developed for use by nonmedical personnel for the screening of large numbers of people. It is a noncontact tonometer in which a jet of compressed air flattens the cornea, and the intensity of a beam of light reflected from the cornea is measured by a photocell. Anesthesia is not essential but adds accuracy when used.

10.23   Gonioscopy

Gonioscopy is the examination of the anterior chamber angle and its trabecular meshwork, which is located where the cornea meets the iris. The opaque tissues of the corneoscleral limbus (the marginal area where the cornea and the sclera overlap) make direct viewing of this region impossible. As a result, gonioscopy must be performed with a contact lens combined with either a mirror or a prism.

Gonioscopy may be direct or indirect. Direct gonioscopy uses a lens to neutralize the light refracted from the cornea; indirect gonioscopy uses a prism. Each method also uses a hand-held microscope and light

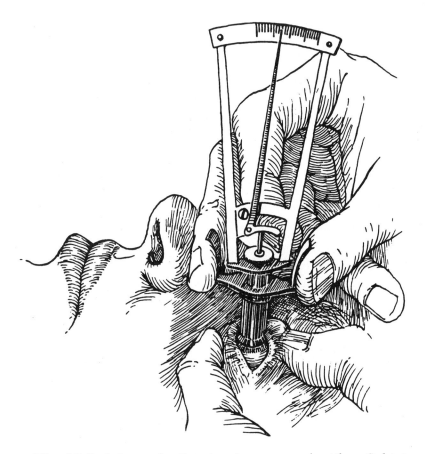

Fig. 10-5. Intraocular tension is measured with a Schiotz tonometer.

source and requires the patient to lie face upward on the examining table. Direct gonioscopy causes less distortion of angle structures and permits a view of deeper structures within a narrow chamber angle. Indirect gonioscopy provides better illumination and magnification (Newell, 1992).

Inspection of the anterior chamber angle is essential to the diagnosis of both angle-closure glaucoma and open-angle glaucoma. Diagnosis of an angle-closure mechanism can be made only when the intraocular pressure is abnormally high and the angle is observed to be closed. Gonioscopy has also been used to develop an effective surgical procedure for congenital glaucoma, and in the evaluation and treatment of many forms of glaucoma.

10.24 Perimetry

Perimetry measures visual function in the field of vision, an assessment that is then compared with the appearance of the optic disk. Used together, these measurements are helpful in diagnosing early glaucoma and in documenting the progression of the disease. In the early stages of glaucoma, visual field defects may be fleeting and seen only when intraocular pressure is abnormally high. In later stages of the disease, the changes become permanent.

Visual fields may be measured by using fixed or moving objects. When moving objects are used, the test object moves from a nonseeing area to a seeing area, and the patient signals when he or she sees the object. When fixed objects are used, a target is shown for 0.5 to 1.0 second, and the targets the patient fails to see are recorded. The fixed target may also be enhanced with an emission of light, which is increased in brightness until the patient is just able to see it. Whether perimetric testing uses fixed or moving targets, and whether or not the objects are enhanced by light, the results are mapped and compared with findings obtained with the Goldmann applanation tonometer. Many different computer-assisted perimeters are now in use, and most of these programs use fixed targets.

10.30 PRIMARY OPEN-ANGLE GLAUCOMA

Primary open-angle glaucoma is the most common of the glaucomas and a leading cause of blindness in the United States. This form of glaucoma usually occurs in both eyes, although onset of glaucoma in each eye is not necessarily simultaneous. There is usually a family history of the disorder. Primary open-angle glaucoma is inherited as an autosomal-dominant trait, that is, as a single-gene defect carried on a chromosome that is not a sex chromosome (Apple and Rabb, 1991). In a typical inheritance pattern, every affected person has at least one affected parent; an affected person marrying a normal person usually has an equal number of affected and normal children; and males and females are equally likely to be affected. The genetic trait causing primary open-angle glaucoma can appear in every generation. However, children born to normal parents will also be normal.

Primary open-angle glaucoma is characterized by two abnormalities: atrophy of the optic nerve, manifesting as a decrease in the surface area of the nerve head known as cupping; and defects in the visual field. It is thought that elevated intraocular pressure decreases blood flow to the optic nerve, which eventually leads to atrophy of the optic nerve and visual field defects, particularly in peripheral vision. According to one investigator (Newell, 1992), open-angle glaucoma occurs because of an abnormality in the aqueous outflow system between the anterior chamber and the canal of Schlemm. The trabecular meshwork in affected individuals becomes sclerotic (densely fibrous), obliterating the pores of the meshwork and making normal drainage of aqueous humor difficult or impossible. However, many types of glaucoma create the same picture, making that description alone nonspecific for open-angle glaucoma. There are varying degrees of severity, and undoubtedly many people have mild forms of the disease without knowing it.

10.31   Signs and Symptoms

Open-angle glaucoma is almost completely without signs and symptoms. The disorder tends to become more evident in patients over the age of 35, and it is found equally in both sexes. It is a disease with a chronic, insidious course; many patients never have visual symptoms. The intraocular pressure slowly increases over several years, and although it may reach a high level, swelling of the cornea and eye pain do not occur. In the early stages of the disease the peripheral vision is not affected. It is not until the disease is very advanced that visual field defects can be estimated accurately. As noted, cupping of the optic disk is characteristic of primary open-angle glaucoma.

10.32   Normal Pressure Glaucoma

Some people with intraocular pressure in the normal range may have a loss of eye tissue and suffer a loss of eye function, presumably because of an increased susceptibility of the ocular tissues. This condition, which is also called low-tension glaucoma (Apple and Rabb, 1991), is usually seen in women over age 60. Patients with this disorder have intraocular pressure at the high end of normal and cupping of the optic disks with changes in the visual field. The anterior chamber angles appear normal, and there are no contributing eye disease or systemic disorders. Normal-pressure glaucoma may result from temporary blood circulation irregularities such as vascular collapse during surgery, excessive bleeding during childbirth, myocardial infarction (heart attack due to a blocked artery) or bleeding ulcer.

Treatment is directed to the primary medical condition and the consequent reduction in intraocular pressure (Newell, 1992).

10.33   Ocular Hypertension

Ocular hypertension is a condition in which the intraocular pressure is consistently 21 mm Hg or more in both eyes in individuals who have open angles, normal optic disks and no abnormalities in the visual field. These individuals are more likely than the average person to develop primary open-angle glaucoma, but that likelihood is greater with higher tension, increased age or higher cup-disk ratios. When all these factors are unfavorable, around 15 percent of such patients develop a visual field defect within five years. Patients with pressure of more than 30 mm Hg are usually treated with a beta-adrenergic antagonist; those with intraocular pressure below that are treated if they have unfavorable factors, such as diabetes mellitus, blood circulation disorders or a family history of glaucoma (Newell, 1992).

10.40   SECONDARY OPEN-ANGLE GLAUCOMA

Most cases of secondary open-angle glaucoma occur when the trabecular meshwork of the eye becomes clogged with particles of blood or various bodily cells, arising from tumors or inflammatory processes, which block the outflow of aqueous (Apple and Rabb, 1991). When this happens, intraocular pressure remains persistently high in one or both eyes. In the early stages, the optic disk and visual fields appear normal; the anterior chamber angle is open and the aqueous has access to the trabecular meshwork but cannot drain normally. The signs and symptoms are the same as those of primary open-angle glaucoma. Secondary open-angle glaucoma may arise from many different mechanisms, including blunt trauma, surgical injury and eye disorders other than glaucoma.

10.41   Trauma

Trauma to the eye can cause dislocation of structures of the eye and mechanical damage to the trabecular meshwork. Where intraocular structures are forced against the meshwork or Schlemm's canal, a disruption in aqueous drainage may result; the anterior chamber angle or the trabecular meshwork may become deformed or fused and block the outflow. The damage may be worsened by the formation of scar tissue within the meshwork.

If traumatic injury to the eye damages the ciliary body, the trabecular meshwork may be compromised by losing the support of the ciliary muscle. Some traumatic insults cause a piercing wound in the limbus, the corner of the eye where the cornea meets the sclera. If such an injury causes the tough tissues of the sclera to be forced into the trabeculum, aqueous drainage is significantly compromised. Increased intraocular pressure may sometimes be evident within a short period following trauma, although it is not unusual for the glaucoma to appear after a delay of many years.

10.42   Hemorrhage Within the Eye

The presence of blood in the anterior chamber of the eye may in some cases block the flow of aqueous and lead to increased intraocular pressure. The blood can come from a variety of causes, including blunt trauma and systemic diseases, and may be an aftermath of surgery. Small amounts of blood from a recent injury are usually cleared easily from the anterior chamber and are not likely to cause a serious drainage problem. However, when particularly large quantities of blood combine with the aqueous, the trabecular meshwork can be overwhelmed and cease to function normally.

Clotted or partially clotted blood is a more serious problem. Clotted blood cells have a tendency to become rigid and are frequently incapable of passing through the meshwork. Further, the breakdown of clotted blood often produces macrophage cells, or phagocytes, which clean up the body by consuming the debris from a hemorrhage. Phagocytes are often too large to clear the trabecular meshwork and often end up as trabecular obstructions.

Another form of hemorrhagic glaucoma is ghost cell glaucoma, so called because of the shape and appearance of the cells. In these cases, debris from old hemorrhages remains in the eye in the form of hollow cells with rigid walls. These ghost cells are large and tough. Unable to pass through the trabecular meshwork, they remain in the anterior chamber and lead to increased intraocular pressure. Medical therapy is often effective. Sometimes, however, repeated irrigation of the anterior chamber is necessary to wash away the cells (McNamara and Benson, 1990).

When blunt injury causes contusion (bruising) of the eye, an immediate increase in intraocular pressure may result and persist for 30 to 45 minutes. If a hemorrhage follows the contusion, a secondary glaucoma may ensue when the meshwork is clogged with blood. In the majority of these cases, glaucoma does not develop. When it does, open-angle glaucoma may appear in one eye anytime from one month to ten years after the injury (Newell, 1992).

10.43   Uveitis (Inflammatory Glaucoma)

The most common form of inflammatory glaucoma arises from uveitis, the swelling and inflammation of the uveal tract (the iris, ciliary body and choroid). Uveitis is classified according to its location in the uvea: the terms *iritis* (in the iris), *cyclitis* (in the ciliary body) and *iridocyclitis* (in both the iris and the ciliary body) all refer to inflammation in the front part of the uveal tract, while *choroiditis* (in the choroid) and *chorioretinitis* (in both the choroid and the retina) refer to the posterior part.

The symptoms of uveitis are eye pain, sensitivity to light, and redness and watering of the eye. Inflammation in the uveal tract may hamper normal outflow of the aqueous and lead to increased intraocular pressure. Iridocyclitis causes secondary glaucoma by blocking the trabecular meshwork with inflammatory cells and other particles. The causes of uveitis, which are varied and sometimes difficult to identify, include spread of infection from other sites in the body, viral infection and allergic reactions. Repeated episodes of uveitis often cause permanent damage to the aqueous outflow channels even after the uveitis has been treated successfully.

The phrase "glaucomatocyclitic crisis" refers to an acute inflammation of the uveal tract, with a buildup in intraocular pressure so rapid that the patient's early symptoms will often resemble symptoms of angle-closure glaucoma. The condition is distinguished from angle-closure glaucoma in that the anterior chamber angle is open. Indomethacin, an anti-inflammatory drug, administered systemically, may end the attack (Newell, 1992).

10.44   Exfoliation Syndrome (Pseudoexfoliation of the Lens)

In the exfoliation syndrome, lens material sloughs off and floats freely in the anterior chamber. The source of this material, which is translucent, flaky and fibrous, is not well understood. Because the lens material resembles the fibers within the basement membrane of the eye, some authors suggest that it originates there, although the same material forms in the eyelids and in some tissues outside the eye as well. Regardless of its source, once the sloughed material enters the anterior chamber, it becomes trapped in the trabecular meshwork and impedes the drainage of aqueous. When exfoliation syndrome glaucoma occurs, it is similar to primary open-angle glaucoma but much more difficult to treat medically. Trabeculoplasty is often successful but may have to be followed with a filtration procedure.

Whether a possible association exists between pseudoexfoliation and angle-closure glaucoma is a matter of controversy. Many authors believe that such a relationship is coincidental, while others believe that pseudoexfoliation patients are more likely to develop angle-closure glaucoma than are those without the condition. One study suggests strongly that pseudoexfoliation patients constitute a high-risk group for the development of angle-closure glaucoma. This study also supports the widely held belief that the use of strong miotics (drugs that contract the pupil of the eye) to treat pseudoexfoliation patients may be responsible for the higher-than-normal incidence of narrowed anterior chamber angles and angle closure in this group (Gross, et al., 1994). This suggests that strong miotics should not be used in pseudoexfoliation patients.

10.45 Pigment Dispersion Syndrome

In the pigmentary dispersion syndrome, the pigment layer epithelium (covering) of the iris becomes detached and withered. Loss of pigment from the iris causes spokelike defects in the iris. If the iris is dilated with mydriatics in the course of an eye examination, or if the affected patient exercises vigorously, pigment material is released into the anterior chamber, where it floats freely, eventually becoming trapped in the trabecular meshwork. Pigment dispersion glaucoma appears identical to primary open-angle glaucoma except for the pigment abnormality, and treatment for the two disorders is the same. Some individuals with pigment dispersion syndrome never develop glaucoma, while other individuals acquire the disorder 10 to 20 years after pigment dispersion is first diagnosed.

10.46 Corticosteroid Glaucoma

Corticosteroid glaucoma is an occasional side effect of topical or systemic treatment with corticosteroids in susceptible individuals. The effects of this type of glaucoma may be limited and of short duration, or they may extend to severe cupping of the optic disk, withering of the optic nerve and a persistent increase in intraoptic pressure.

Although the mechanism of this disorder is not known, some authors believe it may come about as a result of decreased phagocyte activity in the aqueous. When these large scavenger cells fail to break down debris cells, the waste material becomes trapped in the meshwork.

Some groups of individuals are more susceptible than others to corticosteroid glaucoma: some patients with primary open-angle glaucoma and their close relatives, patients with diabetes mellitus and patients with severe myopia (nearsightedness) (Newell, 1992). When patients being treated with corticosteroid therapy do develop secondary glaucoma, the condition usually appears within six to eight weeks from the time the treatment began. However, some patients will react in two or three weeks, while others will not react for several months.

Corticosteroid therapy should be started only after a careful history is taken to determine whether a patient is at high risk for secondary glaucoma. If corticosteroid therapy is chosen, it should be monitored carefully, with regular checks of intracellular pressure. However, diagnosis of secondary glaucoma can be difficult, since clinical signs are identical to primary open-angle glaucoma; this glaucoma may also wrongly be assumed to be a complication of the disease for which corticosteroid therapy was prescribed. When corticosteroid glaucoma is diagnosed, the administration of those drugs must be stopped.

10.47 Lens-induced Glaucoma

Lens-induced glaucoma can be of two types: lens particle glaucoma or phacolytic glaucoma.

[1] Phacolytic Glaucoma

During the formation of cataracts,[1] the lens sometimes deteriorates and liquefies. When this happens, lens elements in liquid form leak into the anterior chamber. This mostly protein material causes inflammation of the structures of the anterior chamber. The damage from this inflammation is similar to that of secondary glaucoma arising from uveitis, with the protein and cellular debris lodging in the drainage system and obstructing the flow of aqueous. Known as phacolytic glaucoma, this cataract-related disorder requires removal of the cataract to correct the inflammation and the glaucoma.

---

[1] *See also* ch. 11.

[2]   Lens Particle Glaucoma

When the lens capsule is accidentally disrupted by trauma or cataract surgery, the resulting severe inflammation and swollen cornea disrupt the flow of aqueous and cause abnormally high intraocular pressure. Immediate relief of pressure can be achieved with paracentesis, a procedure that entails puncturing the anterior chamber and aspirating (removing with a hollow needle) the aqueous fluid. But if the inflammation and glaucoma do not respond to conservative measures, surgical removal of the lens debris is necessary (Newell, 1992).

10.50   PRIMARY ANGLE-CLOSURE GLAUCOMA

Primary angle-closure glaucoma occurs in individuals whose eyes have small anterior structures and shallow anterior chambers. Because the iris is almost in contact with the disproportionately large lens behind it, the anterior chamber is narrowed enough to cause resistance to the flow of aqueous from the posterior chamber to the anterior chamber (Ghezzi and Renner, 1992). Patients with this condition who develop glaucoma do so when the anterior surface of the iris is thrust against the posterior surface of the cornea, a condition referred to as primary angle-closure glaucoma with pupillary block.

Plateau iris, another structural anomaly in the anterior portion of the eye, can also lead to primary angle-closure glaucoma. A fairly uncommon condition, plateau iris is distinguished by an iris which is flat and bends sharply where the edges join the ciliary body, thus creating a narrow angle in the anterior chamber and lessening the rate of aqueous outflow. Individuals with plateau iris who develop glaucoma, do so when the iris bunches and folds over the anterior angle and blocks the trabecular meshwork, a condition known as primary angle-closure glaucoma without pupillary block.

Primary angle-closure glaucoma occurs because of inherited anatomic defects that create a shallow anterior chamber. Both eyes are involved, but they may develop symptoms several years apart. The primary form of angle-closure glaucoma does not follow accidental trauma, eye surgery, systemic diseases or other eye diseases.

10.51   Epidemiology

In the United States and Europe, primary angle-closure glaucoma occurs a quarter as frequently as primary open-angle glaucoma.

Among whites, it is approximately three times more common in women than in men, but among blacks, the incidence is equal in men and in women. Among Japanese, Southeast Asians and Eskimos, primary angle-closure glaucoma is more common than open-angle glaucoma (Newell, 1992).

10.52   The Role of the Anterior Chamber

All individuals with narrow anterior chambers are vulnerable to angle-closure glaucoma. Those who have an anterior chamber with a depth of 2.5 mm or less are very likely to develop angle-closure glaucoma with pupillary block. A shallow anterior angle may be recognized by the decreased distance between the posterior surface of the cornea and the anterior surface of the iris (Newell, 1992).

When there is a narrow angle, there is often a shortened globe, causing the visual image passing through the pupil to be projected to a point behind the retina. This condition is typical in the farsighted eye, and in fact, angle-closure glaucoma occurs more frequently in farsighted individuals. As compensation for the effects of the shortened globe, the lens of the eye thickens, narrowing the anterior chamber even further. Lens thickening also occurs naturally as a person ages, which leads to a higher likelihood of angle-closure glaucoma in the later years.

10.53   Mechanism of Disease

In angle-closure glaucoma, the normal outflow of aqueous is blocked mechanically. This can happen in one of two ways: In patients with small anterior structures and a shallow anterior chamber angle, the iris comes in contact with the cornea to block the flow; and in patients with plateau iris, the iris bunches and blocks the trabecular meshwork, much as a washcloth blocks a bathtub drain. Blockage is most likely to occur when the pupil is dilated halfway, since this is the stage of dilation that produces maximum lens-iris contact.

Many attacks of acute angle-closure glaucoma happen at dusk or when entering a darkened theater. Emotional upset can trigger an attack, as can recovery from the dilation of the pupil after an eye examination. A blocked anterior chamber is sometimes a result of atrophy of the dilator muscles and slackness of the periphery of the iris, a condition found in older patients. In these cases, the iris appears to bow forward, so that it seems to be parallel to the convex posterior surface of the cornea.

When the flow of aqueous becomes blocked by any of these means, intraocular pressure rises dramatically. This rise in pressure may promote damage to the optic nerve and disturbances in the field of vision, both of which are typical of glaucoma. Many individuals whose eyes have shallow anterior angles may never experience the symptoms of angle-closure glaucoma. Others may experience occasional, chronic attacks, but some will experience an acute attack, which is one of the true emergencies in the practice of ophthalmology.

10.54   Classification of Primary Angle-Closure Glaucoma

Primary angle-closure glaucoma may be divided into four phases, according to the severity of the symptoms and the duration of the attack. The phases do not necessarily follow one another; an affected individual may experience one phase only or skip from asymptomatic immediately to acute. There is no typical pattern of progression.

Phase one is asymptomatic. The patient has a shallow anterior chamber but no symptoms. He or she is at risk of developing glaucoma later in life and should be monitored regularly by an ophthalmologist and warned to heed the signs of glaucoma, particularly blurred vision combined with iridescent vision and pain. Some patients who are asymptomatic have occasional angle closure that causes the formation of synechiae (adhesions) between the root of the iris and the cornea that block the flow of aqueous and cause chronic angle-closure glaucoma (Newell, 1992).

In phase two, angle closure occurs occasionally following activities that cause the pupil to dilate, such as watching movies, walking outdoors at night or becoming emotionally upset. These are glaucoma attacks in which the intraocular pressure rises rapidly; there is eye pain, possibly severe, and the patient experiences the "halo vision" characteristic of glaucoma. The symptoms usually disappear when the patient is exposed to light or goes to sleep, both of which cause the pupil to contract.

Phase three is acute angle-closure glaucoma. This is a true emergency that requires prompt treatment. An acute episode begins with a sudden rise in intraocular pressure, which is usually much higher than in open-angle glaucoma. This brings on a number of alarming symptoms within the eye, as well as abdominal symptoms and all-over weakness. Without prompt treatment, adhesions will develop between the root of the iris and the trabecular meshwork that will permanently close the anterior chamber angle.

In phase four, if repeated episodes of angle closure are not treated or do not respond to treatment, the drainage angle becomes permanently closed. This may result in absolute glaucoma, in which the eye becomes irreversibly marble-hard and sightless.

10.55 Signs and Symptoms

Symptoms and signs vary according to whether the attack is acute or subacute.

[1] Subacute Attack

Even an early subacute attack of angle-closure glaucoma brings on a sudden rather than a gradual increase in intraocular pressure. Abrupt onset of symptoms is a hallmark of angle-closure glaucoma, setting it apart from open-angle glaucoma, which features a gradual buildup of intraocular pressure. The suddenness of the increase in pressure produces discomfort ranging from mild to moderately severe. Among the symptoms may be headache or eye ache. Treatment often is not sought for a subacute attack, since the patient attributes the symptoms to routine headache, an assumption seemingly confirmed by the transitory nature of the attack. In most cases, the pain will be gone by morning, because sleep causes the pupil to contract.

Blurred vision and iridescent vision (the appearance of halos and rainbows around light sources) are symptoms of particular concern that should prompt the patient to seek treatment. These disturbances of vision are caused by swelling of the cornea, which causes a hazy appearance of the cornea that is sometimes called steamy cornea. The iridescent vision is most apparent when the patient views a bright light in a dark room and usually takes the form of two colored rings—an outer blue-violet ring and an inner ring of yellow-red.

Not all angle-closure glaucoma patients experience iridescent vision. But when the symptom does appear, it is a strong indication of possible angle-closure glaucoma and should prompt the affected individual to undergo a full ophthalmologic examination.

[2] Acute Attack

Acute angle-closure glaucoma is the most dramatic form of glaucoma; it has a very sudden onset marked by alarming elevations in intraocular pressure, which can run as high as 50 to 80 mm Hg (millimeters per level of mercury, a measurement of atmospheric pressure) (Pederson, 1991). To put these figures into perspective, it helps to remember that an individual with normal (nonglaucomatous) eyes has a mean pressure of 15 mm Hg, plus or minus 3 mm Hg, while an individual with untreated open-angle glaucoma and changes in the visual field has a mean intraocular pressure of at least 22 mm Hg (Newell, 1992). Intraocular pressure tends to increase with age and to be higher in women than in men.

The rapid rise in intraocular pressure brings on severe ocular symptoms, which include blurred vision and iridescent vision. Relief does not occur spontaneously, as it does in a subacute attack. In fact, as intraocular pressure increases, the symptoms become more severe. Routine examination of the patient will reveal a reddened eye, with swelling of the eyelids and conjunctiva (the inner surface of the eyelids). The eyes may give off a large amount of tears; the cornea will appear swollen and cloudy, with droplets of epithelial cells scattered on the surface. The pupil will be in mid-dilation and will not respond to light.

Systemic symptoms include severe, prostrating head pain plus severe nausea and vomiting, all of which may be aggravated by drugs used to treat the attack. There may even be bradycardia (a slow, irregular heartbeat) (Ghezzi and Renner, 1992). The headache is a boring type of pain, with special intensity in and around the eye, and may be distinguished from other headache syndromes by physical examination of the eye.

The eyeball may be firm when palpated, but this is not definitive. Proper diagnosis can only be made with the Schiotz tonometer (Henry, 1992). Acute angle-closure glaucoma is included in the differential diagnosis of the acute abdomen, and if symptoms of this ocular condition are overlooked in acute abdominal cases, unnecessary abdominal operations may be performed.

If the attack persists, adhesions will form between the root of the iris and the cornea. Within the space of several days, these adhesions almost entirely destroy the drainage meshwork (Newell, 1992). Further, the pupil may become semi-dilated and fixed, and withering of the iris may become noticeable. Prompt treatment is essential if sight in the affected eye is to be saved.

10.60   SECONDARY ANGLE-CLOSURE GLAUCOMA

In secondary angle-closure glaucoma, the drainage angle in the anterior chamber closes down when the iris comes in contact with the trabecular meshwork or with the edge of the cornea. In contrast to open-angle glaucomas, which occur when the trabecular meshwork becomes blocked by loose cellular material too large to pass through normally, this comes about by way of a mechanical blockage.

Secondary angle-closure glaucoma may arise from inflammation or other eye disorders, accidental trauma or as a complication of eye surgery, all of which may cause displacement of the structures of the eye. Secondary angle-closure glaucoma may also be triggered by intranasal cocaine abuse (Mitchell and Schwartz, 1996). Cocaine causes the pupil to dilate and can induce angle closure in susceptible individuals. Additionally, there are case reports of angle-closure glaucoma as a complication of inhaled ipratropium bromide therapy for asthma (Hall, 1994).

10.61   Neovascular Glaucoma (Rubeosis Iridis)

Neovascular glaucoma ensues after a fibrous, blood-rich membrane develops over the anterior chamber surface of the trabecular (drainage) meshwork. The membrane derives from the formation of new blood vessels on the surface and the framework of the iris. These new vessels form when the blood supply to the eye is compromised and new vessels are needed to take over the role of the damaged or diseased vessels. The process of growing new blood vessels frequently results from diabetes mellitus and closure of the central eye veins. It may also be an outgrowth of a number of blood disorders, inflammatory conditions and cancer.

The new blood vessels formed in this way are often highly permeable and fragile. The damage they cause results from a vascular membrane growing over the anterior surface of the iris, across the meshwork and across the pupil. Treatment is difficult, especially since the eyes are often blind from the disease that caused neovascularization. Topical application of 1 percent atropine and corticosteroids may relieve pain. An injection of alcohol behind the eyeball relieves pain for several months (Newell, 1992).

10.62   Lens-induced Closed-Angle Glaucoma

Swelling, or intumescence, of the lens is one of the by-products of cataract formation. As cataracts develop and become very mature, the lens takes on a significant amount of fluid. The swelling of the lens causes it to crowd the anterior chamber, and it may eventually close the drainage angle completely.

Another mechanism involving the lens occurs when a dislocated lens blocks the passage of aqueous through the pupil.

10.63   Trauma

Secondary angle-closure glaucoma with pupillary block (when the front of the pupil is in contact with the back of the lens) occurs most commonly following trauma and eye inflammation. Contusion (bruising) of the eye results in an immediate sharp increase in intraocular pressure, which may last for 30 to 45 minutes. Contusion may cause cuts in the ciliary body, the structure that produces aqueous, and may also result in recession of the anterior chamber angle. If angle-recession glaucoma comes about as a result of accidental bruising, it may heal spontaneously before symptoms become apparent. The majority of these injuries do not produce glaucoma and only rarely cause late traumatic glaucoma.

Following penetrating injuries, a membrane composed of scar tissue may develop. This membrane may gradually cover the anterior chamber and close off the drainage angle.

Dislocation of the lens following trauma may result in angle-closure glaucoma. In this case, the lens is pushed into the anterior chamber, blocking the drainage angle. A partially dislocated lens may sometimes be moved to a more posterior position, thus opening the angle. However, when the entire lens is thrust into the anterior chamber, the only alternative in most cases is surgical removal of the lens. Dislocation of the lens and pupillary block may also arise from advanced cases of detached retina.

10.64   Glaucoma Following Ocular Surgery

Because surgery causes trauma to the tissues involved, angle-closure glaucoma secondary to ocular surgery is closely related to the trauma-induced form of the disorder. The angle-closure form of glaucoma associated with surgery is frequently produced by the formation of adhesions that close the anterior chamber angle. These adhesions frequently result in pupillary block, one of the most common disorders leading to angle-closure glaucoma. Pupillary block causes the buildup of aqueous behind the iris, which causes the iris to billow forward, crowding the anterior chamber. This condition is known as iris bombé, which can be rapidly blinding if intraocular pressure is unrelieved.

Surgery may also encourage the anterior surface of the iris to adhere to the posterior surface of the cornea, a condition known as anterior synechia. Synechiae may be caused by the presence of small amounts of blood and other ocular debris in the eye following surgery; this debris blocks the trabecular meshwork. When the aqueous is unable to drain from the eye, the debris fosters the formation of adhesions. This may be avoided by careful wound closure.

If the surgeon believes there is a risk for postsurgical adhesions, he or she may choose to perform one or more iridectomies following the primary surgery. In iridectomy, a small area of the iris is cut away, usually on the periphery, to permit aqueous to flow through the newly created opening. Many surgeons perform iridectomies routinely after trabeculectomy and certain other surgical procedures.

In the aftermath of surgery, epithelial (cellular material that lines hollow organs) or fibrous tissue may grow into the anterior chamber. The tissue usually bulges through a fistula (opening) left in the surgical wound. Unwanted openings allow tissues to escape from the immediate area of the wound and into the anterior chamber, where it may either close off the drainage or block the pupil. In rare cases, vitreous material escapes into the anterior space during cataract surgery, causing a secondary angle-closure glaucoma.

[1] Complications of Cataract Surgery

Most of the complications of cataract surgery are related to wound leakage, which may lead to a flat anterior chamber or detachment of the choroid. The wound leak may be too small to be demonstrated, but it may still be responsible for changes in the anterior space.

Detachment of the choroid as a result of wound leak is much less common now that secure wound closure has become routine. Even when there is a leak from a surgical incision, it is usually self-healing. When it occurs, the onset of choroidal detachment is ordinarily one or two weeks after surgery and is usually resolved one or two weeks later. At that time, the choroidal detachment and shallow anterior space disappear.

Flat anterior chamber following cataract surgery is also related to surgical wound leak but usually appears earlier in the postoperative period than detachment of the choroid.

Initial management for both conditions is conservative. If the anterior chamber flattening resolves spontaneously in a few days, it may not be necessary to do anything further. However, if flat anterior chamber is combined with extremely low intraocular pressure, it may be necessary to explore the surgical site and possibly even retie sutures. The anterior chamber space may then be re-formed with an air bubble. It may also be helpful to evacuate fluid from the space between the choroid and the sclera, which will allow the choroid to resume its normal placement adjacent to the sclera.

Pupillary block following cataract surgery is another possible cause of flat anterior chamber. In this case, the intraocular pressure will be high. Ordinarily the front surface of the vitreous body pushes forward to block the pupil as well as the surgical openings. Medical management involves administration of drugs to promote the flow of aqueous, as well as vigorous efforts to dilate the pupil. If the condition does not resolve, it may be necessary to re-operate.

The invasion of epithelial tissue into the anterior chamber is a possible complication of cataract surgery related to inadequate wound closure. Epithelium, the cellular tissue that lines body cavities, has the ability to cover raw wound surfaces in a few days. Once this tissue enters the anterior chamber, it may spread to cover all available surfaces, or it may form epithelial cysts, which may spread readily throughout the anterior space. The progress of this tissue growth must be stopped by surgical excision, cauterization (burning with heat) or cryotherapy (freezing). As the epithelium proceeds to line the anterior chamber, intractable glaucoma may develop, and the prospect of recovering vision in that eye is not good.

[2]   Complications of Retinal Detachment Surgery

Acute angle-closure glaucoma is an early complication of this surgery. This potentially disastrous form of glaucoma is a result of congestion in the choroid, which causes a forward rotation of the ciliary body and closure of the anterior chamber filtration angle.

Misdiagnosis of this complication is possible because the central portion of the anterior chamber may remain open. Proper diagnosis is made by applanation tonometry. Management includes the use of acetazolamide, timolol, corticosteroids and mannitol (Benson, 1990).

[3] Complications of Vitrectomy

Vitrectomy—surgery on the vitreous body—has been used to restore sight in many diabetics and in many cases of "inoperable" retinal detachments. Vitrectomy is also valuable in the management of endophthalmitis, a serious infection that sometimes complicates ocular (and other) surgeries. However, vitrectomy is a high-risk procedure and should not be undertaken without very careful evaluation.

One important criterion for the patient being screened for vitrectomy is the ability of the affected eye to perceive light. The usual visual examination is not sufficient and must be supplemented with ultrasound and specialized x-ray procedures. Neovascular glaucoma is a frequent complication of vitrectomy in diabetic patients, occurring in 10 to 26 percent of cases (McNamara and Benson, 1990). Once neovascular glaucoma is established, it is very difficult to control intraocular pressure without vision loss.

10.70 DIFFERENTIAL DIAGNOSIS OF ANGLE-CLOSURE GLAUCOMA

The presenting symptoms of acute angle-closure glaucoma bear similarity to other eye disorders that cause pain and redness. These include inflammation of the structures of the eye, ulcers of the cornea and infections such as conjunctivitis. Affected individuals may first experience prostrating systemic symptoms, especially headache, nausea and vomiting. Head pain may be poorly localized, which leads to the consideration of primary problems within the cranium, such as tumors or acute hemorrhage, cavernous sinus thrombosis or vascular headache syndromes such as cluster or migraine. Abdominal symptoms may predominate, imitating acute abdominal or cardiac disease (Ghezzi and Renner, 1992; Arora, et al., 1991). All these disease entities must be differentiated carefully in the effort to reach an accurate diagnosis.

The headache in acute angle-closure glaucoma is a boring type of pain with acute onset (Henry, 1992). The pain is usually most intense in and immediately around the eye. The patient may complain of hazy vision or loss of vision. On examination, the cornea will appear swollen and hazy, and the pupil will be dilated in mid-position. The eyeball may be firm when it is touched, but this is not definitive. Proper diagnosis can be made with a Schiotz tonometer.

Rarely, in an atypical case of acute angle-closure, the patient will not complain of head pain. Rosenberg and Adams (1991) report the case of a woman who appeared in the emergency room complaining of blurred vision after bending over, but denied any other symptoms. On examination, she registered very high intraocular pressure; treatment for acute angle-closure glaucoma was begun, and normal vision returned.

10.80   TREATMENT OF GLAUCOMA

Treatment of open-angle glaucoma consists of medical therapy, laser therapy or surgery.

10.81   Medical Treatment of Open-Angle Glaucoma

Medical treatment is directed toward increasing the outflow of aqueous humor, decreasing the secretion of aqueous or both. The need for medical treatment becomes obvious when increased intraocular pressure occurs with optic disk cupping[2] and characteristic visual field defects. Management of patients with these symptoms must be individualized: Patients with diabetes mellitus, a family history of glaucoma, a large optic cup, any cardiovascular abnormality and advancing age are especially at risk for developing damage from glaucoma. African-American patients are particularly vulnerable (Newell, 1992).

Medical management of open-angle glaucoma presents the same difficulties as treatment of any chronic disease. Glaucoma medications may be absorbed systemically, which can result in a number of side effects. Moreover, many elderly patients take medications for other disorders, and these drugs add to the effects of glaucoma medication. Since drug therapy for glaucoma is usually a lifelong regimen for the patient, patient compliance becomes a problem, especially when several different medications are prescribed for daily use.

Long-term medical management for well-controlled glaucoma includes examination three times a year. The examination should include measurement of intraoptical tension[3] and the charting of any changes in the optic disks. Perimetry and gonioscopy should be repeated at least once a year, depending on the progression or lack of progression of the disease.

---

[2] *See* 10.12 *supra.*

[3] *See* 10.33 *supra.*

If medical treatment fails to control the condition, laser treatment or surgery may be considered. Recent studies indicate that when the goal of therapy is to control intraocular pressure in chronic open-angle glaucoma, both filtration surgery and medical therapy appear to be equally effective in maintaining long-term visual function and a stable optic disk (Stewart, et al., 1996; The Glaucoma Laser Trial [GLT] and Glaucoma Laser Trial Follow-up Study: 7, 1995).

Medical treatment of open-angle glaucoma consists of the use of one or more different classes of drugs, each of which includes a number of different compounds. Treatment should begin with the minimal concentration and frequency of use that will control intraocular pressure and prevent optic nerve atrophy.

[1] Beta-Blockers

Also referred to as beta-adrenergic blockers or as beta-1 and beta-2 antagonists, these drugs decrease the production of aqueous humor without excessively altering the size of the pupil. Beta-blockers are usually better tolerated than carbonic anhydrase inhibitors, which produce similar results. However, beta-blockers can be absorbed systemically and should be used with care when treating patients with asthma, cardiovascular disorders or diabetes. Some patients will experience central nervous system disorders such as anxiety, depression or confusion. Side effects involving the eye are rare, although anesthesia of the cornea has been reported (Ghezzi and Renner, 1992).

Timolol maleate (Timoptic®), the first commercially available drug of this type, is used twice daily in a concentration of either 0.25 percent or 0.5 percent (Newell, 1992). Timolol is a liquid that is applied directly to the eye. Ocular side effects are minimal, and it does not produce the burning or allergic reactions in the eye that are sometimes found with other eyedrops. A newer beta-blocker of this class is betaxolol (Betoptic®), which is nearly as effective as timolol and is less likely to aggravate cardiac and pulmonary symptoms.

[2] Cholinergic Agents

Cholinergic agents mimic the action of the parasympathetic nervous system by chemically stimulating the outflow of bodily fluids and increasing smooth muscle activity. The best-known cholinergic is pilocarpine, the traditional drug of choice for initial treatment of primary open-angle glaucoma. Although it is still in use, it has been largely replaced by beta-blockers. Pilocarpine is usually prescribed in concentrations of 1 percent to 4 percent, three or four times a day, in the form of eyedrops. It is a miotic drug, which means that it causes extreme contraction of the pupil of the eye. It is this action that aids outflow of aqueous humor in primary open-angle glaucoma.

Constriction of the pupil has side effects: Since it reduces the amount of light entering the eye, the patient's vision becomes dim and in shadowy surroundings may be impaired significantly for a few hours. Older patients may experience very decreased vision, especially if they have early-stage cataracts. There are other side effects as well: Approximately a half-hour after taking pilocarpine, many patients report a headache over the eye and an ocular spasm resulting in blurred vision; this effect is more common in patients under age 40. Because of this, timolol, a beta-blocker, is preferred.

Some patients may develop a tolerance to pilocarpine, and carbachol, another cholinergic drug, may be substituted. Carbachol is prescribed in strengths from 0.75 percent to 3.0 percent and is administered every eight hours, which gives it a small advantage in patient convenience over pilocarpine, which is taken more often. In addition, it may be tolerated more easily than pilocarpine by some patients. The molecular structure of carbachol does not permit it to penetrate the cornea as readily as pilocarpine, and as a result, it may not be as effective for some patients. Carbachol may produce the side effects common to all miotic (pupil-contracting) drugs.

[3]   Adrenergic Agents

Adrenergic drugs, as the name implies, have an action resembling that of adrenaline. Adrenergics stimulate sympathetic nervous system reactions by directly activating the adrenergic nerve receptors, and they may decrease secretion of aqueous humor and improve outflow.

Epinephrine, applied directly to the eye in a 0.5 percent to 2 percent solution, is a widely used adrenergic. This drug is mildly irritating to the eye and may cause systemic reactions such as hypertension (abnormally high blood pressure) and tachycardia (irregular heartbeat). Another adrenergic drug, divipefrin (Propine®) used topically in a 0.1 percent concentration, undergoes local transformation to epinephrine and produces fewer side effects than epinephrine (Newell, 1992; Ghezzi and Renner, 1992).

Epinephrine solutions are used either alone or in combination with a cholinergic drug such as pilocarpine.

[4] Cholinesterase Inhibitors

Cholinesterase inhibitors have a very powerful miotic effect; that is, they dramatically contract the pupil of the eye. Because of this action, cholinesterase inhibitors are very effective in reducing intraocular pressure.

Echothiophate iodide (phospholine iodide) is a cholinesterase inhibitor that, despite strong contraindications, is used in the treatment of primary open-angle glaucoma and some secondary glaucomas. It is used twice daily, usually in 0.03 percent to 0.06 percent concentrations. Higher concentrations of 0.125 percent and 0.25 percent are also available. Echothiophate iodide causes intense miosis (pupil constriction), with a maximum effect in four to six hours that lasts for two hours.

Cholinesterase inhibitors should not be used to treat patients with angle-closure glaucoma, bronchial asthma, gastrointestinal spasm, vascular hypertension, myasthenia gravis and Parkinson's disease (Newell, 1992). If cholinesterase inhibitors are taken along with general anesthesia using succinylcholine chloride, systemic side effects include apnea (prolonged suppression of breathing) and possible cardiovascular collapse (Pederson, 1991). Toxic reaction may also follow the use of procaine (also called Novocaine®). Particularly in children, cholinesterase inhibitors may cause cysts on the iris, which sometimes disappear if use of the drugs is stopped. However, the cysts may also break free, rupture and enter the aqueous humor.

Cholinesterase inhibitors are known to foster the formation of cataracts, usually in the form of small vacuoles (cavities) on the lens, particularly when the drug has been used habitually. Moreover, the strong contraction of the ciliary body caused by the drug may exert force on the peripheral retina, creating a risk of retinal detachment. To prevent these potential side effects, a thorough examination, including gonioscopy, is required to confirm the absence of cataracts and to assess the condition of the anterior chamber angle, the retina and surrounding structures.

Cholinesterase inhibitors may cause significant eye irritation as well as stinging, burning and excessive tearing. They may also cause sweating, bronchial spasm, abdominal pain and diarrhea.

[5] Carbonic Anhydrase Inhibitors

Carbonic anhydrase, an enzyme in living tissues, aids the passage of carbon dioxide from the tissues and its outward flow from the blood in the lungs. When carbonic anhydrase inhibitors are used in the treatment of primary open-angle glaucoma, they reduce the secretion of aqueous humor by the ciliary process.

These drugs are taken orally, and their action is systemic; they have the ability to inhibit aqueous flow for at least 24 hours and to lower resistance to aqueous outflow. Carbonic anhydrase inhibitors may be taken alone or in various combinations of other drugs.

Acetazolamide (Diamox®) and methazolamide (Neptazane®), the carbonic anhydrase inhibitors most often used in the treatment of primary open-angle glaucoma, are powerful drugs with unpleasant side effects. Patients who are allergic to sulfa should not take these drugs. Patients who take this class of drug over the long term may have difficulty tolerating them because of side effects such as nausea, abdominal cramping, feelings of depression, and numbness and tingling in the extremities (paresthesias). If dosages are reduced or another carbonic anhydrase inhibitor is substituted, these side effects may be reduced or relieved altogether.

Carbonic anhydrase inhibitors can cause the formation of kidney stones. More rarely, this class of drugs can cause idiosyncratic aplastic anemia, a defect in the formation of new red blood cells.

10.82 Surgical Treatment of Open-Angle Glaucoma

Primary open-angle glaucoma is treated medically if normal intraocular pressure can be maintained by drugs, if there is no progression in the severity of the disease when changes to the optic disk are monitored by ophthalmoscopy, and if there are no visual field defects (Newell, 1992). On the other hand, when primary open-angle glaucoma is progressive, surgery should not be considered a last resort but the treatment of choice (Spaeth, 1990).

Surgery for primary open-angle glaucoma is indicated when there is documented or anticipated damage to the optic nerve or visual field, despite maximum tolerated medical therapy. In a large study reported in 1995 (Glaucoma Laser Trial [GLT]: 6), open-angle glaucoma patients were followed for 3½ years to compare differences in visual fields in one group of patients treated first with trabeculoplasty with another group of patients treated first with topical medication. Eyes treated first with trabeculoplasty were judged to have slightly more improvement in visual fields than the medically treated group.

[1] Laser Trabeculoplasty

Laser trabeculoplasty is a noninvasive procedure to open drainage holes in the trabecular meshwork (the sievelike structure located in the anterior chamber recess). As a preventive measure to reduce or eliminate swelling in the anterior chamber space during and after trabeculoplasty, some surgeons apply fluorometholone, a topical anti-inflammatory, to the tissues involved. Fluorometholone has been shown to be effective in controlling inflammation, and its use has no significant impact on the results of trabeculoplasty (Shin, et al., 1996).

This operation can be done only when the trabecular meshwork is clearly visible. The patient's eye is anesthetized with a topical anesthetic, and the trabecular meshwork is viewed through a nonreflective prism. The argon laser is ordinarily used, with a 50 μ (micrometer) spot size and a 0.1-second duration. An initial power, usually 400 mW (milliwatts), can be upped in 200 mW increments until an observable change occurs. The power is then reduced 100 mW, and that level of power is used for treatment. Generally 20 to 25 holes are spaced evenly in each quadrant of the anterior meshwork, and only two quadrants are initially treated. If that amount of treatment is successful, the congestion in the trabecular meshwork will be relieved, the aqueous will flow through the newly created openings and the intraocular pressure will be reduced. If it is not successful, the remaining two quadrants may be treated four to six weeks later (Newell, 1992).

The main complication is a temporary increase in intraocular pressure; other complications are minor. Laser trabeculoplasty is successful in controlling intraocular pressure in about 85 percent of patients, but most of these continue to need medical therapy.

[2] Trabeculectomy

Trabeculectomy is what is known as a filtering operation, and it is the operation of choice in many hospitals when trabeculoplasty fails to control the intraocular pressure or when the patient's trabecular meshwork cannot be seen. In some centers, trabeculectomy is the surgical procedure of choice for primary open-angle glaucoma.

Trabeculectomy is a microsurgical procedure done with a magnification of 8x. In this operation, a superficial flap is created from the sclera, through which a small portion of the trabecular meshwork is removed. The flap is then replaced, and the edges of the wound are cauterized so that scarring during the healing process will not close the opening. The aqueous may then flow freely.

Trabeculectomy is routinely accompanied by a complete or partial iridectomy, in which a portion of the iris is removed. This procedure reduces the chance that a segment of the iris will adhere to and block the opening created by trabeculectomy.

The most frequent complication following trabeculectomy is the formation of blebs (nodules filled with liquid) that frequently form around draining surgical wounds. If there is leakage of a bleb after trabeculectomy, it must be sealed by covering it with a flap of tissue formed from the sclera. According to one researcher (Pederson, 1991), trabeculectomy is successful in more than 90 percent of patients, but it sometimes leads to later cataract formation.

[3]   Cyclocryotherapy

Cyclocryotherapy is a procedure that destroys cells in the ciliary body by freezing; this may reduce inflow of aqueous humor and lower intraocular pressure. The destruction of tissue is the explanation for the side effects and complications of cyclocryotherapy as well as for its benefits. Cyclocryotherapy has played an important part in the management of glaucoma in the past, but the procedure has been somewhat replaced by laser cyclophotocoagulation. When laser cyclophotocoagulation is not available, cyclocryotherapy still plays an important role in the management of selected glaucoma patients.

Elderly patients with advanced visual damage and a history of failure with other glaucoma procedures may be candidates for cyclocryotherapy. In approximately 80 percent of cases, successful regulation of intraocular pressure will occur. The incidence of serious complications is at least 5 percent and include a possibly excruciating headache.[4]

[4]   Cyclophotocoagulation

For the substantial number of patients who do not respond to medical therapy or to filtration surgery, cyclophotocoagulation is the

---

[4] See 10.90 infra.

treatment of choice. Laser cyclophotocoagulation destroys tissue in the ciliary body, as does cyclocryotherapy, but with less discomfort and fewer complications afterward. The complications that do appear are not as severe as those following cyclocryotherapy.

10.83 Medical Treatment of Angle-Closure Glaucoma

Acute angle-closure glaucoma is an emergency that requires prompt attention. If intraocular pressure is not lowered within 24 to 48 hours of an acute attack, irreversible loss of vision is likely. Initial emergency management includes the use of a miotic (pupil-contracting) agent to pull the periphery of the iris away from the trabecular meshwork.[5] Some researchers (Ghezzi and Renner, 1992) recommend the administration of pilocarpine in a 2 percent concentration, one drop every 15 minutes, for two hours, then every four hours as needed; they further recommend that more frequent or higher doses should be avoided. Pilocarpine should then be placed in the unaffected eye every six hours to prevent a similar attack.

In very severe cases, miotics may not be effective until the pressure is reduced by other agents. In these cases, topically administered timolol[6] causes intraocular pressure to fall within 30 to 60 minutes, with peak effects in two hours. Timolol may also help the cornea absorb pilocarpine when it is then administered.

Oral glycerine in a 50 percent solution can be administered as a hyperosmotic agent to drain water from the eye as well as to decrease aqueous production. Drugs to control vomiting and sedatives may also be indicated. If nausea and vomiting prohibit oral administration of glycerine, mannitol given intravenously in a 20 percent concentration may be used (Pederson, 1991). However, high-dosage infusions of mannitol may sometimes result in acute renal (liver) failure, with a high dose described as more than 200 grams a day or a cumulative dose of more than 400 grams in 48 hours. Acute renal failure may occur after mannitol infusion for the treatment of narrow-angle glaucoma; one patient in whom this developed readily responded to immediate hemodialysis (a process for purifying the blood) (Gadallah, et al., 1995). Patients who do not receive hemodialysis have increased morbidity and a much longer hospital stay.

---

[5] *See* 10.81[2] *supra.*

[6] *See* 10.81[1] *supra.*

10.84 Surgical Treatment of Angle-Closure Glaucoma

The definitive treatment of acute angle-closure glaucoma is surgical, once the intraocular pressure has been relieved medically. The procedures of choice involve surgery on the iris, and a number of approaches are available, depending on the therapeutic goal for the patient in question. In the literature, terms for surgical procedures on the iris begin with the prefix *irid-* to indicate the anatomic location of the surgery in the iris.

Two types of iris surgery are used in the treatment of angle-closure glaucoma: iridectomy, an incision into the iris by laser or surgical cutting; and iridotomy, removal of part of the iris. Both procedures create an opening in the peripheral portion of the iris that allows free flow of the aqueous between the posterior and anterior chambers, bypassing the pupil (Ghezzi and Renner, 1992). Iridectomy is curative if it is performed within one week of the attack, before adhesions develop. Because angle-closure glaucoma is bilateral, preventive iridectomy is always recommended for the asymptomatic eye also (Pederson, 1991).

[1] Iridectomy

The main reason to perform iridectomy is to eliminate pupillary block, a condition that results when the anterior surface of the pupil comes in contact with the posterior surface of the cornea. When pupillary block occurs, the drainage angle in the anterior chamber closes down, making it impossible for aqueous to flow normally. One way to correct this problem is to cut a hole in the iris so that there will be an uninterrupted connection between the anterior and posterior chambers to allow free flow of aqueous.

At present, when iridectomy is indicated, laser iridotomy is the usual procedure of choice. However, there are instances when laser iridotomy is inadvisable, as in eyes with flat anterior chambers, or impossible, as in eyes with cloudy corneas. Consequently surgical iridectomy is still an important procedure (Spaeth, 1990). If all efforts to control intraocular pressure before surgery have failed, paracentesis may be needed immediately before surgery.[7]

---

[7] *See* 10.84[3] *infra.*

[2] Laser Iridotomy

When discussing laser surgery, it is important to bear in mind that treatment with a laser is indeed surgery and that a laser is only somewhat less invasive than traditional surgery with a scalpel. The laser beam of light has the ability to pass through some tissues without apparent damage as well as the ability to alter, and possibly damage, other tissues. Laser surgery on the iris is an important advance in ophthalmic surgery, but it is not without complications. Several types of lasers are suitable for performing iris surgery, no one of which is usable in every case.

The known complications of laser iridotomy include laser burns on the cornea, in addition to the complications of glaucoma surgery.[8] Furthermore, laser iridotomy for pupillary block angle closure is sometimes followed by a flattening of the iris, which increases contact between the iris and the lens, narrowing the anterior drainage angle (Caronia, et al., 1996).

[3] Paracentesis

If all measures to reduce intraocular pressure before iridectomy have failed, paracentesis may be needed immediately before surgery. In this procedure, a nonleaking opening into the anterior chamber space is created, which may allow the space to be re-formed, with the introduction of air or a saline solution. It may also be possible to irrigate the anterior space and to restore intraocular pressure to normal. When paracentesis is correctly performed, the risks are very slight, especially when compared to the possible benefits. Paracentesis may also be performed after surgery to re-form the anterior chamber.

[4] Trabeculectomy

Trabeculectomy[9] is the procedure of choice in cases of acute primary angle-closure glaucoma when iridectomy is considered inadequate. Trabeculectomy is also the procedure of choice in uncontrolled chronic angle-closure glaucoma.

10.90 COMPLICATIONS OF GLAUCOMA SURGERY

Specific complications of glaucoma surgery include flat anterior chamber, failure to filter, suprachoroidal hemorrhage, problems related

---

[8] *See* 10.90 *infra.*

[9] *See* 10.82[2] *supra.*

to repair of blebs (blood blisters) and endophthalmitis, an infection starting in the bleb (Spaeth, 1990).

10.91   Flat Anterior Chamber

Many surgical operations are designed to enable the aqueous to leave the eye more easily. The complication that may occur in all these procedures is the flat anterior chamber, a condition that is very difficult to define. A flat anterior chamber may mean different things to different physicians and may come about for many different reasons. Moreover, a flat anterior chamber in one patient may never cause problems, while the same circumstance in another patient may be very troublesome.

In the effort to define flat anterior chamber, its diagnosis and treatment, the condition should be divided into three types, since treatment differs for each type. In type one, there is contact between the edge of the iris and the surface of the cornea, with some preservation of the anterior space adjacent to an iridectomy, if that procedure had been done. In type two, the front surface of the iris touches the rear surface of the cornea, with no preservation of anterior space but some space between the cornea and the lens surface. In type three, the iris and the cornea are completely in contact and the lens is in contact with the cornea, with no anterior space at all. These three types behave differently and require different treatment. Furthermore, the condition of the eye changes gradually after surgery and may be quite different two weeks or four weeks postoperatively.

Diagnosis of flat anterior chamber as a complication of eye surgery includes monitoring the level of intraocular pressure and the nature of aqueous flow, which may be done by intravenous injection of fluorescein dye. The condition of the pupil and the iridotomy must also be watched for signs of obstruction, using diagnostic ultrasound.

Treatment of flat anterior chamber is surgical, with the goal of reforming the anterior chamber. Many possible procedures may accomplish the task, and each of those is designed to reconstruct the anterior chamber using a viscoelastic substance, which both stretches and adheres to ocular structures. If the anterior chamber space is successfully reopened, intraocular pressure can be maintained at a normal level.

10.92 Failure to Filter

After a filtering operation for glaucoma, the intraocular pressure may remain elevated, which usually means that there is still a stubborn resistance to the outflow of aqueous. This development does not necessarily mean that the surgery has failed. In some cases, one or more sutures in the surgically created flap of skin may be too tight and need to be released, usually by means of an argon laser. In other cases, the trabecular meshwork may be functioning poorly as a result of the trauma of surgery. As healing proceeds, the meshwork may resume its normal function, and additional filtering of aqueous comes about as a result of the trabeculotomy. These two mechanisms together may mean that intraocular pressure is then lower than it was before surgery.

If, in the immediate period after surgery, normal outflow of aqueous still does not take place, gentle compression of the globe—in highly selected cases—may sometimes be helpful. However, this is a controversial issue. In the literature, compression is sometimes called massage, a term usually thought to imply motion rather than pressure. Motion combined with compression of the eye can do a great deal of damage, such as ruptured incisions and significant bleeding. When compression is used, the goal is to force aqueous to flow through the fistula (opening) that was created surgically as another outflow channel for aqueous. If the fistula is temporarily blocked, gentle pressure on the globe may, in some cases, momentarily raise intraocular pressure enough to expel the blockage and open the fistula.

10.93 Suprachoroidal Hemorrhage

The term suprachoroidal hemorrhage refers to excessive bleeding between the choroid (the middle layer) and the sclera (the outer protective layer) of the globe. Suprachoroidal hemorrhage is one of the most dreaded complications of eye surgery. Fortunately the causes and treatment of this complication are better understood now than in the past, and appropriate preventive measures can now be used to limit the development of these hemorrhages during or after surgery.

Factors that predispose a patient to suprachoroidal hemorrhage include the presence of glaucoma, systemic hypertension (higher than normal blood pressure), many years of very high intraocular pressure and advancing age of the patient. Glaucoma patients are ten times as likely as other patients to experience suprachoroidal hemorrhage as a result of eye surgery.

Before eye surgery is attempted in a high-risk patient, intraocular pressure should be brought down and kept down, if possible, for an extended period. During surgery, blood pressure should be well controlled and monitored carefully, and a general anesthetic should be used. After surgery, a high-risk patient should be strongly warned against strenuous activity, which can bring on hemorrhage.

10.94   Repair of Leaking or Excessive Conjunctival Blebs

Repairing a leaky bleb (blood blister) on the conjunctiva (the inner lining of the eyelid) is difficult, though not impossible, and may lead to further complications if it is attempted. The surgeon's main goal in these cases is to maintain the health of the optic nerve. If the optic nerve is already severely damaged, it may be preferable for the patient to bear with the side effects of the leaking bleb, with medical management that includes antibiotic ointment to guard against infection, and careful monitoring. If, however, the optic nerve is healthy, it may be preferable to repair the bleb in an effort to prevent damage. Surgical repair is also recommended when filtering blebs cause recurrent infection. In all cases of leaking blebs, the first approach is medical.

10.95   Endophthalmitis

Endophthalmitis is a severe inflammation affecting the uveal tract, vitreous body and retina, characterized by suppurating (pus-producing) sores. The organism responsible for the inflammation may be introduced by accidental or surgical trauma as well as by some systemic and ocular diseases (Burchfield, et al., 1996; Rosenberg and Siegfried, 1996).

Endophthalmitis spread from a leaking bleb and treated early in its course has a good outlook. On the other hand, some late cases of bacterial endophthalmitis cause rapid and permanent damage. The more serious form of the inflammation occurs when there is direct touching of an infected bleb and the vitreous. This extremely damaging type of inflammation must be treated aggressively if sight in the affected eye is to be saved.

Treatment of endophthalmitis is accomplished with antibiotics injected into the vitreous body. Some physicians use a combination of antibiotics administered systemically and intraocularly, and others use only intraocular injection. Vitrectomy, a surgical procedure that involves incision(s) into the vitreous for the purpose of removing foreign bodies, areas of dead cells or infection, is advocated by some authors as an adjunct to antibiotic therapy.

Vitrectomy may help control the infection in several ways: by removing live bacteria from the eye, by washing out bacterial enzymes and necrotic (dead or dying) inflammatory cells, and also by allowing for better diffusion of antibiotics throughout the vitreous cavity (McNamara and Benson, 1990). However, the role of vitrectomy in the treatment of endophthalmitis remains a matter of controversy. Antibiotics alone have cured some cases of endophthalmitis, as have the combination of vitrectomy and antibiotics.

10.100 BIBLIOGRAPHY

Text References

Apple, D. J. and Rabb, M. F.: Glaucoma. In: Apple, D. J. and Rabb. M. F.: Ocular Pathology, Clinical Applications and Self-Assessment. St. Louis: Mosby-Year Book, 1991.

Arora, R., et al.: Renal Hypertension Presenting as Acute Angle Closure Glaucoma [letter]. Arch. Ophthalmol. 109(6):776, June 1991.

Benson, W. E.: Retinal Detachment. In: Spaeth, G. L.: Ophthalmic Surgery: Principles and Practice. Philadelphia: Saunders, 1990.

Burchfield, J. C., et al.: Endophthalmitis following Trabeculectomy with Releasable Sutures [letter]. Arch. Ophthalmol. 114(6):766, June 1996.

Caronia, R. M., et al.: Increase in Iris-Lens Contact after Laser Iridotomy for Pupillary Block Angle Closure. Am. J. Ophthalmol. 122(1):53-57, July 1996.

Gadallah, M. F., et al.: Case Report: Mannitol Nephrotoxicity Syndrome: Role of Hemodialysis and Postulate of Mechanisms. Am. J. Med. Sci. 309(4):219-222, Apr. 1995.

Ghezzi, K. and Renner, G. S.: Ophthalmic Disorders. In: Rosen, P. and Barkin, R. M.: Emergency Medicine, Concepts and Clinical Practice, Vol III. St. Louis: Mosby-Year Book, 1992.

The Glaucoma Laser Trial (GLT) and Glaucoma Laser Trial Follow-up Study: 7. Results. Glaucoma Laser Trial Research Group. Am. J. Ophthalmol. 120(6):718-731, Dec. 1995.

The Glaucoma Laser Trial (GLT): 6. Treatment Group Differences in Visual Field Changes. Glaucoma Laser Trial Research Group. Am. J. Ophthalmol. 120(1):10-22, July 1995.

Gross, F. L., et al.: Increased Prevalence of Occludable Angles and Angle-Closure Glaucoma in Patients with Pseudoexfoliation. Am. J. Ophthalmol. 117(3):333-336, Mar. 1994.

Hall, S. K.: Acute Angle-Closure Glaucoma as a Complication of Combined Beta-agonist and Ipratropium Bromide Therapy in the Emergency Department. Am. Emerg. Med. 23(4):884-887, Apr. 1994.

Henry, G. L.: Headache. In: Rosen, P. and Barkin, R. M.: Emergency Medicine, Concepts and Clinical Practice, Vol III. St. Louis: Mosby-Year Book, 1992.

McNamara, J. A. and Benson, W. E.: Vitrectomy. In: Spaeth, G. L.: Ophthalmic Surgery: Principles and Practice. Philadelphia: Saunders, 1990.

Mitchell, J. D. and Schwartz, A. L.: Acute Angle-Closure Glaucoma associated with Intranasal Cocaine Abuse. Am. J. Ophthalmol. 122(3):425-426, Sept. 1996.

Newell, F. W.: The Glaucomas. In: Newell, F. W.: Ophthalmology, Principles and Concepts. St. Louis: Mosby-Year Book, 1992.

Oram, O., et al.: Picosecond neodymium:yttrium Fluoride (Nd:YLF) Laser Peripheral Iridotomy. Am J. Ophthalmol. 119(4):408-414, Apr. 1995.

Pederson, J. E.: Glaucoma, A Primer for Primary Care Physicians. Postgrad. Med. 90(7):41-45, 48, Nov. 1991.

Quigley, H. A., et al.: Rate of Progression in Open-Angle Glaucoma Estimated from Cross-sectional Prevalence of Visual Field Damage. Am. J. Ophthalmol. 122(3):355-363, Sept. 1996.

Rosenberg, C. A. and Adams, S. L.: Narrow-Angle Glaucoma Presenting as Acute, Painless Visual Impairment. Ann. Emerg. Med. 20(9):1020-1022, Sep. 1991.

Rosenberg, L. F. and Siegfried, C. J.: Endophthalmitis associated with a Releasable Suture [letter]. In: Arch. Ophthalmol. 144(6):767, June 1996.

Shin, D. H., et al.: Effect of Topical Anti-inflammatory Treatment on the Outcome of Laser Trabeculoplasty. The Fluorometholone-Laser Trabeculoplasty Study Group. Am. J. Ophthalmol. 122(3):349-354, Sept. 1996.

Spaeth, G. L.: Glaucoma Surgery. In: Spaeth, G. L.: Ophthalmic Surgery: Principles and Practice. Philadelphia: Saunders, 1990.

Stewart, W. C., et al.: Surgical vs. Medical Management of Chronic Open-Angle Glaucoma. Am. J. Ophthalmol. 122(6):767-774, Dec. 1996.

CHAPTER 11

CATARACT

SCOPE

Age-related cataract can be divided into two basic types—nuclear, which occur deep in the lens, and cortical, which are more superficial—although both forms may occur together. Varying degrees of age-related change can be found in more than half of individuals between the ages of 50 and 60; past the age of 60, changes are apparent in well over three fourths of people. A genetic component appears to be involved in the development of age-related cataract, but the multifactorial nature of cataractogenesis makes it generally difficult to isolate individual factors.

SYNOPSIS

11.00   INTRODUCTION

A cataract is a loss of the natural transparency of the crystalline lens of the eye due to opacification (clouding). The opacities may be small and local, or involve the entire lens; they may be of various shapes, sizes, forms, colors and intensities (Olson, 1991). The shape and appearance of one of the earliest lens opacities to be described resembled a waterfall (in Latin, *cataracta*), hence the name.

Opacification of the lens may be caused by hereditary factors, trauma, inflammation, metabolic or nutritional disorders or defects, radiation or, most commonly, the effects of aging (Murrill, et al., 1994). There are many different forms of cataract; each differs with respect to its etiology and the biochemical mechanisms of formation (Datiles and Kinoshita, 1991). The most common anatomic types are *nuclear* (deep in the lens), *cortical* (more superficial) and *subcapsular* (beneath the capsule, or the thin membrane surrounding the lens) (Murrill, et al., 1994).

The eye that contains its original crystalline lens is termed a *phakic* eye. The eye from which the biologic lens has been removed or lost due to trauma is termed an *aphakic* eye. The eye in which a prosthetic (intraocular) lens has been implanted to replace the natural lens is termed a *pseudophakic* eye. Aphakia and pseudophakia may be unilateral or bilateral, depending on whether one or both eyes are affected.

Cataract is the most common cause of visual impairment and blindness throughout the world; however, technical advances of the past two decades, coupled with the availability of improved training opportunities for specialists in industrialized countries, has improved operative results and tremendously decreased the incidence of visual impairment and blindness in these countries (Douthewaite, 1993a). At the same time, it must be kept in mind that the success of surgery or any other treatment for cataract depends on the integrity of other ocular structures. For example, the most flawless cataract surgery will be of little value for a patient whose eye has a damaged retina.

The chances that such damage will exist are much greater in cases of traumatic eye injury, so that in these cases, the prognosis for the outcome of cataract surgery is immediately more guarded. Moreover, postoperative complications, early or late, may occur following even the most perfect surgery. The increasing trend to co-management of the patient by optometrist and ophthalmic surgeon may provide the patient with improved care (Revicki, et al., 1993; Murrill et al., 1994; Bettman, 1990).

In cases of decreased vision, it is important to evaluate not only the decrease in vision as measured by the Snellen chart (the standard "E" eye chart) but to take into account ancillary factors as well, such as loss of visual field, loss of depth perception, loss of binocular vision and psychological impairment. The responsibility of the optometrist and ophthalmologist to diagnose co-existing eye disease and to warn the patient of the adverse effects of eye disease on his or her life generally is now being codified in federal and professional guidelines for the delivery of eye care (Murrill, et al., 1994b).

11.10 EFFECTS OF LENS OPACIFICATION ON VISION

Cataract, or lens opacification, is the cause of blindness in 13 million people worldwide, accounting for 50 percent of all cases of blindness (Douthwaite, 1993a). Lens opacification is not synonymous with blindness, however; rather, cataract is usually regarded more broadly as producing a reduction in visual performance. Visual performance may be reduced in numerous ways and to varying degrees by various types of lens opacities. Worldwide, approximately 50 million people experience cataract-related reduction in visual performance (Douthwaite, 1993a).

To understand these lens changes and their effects, the optometrist and/or ophthalmologist must be thoroughly familiar with the structure and function of the eye. Depending on its location within the lens, a cataract can cause loss of visual acuity (sharpness of vision), visual field changes (changes in the entire area the eye can see while looking straight ahead), monocular diplopia (double vision in which one object is seen as two with one eye), binocular diplopia (in which a single object is seen as two by both eyes, the eyes being unable to fuse the visual stimuli into a single image) and loss of coordination of binocular vision (ability of the brain to integrate images seen by both eyes).

11.11   In General

The initial complaint of a patient with cataract is typically that of impaired vision; most commonly, this involves a slow, progressive, painless deterioration in visual acuity that is described as a film, fog or grease mark over the eye. In some instances, the question may arise whether a cataract is causally related to or aggravated by an injury. It is the physician's responsibility to identify all possible sources of this complaint and to determine which of them are contributing to it and to what extent. If the impaired vision is found to be due to cataract, the physician must further determine whether there is a disability that prevents the person from performing daily activities that are either desired by or required of him or her.

In approaching the patient with a complaint of impaired vision, both subjective and objective findings must be obtained and combined. Many physicians use the SOAP formula: obtain the patient's Subjective complaints and history, collect Objective data, combine subjective and objective findings to make an Assessment and formulate a treatment and management Plan. Subjective findings should include the chief complaint, ocular history and general medical history. A careful and detailed history of the claimant's visual symptoms can be helpful and sometimes crucial in pinpointing the inception and progression of cataract. It is therefore important to review these symptoms and then question the claimant in great detail regarding the sequence and overall chronology of symptoms.

Objective findings should include tests of vision, pupils, refraction, intraocular pressure, slit lamp evaluation (SLE), dilated fundus examination (DFE) and other neurologic and binocular testing. The assessment should include an evaluation of all significant potential causes of the complaint, including relevant co-existing conditions. The treatment plan should include provisions for all contributing conditions.

The general sequence of cataract formation proceeds from an initial disturbance of vision, to a reduction of vision, to a loss of vision. The ultimate degree of visual impairment produced, however, is largely influenced by the location of the opacity (Hesler, 1993). A posterior opacity (on the back of the lens) causes greater reduction of vision, since it is located closer to the retina (layer of light-sensitive nerve endings lining the back of the eye) and forms a larger shadow than an anterior opacity (at the front of the lens) or peripheral opacity. An axial opacity (at the center of the lens) causes less impairment in dim light, when the pupil is dilated, as the patient is able to see around the opacity through the clear portion of the lens.

In the case of a peripheral opacity, a bright light contracts the pupil, eliminating the opacity from view and causing a pinhole effect, thus improving vision. In opacities in the nucleus of the lens (inner layer), the increasing density increases the refractive (light-bending and focusing) power of the lens, thus increasing myopia (nearsightedness) or decreasing hyperopia (farsightedness). It is relatively common for such patients, particularly older ones, to eventually develop what is known as second sight, the ability to see at close range to the extent that they no longer need reading glasses.

11.12 Specific Symptoms of Cataracts

Beyond the general complaint of deterioration of visual performance, there are nine specific ocular signs and symptoms of cataract formation: myopic shift, monocular diplopia, astigmatism, contrast sensitivity reduction, glare, color shift, light transmission reduction, visual field loss and visual acuity reduction (Hesler, 1993). Some of these occur in other eye disorders as well (e.g., glaucoma[1]); sometimes two or more disorders, such as cataract and glaucoma, co-exist. There is thus considerable potential for confusion in making the differential diagnosis.

---

[1] *See also* ch. 10.

[1]   Myopic Shift

Normal aging of the crystalline lens causes a shift to hyperopia (farsightedness). During the progression of nuclear cataract, in contrast, the hardening and compacting of the lens causes an increase in the refractive index (light-bending and focusing properties) of the lens and a shift to myopia (nearsightedness). A shift of 0.50 diopter (D; a measurement of refractive power) measured two years apart more than offsets the normal hyperopic shift and indicates that a cataract is developing in the nuclear (core) region of the lens. At first, patients are often delighted that they are able to see well with weaker glasses, but eventually the light-scattering effect of the cataract causes degradation of the image projected onto the retina and other deficiencies in visual performance.

[2]   Monocular Diplopia

Seeing two images with the same eye is due to the uneven changes in the refractive index that occur in a cataractous lens. A localized area of differing refractive index acts like a prism and splits the incoming light rays into two images. Various disorders of the retina can also cause monocular diplopia. Differentiation can be made with a pinhole. If the diplopia is due to cataractous refractive changes in the lens, the diplopia will be eliminated when the pinhole is in place; if due to retinal pathology, the double vision will remain. Correction of monocular diplopia with spectacles is very difficult, but the patient may at least be made less aware of the double image.

[3]   Astigmatism

Refractive changes in the lens during cataract progression cause fluctuations in the eye with astigmatism (blurred vision due to irregularities in the surface of the cornea). Objective methods are generally unhelpful in determining astigmatic correction in patients with cataract. Spectacle correction can often correct all or most astigmatic shifts due to cataract progression (Steinert, et al., 1991b).

[4]   Contrast Sensitivity Reduction

The increasing light scattering effect of a cataractous lens causes a progressive reduction in the ability of the person to perceive objects with low contrast relative to their background. On a practical note, this calls into question the ability of a person with cataract to drive safely in foggy and rainy conditions, when visual performance is likely to be below legal levels.

Contrast sensitivity assessment is now regarded as a more thorough evaluation of visual performance than visual acuity (sharpness) (Elliott, et al., 1990a). It can be measured quickly and inexpensively by means of a number of contrast sensitivity charts, such as the Pelli-Robson chart and the Cambridge low-contrast gratings test (Elliott, 1993a; Elliott and Whitaker, 1992). Because the reduction in contrast sensitivity in patients with uniocular cataract is more impaired than measurements on the better eye alone would indicate, it is important to test binocular contrast sensitivity in these individuals (Pardhan and Gilchrist, 1991).

[5] Glare

Glare is caused by forward scattering (i.e., toward the retina) of light by a cataract. This causes objects to be perceived poorly, particularly in low light, such as at dusk or at night (van den Berg, 1991). If the pupil dilates normally, visual acuity may test as satisfactory. It should be noted that aging of the normal lens in middle-aged individuals also produces light scattering and poor visual performance due to glare (Lasa, et al., 1992).

Glare can be tested using a number of clinical instruments, such as the brightness acuity tester (Elliott, 1993a; Elliott, 1993b). A simple and effective glare test is to shine a penlight into the eye being evaluated, at a distance of about a foot, while the patient reads a Snellen chart (standard eye chart used to examine visual acuity, in which the lines of print are arranged so that each lower line is progressively smaller than the one above). A normal eye will be unaffected by the light, but an eye with cataract will manifest impaired performance (Elliott and Bullimore, 1993).

[6] Color Shift

With aging, the normal lens progressively absorbs more light at the blue end of the spectrum. As a result, less blue light reaches the retina, and the person experiences diminished blue color perception. Cataract further increases blue light absorption and the resultant effect. Cataractous changes (e.g., amber to black coloration of the lens nucleus) can be seen using a slit lamp (a microscopelike instrument used to examine the eye). With this instrument, the exact location and position of the lens opacity can be ascertained. After cataract removal, some individuals experience a fleeting blue vision called cyanopsia. Many patients are delighted at the depth and vividness of colors, having become accustomed to dull hues, often for years.

[7]   Light Transmission Reduction

Thickening of the crystalline lens with age causes reduced light transmission due to increased absorption and light scattering. The pupil also has reduced capacity for dilating in low light. Although the retina in a normal eye has considerable capacity to adapt with respect to its sensitivity to light, absorption and light scattering by a cataract will overwhelm this capacity; much less light reaches the retina, and vision is reduced, especially under poor lighting conditions. Vision can be improved if the pupil is allowed to dilate (i.e., by avoiding medications, if possible, that prevent this or cause pupillary constriction).

[8]   Visual Field Loss

Visual field loss or reduction is produced when a cataract casts a shadow on the retina. Visual field changes also occur in glaucoma (condition involving buildup of pressure within the eye). A developing cataract can be misdiagnosed as an increasing glaucomatous field defect in a patient already diagnosed with glaucoma. Increasing the illumination of the test stimulus during perimetry (quantitative assessment of visual acuity in all sectors of the visual fields) can help distinguish the two conditions.

[9]   Visual Acuity Reduction

The measurement of visual acuity, which is done under ideal conditions in the clinic, provides a poor assessment of visual performance under conditions that prevail in the real world (Geddes, et al., 1990). Specifically, it tends to overestimate the patient's true visual performance. The letters on the Snellen chart, for example, have a contrast of nearly 100 percent, whereas the contrast of newsprint is considerably less (Hesler, 1993). In the examination room, lighting is bright and generally free from glare; when driving at night, on the other hand, lighting is poor and there is a lot of glare from oncoming headlights. Under the latter condition, the visual performance of a person with cataract would most likely be below legal levels.

11.13 Progression of Cataracts

With the exception of traumatic cataract, in which the lens capsule is damaged and progression is very rapid, most cataracts develop and progress slowly. The rate of progression varies with each case, however, and is unpredictable, as is the need for surgery; not all cataracts require surgical treatment (Albert and Jakobiec, 1993).

A cataract may progress rapidly for several months and then slow for an unpredictable length of time. In some cases, progression of a cataract may cease altogether. In some of these cases, the condition may remain arrested for the rest of the person's life; others may resume after months or years and progress at an unpredictable rate.

Both the patient and the physician will be aware when progression is occurring, through subjective and objective measures of visual performance. It is important to incorporate into the patient assessment protocol methods that assess retinal and neural function as well as cataract, since deterioration of visual function can be caused by a deterioration of retinal or optic nerve function as well as by cataract (Hurst, et al., 1993b).

The doctor should be sure that the patient understands the foregoing facts of the situation in order to prevent the person from becoming fatalistic and depressed, especially in the early stages of cataract.

11.14 Cataract-induced Glaucoma

Perhaps the most important complication of cataract progression, in addition to diminishment of visual acuity, is the development of glaucoma. Glaucoma is characterized by increased intraocular pressure due to restriction of the normal outflow of the aqueous fluid from the anterior chamber of the eye into the angle between the iris (pigmented part of the eye) and the cornea (transparent dome in front of the lens) and thus into Schlemm's canal. As the condition progresses, it is accompanied by excavation and degeneration of the optic disk (the region where the nerve fibers converge and leave the eye to form the optic nerve), nerve fiber damage, visual field defects (blind spots) and eventual blindness. In cataract-induced glaucoma, the normal drainage of aqueous is obstructed by the increasing size of the lens, which results from the continual laying down of new lens fibers by the epithelial (outer layer) cells of the lens.

It is therefore necessary for the cataract patient to be examined every four to six months for the development of glaucoma. If glaucoma is found, it must be treated medically or surgically in order to prevent permanent loss of vision from this condition.

When glaucoma co-exists with cataract, whether it has been induced by cataract or was pre-existing, two important questions must be answered (Weatherill, 1993):

1. Has glaucoma destroyed the visual field of the eye to the extent that cataract surgery would be useless or dangerous? Surgery within the eye in patients with severely restricted visual fields can lead to complete blindness. On the other hand, cataract removal in patients with glaucoma makes it easier to see and monitor the optic disk, increases the reliability of diagnostic perimetry and allows miotic (pupil-contracting) drops to be used without impairing visual acuity.

2. Is the glaucoma well controlled, or is surgical treatment (trabeculectomy) necessary? Open-angle glaucoma that has been well controlled with medication usually remains well controlled following cataract surgery. Closed-angle glaucoma, on the other hand, is unpredictable and requires close monitoring. If surgical treatment of glaucoma is required, several options must be considered. Glaucoma and cataract surgery may be performed at the same time, or they may be done in sequence, with the more urgent problem being treated first. Cataract surgery is more difficult following glaucoma or other drainage surgery, and therefore more risky. Nevertheless, it should be done when indicated, for the reasons just enumerated.

11.20 CATARACTS CAUSED BY MECHANICAL TRAUMA

Traumatic cataracts develop secondary to blunt or penetrating injury of the eye. There may be frank structural damage to the lens as well as to the zonules (threadlike suspensory ligaments arranged like wheel spokes around the circumference of the lens, holding it in place).

11.21 Concussion and Contusion of the Eyeball

Cataract formation or lens subluxation (partial dislocation) occurs in 25 percent of all cases of blunt trauma to the eye, being more common in cases of severe trauma (Kwitko and Kwitko, 1990). Cataracts due to blunt trauma are most commonly star-shaped. Complete opacification of the lens (uniform milky appearance) may occur with blunt trauma but is more typical of penetrating trauma (Young, 1993a).

[1] Mechanism of Injury

The mechanism of these injuries is mechanical. In essence, the rigidity of the lens and the capsule (thin membrane) result in most of the energy of a blow being dissipated almost entirely within these structures. The resulting disruption of lens fiber junctions produces layers of optical discontinuity, lens fiber necrosis (tissue death) and opacity (Hurst, 1993a). The capsule may be torn or separated from the lens. In some cases, a tear in the anterior aspect of the capsule may be sealed off by fibrin (a protein substance involved in clotting), preventing absorption of fluid by the lens. The result can be a local opacification with no visual loss, provided the opacity is not in the optical center of the lens (Young, 1993a).

[2] Evolution of the Lesion

The cataract may develop quickly (over hours, weeks or months) or slowly (over years). In individuals under 40 years of age, lens opacities are usually localized and stationary. In many cases, there is no associated vision loss (Murrill, et al., 1994). The lesions are in the subcapsular zone (below the capsule, the thin membrane surrounding the lens), and usually anterior. As time goes by, the opacities become buried by the formation of new clear lens fibers so that they eventually lie deeply within the lens and are separated from the capsule by an optically clear zone. In people older than 40, similar opacities may be followed by progressive changes typical of what is known as senile cataract. These cases have a guarded prognosis, as the cataract could develop to the point of complete vision loss, requiring cataract surgery (Young, 1993a). An eye that has sustained blunt trauma should be examined with a gonioscope (instrument for direct observation of the angle of the anterior chamber of the eye) to ascertain if there has been any damage to the anterior chamber angle, particularly angle recession, which is associated with an increased risk of traumatic glaucoma (Murrill, et al., 1994).

11.22 Classification of Concussion-related Cataracts

Concussion-related lens opacities can be recognized and classified on the basis of their appearance and location within the lens (Chylack, et al., 1992). The location, as well as the density, of the opacities also determines the degree of visual impairment that will exist (Luntz, 1991). Vision is reduced most by axial opacities (i.e., those lying on an imaginary line or axis running from the center of the pupil to the center of the retina). Posterior opacities (toward the back of the lens, closer to the retina) cause more visual loss than anterior opacities, owing to the larger shadow cast on the retina by posterior opacities.

[1]   Vossius' Ring Opacity

This is a ring of iris pigment that results from imprinting of the pupillary border on the anterior lens capsule during a concussion. It appears only in young individuals and tends to disappear slowly over several weeks or months.

[2]   Subepithelial Opacities

Discrete subepithelial opacities may be few or numerous, transient or permanent, depending on the magnitude of the trauma. Subepithelial disseminated traumatic opacities are small, flat, discrete, punctate or flaky opacities that are adjacent to the anterior lens capsule, axial (center of the lens) or equatorial (periphery of the lens) in distribution. They may appear and disappear within a few days or weeks after the injury, or their appearance may be delayed for up to two years. In rare cases, the opacities may be dense, round and discrete, resembling a small anterior polar cataract (cataracta nodiformis). A diffuse subcapsular cobweb opacity, which may be centrally or eccentrically located, has also been described. The latter follow a sudden, violent concussion and are permanent.

[3]   Traumatic Rosette-shaped Opacity

This is the most typical type of traumatic cataract and follows both blunt and penetrating eye trauma. Rosette-shaped (stellate) opacities may be classified as fresh or late. Fresh rosette opacities are evident a few hours, weeks or months after the trauma; they are usually located anteriorly after blunt trauma and posteriorly after penetrating trauma. They may disappear completely within a few days or weeks. Late rosettes are seen several years after the trauma, located deep in the lens cortex (outer layer) or in the adult nucleus, separated from the lens capsule by a clear zone of varying thickness.

[4]   Post-traumatic Atrophy of the Lens

Blunt trauma can result in atrophy (wasting) of the lens. This can affect visual performance by affecting the refractive (focusing) power of the lens.

[5]   Presenile and Senile Lens Changes

These changes occur following blunt trauma in individuals 40 to 45 years of age. The changes consist of coronary cataract, sclerosis (hardening) of the lens nucleus, punctate opacities of the lens cortex and water clefts. The changes are progressive, and, as with all cataracts, the rate of progression will vary unpredictably; progression may stop intermittently or even permanently.

[6]   Diffuse Concussion Cataract

These opacities are rare, except when associated with rupture of the lens capsule. A rapidly spreading milkiness of the lens occurs due to uptake of aqueous by the lens. In young people, the lens material may absorb completely, leaving a transparent lens capsule. In older persons, complications such as iritis (inflammation of the iris) and glaucoma occur with degenerative changes, and the lens must be removed. The prognosis is guarded.

11.23   Treatment of Concussion Cataracts

Treatment of an eye that is already injured must be based on careful assessment of the injury and its effect on vision, since the risk of operative complications may be increased by the existing damage. When there is disabling obstruction of vision and/or uncontrollable glaucoma caused by the cataract, the damaged lens should be removed immediately and replaced with an intraocular lens (IOL) implant.[2] Any infection must be controlled prior to surgery. The presence of uveitis (inflammation of the uvea, the middle coat of the eye), is no longer considered a contraindication to IOL implantation, due to the availability of modern surgical techniques and heparin-coated lenses (Weatherill, 1993).

Disruption of the zonules (suspensory ligaments of the lens) and recession (widening) of the anterior chamber angle (angle between the iris and the cornea, which provides drainage for the aqueous humor in the front part of the eye) may complicate removal of the cataract.

---

[2] *See* 11.44 *infra.*

Implantation of an anterior chamber IOL may be contraindicated if there is significant recession of the anterior chamber angle, particularly in the presence of elevated intraocular pressure (Balyeat, 1990).

11.24   Displacement of the Crystalline Lens

Displacement of the lens can involve partial dislocation (subluxation) or complete dislocation (luxation). These injuries result from traumatic tearing of part or all of the suspensory ligaments (zonules) of the lens. The lens can be displaced in any direction, depending on which area of the zonules has been affected.

A characteristic sign of subluxation is trembling of the iris on movement of the eye (iridodonesis). A predisposition to subluxation of the lens due to atrophy of the zonules can be caused by a congenital defect in the zonules as well as diseases such as Marfan's syndrome, mature cataract, high myopia (severe nearsightedness), old uveitis and syphilis. In these cases, subluxation may be produced by a much less forceful trauma than in a normal eye.

The decision to remove a subluxated lens is based on the needs of the patient (Gressel, 1991). Some patients retain good vision with subluxation. Others may develop myopia (nearsightedness), often with marked astigmatism and impairment of accommodation (alteration of the lens shape) or monocular or binocular diplopia (double vision). Some patients will do well with spectacle or contact lens correction. Other patients will develop lens opacities; while most of these are localized, stationary and not associated with significant loss of vision, some people will develop opacities requiring cataract extraction within 12 months of injury. Some patients will develop retinal detachment, before or after surgical removal of the subluxated lens.

Because lens displacement is a zonular injury, intracapsular cataract extraction (ICCE; removal of the entire lens, including the capsule or outer membrane) is usually required. The lens implant is placed in the sulcus (groove) and sutured, or an anterior chamber implant is used (Murrill, et al., 1994).

Damage to the anterior chamber angle commonly results in a slow rise in intraocular pressure. Angle-recession glaucoma may develop. These angle changes are diagnosed by gonioscopy, a procedure in which a contact lens with mirrors is placed on the eyeball, enabling the physician to view the anterior chamber angle. Decreased vision of the affected eye can lead to binocular diplopia (double vision), loss of depth perception, loss of binocular vision and, eventually, to turning in or out of the affected eye (internal or external strabismus).

Total dislocation of the lens can occur primarily, following blunt trauma to the eyeball, or it can result from the conversion of a subluxation into a total dislocation, either spontaneously or following additional trauma. In total dislocation, with rupture of all the zonules, the lens can drop into the vitreous (gelatinous fluid filling the back part of the eye). This may cause no complications, or it may lead to uveitis, glaucoma or detachment of the retina. Alternatively, the lens may drop into the anterior chamber, where it usually causes acute glaucoma, necessitating immediate removal. Pathologic degenerative changes occur in a lens that has been dislocated.

11.25　Lens Changes due to Perforation of the Eyeball

Penetrating trauma is an ocular emergency. If the lens itself is penetrated, the lens fibers will imbibe aqueous fluid, and opacification will develop rapidly (Murrill, et al., 1994). Penetrating injuries are usually due to a sharp object, such as a knife, piece of glass or wire, or an intraocular foreign body. A mass of copper within the eye can give rise to a yellowish lens opacity or sunflower cataract; a mass of steel or iron can give rise to cataract and a brown discoloration of the lens.

Occasionally the globe can be ruptured by a direct blow, especially if there is a pre-existing weak point due to a congenital defect or previous injury. The lens changes in these cases resemble those following blunt trauma of the eyeball (Chawla, 1993).

[1]　Localized Nonprogressive Changes

Localized nonprogressive changes are usually due to small puncture injuries caused by a small foreign body such as a thorn or needle piercing the lens. The capsule is damaged but seals, occasionally with a bulge into the anterior chamber and/or the vitreous. Dots or linear opacities along the track of the wound may appear in many shaped and sizes.

[2]　Rosette (Star-shaped) Cataract

This type of cataract may appear at the anterior pole of the lens (the center of the front surface of the lens), but it appears more commonly at the posterior pole (the center of the back surface of the lens), within a few hours or days following the injury. It begins in the center of the lens but radiates rapidly to the periphery. In some cases, the cataract fades and even disappears, while in other cases, it remains and becomes buried by new layers of lens fibers, which are laid down more superficially. As time goes by, the star shape of the opacity changes to a lacework of vacuoles (small cavities) that gradually become smaller and more discrete.

[3]   Total Traumatic Cataract

In some cases, instead of forming a localized opacity, a perforated lens may rapidly imbibe aqueous and become swollen, milky and opaque; this is known as intumescent cataract. In younger individuals, the lens can be completely absorbed, leaving a clear capsule. After age 30, secondary glaucoma or recalcitrant iridocyclitis (inflammation of the iris and ciliary body) may make operative removal of the lens mandatory.

In severe cases, the capsule may be widely lacerated, and cortical material may pour into the anterior chamber. An eye with this condition is severely damaged and has a guarded prognosis. In recent years, the prognosis in many of these cases has improved enormously, due to advances such as computerized instruments and methods of cortical cleanup, vitrectomy (removal of vitreous), better sutures and microsurgery (Kwitko and Kwitko, 1990).

[4]   Displacement of the Lens under the Conjunctiva

A dislocated lens can also enter the area under the conjunctiva (membrane lining the inner surface of the eyelid and the front surface of the eye). As this cannot happen unless the eyeball has been perforated, it indicates a severely injured eyeball. It is frequently prudent not to remove the lens, since it may be acting as a plug in the hole in the eyeball. The lens will often disintegrate on its own, without having to be removed. When this occurs, damage to the interior of the eyeball caused by removal of the lens is avoided (Murrill, et al., 1994).

11.26   The Relationship Between Trauma and Cataract Formation

A complete and accurate history is mandatory for establishing or eliminating a given trauma as the cause of a cataract. Vital information to be collected include the date, time and place of the injury; the speed, size and configuration of any moving object or blunt instrument; and the patient's ocular status prior to the injury.

The responsibilities of optometrists and ophthalmologists are considered to be the following (O'Day, et al., 1993; Foreman, 1990a,b,c):

1. To accurately diagnose ocular disease other than cataract.

2. To warn the patient of the risk of cataract formation secondary to the use of some topical drugs (e.g., topical steroids) and of the consequences of visual impairment due to cataract (e.g., loss of legal privilege to drive).

3. For the optometrist, to refer the patient to an ophthalmologist when the diagnosis of cataract is made. Although this is a subjective decision and a controversial point, a sensible rule of thumb is to refer the patient when the cataract is impairing the person's ability to function and affecting his or her quality of life.

In the past, the role of the optometrist was to refer a patient who needed cataract surgery to an ophthalmologist and then to provide spectacle or contact lenses for visual correction after surgery. Today the optometrist is much more involved, and the optometrist and ophthalmologist may actually co-manage the patient preoperatively, intraoperatively and postoperatively (Murrill, et al., 1994).

11.30 OTHER ETIOLOGIC CONSIDERATIONS

The development of cataract may be a result of a wide variety of factors. Some of these are environmental (e.g., various types of trauma), some are genetic and others are related to metabolic changes or aging. There are also many different forms of lens opacification (clouding), with varying effects on vision.[3]

11.31 Toxic Drugs

In addition to accidental exposure to a chemical in the external environment, the development of cataract may also be due to excessive use, abuse or prolonged administration of several pharmacologic agents.

---

[3] *See* 11.10 *supra.*

[1] Corticosteroids

The administration of corticosteroids, either systemically or topically to the eye, is associated with the development of axial posterior subcapsular cataracts (in the rear region beneath the capsule, or the thin membrane surrounding the lens), within several months; the cataracts may later spread to the central posterior cortex of the lens. The development and size of these cataracts is dependent on the dose and duration of administration (Young, 1993b). Once formed, the opacity is usually irreversible, although there have been reports of very early reversibility with cessation of corticosteroid therapy; individual susceptibility may be involved (Young, 1993a).

Accordingly, all individuals requiring prolonged corticosteroid therapy should receive careful lens evaluations as part of their care. Corticosteroids are commonly used to treat inflammatory reactions. Ophthalmologic conditions commonly treated with corticosteroids include chronic iritis (inflammation of the iris), uveitis (inflammation of the uvea, the middle coat of the eye) and prophylaxis of cystoid macular edema (swelling of the macula, the portion of the retina responsible for sharp vision). Nonsteroidal anti-inflammatory drugs (NSAIDs) may provide a satisfactory alternative in problem cases (Murrill, et al., 1994).

[2] Miotic Agents

Miotic agents are drugs that cause the iris to constrict and the size of the pupil to decrease. They are used as eyedrops in the treatment of glaucoma and, less often, in the treatment of postsurgical corneal edema (swelling of the cornea) and monocular diplopia (a condition in which a single object appears as two, when looking with one eye) (Murrill, et al., 1994).

Prolonged use (12 to 24 months) of miotic agents is associated with the appearance and growth of anterior subcapsular lens opacities and vacuoles (small cavities), as well as cysts of the iris. Later there are changes in the cortical and nuclear regions of the lens, with consequent myopia.

The long-acting cholinesterase inhibitor echothiopate is most likely to cause these adverse effects. Standard dosing is by solutions of 0.03 percent to 0.25 percent twice a day. Another miotic agent, pilocarpine, administered four times a day in solutions of 1 percent to 4 percent, is associated with a lower incidence of drug-induced cataract. Nevertheless, the use of miotics has declined in light of these findings (Young, 1993b).

[3]   Chlorpromazine (Thorazine®)

Thorazine® is an antipsychotic drug used in the treatment of psychiatric disorders, especially schizophrenia. Large does (total dose of 2500 grams) over a prolonged period of time have been shown to produce bilateral axial anterior subcapsular deposits in 90 percent of patients. The exact nature of these white star-shaped opacities is not yet known. In most cases, they do not appear to have an adverse effect on vision. A small number of patients show more severe ocular changes and visual impairment. Because these changes are related to dose and duration, patients taking moderate to high doses (300 mg per day) over a long term (two years or more) should have regular eye exams (Physicians' Desk Reference, 1995).

[4]   Antimitotic Agents

Cataractous changes in the lens have been associated with the extensive use of antimitotic medications, which are substances that inhibit cell division. Antimitotic agents must therefore be considered and ruled out as a cause of cataract in patients who have undergone chemotherapy.

[5]   Other Toxic Drugs

Other substances implicated in causing cataracts are dinitrophenol, once a popular weight reducing agent; paradichlorobenzene, a moth repellant; and triparanol, a cholesterol-lowering agent. These substances are no longer in use.

Chloroquine and related substances used in the prophylaxis and treatment of malaria, lupus erythematosus, rheumatoid arthritis, ankylosing spondylitis, hepatic amebiasis and leishmaniasis have been associated with the deposition of pinpoint flakes beneath the posterior capsule in the axial region in 40 percent of cases (Newell, 1992). These changes appear to be nonprogressive and do not cause a significant decrease of vision.

An association between ethanol, alcoholism and cataract has also been reported (Newell, 1992). Alkali burns of the eye, which are very destructive, cause cataract secondary to ischemia (deficiency of the blood supply) of the anterior segment; these cataracts may become intumescent (swollen and enlarged).

11.32   Environmental Causes

Several physical agents and factors in the external environment can cause lens damage and cataract as a result of energy transfer to the lens.

[1]   Electricity

In general, the aftermath of electric shock is quite variable as far as cataract formation is concerned (Young, 1993a). Significant eye injuries have not occurred at less than 200 volts, but otherwise the degree of lens change bears no relation to the strength of the current. Changes tend to be bilateral in lightning cataract and unilateral in industrial accidents, but this rule is not absolute. The onset of electrically induced cataract varies tremendously, from 2 to 6 months to up to 11 years. The cataracts can be anterior subcapsular (in the front region beneath the capsule, or the thin membrane surrounding the lens), posterior subcapsular (in the back region beneath the capsule) or cortical (more superficial).

Regression, partial disappearance or complete disappearance of the opacity may occur. Frequently vacuoles (tiny bubbles) form beneath the capsule; gray opacities form beneath the capsule as well as in the capsule and subcapsular regions. The opacities may take the form of straight and/or winding linear streaks as well as other configurations.

In some cases, vision remains quite good, while in others, maturation of the cataract occurs in about six months.

[2]   Heat and Cold

Lens changes due to exposure to heat (infrared radiation) typically follow chronic exposure to subclinical doses (so small as to remain unnoticed or undetectable). The earliest change is failure of accommodation with premature presbyopia (diminished power of the eye to accommodate for close vision, which usually occurs in middle age). The cataract that eventually forms is characteristically a posterior subcapsular one. There is frequently a thickening of the lens capsule and exfoliation (sheets of lens capsule floating in the anterior chamber) (Young, 1993a).

Once a common condition among glass blowers, furnace workers and others exposed to extreme heat, heat cataract is now rare. This is due to automation and to preventive measures such as workers wearing goggles with heat-absorbing or heat-reflecting glass.

Exposure to microwave, radar and laser radiation have been implicated as causes of cataract, but definitive evidence is still lacking (Young, 1993a).

Exposure to extreme cold can also lead to lens opacification, although it is apparently not a widespread problem, and little has been written about it (Newell, 1992).

[3]   Ionizing Radiation

Ionizing forms of radiation, which form harmful charged particles in biological tissue as they pass through it, include x-rays, gamma-rays, beta rays, alpha beams and neutron beams. In the lens, these forms of radiation affect the germinal epithelium (thick covering membrane) at the lens equator. After a variable period that lasts from several months to several years, the damaged epithelium gives rise to granular material that moves outward in the subcapsular region toward the poles of the lens. The opacities are more severe in younger individuals, because of the greater cell division occurring in the epithelium of their lenses (Young, 1993a).

A high incidence of radiation cataract follows therapeutic radiation by x-rays, gamma rays or cobalt beam. The latent period is from 6 to 24 months (Young, 1993a).

Beta rays, because of their lack of penetration, have been used in ophthalmology near the margin of the cornea (limbus). This has caused lens opacifications, although in general, they are localized, do not progress and do not interfere with vision.

Neutron and alpha-particle beams produce the greatest degree of ionization and thus carry the greatest risk of cataract formation; a single small dose may be sufficient to result in posterior capsular opacities (Young, 1993a).

The most effective way to deal with ionizing radiation cataract is to prevent it by the use of appropriate shielding consisting of lead, concrete, water, earth or paraffin, depending on the type and energy level of the radiation. This applies to workers exposed to ionizing radiation as well as to patients receiving therapy. In some cases, deep radiation must be used to save a patient's life, even with the knowledge that cataract formation is almost inevitable. In all cases, detailed informed consent regarding this potential effect of radiation is mandatory.

Nonionizing radiation can also cause cataract formation. Common forms include ultraviolet (UV), infrared, microwave and laser radiation. The most common source of UV radiation is sunlight. Tanning beds are another source today. While it has not been definitively proven that UV radiation causes lens damage, there is some evidence for a positive correlation between length of exposure to sunlight and the prevalence of age-related cataract (Young, 1993b). The lens absorbs UV at wavelengths of 320 to 400 nanometers (nm) and is thought, thereby, to provide a protective effect for the retina. UV filters that block transmission of light below 400 nm are routinely added to spectacles, contact lenses and intraocular lens (IOL) implants as a possible means of preventing putative UV cataract. For the same reason, people should be advised to wear protective filters when using tanning beds.

[4] Sudden Barometric Decompression

Rapid barometric decompression can result in bubbles of gas entering the bloodstream, a condition known as the bends. Cataract has been reported as one ocular effect of this condition. Those at risk of sudden barometric decompression include deep-sea divers, workers in a compressed atmosphere who undergo decompression too rapidly, and airplane pilots and passengers.

11.33 Metabolic Factors

Cataract may also be a consequence of any of a wide variety of inherited or acquired derangements of the body's physiologic chemistry.

[1] Diabetes Mellitus

A link between diabetes mellitus and cataract has been suspected for the past two centuries. Although research on this association has produced controversial literature, the existence of a connection is generally accepted (Young, 1993a).

Two groups of patients are distinguished: (1) those with diabetes- and age-related cataracts, and (2) those with "true" diabetic cataract. The largest group is individuals with diabetes who develop age-related lens changes. These occur at an earlier age than in nondiabetic individuals, occur more frequently and progress to maturity more rapidly.

Three mechanisms have been proposed to explain the formation of age-related diabetic cataracts (Young, 1993a). According to the *polyol* theory, the accumulation of sorbitol in the lens produces an osmotic imbalance, which leads to excessive hydration of and damage to the lens. According to the theory of *nonenzymatic glycosylation,* the reaction of glucose and glucose-6-phosphate with lens proteins produces an altered conformation of the proteins and a resulting opalescence. The theory of *auto-oxidation of sugars* holds that the by-products (especially free radicals) of spontaneous oxidation of sugars in the lens react with lens proteins and alter the conformation of the lens. None of these theories is completely satisfactory: the polyol and nonenzymatic glycosylation theories are considered to be important, while the auto-oxidation theory is still lacking proof.

"True" diabetic cataract is a rare complication of diabetes mellitus in the young. It generally develops rapidly and bilaterally and is characterized by myopia and by white, flaky, punctate (covered with small dots) opacities in the superficial anterior and posterior layers of the lens cortex. Progression leads to intumescent (marked by swelling) cataract and finally to total uniform opacification. The rate of progression is greater in younger individuals, but it may be reversible in the early stages, regardless of the patient's age (Young, 1993a).

The factors involved in the production of true diabetic cataract are osmotic hydration of the lens secondary to its high sugar content, acidosis (high acid content of blood) associated with diabetes and disturbances of carbohydrate metabolism in the lens. Hydration may lead to the formation of water clefts and vacuoles (tiny bubbles) deep in the cortex.

All diabetic cataracts are treated by surgical removal. The risk of hemorrhage and infection is greater in people with diabetes but must be assumed. Control of blood glucose levels by the judicious use of insulin and prophylaxis for infection with local and/or systemic antibiotics have dramatically lowered the incidence of these two complications.[4]

---

[4] *See also* ch. 9 for a complete discussion of diabetes.

[2]   Hypocalcemia

Cataract associated with hypocalcemia, or low blood level of calcium, is one of the systemic conditions that must be ruled out in determining the etiology of cataract, particularly when trauma is implicated. Lens changes in cataract associated with hypocalcemia consist of discrete white punctate spots, flakes and iridescent crystals in the anterior and posterior cortex, separated from the capsule by a clear zone.

The rate of progression is variable. The opacities may remain stationary indefinitely and give rise to little disturbance of vision, or they may progress to intumescence and finally to opaque cataract. Following thyroid surgery, this may occur in a short time. Following thyroidectomy (surgical removal of the thyroid), hypocalcemic cataracts may occur within a few days or not for as long as two decades (Newell, 1992).

Associated eye abnormalities that may develop include conjunctivitis, pigmentation of eyelid skin, loss of eyebrow hair or eyelashes, diplopia (double vision), strabismus (inability of the two eyes to be directed at a given object at the same time) and photophobia (extreme sensitivity to light). Low blood level of calcium is also associated with high serum phosphate level and hyperexcitability of the nervous system.

Cataracts do not always develop in the presence of low calcium levels, and the mechanism of their development remains unknown (Newell, 1992). The etiology is associated with hypoparathyroidism (diminished function of the parathyroid glands), thyroid deficiency disorders, chronic renal failure with inability to synthesize calcitriol, alcoholic liver disease associated with magnesium depletion resulting in impaired metabolism of the parathyroid glands, malabsorption syndrome, rickets and some malignant disorders.

Because hypocalcemic cataracts are not reversible, attempts should be made to prevent their development or progression. Blood serum calcium levels should be maintained at 8.5 to 9.0 milligrams per 100 milliliter by administration of calcium and vitamin D.

On the other hand, hypercalcemia and hypercalciuria (excess calcium in the urine) can lead to kidney damage due to the accumulation of calcium in renal tissues (nephrocalcinosis) and the consequent formation of kidney stones (nephrolithiasis). In addition, digitalis intoxication with cardiac arrhythmias (irregular heartbeats) and toxic effects of thiazide diuretics must be avoided.

[3]   Hypothyroid Cataract

This type of cataract has only rarely been reported. It is described as small, flaky deposits in the superficial anterior and posterior cortex of the lens, interspersed with iridescent crystalline deposits. The relationship to hypothyroidism (deficient activity of the thyroid gland) is questionable and not generally confirmed, since case reports are so rare and hypothyroidism is so common (Newell, 1992).

[4]   Hepatolenticular Degeneration (Wilson's Disease)

This disease is characterized by the corneal deposition of copper in the form of a rust-colored ring, cirrhosis of the liver and progressive central nervous system damage (Newell, 1992). It arises from an inborn error in the synthesis of ceruloplasmin, resulting in the excessive absorption of copper and other metals from the intestine and their deposition in various organs when they are bound to protein.

The lens changes consist of a thick, powdery deposit in and beneath the anterior capsule, with brilliant colors varying from green to red to brown in the form of a central round deposit from which spokes run outward toward the periphery. These lens changes do not seriously impair vision. The most serious consequences of the disease are the hepatic (liver) and neurologic sequelae (Newell, 1992).

Diagnosis is made by measuring the copper content of a liver biopsy. Treatment is by copper chelation (to remove the copper from participation in biological reactions) or, in cases of irreversible liver damage, liver transplantation.

[5]   Deficiency Cataract

While deficiency in certain vitamins, such as vitamin A, and protein malnutrition have been postulated to be involved in cataract formation, the evidence has not been conclusive (Newell, 1992). Cataract may develop in association with anorexia nervosa (abnormal loss of appetite), but this is not common.

[6]   Bone Disease

Although cataract has been associated with diseases and deformities of bone, the connection may be coincidental in many cases.

11.34 Complicated Cataract

Complicated cataract refers to those that occur secondary to local eye disease or inflammatory, degenerative and ischemic (oxygen deficient) conditions. They may also occur following local eye surgery, especially retinal detachment surgery and glaucoma operations on the filtering network of the eye. Complicated cataract opacifications usually progress to mature cataracts unless the underlying disease process can be treated (Young, 1993a).

[1] Uveitis

Uveitis is an inflammation of the entire uveal tract (iris, ciliary body and choroid); iridocyclitis is an inflammation of the iris and ciliary body; choroiditis is an inflammation of the choroid. A persistent iridocyclitis or the steroids used to treat it often results in a posterior subcapsular cataract (in the back region beneath the capsule). Opacities are initially seen beneath posterior synechiae (adhesions of the iris to the lens), but in time, the entire lens becomes opacified and can ultimately become infiltrated with crystalline and calcareous deposits as well as blood vessels. Eventually liquefaction, shrinkage and subluxation (partial dislocation) of the lens occur.

Much less commonly, a somewhat different type of cataract can result from choroiditis (also called posterior uveitis). In these instances, opacities begin as iridescent, polychromatic punctate deposits under the posterior lens capsule and in the posterior cortex of the lens. As they increase, the opacities commonly assume a rosette formation. The opacities are never clearly demarcated from the surrounding tissue but are submerged in a cloudy haze. Because a rosette shape is the most common configuration of traumatic cataracts, it can be difficult to make the differential diagnosis between cataract due to uveitis and that due to trauma. The problem is compounded by the fact that some cases of uveitis are traumatic in origin. Most cases of traumatic uveitis are anterior.

Treatment of cataract secondary to uveitis is surgical removal by the intracapsular method combined with sector iridectomy. The intracapsular method is associated with a lower incidence of uveitis than is the extracapsular extraction method. In addition, the extracapsular technique leaves the posterior capsule, on which a thick, opaque inflammatory membrane is more likely to form. Iridectomy prevents distortion of the pupil and adhesions (synechiae) in any future episodes of uveitis. Narrow sector iridectomy is still preferred by many ophthalmologists because it gives the surgeon a better view of the back of the eye and prevents further synechiae. If cyclitic membranes are present behind the lens, they should be removed. Although intraocular lens (IOL) implantation was formerly contraindicated in cases of uveitis, the use of heparin-coated lenses and modern surgical techniques now gives good results, provided the uveitis is under control (Wetherill, 1993).

[2]　Heterochromia and Cataracts

Cyclitis (inflammation of the ciliary body) in eyes with different color irises can result in the development of a cataract known as heterochromic cataract. The opacities begin as fine dots in the posterior cortex and striae in the periphery of the lens. Progression is rapid, until the entire lens is opaque. The inflammation, referred to as Fuch's heterochromic iridocyclitis, does not respond to treatment with steroids as do other types of cyclitis, but extraction of the cataracts can be quite successful.

The incidence of chronic glaucoma is increased in these patients. Patients do very well with extracapsular lens extraction with posterior chamber intraocular lenses.

[3]　Degeneration

The lens may be affected by a number of degenerative disorders, although it is not the primary site affected.

[a]　High Myopia

Posterior cortical (superficial) and nuclear (deep in the lens) cataracts may develop in mid-life or earlier in a highly myopic (nearsighted) eye. In such an eye, it is reasonable not to implant an intraocular lens (IOL). However, many surgeons prefer to do so in order to "stabilize" the architecture of the eye and possibly reduce the risk of retinal detachment, which is increased by high (severe) myopia (Murrill, et al., 1994).

[b]　Retinitis Pigmentosa

Pigmentary degeneration of the retina, with severe restriction of the visual field and night blindness, is frequently accompanied by the development of cataract in the central posterior part of the lens cortex.

Surgical extraction of these cataracts does not entail greater than normal risk and can be performed successfully. Even though cataract removal does not correct the retinal pathology, removal of the opaque lens does restore remaining central vision by eliminating the obstruction; it also may stimulate the remaining functioning retina, increasing the time it continues to function.

[c]   Retinal Detachment

A long-standing retinal detachment or break will result in a posterior subcapsular cataract with sclerosis of the lens nucleus; in time, the cataract will mature. These cataracts imply that a retinal detachment is long standing and pre-existing in cases of relatively recent accidental trauma. These cataracts are often not operated on, as removal of the cataract will not restore vision lost to retinal pathology. All cases of retinal detachment, however, including long-standing ones, must be referred immediately to a retinal specialist for consultation. The prognosis for restoration of vision depends on the duration of detachment, whether or not the macula (part of the retina that represents the area of keenest vision) has been involved (Murrill, et al., 1994).

[d]   Absolute Glaucoma

In absolute glaucoma, the eye is incapable of light perception due to uncontrolled elevated intraocular pressure and optic nerve damage. A cataract develops in the nucleus of the lens but is not extracted, because removal of the cataract will neither restore vision nor relieve the glaucoma.

[e]   Ocular Tumors

Pressure from eye tumors can result in cataracts. If clinical visualization of the tumor is prevented by the density of the cataract, the tumor may be demonstrated by ultrasonography and documented by photographs of the ultrasonography screen output.

[4]   Ocular Ischemias

Lens opacification develops in association with a number of conditions that involve ischemia, or compromise of the blood supply to the eye. Acute angle closure glaucoma can result when a rapidly developing age-related cataract absorbs a lot of fluid, becomes intumescent (swollen) and blocks the angle of the anterior chamber (angle between the iris and the cornea, which provides drainage for the aqueous humor in the front part of the eye). Traumatic glaucoma may occur by a similar process.

On the other hand, a narrow anterior angle and an acute angle closure episode with a significant elevation of intraocular pressure (IOP) over several hours can produce nuclear and posterior subcapsular cataracts. The risk of this is increased the longer the IOP remains elevated.

In pulseless disease, obliteration of the large arteries arising from the aorta results in a lowering of blood pressure and decreased blood supply to the organs, including the eyes, that are supplied by these vessels. The resulting hypoxia (oxygen deficiency) makes cataract development common in the later stages of pulseless disease. Early opacities are subcapsular and cortical; eventually the entire lens becomes completely opaque.

Buerger's disease is a vascular inflammation that results in obliteration of vessels. If the retinal vessels are affected, a rapidly maturing cataract occurs. Surgical removal is fraught with danger of loss of the eye and phthisis (shrinking of the eyeball) because of poor healing secondary to poor blood supply.

Necrosis (tissue death) of the anterior segment (front part of the eyeball) can occur after surgery for retinal detachment where the buckle is too tight and cuts off the blood supply to the anterior segment. Cataract is a relatively common complication of this condition due to interference with the nourishment of the lens.

11.35 Age of the Patient

Cataracts occur most often at the extreme ends of the life cycle. Cataracts that develop in the elderly are called age-related cataracts.

Age-related cataract can be divided into two basic types—*nuclear,* which occur deep in the lens (25 percent) and *cortical,* which are more superficial (75 percent)—although both forms may occur together in a single lens (Young, 1991). Lens changes begin in individuals between the ages of 50 and 60 years, when varying degrees of change can be found in about 60 percent of individuals; past the age of 60, changes are apparent in about 85 percent of people (Young, 1991). A genetic component appears to be involved in the development of age-related cataract, but the multifactorial nature of cataractogenesis makes it generally difficult to isolate individual factors (Murrill, et al., 1994).

[1]   Nuclear Cataract

Nuclear cataract consists of progressive sclerosis (hardening) of the lens nucleus. Clinically it is the most frequently encountered age-related cataract (alone or in combination with other lens changes) and the one that most often causes reduced central visual acuity (Young, 1993a). Nuclear sclerosis may also occur secondary to trauma or uveitis.

Even though the water content of the lens may decrease by 50 percent, the weight and size of the lens may increase by a third as new lens fibers are continually laid down. The increased lens size crowds the anterior angle and can give rise to glaucoma (increased intraocular pressure). There may be a gradual reduction in visual acuity, especially in bright light, as well as distortion of objects and progressive myopia (nearsightedness).

These cataracts usually progress slowly. The opacity may spread toward the periphery of the lens and eventually occupy almost all of the lens tissue, although a little cortical substance always remains. As progression proceeds, the brown color of the opacity becomes deeper (cataracta brunescens) until it is finally black (cataracta nigra).

In some cases, sclerosis is initially limited to the fetal nucleus, spreading finally to the entire adult nucleus, but the remaining cortex remains clear and hyperopic (farsighted). This results in what is known as a false cataract or lens with a double focus. The refractive difference (focusing power) between the two regions of the lens can be 10 to 12 diopters (unit of refractive power) or greater. The double vision (diplopia) that results must be distinguished from diplopia due to trauma.

[2]   Cortical Cataract

The formation of cortical cataract is characterized by lens hydration, the formation of vacuoles (tiny bubbles) and splitting of the lens sutures with the formation of water clefts. As hydration increases, the size of the lens grows to the point of intumescence (swelling). The crowding of the anterior chamber angle by the enlarged lens often causes angle-closure glaucoma. This is a surgical emergency, requiring removal of the lens to avoid loss of vision or blindness due to optic nerve damage.

Cortical cataract is also referred to as soft cataract, in contrast to the hard character of nuclear cataract. The cortical opacities assume various shapes and configurations. Cataracts deep within the cortex are sometimes classified separately as supranuclear cataracts.

[3] Cuneiform Cataract

This is a form of cortical cataract consisting of wedge-shaped opacities that begin as radial spokes pointing to the center of the lens from its periphery. Since the bases of the wedges are on the periphery of the lens, vision is not affected until the apices of the wedges approach the center, fuse and cross the visual axis. The anterior cortex is usually more affected then the posterior cortex (Young, 1993a). When it is associated with hydration of the lens, the progression of these cataracts can be rapid and acute; otherwise, progression may be very slow.

Ultimately the entire lens becomes bright silver-white to dark gray or yellow, opaque and intumescent. At this stage, the cataract is referred to as mature or ripe. Light perception itself is reduced, and spectacle or contact lens correction produces no improvement. The cataract must be surgically removed at this stage to prevent the next stage of hypermaturity and fluid absorption.

Hypermaturity and fluid absorption are to be avoided, as they are frequently complicated by anterior uveitis and finally complete degeneration of the eyeball. The eye is then permanently blind. It is often also painful and may have to be removed for that reason. The opportunity for restoration of vision by cataract surgery, which has a high rate of success, is thus lost forever. Another reason to remove a mature cataract before it reaches the stage of hypermaturity is that a hypermature lens is more difficult to remove, and its removal is associated with more complications.

In some cases, absorbed fluid is retained in a hypermature lens. In this event, the solid nucleus floats in a white, milky fluid cortex, a condition known as Morgagnian cataract. The same problems exist with Morgagnian cataract as with a dehydrated hypermature cataract.

[4] Perinuclear Cataract

Perinuclear cataract is characterized by a thickening of the anterior and posterior bands of the adult nucleus, multiple small opaque dots and larger plaques that form small foci, concentrated lines and large patches in the deeper layers of the cortex. They may remain unchanged for a long time, but complete opacification eventually results as other types of cortical cataract changes intervene.

[5]   Subcapsular (Cupuliform) Cataract

This opacity has a concave disk-shaped appearance, is yellow in color—especially when it is located posteriorly—and appears as a thin line of opacification on slit lamp examination (a microscopelike instrument used to examine the eye). Most of these opacities can also be visualized with the ophthalmoscope, but not with as much accuracy and definition. Cortical and/or nuclear sclerotic opacities may co-exist with subcapsular cataract. It is much more common for subcapsular opacities to be posterior rather than anterior in location, although both may sometimes occur, with or without cortical and/or nuclear lens changes.

Subcapsular cataracts are usually located centrally as well, in the pupillary area. The combination of pupillary and posterior subcapsular location causes a great reduction in visual acuity. These cataracts progress and mature over a period of months when the insult (e.g., trauma, radiation, eye disease) is severe or is not removed or corrected. Whatever the cause, damage to the subcapsular epithelium (outer layer) followed by proliferation of epithelial cells is the common underlying histopathologic change. When the opacities are located anteriorly or peripherally, which is far less common, they may not affect vision at all, and their progression is very slow.

11.40   TREATMENT OF CATARACTS

The only effective treatment currently available for cataracts is surgical removal of the opacified (clouded) lens. Removal of discrete, punctate opacities while leaving the unaffected clear part of the lens in place is not possible; as soon as the lens capsule is broken, the lens will undergo general opacification.

Work on the biochemical mechanisms of lens opacification over the past few decades has given rise to research aimed at finding pharmacologic agents that might normalize the biochemistry of the lens and thus prevent, slow or reverse cataracts (Harding, 1991). Agents under investigation include aldose reductase inhibitors (e.g., sorbinil); nonsteroidal anti-inflammatory agents (NSAIDs; e.g., aspirin, bendazac lysine); sulfur-containing agents (e.g., fluorenone derivatives); inorganic salts (e.g., strontium, potassium, sodium, calcium); natural plant and animal extracts (e.g., digitalis, hormones); and vitamins (e.g., B, C and E). The aldose reductase inhibitors are considered among the most promising. However, there is presently an almost complete lack of well-controlled efficacy studies for anticataract agents, and most optometrists and ophthalmologists are of the opinion that no medical treatment currently exists for cataract. Anticataract medications may be prescribed to patients as placebos in order to reassure them that their condition is being treated prior to surgery (Young, 1993b).

11.41 Early Observation of Cases of Cataract

Penetrating eye trauma is an ophthalmologic emergency that requires stabilization, shield protection of the eye and immediate referral (Murrill, et al., 1994). Apart from this, the development of cataract is usually not an emergency. Although the status of the cataract must be monitored carefully, ample time is characteristically available to allow a thorough assessment of the cataract, retinal and neurologic status, and any co-existing eye or relevant medical conditions.

11.42 Indications for Surgery

The indications for cataract surgery are not rigid and depend on both medical and patient factors (Murrill, et al., 1994). Until the early part of the twentieth century, cataract surgery was performed only when the cataracts had "ripened" (turned steel gray or blue) and the person had no light perception. Under these conditions, cataract surgery was often unsuccessful, because vision had been destroyed by underlying ocular disease. In the intervening years, tremendous improvements in anesthesia, antisepsis and surgical technique (including the development of intraocular lens implants and the operating microscope) made cataract surgery both safer and more successful. This led to a more favorable attitude toward cataract surgery among patients and increased patient demand for the operation.

Increased longevity has also led to an increased need for better vision among the elderly. In general, the impact of cataract on the person's ability to function normally has become a criterion for making the decision to operate. As a result of all this, cataracts are being surgically treated at earlier stages of development in increasing numbers of people.

There are two general criteria for deciding whether to perform cataract surgery:

  • if the cataract is interfering with the person's ability to perform as he or she would like to or is required to; and

- if other eye disease is present.

The patient must be fully informed about the benefits and risks of surgical treatment. As with any procedure, surgery is only justified if the patient will benefit. A complete assessment of benefit to the patient must include considerations of the patient's psychology, lifestyle and visual requirements as well as his or her beliefs and expectations about cataract surgery (Bartley and Narr, 1991). Some individuals will be genuinely unconcerned about visual impairment, while others will be made unbearably anxious by anything less than perfect vision. Some individuals may appear unconcerned about visual impairment when they are really using the defense mechanism of denial to mask a fear of surgery or blindness. Many people still mistakenly believe that cataracts cannot be removed until they are "ripe" and the person has gone completely blind (Weatherill, 1993).

With regard to medical factors, in general, the elderly are more likely to have pre-existing ocular conditions (especially macular degeneration and diabetic retinopathy), putting them at higher risk for a poorer outcome than younger individuals (Davis, et al., 1991).

11.43   Surgery to Remove Cataract

In essence, the operation involves removing the lens containing the opacity in order to provide an unobstructed path for light rays to enter the eye. This alone will cause improved vision in the case of mature cataract, to the point that the person will be able to count fingers at a distance of three feet.

The earliest method of accomplishing this, called couching, dates back thousands of years to India, Egypt and other ancient civilizations (Elliott, 1993a). Couching was performed by simply pushing the lens inward and allowing it to fall into the posterior area of the eye; sometimes a small incision was made in the eyeball; sometimes the lens was simply pushed in with the thumbs. Although no statistical data are available, the complication rate was undoubtedly high.

Today, for example, dislocation of the lens onto the floor of the posterior segment of the eye is recognized as a complication of cataract, although cases have been reported in which the eye has been undamaged by this and vision has been restored, provided the capsule has remained intact. In such cases of lens dislocation occurring after trauma or surgery, attempts to remove the lens are often contraindicated, as they may result in more complications than leaving the lens where it is. In recent years, recovery of a dislocated intraocular lens with vitrectomy a day or two after the original operation has been done with success in the majority of cases.

Restoration of acceptable vision, however, requires replacement of the removed lens with an optical substitute: spectacles, contact lenses or an intraocular lens implant.

11.44 Lens Extraction

Modern methods for surgically removing the opacified lens fall into two basic categories: intracapsular and extracapsular extraction. Within these two broad categories, dozens of specific operative techniques have been developed, with new techniques being introduced all the time, particularly for extracapsular extraction. Although intracapsular techniques are still considered acceptable and are preferred by some ophthalmic surgeons, they have been almost completely supplanted by extracapsular techniques (Murrill, et al., 1994).

[1] Intracapsular Lens Extraction

Intracapsular cataract extraction (ICCE) involves removal of the whole lens along with its intact capsule. If the anterior hyaloid (front part of the membrane surrounding the vitreous humor, the material filling the posterior part of the eye) remains intact, it forms the posterior wall of the anterior chamber of the eye in the region of the pupil; otherwise, vitreous fluid fills the anterior chamber, and the anterior and posterior chambers become one common chamber.

[2] Extracapsular Lens Extraction

In an extracapsular cataract extraction (ECCE), the anterior lens capsule is opened and removed; the nucleus (core) and cortex (outer layer) of the lens are then removed, but the posterior capsule is left intact. The posterior lens capsule in this case maintains the separation of the anterior and posterior chambers of the eye. *(See Figure 11-1.)*

[3] Changes of Preference in Extraction Technique

Techniques for extracting cataracts have undergone considerable evolution over the years, and that evolution continues today, with new techniques and variations being introduced all the time. The highlights of these changes since the 1950s are presented in the following discussion, as they have clinical relevance to many cataract surgical patients who are still living (Murrill, et al., 1994).

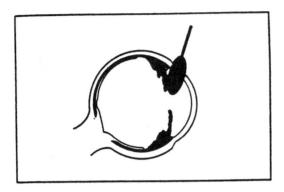

Fig. 11-1. In extracapsular cataract extraction (ECCE), the posterior capsule is left in place.

Extracapsular cataract extraction (ECCE) predominated in the 1950s. The procedure involved grasping and tearing the anterior lens capsule with a toothed forceps inserted through a 120-degree, 10-mm incision in the cornea. The nucleus of the lens was then manually expressed, and the cortex was removed by irrigation. The posterior capsule was left intact, and the incision was closed with a single silk suture. The major disadvantage of ECCE by nuclear expression as performed in the 1950s was that a nearly mature cataract was required, since the nonopacified clear portions of the lens were difficult to extract. This meant that patients were severely visually disabled before surgery was performed.

In the late 1960s and early 1970s, intracapsular cataract extraction (ICCE) became the preferred method, since it involved removal of the entire lens within its intact capsule and thus avoided the difficulties encountered with ECCE. ICCE produced excellent results, especially with contact lenses. The method also had several serious shortcomings, however. A major disadvantage was that removal of the posterior capsule left no support for the intraocular lens and also permitted vitreous to leak forward into the anterior chamber of the eye. A variety of lenses were devised that could be implanted in the anterior chamber, but all had disadvantages. A major one was that the excessive mobility of the implant caused corneal decompensation,[5] which required corneal grafting. In addition, the requirement for a large incision is

---

[5] *See* 11.54 *infra.*

associated with an increased rate of complications,[6] some of them serious.

In 1967, Kelman developed an extraction method called phacoemulsification (Weatherill, 1993). This involved breaking up the lens with an ultrasonic probe and aspirating it through a cannula, all through a small (3 mm) incision. Because the technique was somewhat difficult to perform and was associated with a relatively high risk of rupture of the posterior capsule, many surgeons were reluctant to adopt phacoemulsification at the time. *(See Figure 11-2.)*

Throughout this period, meanwhile, surgeons had been experimenting with placement of the intraocular lens (IOL) implant, which had been introduced following World War II. *(See Figure 11-3.)* Anterior chamber, posterior chamber and iris-fixation placement were all tried. All involved a large incision and various complications. In the late 1970s, a posterior chamber IOL that could be inserted through a small incision was perfected. In the 1980s, a method of continuous-tear capsulotomy (called capsulorhexis) was devised that allowed a smooth rather than a jagged opening of the anterior capsule; this prevented capsular tears and allowed clear visualization of the lens through the operating microscope (Casteneda, et al., 1992).

Today more than 90 percent of IOLs are implanted in the posterior chamber; approximately 95 percent of all cataract extractions in the United States are performed by extracapsular extraction, with 50 percent of them being done through a small incision by phacoemulsification (Busin, et al., 1993). In the opinion of Murrill and colleagues

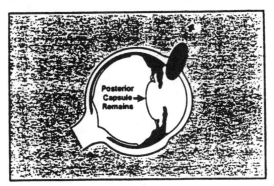

Fig. 11-2. In phacoemulsification, high-frequency ultrasound is used to break up the lens, which is then extracted by aspiration.

---

[6] *See* 11.50 *infra.*

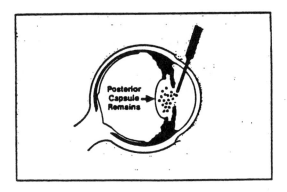

Fig. 11-3. An intraocular lens (IOL) implant.

(1994), this is the preferred way to perform cataract surgery, allowing for rapid restoration of stable visual acuity with a minimum of intra- and post-operative complications.

11.45   Postoperative Visual Correction

Removal of the lens represents the loss of an optical component with a dioptic (refractive or focusing) power of about 20 diopters (D; unit of refractive power); there is also typically an induced astigmatism on the order of 2 D (Douthwaite and Tunacliffe, 1993). These losses must be compensated for in order to allow the eye to see objects in focus. Three methods of postoperative visual correction are available: spectacles, contact lenses and intraocular lens implants.[7] Regardless of the method used, ultraviolet filters should be incorporated into the prosthetic lens to avoid damage to the retina.

[1]   Spectacle Correction

Although intraocular lens (IOL) implants are used increasingly to correct aphakia (absence of a lens) following cataract removal, a small number of patients who are not suitable candidates for IOLs (or contact lenses), such as those with severe myopia, may have their vision corrected by means of spectacles. Spectacle lenses can restore distance and reading vision satisfactorily in patients who have had bilateral cataract removal. *(See Figure 11-4.)* Spectacles are not practical for those who have been operated on for monocular cataract, because the retinal image formed by the aphakic eye is 30 percent larger than the

---

[7] *See* 11.60 *infra.*

retinal image formed by the unoperated eye. The person cannot fuse these two images, and intolerable double vision results. A new, ultrathin lens has been developed that markedly reduces the discrepancy in the size of the two images, but still not enough for the majority of patients to tolerate (Douthwaite and Tunnacliffe, 1993).

[2]   Contact Lenses

The advent of contact lenses solved the problem of image size discrepancy in monocular aphakia. Because the contact lens is closer to the nodal point of the eye than the spectacle frame lens, the discrepancy in image size between the aphakic and unoperated eye is reduced sufficiently to allow fusion of the two images and avoidance of double vision (Douthwaite, 1993b). A number of problems may be associated with wearing contact lenses, however, which may make them unsuitable for some patients.

[3]   Intraocular Lens (IOL) Implants

The problem of image size discrepancy is solved even more ideally by intraocular lens (IOL) implants, because the implant is located even closer to the nodal point and produces a retinal image that is nearly equal in size to that produced by the unoperated eye (Douthwaite, 1993c). Moreover, the problems involved in wearing contact lenses are avoided. IOLs can have their own complications, however, which may make them unsuitable for some patients (Noble and Hayward, 1991).

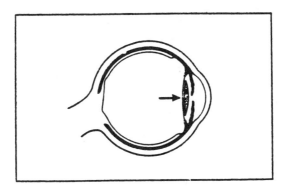

Fig. 11-4. (A) Cataract spectacle. Note the thick central portion of the lens. (B) Contact lens. This correction is visually more comfortable than a spectacle lens.

An intraocular lens consists of a lens of a certain power and haptics, usually C-shaped loops, for fixing the lens to the eye (Atchison, 1990). *(See Figure 11-5.)* There are three basic types of IOL: posterior chamber, anterior chamber and iris supported implants. These are briefly described in the following sections (Murrill, et al., 1994).

[a] Posterior Chamber Implants

The most popular IOL is the posterior chamber implant, which is placed behind the iris and fixed by haptics extending into the capsule. The lens becomes fixed by fibrosis (overgrowth of fibrous tissue) within two months of the operation. Posterior implants can be used only if the posterior lens capsule has remained intact during the operation, because if it is not intact, the implant can sink to the bottom of the eye. This lens has the advantage of being located in the same

A.

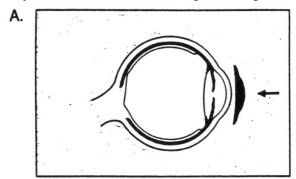

B.

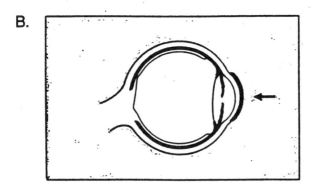

Fig. 11-5. The posterior chamber IOL, with haptics in the ciliary sulcus, the groovelike space posterior to the iris, and anterior to the ciliary body (muscle).

area of the eye as the natural lens; it is thereby optically most efficient, and its haptics do not traumatize or affect the anterior chamber angle, as can occur in anterior chamber and iris supported implants. The posterior chamber implant is the most difficult to remove, however, should this be necessary.

[b] Anterior Chamber Lens Implants

This is the second most popular IOL implant; it is located in front of the pupil, and the haptics are placed in the anterior chamber angle. *(See Figure 11-6.)* The advantages of the anterior chamber IOL are that it can be implanted after either extracapsular or intracapsular cataract extraction, rarely dislocates and is easier to remove, should this become necessary.

[c] Iris Clip Implants

The haptic loops of the iris fixated IOL straddle the iris, one set over the posterior surface of the iris and the other set over the anterior surface, so that the lens is "clipped" in place. Because of a tendency to dislocate, it was once the practice to suture one of the haptics to the iris. The iris fixated IOL is now considered outdated and is rarely used today, due to the high incidence of complications it causes. *(See Figure 11-7.)* These include irritation, inflammation, bulbous keratopathy (edema of the cornea) and atrophy of the iris as well as cystoid macular edema.

[d] Preferences in Choice of Lens Implant

More than 90 percent of IOL implants are now of the posterior chamber type (Jaffe, et al., 1990).

[4] Secondary Lens Implantation

The insertion of an IOL at the time a cataract is removed is referred to as primary implantation. The insertion of an IOL into an aphakic eye at a later time is referred to as secondary lens implantation. Prior to the 1980s, it was common to perform intracapsular cataract extractions (ICCE) without primary IOL implantation. Now that ICCE has all but disappeared, secondary lens implants are almost never performed. They are still performed, however, for patients who were unable, for various reasons, to receive an implant at the time of primary cataract surgery or who have developed problems with their original IOL (Murrill, et al., 1994).

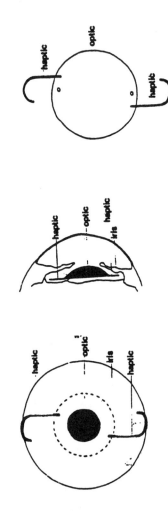

Fig. 11-6. An anterior chamber lens with flexible haptic in the anterior chamber angle, in cross section (left) and frontal view (right).

11.50 COMPLICATIONS OF CATARACT SURGERY

With modern advances in surgical methods, complications of cataract surgery have become rare (Patorgic, 1991). Because the number of cataract procedures being performed has increased dramatically, with several million operations now being performed each year, a considerable variety of complications has inevitably been reported (Weatherill, 1993). Some of these are due to the newer methodologies

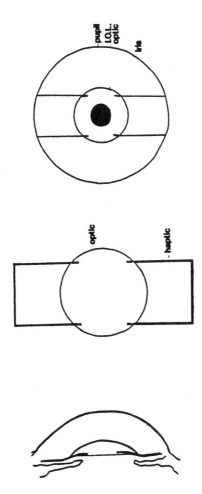

Fig. 11-7. The 4-loop lens, an iris clip implant, with haptics straddling the iris, in cross-section (left) and frontal (right) views.

themselves, such as intraocular lens (IOL) implantation. Although complications have become rare, they still merit serious consideration by both surgeon and patient when weighing the risks and the benefits of the operation.

11.51 Operative Complications

The most common and clinically important complications of cataract surgery are described.

[1]   Rupture of the Lens Capsule

Rupture of the posterior capsule may result in leakage of vitreous through the tear into the anterior chamber of the eye, with its consequent risk of complications. Posterior capsule rupture is most likely to be associated with phacoemulsification (cataract extraction in which ultrasonic vibrations are used to break up the cataract),[8] and fear of this complication remains one of the main barriers to surgeons' acceptance of the technique (Murrill, et al., 1994).

The likelihood of capsular rupture increases directly with the density of the cataract (especially sclerosis of the lens nucleus) and inversely with the experience and expertise of the surgeon. An experienced surgeon can perform phacoemulsification with less structural damage to the eye. An extremely dense sclerotic nuclear cataract may have to be removed by extracapsular nuclear expression[9] rather than by phacoemulsification.

Rupture of the lens capsule is also a complication of intracapsular extraction methods (in which the lens and capsule are both entirely removed).[10] Techniques have been developed to minimize the risk of this complication, but, more to the point, intracapsular techniques have been largely supplanted by extracapsular extraction methods.

[2]   Expulsive Hemorrhage

Expulsive (choroidal) hemorrhages are rare with current surgical methods, especially phacoemulsification and its small incision; the use of smaller incisions generally in cataract surgery has contributed significantly to a reduction in the incidence of this complication (Murrill, et al., 1994). The severity of hemorrhaging ranges from barely perceptible to so profuse that the intraocular contents, including the vitreous and the lens, are expulsively pushed out of the eye. Although this complication is rare, when expulsive hemorrhaging occurs, it almost always results in total loss of the eye. It is thus the most serious intraoperative complication of cataract surgery. It is thought that expulsion occurs when the sudden drop in intraocular pressure due to the incision results in rupture of presumably fragile blood vessels in the choroid.

---

[8] *See* 11.44[3] *supra.*

[9] *See* 11.44[2] *supra.*

[10] *See* 11.44[1] *supra.*

The risk of expulsive hemorrhage is greatest in elderly patients with glaucoma, atherosclerosis and/or systemic hypertension, and with longer, more complicated surgical procedures and larger incisions. The occurrence of expulsive hemorrhage is virtually impossible to predict, and various preoperative and intraoperative measures routinely taken to prevent or control it (e.g., osmotic therapy, massage) are usually unsuccessful.

[3] Operative Loss of Vitreous

Loss of vitreous following rupture of the posterior capsule is one of the most common intraoperative complications associated with phacoemulsification (Murrill, et al., 1994). When it occurs, vitrectomy (clearing the anterior chamber and wound of vitreous) may have to be performed in order to avoid the risk of vitreous traction and incarceration in the wound and their sequelae. Under the most favorable circumstances, the anatomy of the eye can be restored, an intraocular lens can be implanted, and excellent visual results achieved (Weatherill, 1993).

Complications of vitreous loss include a marked increase in the incidence of retinal detachment, bullous keratopathy, secondary glaucoma, vitreous opacities, vitreous hemorrhage, misshapen pupil, iris prolapse, endophthalmitis and wound infection, chronic ocular inflammation, cystoid macular edema and iritis, and defects of wound healing with resultant excess astigmatism, fibrous ingrowth and iris prolapse. Vitrectomy can prevent most of these complications, but the risks of chronic inflammation, retinal detachment and macular edema remain (Jaffe, et al., 1990).

11.52 Retinal Detachment

Detachment of the retina is usually a late complication of cataract surgery, occurring most often within six months of surgery and often within the first two weeks. However, it may occur at any time later than six months, especially in patients with predisposing conditions, which include axial myopia, and a history of retinal detachment in the other eye. The peripheral fundus (back part of the interior of the eyeball) must be examined preoperatively in all patients for the presence of these risk factors, especially retinal tears. All patients must be given a periodic dilated fundus examination during the early postoperative period and thereafter must be examined annually. Education about the symptoms of retinal tears and detachment is also of paramount importance. Patients at heightened risk must be monitored for life with regular dilated fundus examinations.

Overall estimates of the incidence of retinal detachment following cataract surgery range from 0.02 percent to 3.60 percent (Weatherill, 1993). Extracapsular cataract extraction (ECCE) with nuclear expression or phacoemulsification is associated with a low incidence of retinal detachment, averaging about 1 percent (Javitt, et al., 1991b). The incidence is higher with intracapsular cataract extraction (ICCE) and in the presence of vitreous loss (Sorensen and Baggesen, 1990). Intraocular lens implants do not appear to have an effect on the incidence of retinal detachment (Murrill, et al., 1994).

Detachment of the retina occurs due to traction (pulling) of the vitreous in the presence of strong adhesions between the vitreous and the retina, usually in a thin or weak area of the retina. The majority of retinal tears do not immediately cause detachment, but any tear may eventually result in detachment of the involved retinal flap. Any asymptomatic retinal tears found during preoperative peripheral fundus examination should be considered for prophylactic treatment prior to cataract surgery (Jaffe, et al., 1990).

11.53   Cystoid Macular Edema

The macula lutea is a shallow oval depression in the retina about the same size as the optic disk (the region where the nerve fibers converge and leave the eye to form the optic nerve). It is the zone of the retina that is responsible for color vision and visual acuity (sharpness). The macula has the ability to absorb large quantities of fluid, thus making it more prone to edema (swelling) than other areas of the retina. A result of macular edema is a decrease in visual acuity, which, in the vast majority of cases, is reversed as the fluid is absorbed and the swelling subsides.

Cystoid macular edema (CME) is one of the most common causes of postoperative loss of visual acuity. Visual loss from CME occurs in approximately 3 percent to 5 percent of cases following uncomplicated extracapsular cataract extraction (ECCE) and intraocular lens (IOL) implantation. In most cases, the condition resolves and vision improves spontaneously; in 1 percent of cases, edema and visual loss persist (Murrill, et al., 1994).

The exact cause and mechanism of CME remain uncertain. However, CME that occurs following cataract surgery is most likely due to intraoperative trauma and/or postoperative inflammatory reaction. In brief, the trauma of surgery is thought to release inflammatory mediators such as prostaglandins and leukotrienes (Flach, 1992). Direct trauma to the macula from vitreous traction on it may also contribute to the development of CME. CME is more common in patients with intraocular complications such as loss of vitreous, incarceration of vitreous in the surgical wound, uveitis, posterior capsule rupture and postoperative rupture of the anterior hyaloid membrane (Murrill, et al., 1994).

The definitive diagnostic test for CME is fluorescein angiography (in which a photograph of the retina is taken after injecting fluorescein dye into a vein). Other potential causes of decreased vision that need to be ruled out include corneal edema, uveitis, capsular clouding and retinal disease or detachment. Other causes of CME, besides intraoperative trauma and postoperative inflammatory reaction, that must be ruled out include retinal vascular disease, subretinal neovascularization and uveitis. When CME is associated with uveitis, other causes of the inflammation must be ruled out, including pupillary capture, retained lens material and/or a history of chronic iritis (Murrill, et al., 1994).

While most cases of CME will resolve spontaneously, some patients will require treatment for various situations. The treatment of CME has been reviewed recently by Jaffe and colleagues (1990). CME in the presence of complications such as posterior capsular rupture, especially with vitreous loss and vitreous to the wound, has been shown to respond to various treatments. Topical steroids (e.g., prednisolone acetate) or nonsteroidal anti-inflammatory drugs (NSAIDs, e.g., suprofen, diclofenac) may be tried for a period of four to six weeks. If there is no improvement, a combination of betamethosone acetate and sodium may be added subconjunctivally. If there is still no improvement, oral steroids may be considered. If both topical and oral steroids fail, Nd:YAG laser vitreolysis may be effective. Finally, anterior vitrectomy and/or lens exchange with vitrectomy may be considered.

In uncomplicated CME, topical steroids alone are often beneficial in acute cases (Melberg and Olk, 1993). Topical ketorolac has shown some promise in chronic CME, but orally administered nonsteroidal agents such as indomethacin appear to have no effect on the resolution of chronic macular edema (Flach, et al., 1991). In some cases, Dolabod®, 500 mg twice a day by mouth, is effective after one to two weeks of use.

Administration of corticosteroids postoperatively to reduce inflammation from surgical trauma is the standard method of prophylaxis for CME; anecdotal reports have indicated some success with the use of NSAIDs preoperatively or in combination with topical steroids postoperatively, but no large controlled clinical trials support this practice as yet (Flach, et al., 1990).

11.54   Corneal Decompensation

Corneal decompensation is the most common visually disabling complication of cataract surgery. The cornea is a major component of the refractive (light-focusing) power of the eye and must remain transparent if an optically clear image is to be formed on the retina. The transparency of the cornea is dependent on its hydration, which, in turn, is dependent on the integrity of its endothelial (inner) cell layer. These cells serve as a barrier against the flow of fluid into the cornea and also contain a dehydrating mechanism to pump fluid out to maintain normal hydration. The density of the corneal endothelial cells tends to decrease with age, from about 3,000 cells square mm in young children to 2,000 per mm in individuals past 50 years of age (Murrill, et al., 1994).

Damage to the endothelial cells results in edema (swelling due to accumulation of fluid) of the cornea. When a sufficient number of cells are lost, the endothelial layer loses its ability to keep the cornea properly hydrated and clear; aqueous enters the cornea, and it becomes translucent. As this process, called corneal decompensation, continues, bullae (blebs or blisters) form. When bullae are present, the condition is called pseudophakic bullous keratopathy (PBK). Complications of PBK include severe vascularization of the cornea as well as scarring, ulceration, corneal melting and perforation, and endophthalmitis. As corneal decompensation progresses, the patient experiences gradually diminishing vision, the sensation of a foreign body in the eye, acute pain and other symptoms.

Damage to the endothelial cells of the cornea may occur intraoperatively or postoperatively and may be direct or indirect.

Direct damage during cataract surgery may be due to contact with surgical instruments, the IOL or fragments of the biological lens being removed. Indirect damage may be caused by changes in pH or chemical composition of the aqueous resulting from irrigating solutions or by hydraulic forces during irrigation. Surgical trauma to the corneal endothelium can be limited in patients with pre-existing damage by the use of viscoelastic agents and endocapsular rather than anterior chamber phacoemulsification (Glasser, et al., 1991).

Postoperatively direct damage to the corneal endothelium may be due to intermittent or constant contact with the IOL. This is common with iris-fixated IOLs, less so with anterior chamber IOLs with their support in the anterior angle, and rare with posterior IOL implants (Murrill, et al., 1994). Indirect damage may be due to chronic inflammation or chronic elevation of intraocular pressure; the latter may also produce optic nerve damage.

Other sources of vision loss and pain that must be ruled out include acute corneal edema and keratitis (inflammation of the cornea) secondary to topical postoperative medications (medicamentosa). Although any topical drug may cause medicamentosa postoperatively, it is most commonly found to be due to beta-blockers and aminoglycosides.

Initially corneal edema is treated with topical steroids to control inflammation and with antiglaucoma medication to lower IOP. Bullae are treated with topical hyperosmotic drops. Miotic agents can be used following cataract surgery to treat corneal edema due to elevated intraocular pressure. They are seldom used in the early postoperative period, however, because of their tendency to increase the intraocular inflammation that already exists (Murrill, et al., 1994).

If symptoms are not controlled or progress, consultation or return to the cataract surgeon is necessary to avoid corneal decompensation and its sequelae. During the early stages of decompensation, progression may be halted by IOL exchange. In a recent series, 71 percent of patients had the same or improved vision following IOL exchange (Coli, et al., 1993). Of the 29 percent of cases in which the operation failed, 75 percent of patients had corneal endothelial cell counts of 500 cells per mm or less at the time of surgery (Coli, et al., 1993).

The ultimate treatment for corneal decompensation is penetrating keratoplasty (corneal transplant) (Hassan, et al., 1991; Kornmehl, et al., 1990).

The prognosis for success is very good (Murrill, et al., 1994). It must be kept in mind, however, that cystoid macular edema (CME) is closely associated with PBK and corneal decompensation, so that long-standing CME may limit the final visual potential of keratoplasty.

Patients should be advised of this as part of the decision to undergo corneal grafting.

11.55   Infections

The incidence of postoperative infections is lower for the eye than for most other organs. However, infections that do occur tend to be more serious, due to the lack of vascularization by means of which infection-fighting immunologic factors (white blood cells, antibodies, etc.) are normally delivered to a site of infection. Under these conditions, organisms that are benign elsewhere in the body are highly pathogenic when they gain access to the eye.

[1]   Intraocular Infection

Inflammation of the internal structures of the eye (endophthalmitis) is a rare but potentially catastrophic complication of intraocular surgery. Although rates as high as 0.5 percent have been reported (Murrill, et al., 1994), the largest study available to date found rates of 0.17 percent for intracapsular cataract extraction and 0.12 percent for phacoemulsification or extracapsular extraction (Javitt, et al., 1991a; Miller and Glasgow, 1993).

Endophthalmitis results from microbial invasion of the anterior chamber or posterior segment perioperatively or during postoperative follow-up. Specific causes include contaminated intraocular lens implants; viscoelastic and other solutions and medications injected into the eye; airborne contaminants; normal microbial flora of the patient or surgical personnel (skin, lacrimal sac and nose); corneal grafts; vitreous implants; and surgical instruments, appliances and sutures. Late postsurgical endophthalmitis may be associated with wound dehiscence or from an infected filtering bleb when combined cataract extraction and trabeculectomy (creating a channel to relieve fluid buildup) for glaucoma is performed (Alvarez, et al., 1991). The risk of infection is increased by the use of 5-fluorouracil in trabeculectomies (Wolner, et al., 1991). Causative microbes include *Staphylococcus aureus, Staphylococcus epidermidis,* streptococcal and Gram-negative species (Speaker, et al., 1991).

The classic clinical signs of endophthalmitis appear within 24 to 72 hours; they include pain, reduced vision, increased intraocular pressure, edema and redness of the eyelid and conjunctiva, corneal edema, vitreous inflammation and a severe reaction in the anterior chamber, including pus (hypopyon), which must be differentiated from postoperative uveitis without infection. The clinical symptoms, course and prognosis are quite variable, however, and are related to the pathogenicity of the infecting species, with streptococcal and Gram-negative species being the more virulent (Mao, et al., 1992).

A more subtle presentation is produced by *Staphylococcus epidermidis,* for example (Ormerod, et al., 1993c; Mazwell and Baber, 1992). Affected patients present without severe pain or hypopyon (presence of pus in the anterior chamber) from days to weeks following surgery. They are often misdiagnosed as having a noninfectious inflammatory reaction and treated with topical corticosteroids. The condition may improve initially and then worsen again as administration of the steroid medications is tapered (Ormerod, 1993b).

A delayed onset of months or years may be caused by *Propionibacterium acnes,* due to this organism's ability to sequester itself. This type of endophthalmitis is frequently exacerbated following Nd:YAG laser posterior capsulotomy, due to the dispersal of microbes into the vitreous by this procedure (Murrill, et al., 1994). A whitish plaque of capsular infiltrate observed through the dilated pupil is highly suggestive of *P. acnes* endophthalmitis (Fox, et al., 1991).

Because of the potentially catastrophic outcome of endophthalmitis, any patient with a disproportionate inflammatory reaction following cataract surgery must be carefully and promptly examined for this complication, taking care to rule out sterile inflammatory processes (e.g., uveitis). The more promptly endophthalmitis is treated, the better the outcome.

Treatment is by antibiotics. If clinical suspicion is high, the individual is treated with intravitreal, subconjunctival and topical antibiotics while waiting for culture results. A core vitrectomy may also be performed to remove microbes and the debris of inflammation and to enhance distribution of the antibiotics. The benefit of systemic antibiotics is controversial (Murrill, et al., 1994). The effectiveness of systemic antibiotics and vitrectomy is currently under investigation (Doft, 1991). Vitrectomy has contributed a great deal to the successful treatment of this condition, because it gets a more accurate diagnosis bacteriologically and because it can get a high concentration of the antibiotic used in the area affected.

[2] Uveitis

Any surgical technique will produce a certain amount of trauma, which will result in a certain amount of inflammatory reaction. In the case of cataract surgery, uveitis—inflammation of the uvea (which comprises the iris, the ciliary body and the choroid)—is usually transient (one to two weeks), responds well to topical steroids and leaves no permanent sequelae. Moreover, modern advances in surgical methods have dramatically reduced the incidence of uveitis compared with the early days of cataract surgery (Murrill, et al., 1994).

Uveitis may be caused by foreign material in the eye, including airborne particles, drugs and medications used in cataract surgery (e.g., alphachymotrypsin and viscoelastics such as Healon®) and the intraocular lens (IOL) implant. The inflammatory effects of iris-fixated (clip) and rigid anterior chamber IOLs are well known (Chung and Yeh, 1990; Lim, et al., 1991). Posterior chamber IOLs can also cause a disproportionate inflammatory reaction, especially if they are sutured to the iris or placed in the ciliary sulcus (groove) (Busin, et al., 1990). In the early days of IOL use, inflammatory reactions ("toxic lens syndrome") were caused by residual substances from the lens sterilization process; improvements in the sterilization procedure have made this complication rare (Murrill, et al., 1994).

Cataract surgery in patients with pre-existing uveitis should be deferred until the eye has been quiet and stable for several months. These individuals may require more aggressive steroid therapy before, during and after the operation. The use of a continuous tear capsulotomy and placement of the IOL in the capsular bag will provide a greater blood-aqueous barrier and help reduce postoperative inflammation. These patients should be advised before the operation that they may experience a greater than usual inflammatory reaction postoperatively (Hooper, et al., 1990)

The differential diagnosis for uveitis includes infectious endophthalmitis and, in the presence of decreased vision and cells in the anterior chamber, cystoid macular edema and retinal detachment. The goal in managing uveitis is to reduce the inflammatory response in order to prevent scarring and corneal and macular edema. This is accomplished by means of topical corticosteroids, cycloplegic agents and possibly topical nonsteroidal anti-inflammatory drugs (NSAIDs). If intraocular pressure (IOP) is mildly elevated, observation is sufficient if there is no history of glaucoma or occlusive disease of retinal vasculature.

Significant IOP elevations should be treated with antiglaucoma medication.

[3]   Sympathetic Ophthalmitis

Sympathetic ophthalmitis is a rare bilateral inflammation of the entire uveal tract that occurs following penetrating trauma involving that region of the eye. The condition can also occur following cataract surgery, but this is very rare.

[4]   Phacoanaphylactic Uveitis

This condition sometimes occurs following trauma or uncomplicated extracapsular cataract extraction (ECCE) and is due to an immunologic reaction against proteins in residual crystalline lens material. The condition develops within days to weeks following disruption of the crystalline lens. Corticosteroids produce initial improvement, but the condition returns when they are tapered. Removal of the residual lens fragments usually clears up the problem rapidly. This differentiates the condition from sympathetic ophthalmia. Definitive diagnosis of phacoanaphylactic uveitis requires histopathologic examination (Marak, 1992).

In severe cases, hypopyon (pus) may occur, and the intraocular pressure (IOP) may become elevated due to deposition of lens material and debris onto the trabecular meshwork of the anterior chamber. The increased IOP may produce corneal edema. Peripheral anterior synechiae or adhesions of the iris in the angle of the anterior chamber may aggravate the glaucoma (elevated IOP). If this condition is neglected, cystoid macular edema, retinal detachment and permanent corneal edema may occur (Jaffe, et al., 1990).

11.56   Retained Lens Material

The proliferation and migration of lens epithelial cells (and their derivatives) retained in the eye following phacoemulsification and other forms of extracapsular cataract extraction (ECCE) can cause a clouding of the posterior lens capsule (Blodi, et al., 1992). This is known as secondary cataract, aftercataract, capsular fibrosis or epithelial (Elschnig's) pearls. Such posterior capsular opacities (PCOs) generally occur from a few days to a few weeks following cataract surgery. Up to 50 percent of eyes operated on by ECCE techniques develop posterior capsular opacities within five years of surgery; while postsurgical PCOs occur in all age groups, they are more common in younger patients, due to the greater proliferative activity of epithelial cells in the young (Apple, et al., 1992).

Patients usually report that their vision was excellent following surgery but then became as poor as when they had cataract. Chief symptoms are decreased visual acuity and glare in bright light. Examination is similar to preoperative examination. In particular, the capsular opacity and/or other sources of loss of vision should be identified by means of slit lamp and dilated fundus examinations; the integrity of the retina should be assured by peripheral fundus exam; and the probability of improved visual acuity should be ascertained using a potential acuity test (Murrill, et al., 1994).

Once the foregoing determinations are made and the patient has been counseled and given informed consent, treatment is by capsulotomy using an Nd:YAG laser. The objective is to create a hole in the posterior capsule slightly larger than the diameter of the pupil. When the procedure is successful—as it is in most cases—the individual should never experience symptoms again or require additional treatment. On occasion, symptoms may continue due to an off-center capsulotomy or capsular remnant that thickens; in rare cases, the formation of Elschnig's pearls may continue. Repeat Nd:YAG capsulotomy may be performed in all these cases.

In performing capsulotomy, the laser should be focused directly behind the posterior capsule. Focusing the laser at or near the surface of the IOL implant will cause pits to form in the IOL. A few small pits are commonly associated with the procedure; they do not significantly affect vision. Focusing the laser inside the IOL, however, will cause cracks to occur in the IOL, and these may cause significant glare.

The most common complication of laser capsulotomy is transient or late elevation of intraocular pressure (Fourman and Apisson, 1991). Apraclonidine hydrochloride, an alpha-adrenergic agonist, can reduce these IOP spikes by about 40 percent (Silverstone, et al., 1992). Side effects include retraction of the eyelid, blanching of the conjunctiva and mydriasis (pupil enlargement). Beta-blockers have the same effect, but they are less commonly used now. Other complications of Nd:YAG laser capsulotomy include exacerbation of endophthalmitis, dislocation/decentration of intraocular lens implants, cystoid macular edema and retinal detachment (Apple, et al., 1992).

Other causes of posterior capsular opacities include accumulation of protein deposits due to postoperative inflammation; layering of white blood cells on the surface of the capsule; entrapment of residual lens cortex between the posterior capsule and the posterior chamber intraocular lens (IOL) implant, due to incomplete aspiration; entrapment of red blood cells or blood stains from a hyphema (bleeding in the anterior chamber) between the posterior capsule and the posterior IOL; and colonies of slow-growing, low-virulence bacteria such as *Propionibacterium acnes*.

11.57 Loss of Anterior Chamber

A flat or shallow anterior chamber (front part of the eye containing the aqueous humor) accompanied by low intraocular pressure (IOP) following cataract surgery is usually due to wound leakage or choroidal detachment. The condition is rare but requires further evaluation and treatment when it occurs. Wound leakage is usually due to improper surgical technique, poor wound healing or trauma (Jaffe, et al., 1990). A shallow anterior chamber can also occur in the absence of the preceding factors, often in association with choroidal detachment (Murrill, et al., 1994).

Loss of the anterior chamber may be an early or a late (several days to weeks) complication. Causes of early loss include an irregular incision, inadequate suturing, excessive cauterization at the wound edges, incarceration of material in the wound, poor coaptation of the wound margins, accidental trauma (rubbing of the eye or a blow to the eye), poor ocular structure and elevation of intraocular pressure. Late loss may be caused by sloughing of a suture, too rapid absorption of an absorbable suture, necrosis (tissue death) around the suture, early suture removal, or other trauma and interference with aqueous secretion associated with wound leakage. Probably the most common cause of late flattening of the anterior chamber is external pressure against the wound.

The patient may or may not report pain. Slit-lamp examination and instillation of fluorescein should be performed to reveal symptoms such as leakage along the wound edge. Intraocular pressure should be measured to rule out pupillary block. Although all tonometers (instruments used to measure intraocular pressure) are inaccurate at low IOPs, noncontact tonometers such as an air-puff tonometer are particularly inaccurate; a Goldmann applanation tonometer is recommended instead (Murrill, et al., 1994). Malignant glaucoma and choroidal detachment must also be ruled out.

The most important sequelae of wound leak with a shallow anterior chamber are anterior synechiae (adhesions between the iris and the cornea) and pupillary block, both of which can result in glaucoma; recurrent inflammation; intraocular infection; and chronic choroidal detachment. A rare but feared complication is epithelial invasion of the anterior chamber, which is favored by malunion of the wound; this can destroy the eye.

In order to decrease the risk of these complications, surgical consultation and treatment must be swift when a wound leak is identified. It is recommended that the anterior chamber be surgically reformed immediately when flat anterior chamber occurs early (Jaffe, et al., 1990). When the condition occurs within a few days of surgery, surgical reformation of the anterior chamber may be performed, or the eye may be pressure-patched and dilated using a short-acting mydriatic agent (Weinstein, 1991c). An oral hypotensive agent may also be given to slow aqueous production and percolation through the wound. With such treatment, the wound may heal, sealing the leak, and the anterior chamber may reform. If this treatment fails, the anterior chamber can be reformed by introduction of a bubble of air or a viscous agent such as sodium hyaluronate (Healon®) into the anterior chamber. If choroidal detachment is present, further treatment is necessary to correct this condition (Assia, et al., 1991b).

11.58   Hemorrhage

Hemorrhage is a potential complication of virtually all surgery. In cataract surgery, hemorrhage may occur in the anterior chamber (hyphema), in the vitreous cavity or as an expulsive hemorrhage.

[1]   Hyphema

Blood in the anterior chamber of the eye may arise from the operative wound, the iris or the ciliary body. While it usually occurs between the first and seventh postoperative day, it may appear later. It can be caused by defective wound healing, trauma, excessive cauterization of blood vessels near the incision, trauma to the ciliary body, abnormal vascularization of the iris or the anterior chamber angle, blood disorders such as hemophilia, thrombocytopenia and polycythemia, and anticoagulant therapy. Anticoagulant therapy is generally stopped a week or two before surgery is performed.

Hyphema is one of the most unnecessarily alarming sequelae of cataract surgery, for both patient and physician. Although even mild to moderate hyphemas will cause a dramatic loss of vision and slow visual recovery, the majority of hyphemas are benign and resolve within two to six days; even a large hyphema will generally resolve in two to four weeks (Murrill, et al., 1994). Treatment is thus conservative. Prednisone and aminocaproic acid have been administered for inflammation control (Farber, et al., 1991). Occasionally irrigation of the anterior chamber is necessary to evacuate some of the blood, particularly if intraocular pressure (IOP) has been elevated by the hyphema. Elevation of IOP is most often a problem with severe hyphemas.

The retention of an intact posterior capsule in an extracapsular cataract extraction will not necessarily confine a hyphema to the anterior chamber of the eye. Blood may pass into the vitreous chamber and remain there for several months. This condition is also benign and self-limiting in most cases. In some cases, secondary glaucoma due to excessive bleeding may occur, as may blood staining of the cornea. The latter sequela is rare, however, even after significant hyphema (Murrill, et al. 1994).

[2] Vitreous Hemorrhage

Bleeding into the vitreous following cataract surgery can occur by means of a number of mechanisms. The presence of hyphema (blood in the anterior chamber) and a broken lens capsule can result in the accumulation of red blood cells in the vitreous. Traction of the zonules (suspensory ligaments of the lens) may also produce vitreous bleeding in the absence of hyphema or capsular breaks. In the presence of a retinal detachment, bleeding into the vitreous is usually caused by rupture of a diseased blood vessel in connection with horseshoe breaks or lacerations of the retina.

In most cases, bleeding is not significant enough to impair vision seriously, and the blood is rapidly and completely resorbed. In a small number of cases, complications may develop, some of them serious (Murill, et al., 1994g).

Ghost cell glaucoma is a condition due to the accumulation of rigid degenerated red blood cells. Because they do not pass readily through the trabecular meshwork, they tend to clog it and produce elevated IOP. The condition is usually transient, as the ghost cells eventually pass through the meshwork.

[3] Expulsive Hemorrhage

Although expulsive hemorrhage is rare, it is one of the most frightening and devastating complications of cataract surgery. It is most likely to occur in elderly patients with glaucoma, atherosclerosis and hypertension. It is due to the rupture of one of the posterior ciliary arteries when the eye is opened and the intraocular pressure suddenly drops (Weatherill, 1993). In some cases, it may occur several days after surgery.

In most cases, the hemorrhage is so severe that it pushes all of the intraocular contents out through the incision and the eye is lost. In a few cases, hemorrhaging is mild, and the eye can be saved and vision restored.

Modern surgical techniques have greatly reduced the incidence of this complication by permitting excellent control of the intraocular environment. Specifically, choroidal hemorrhage is less likely with small incisions and extracapsular cataract extraction with phacoemulsification, wherein the intraocular pressure remains near normal levels (Murrill, et al., 1994).

11.59 Other Complications

Other complications have been associated with cataract surgery, such as glaucoma and retinal burns. Complications of anesthesia may result from any surgical procedure.

[1] Glaucoma

Glaucoma is characterized by elevated intraocular pressure (IOP), optic nerve damage and visual field restriction. A distinction must be made between individuals who had primary open angle glaucoma prior to cataract surgery and those who did not. Glaucoma in the latter group may be referred to as aphakic glaucoma, implying that the condition arose as a complication of cataractous lens extraction.[11]

[a] Open and Closed Angle Glaucoma

Cataract surgery in the presence of glaucoma may be beneficial or harmful. Various factors need to be considered for each individual patient (Weatherill, 1993). For example, open-angle glaucoma that has been controlled before cataract surgery usually remains controlled after

---

[11] *See also* ch. 10 for a complete discussion of glaucoma.

surgery. Chronic closed-angle glaucoma is always unpredictable and requires close monitoring. Previous filtering (trabecular) surgery for glaucoma makes cataract extraction more difficult. The most common problems are that posterior synechiae (adhesions between the iris and the lens) cause the pupil to dilate poorly; and drainage blebs created in connection with the surgery encroach on the cornea and make it necessary to place the incision more anteriorly or in a different quadrant of the limbus (margin of the cornea).

The advantages of cataract surgery are that removal of a cataract will allow easier visualization of the optic disk, more reliable perimetric evaluations and the use of miotic drops without impairment of visual acuity (Onali and Raitta, 1991). A common disadvantage is that the corticosteroids routinely used following cataract surgery for the control of inflammatory reactions carry a risk of steroid-induced elevation of intraocular pressure (Murrill, et al., 1994).

[b] Aphakic Glaucoma

A transient elevation of intraocular pressure (IOP) is common following cataract surgery with any technique and occurs in about half of all patients (Murrill, et al., 1994). This occurs whether or not patients have pre-existing glaucoma, although those with pre-existing glaucoma are more likely to experience IOP spikes. Phacoemulsification and small corneal incisions are associated with a lesser elevation in IOP, while the use of viscoelastic agents is associated with a greater rise.

Most studies have found that viscoelastics cause a postoperative elevation of IOP if they are not removed by aspiration (removal by suction) at the time of surgery; many surgeons also administer acetazolamide (Diamox®) (Liesegang, 1990). IOP elevation is directly due to blockage of the meshwork by the viscoelastic molecules. It is generally thought that viscoelastics of lower molecular weight may be less likely to elevate IOP (Lane and Lindstrom, 1992). One study, on the other hand, has reported no significant difference in postoperative IOP regardless of whether the viscoelastic is removed (Stamper, et al., 1990).

Elevated intraocular pressure may result from obstruction of the trabecular (filtering) meshwork by inflammatory debris, substances used during the operation, vitreous, red blood cells, lens particles and pigment. The latter three are the most common causes.

Obstruction of the trabecular meshwork due to surgically induced trabeculitis (inflammation) can also produce elevated IOP, as can distortion of the meshwork by sutures that are too tight; the latter situation is most likely to occur with a limbus-based incision (i.e., in the margin of the cornea).

Other causes of early IOP elevation include the use of the enzyme alphachymotrypsin during intracapsular cataract extractions to dissolve the zonules holding the lens in place and vitreous debris following vitrectomy. Topical steroids applied for postsurgical inflammation control can also elevate IOP; this usually does not occur for two to three weeks, but may occur within a few days (Tomey, et al., 1991).

[2] Anesthetic Complications

Complications of anesthesia may be due to iatrogenic (caused by treatment) or physiologic causes (Hamilton and Grizzard, 1993; Jaffe, 1990).

[a] Local Anesthesia

Because most cataract surgery is now done on an ambulatory care basis, local anesthesia is most commonly used, especially a mixture of xylocaine and marcaine. Peribulbar injections (peribulbar block, administered in the lower outer area of the eye) are most often used. Complications are rare. They include hemorrhage, ocular penetration, persistent diplopia (double vision), chemosis (swelling of the conjunctive), ptosis (drooping eyelid) and ecchymosis (bruising) of the eyelid. Hemorrhages tend to be limited to the peribulbar area and do not interfere with surgery.

Idiosyncratic reactions to the agent and cardiac arrest may occur. It has been suggested that postoperative strabismus (lack of eye convergence) may sometimes be due to the muscle toxicity of the anesthetic. Because of the effectiveness and greater safety of peribulbar blocks, retrobulbar and facial blocks are rarely used in an ambulatory care setting (Murrill, et al., 1994; Mieler, et al., 1990). Recently topical anesthesia has become popular and has proven successful when used with small incisions, either tunnel or corneal.

[b] General Anesthesia

The standard complications of general anesthesia may be seen in cataract surgery; lightening of the anesthesia may cause too much pressure behind the eyeball, with possible loss of intraocular contents, especially vitreous. Other possible sequelae include idiosyncratic reactions to the anesthetic agent and cardiac arrest.

[3] Retinal Burns

The introduction of the operating microscope has revolutionized many surgical fields, including ophthalmology. One of the potential complications associated with its use is the possibility of retinal burns from the light source. Burns can occur in some cases in spite of the use of filters and light barriers. Attempts are now made to minimize the occurrence of such burns by covering the cornea with opaque fiber material during as much of the procedure as possible.

[4] Behavioral Disorders

Most surgery engenders a number of psychological reactions in those undergoing it. Fear and anxiety are common prior to surgery; depression is common afterward. In most cases, these reactions are mild to moderate and self-limited. They have been minimized by advances in cataract surgery over the past few decades that have shortened hospital stays and recovery times and have made it possible to perform most procedures on an ambulatory care basis (Jaffe, et al., 1990). Psychological distress can be further minimized by an empathetic staff who encourage the patient to express his or her concerns and who carefully explain the procedure, what to expect and why it is necessary. Anxiolytics and antidepressants can be used if necessary, but care must be taken to avoid overdosage in elderly patients. Psychological distress is the most common complication of postoperative hyphema for both patient and physician (Murrill, et al., 1994).

[5] Complications of Intraocular Lens Implantation

In addition to complications attributable to the intraocular lens (IOL) implant or the implantation procedure, implantation can sometimes exacerbate the complications associated with cataract surgery generally. The type of implant used and the skill and experience of the surgeon are two key factors affecting the rate of complications. Among these complications are hyphema, vitreous loss, endophthalmitis, dislocation of the lens, retinal detachment, cystoid macular edema and glaucoma.

11.60   REHABILITATION OF THE APHAKIC PATIENT

It was once standard for patients to remain aphakic (without a lens within the eyeball) following cataract surgery, but today this is rare for adults (Murrill, et al., 1994). Common reasons for aphakia in adults today include surgical complications, pre-existing disease or high myopia (severe nearsightedness), all of which are contraindications for implantation of an intraocular lens (IOL).

Three methods are available for correction of aphakia: spectacle lenses, contact lenses and intraocular lens (IOL) implants.[12] Whichever method is used, the prosthetic optical device must contain an ultraviolet (UV) filter to protect the retina from UV radiation damage.

In addition to technical optical corrections, the support and encouragement of the ophthalmologist and optometrist are also key factors in facilitating rehabilitation following cataract extraction. When vision has been corrected, the patient should be specifically informed that the prognosis for maintaining restored vision is good (Jaffe, et al., 1990).

11.61   Spectacle Lenses

Spectacle lenses represent the oldest method of restoring vision to an aphakic eye. They have a number of important limitations but are still useful for selected individuals (Murrill, et al., 1994). Most fundamentally, spectacle lenses can only be used by patients who have aphakia in both eyes (or, in the case of cataract removal from a single eye, no vision in the other eye). If the other eye has normal vision and the aphakic eye is corrected with spectacle lenses, the difference in image sizes reaching the retinas will be too great for the brain to fuse, and he or she will experience diplopia (double vision). While newer, ultrathin lenses have been devised to overcome this problem to some extent, they are successful in only a small minority of cases.

Additional disadvantages of spectacle lenses include restriction of the field of view, restriction of peripheral vision and distortions of spatial discrimination and judgment (e.g., a straight line appearing curved). The great majority of individuals eventually accommodate to these problems, however, and actually do very well when the technical parameters of the lenses are properly provided (e.g., vertex distance adjustment and well-placed optical centers) (Murrill, et al.,

---

[12] *See* 11.45 *supra.*

1994). Spectacle lenses also avoid the complications associated with contact lenses and intraocular lens implants.

11.62   Contact Lenses

Contact lenses are generally preferable to spectacle lenses for aphakia, whether monocular or binocular (Murrill, et al., 1994g). Potential problems include infections, foreign bodies and vascularization of the cornea, but these can usually be managed without too much risk or difficulty. Extended-wear soft lenses are the most convenient, but daily-wear soft lenses and rigid lenses are also acceptable options (Douthwaite, 1994b; Garcia, et al., 1990).[13]

11.63   Intraocular Lenses

Except for a small proportion of patients for whom intraocular lens (IOL) implants are contraindicated,[14] IOLs are the ideal method for correcting aphakia. They are the most physiologic solution and require no care or maintenance other than taking care not to rub the eye. IOLs increase the image size to a negligible degree, compared with a 6 percent increase with contact lenses and a 30 percent increase with spectacle lenses (Douthwaite, 1993c).[15]

11.70   AMA EVALUATION OF PERMANENT IMPAIRMENT

The American Medical Association's *Guides to the Evaluation of Permanent Impairment* (AMA, 1993) provides criteria and a method for evaluating permanent impairment of the eyes and relating it to permanent impairment of the whole person. Degrees of impairment are expressed as a percentage representing loss of function.

Evaluation of visual impairment is based on deviation from normal in one or more of the following three functions of the eye: (1) corrected visual acuity for near and far objects; (2) visual field perception; and (3) ocular motility with diplopia (double vision). These three functions are not equally important separately, but if all three are not coordinated, vision is impaired. Other ocular abnormalities are taken into account to the extent that they affect one or more of these three basic

---

[13] *See* 11.45[2] *supra.*

[14] *See* 11.59 *supra.*

[15] *See* 11.45[3] *supra.*

functions. Examples of such abnormalities include opacities of the lens (cataract) or cornea, opacities of the ocular media (aqueous and vitreous) and abnormalities that cause symptoms such as epiphora (watery eye), photophobia (abnormal sensitivity to light) or metamorphopsia (distortion of objects). For each of these conditions, an additional 5 to 10 percent is combined with that for the impaired visual function in the affected eye.

The three basic ocular functions are not impaired by conditions such as permanent deformities of the orbit (e.g., scars, cosmetic defects), but the evaluating physician may add as much as 10 percent to the visual impairment scores due to impairment of the whole person.

The following equipment is needed to evaluate the functions of the eye:

- visual acuity test charts: Snellen test chart, illiterate E chart or Landolt's broken-ring chart for distance vision; charts with print similar to that of the Snellen chart, Revised Jaeger Standard print, American point-type notation for near vision;

- visual field testing: the traditional stimulus III-4e of the Goldmann perimeter or the stimuli and perimeters of the ARC perimeter, Allergan-Humphrey or Octopus; and

- refraction equipment: a phoro-optometer or combination hand-held lens and retinoscope.

11.71   Central Visual Acuity

Central visual acuity is sharpness of vision and the ability to discern fine details. The loss of central vision (acuity) in one eye ranges from 0 percent (Snellen rating for distance in feet of 20/15 and a Snellen rating for near vision in inches of 14/14) to 97 percent (Snellen distance rating of 20/800 and Snellen near rating of 14/140). These figures are for a native lens. Figures are also available to allow for aphakia (absence of a lens) or pseudophakia (intraocular lens implant) of the eye.

For example, a person in his fifties with a native lens and a Snellen distance rating of 20/30 and a Snellen near vision rating of 14/24 would have a 9 percent loss of central vision in that eye.

11.72   Visual Fields

Visual field refers to the ability to see well over a breadth of view. It is characterized by two parameters: the most peripheral point at which a standard object can be detected, and the quality of visual performance at every point within the field. Two different methods for estimating visual impairment may be used, based on one or the other of these parameters. They are described in detail in the *AMA Guides* (1993).

11.73 Ocular Motility and Diplopia

Impaired ocular motility due to diplopia (double vision) rarely causes significant impairment of vision unless the double vision is within 30 degrees of the center of gaze fixation. Details of testing are given in the *AMA Guides* (1993).

11.74 Impairment of the Whole Person

Total visual impairment is determined from a Combined Values Chart, using the values arrived at for loss of central vision, loss of visual field and loss of ocular motility/degree of diplopia (American Medical Association, 1993). A corresponding impairment of the whole person is then determined from another chart, Impairment of the Visual System as It Relates to Impairment of the Whole Person.

For example, a 10 percent impairment of the visual system corresponds to a 9 percent impairment of the whole person; a 90 to 100 percent impairment of the visual system corresponds to an 85 percent impairment of the whole person.

Individuals with mild to moderate visual impairment can usually perform most of their daily tasks independently with the help of low-vision aids (e.g., magnifiers, reading glasses). Those with severe impairment may need help even in reading a personal letter or going to the store. Such loss of privacy and independence can be difficult to adjust to psychologically. For the vast majority of people with cataracts, vision can be restored to a highly satisfactory extent, so that visual impairment is a problem only during the preoperative and early postoperative period.

11.100 BIBLIOGRAPHY

Text References

Albert, D. M. and Jakobiec, F. A. (Eds.): Principles and Practice of Ophthalmology. Philadelphia: Saunders, 1994.

Alvarez, O., et al.: Haemophilus Aphrophilus Endophthalmitis Associated with a Filtering Bleb. Arch. Ophthalmology 109(4):612-620, 1991.

Apple, D. J., et al.: Posterior Capsule Opacification. Surv. Ophthalmology 37(1):73-116, 1992.

Assia, E. I., et al.: Clinicopathologic Study of the Effect of Radial Tears and Loop Fixation on Intraocular Lens Decentration. Ophthalmology 100(2):153-158, 1993.

Assia, E. I., et al.: Mechanism of Radial Tear Formation and Extension After Anterior Capsulotomy. Ophthalmology 98(3):432-437, 1991a.

Assia, E. I., et al.: An Experimental Study Comparing Various Anterior Capsulotomy Techniques. Arch. Ophthalmology 109(4):642-647, 1991b.

Atchison, D. A.: Optical Design of Poly (Methyl Methacrylate) Intraocular Lenses. J. Cataract Refract. Surg. 16(2):178-127, 1990.

Balyeat, H. D.: Secondary Lens Implantation. In: Cangelosi, G. C. (Ed.): Advances in Cataract Surgery: New Orleans Academy of Ophthalmology. Thorofare, N.J.: Slack, 1990.

Bartley, G. B. and Narr, B. J.: Preoperative Medical Examinations for Patients Undergoing Ophthalmic Surgery. Am. J. Ophthalmology 112(5):725-727, 1991.

Bettman, J. W.: Seven Hundred Medi-Legal Cases in Ophthalmology. Ophthalmology 97(9):1379-1384, 1990.

Blodi, B. A., et al.: Retained Nuclei After Cataract Surgery. Ophthalmology 99(1):41-44, 1992.

Busin, M., et al.: Long-Term Results of Sutureless Phacoemulsification with Implantation of a 7-mm Polymethylmethacrylate Intraocular Lens. Arch. Ophthalmology 111(3):333-358, 1993.

Busin, M., et al.: Complications of Sulcus-Supported Intraocular Lenses with Iris Sutures Implanted During Penetrating Keratoplasty After Intracapsular Cataract Extraction. Ophthalmology 97(3):401-406, 1990.

Casteneda, V. E. et al.: Posterior Continuous Curvilinear Capsulorhexis: An Experimental Study with Clinical Applications. Ophthalmology 99(1):45-50, 1992.

Chawla, H. B.: Ophthalmology, 2nd ed. Edinburgh: Churchill Livingstone, 1993.

Chung, Y. M. and Yeh, T.: Intraocular Lens Implantation Following Extracapsular Cataract Extraction in Uveitis. Ophthal. Surg. 21(2):272-276, 1990.

Chylack, L. T., et al.: The Lens Opacities Classification System, Version III (LOCS III). Invest. Ophthalmol. Visual Sci. 33(Suppl.):1096-1099, 1992.

Coli, A. F., et al.: Intraocular Lens Exchange for Anterior Chamber Intraocular Lens-Induced Corneal Endothelial Damage. Ophthalmology 100(3):384-393, 1993.

Datiles, M. B. and Kinoshita, J. H.: Pathogenesis of Cataracts. In: Tasman, E. (Ed.): Duane's Clinical Ophthalmology, vol. 1. Philadelphia: Lippincott, 1991.

Davis, E. T., et al.: Pre-Surgical Prediction of Post-Surgical Visual Function in Cataract Patients: Multivariate Statistical Analyses of Test Measures. Clinical Vision Sciences 6(2):191-207, 1991.

Doft, B. H.: The Endophthalmitis Vitrectomy Study. Arch. Ophthalmol. 109(3):487-488, 1991.

Douthwaite, W. A.: Introduction. In: Douthwaite, W. A. and Hurst, M. A.: Cataract: Detection, Measurement and Management in Optometric Practice. Oxford: Butterworth-Heinemann, 1993a.

Douthwaite, W. A.: Contact Lens Correction. In: Douthwaite, W. A. and Hurst, M. A.: Cataract: Detection, Measurement and Management in Optometric Practice. Oxford: Butterworth-Heinemann, 1993b.

Douthwaite, W. A.: The Intraocular Lens. In: Douthwaite, W. A. and Hurst, M. A.: Cataract: Detection, Measurement and Management in Optometric Practice. Oxford: Butterworth-Heinemann, 1993c.

Douthwaite, W. A. and Tunnacliffe, A. H.: Spectacle Correction. In: Douthwaite, W. A. and Hurst, M. A.: Cataract: Detection, Measurement and Management in Optometric Practice. Oxford: Butterworth-Heinemann, 1993.

Edmonds, S. A.: Contact Lens Management of Aphakic Children. Contact Lens Forum 15(1):15-56, 1990.

Elliott, D. B.: New Clinical Techniques to Evaluate Cataract. In: Douthwaite, W. A. and Hurst, M. A.: Cataract: Detection, Measurement and Management in Optometric Practice. Oxford: Butterworth-Heinemann, 1993a.

Elliott, D. B.: How Useful Is the Vistech MCT8000 for Contrast Sensitivity and Glare Testing? Can. J. Optom. 54(2):194-198, 1993b.

Elliott, D. B. and Bullimore, M. A.: Assessing the Reliability, Discriminative Ability and Validity of Disability Glare Tests. Invest. Ophthalmol. Visual Sci. 24(1):108-119, 1993.

Elliott, D. B. and Whitaker, D.: Clinical Contrast Sensitivity Chart Evaluation. Opththal. Physiological Optics 12(2):275-280, 1992.

Elliott, D. B. et al.: Comparative Clinical Tests of Visual Function in Cataract with the Patient's Perceived Visual Disability. Eye 4(5):712-717, 1990.

Farber, M. D. et al.: Aminocaproic Acid Versus Prednisone for the Treatment of Traumatic Hyphema. Ophthalmology 98(2):279-286, 1991.

Flach, A. J.: Cyclo-Oxygenase Inhibitors in Ophthalmology. 36(3):259-284, 1992.

Flach, A. J., et al.: Improvement in Visual Acuity in Chronic Aphakic and Pseudophakic Cystoid Macular Edema After Treatment with Topical 0.5% Ketorolac Tromethamine. Am. J. Ophthalmol. 112(4):514-519, 1991.

Flach, A. J., et al.: Prophylaxis of Aphakic Cystoid Macular Edema Without Corticosteroids. Ophthalmology 97(8):1253-1258, 1990.

Foreman, J.: Federal Agency to Develop Cataract Management Guidelines by January 1991. Arch. Ophthalmol. 108(10):1391-1392, 1990a.

Foreman, J.: Johns Hopkins Outcome Study for Cataract Management. Arch. Ophthalmol. 108(11):1533-1536, 1990b.

Foreman, J.: The Clinical Appropriateness Initiative—Cataract Management Study. Arch. Ophthalmol. 108(12):1678-1682, 1990c.

Fourman, S. and Apisson, J.: Late-Onset Elevation of Intraocular Pressure After Neodymium-YAG Laser Post Capsulotomy. Arch. Ophthalmol. 109(4):511-513, 1991.

Fox, G. M., et al.: Delayed-Onset Pseudophakic Endophthalmitis. Am. J. Ophthalmol. 111(2):163-173, 1991.

Garcia, G. E., et al.: Extended Wear Rigid Gas Permeable Lenses Used for Correction of Aphakia. CLAO J. 16(2):195-199, 1990.

Geddes, L. A., et al.: A Comparison of Snellen and Interferometer Visual Acuity in an Ageing Noncataractous Population. Optom. Vision Sci. 67(3)361-365, 1990.

Glasser, D. B., et al.: Endothelial Protection and Viscoelastic Retention During Phacoemulsification and Intraocular Lens Implantation. Arch. Ophthalmol. 109(10):1438-1440, 1991.

Gressel, M. G.: Lens Induced Glaucoma. In: Tasman, W. T. (Ed.): Duane's Clinical Ophthalmology, vol. 3. Philadelphia: Lippincott, 1991.

Hamilton, R. C. and Grizzard, W. S.: Complications. In: Gills, P., et al. (Eds.): Ophthalmic Anesthesia. Thorofare, N.J.: Slack, 1993.

Harding, J.: Cataract. Biochemistry, Epidemiology and Pharmacology. London: Chapman and Hall, 1991.

Hassan, T. S., et al.: Implantation of Kelman-Style, Open Loop Anterior Chamber Lenses During Keratoplasty for Aphakic and Pseudophakic Bullous Keratopathy. Ophthalmology 98(5):875-880, 1991.

Hesler, R.: Signs, Symptoms and Patient Management. In: Douthwaite, W. A. and Hurst, M. A.: Cataract: Detection, Measurement and Management in Optometric Practice. Oxford: Butterworth-Heinemann, 1993.

Hooper, P. L., et al.: Cataract Extraction in Uveitis Patients. Surv. Ophthalmol. 35(2):120-144, 1990.

Hurst, M. A.: Lens Structure, Biochemistry, and Transparency. In: Douthwaite, W. A. and Hurst, M. A.: Cataract: Detection, Measurement and Management in Optometric Practice. Oxford: Butterworth-Heinemann, 1993a.

Hurst, M. A., et al.: Assessment of Retinal and Neural Function Behind a Cataract. In: Douthwaite, W. A. and Hurst, M. A.: Cataract: Detection, Measurement and Management in Optometric Practice. Oxford: Butterworth-Heinemann, 1993b.

Jaffe, N., et al.: Cataract Surgery and Its Complications, 5th ed. St. Louis: Mosby, 1990.

Javitt, J. C., et al.: National Outcomes of Cataract Extraction/ Endophthalmitis Following Inpatient Surgery. Arch. Ophthalmol. 109(7):1085-1089, 1991a.

Javitt, J. C., et al.: National Outcomes of Cataract Extraction. Ophthalmology 98(5):895-502, 1991b.

Kornmehl, E. W., et al.: Penetrating Keroplasty for Psuedophakic Bullous Keratopathy Associated with Closed Loop Anterior Chamber Intraocular Lenses. Ophthalmology 97(3)407-414, 1990.

Catch, M. L. and Catch, G. M.: Management of the Traumatic Cataract. Current Opinion in Ophthalmology 1(1):25-27, 1990.

Lane, S. S. and Lindstrom, R. L.: Viscoelastic Agents: Formulation, Clinical Applications, and Complications. Seminars in Ophthalmology 7(2):253-270, 1992.

Lasa, M. S. M., et al.: Contrast and Glare Sensitivity: Association with the Type and Severity of the Cataract. Ophthalmology 99(7):1045-1049, 1992.

Liesegang, T. J.: Visoelastic Substances in Ophthalmology Survey of Ophthalmology 34(3):268-293, 1990.

Lim, E. S., et al.: An Analysis of Flexible Anterior Chamber Lenses with Special Reference to the Normalized Route of Lens Explantation. Ophthalmology 98(2):243-246, 1991.

Luntz, M. H.: Clinical Types of Cataracts. In: Tasman, E. (Ed.): Duane's Clinical Ophthalmology, vol. 1. Philadelphia: Lippincott, 1991.

Mao, L. K., et al.: Endophthalmitis Caused by Streptococcal Species. Arch. Ophthalmol. 110(5):798-801, 1992.

Marak, G. E.: Phacoanaphylactic Endophthalmitis. Surv. Ophthalmol. 36(2):325-339, 1992.

Mazwell, D. P. and Baber, W. B.: Acute Postoperative Endophthalmitis Associated with Dual Strains of Staphylococcus Epidermidis. Ophthal. Surg. 23(2):222-224, 1992.

Melberg, N. S. and Olk, R. J.: Corticosteroid-Induced Ocular Hypertension in the Treatment of Aphakic or Pseudophakic Cystoid Macular Edema. Ophthalmology 100(2):164-167, 1993.

Miller, K. M. and Glasgow, B. J.: Bacterial Endophthalmitis Following Sutureless Cataract Surgery. Arch. Ophthalmol. 111(2):377-379, 1993.

Mieler, W. F., et al.: Localized Retinal Detachment with Combined Central Retinal Artery and Vein Occlusion After Retrobulbar Anesthesia. Retina 10(2):278-283, 1990.

Murrill, C. A., et al.: Trends in Cataract Care. In: Murrill, C. A., et al.: Primary Care of the Cataract Patient. Norwalk, Conn.: Appleton & Lange, 1994.

Newell, F. W.: Ophthalmology: Principles and Concepts, 7th ed. St. Louis: Mosby, 1992.

Noble, B. and Hayward, M.: Contraindications to Intraocular Lens Implantation. In: Percival, P. (Ed.): Color Atlas of Lens Implantation. St. Louis: Mosby Year Book, 1991.

O'Day, D. M., et al.: Cataract in Adults: Management of Functional Impairment. Clinical Practice Guideline No. 4. USDHHS, PHS. Agency for Health Care Policy and Research, p. 21, 1993.

Olson, L.: Anatomy and Embryology of the Lens. In: Tasman, E. (Ed.): Duane's Clinical Ophthalmology, vol. 1. Philadelphia: Lippincott, 1991.

Onali, T. and Raitta, C.: Extracapsular Cataract Extraction and Posterior Chamber Lens Implantation in Controlled Open-Angle Glaucoma. Ophthal. Surg. 22(3):381-387, 1991.

Ormerod, L. D., et al.: Scleral Flap Necrosis and Infectious Endophthalmitis After Cataract Surgery with a Scleral Tunnel Incision. Ophthalmology 100(2):159-163, 1993a.

Ormerod, L. D., et al.: Endophthalmitis Caused by the Coagulase-Negative Staphylococci. Disease Spectrum and Outcome. Ophthalmology 100(5):715-723, 1993b.

Ormerod, L. D., et al.: Endophthalmitis Caused by the Coagulase-Negative Staphylococci. Factors Influencing Presentation After Cataract Surgery. Ophthalmology 100(5):724-729, 1993c.

Pardhan, S. and Gilchrist, J.: The Importance of Measuring Binocular Contrast Sensitivity in Unilateral Cataract. Eye 5(1): 31-35, 1991.

Patorgic, C. G.: Complications of Cataract and Implant Surgery Optometry Clinics 1(2):81-113, 1991. Physicians' Desk Reference, p. 2409. Montvale, N.J.: Medical Economics, 1995.

Revicki, D. A., et al.: Patient Outcomes with Co-Managed Post-Operative Care After Cataract Surgery. J. Clin. Epidemiol. 46(1):5-15, 1993.

Roberts, C. W., et al.: Cataract Surgery in Anticoagulated Patients. J. Cataract Refract. Surg. 17(Suppl.):309-312, 1991.

Silverstone, D. E., et al.: Prophylactic Use of Apraclonidine for Intraocular Pressure Increase After Nd:YAG Capsulotomies. Am. J. Ophthalmol. 113(3):401-405, 1992.

Sorensen, K. E. and Baggesen, K.: Retinal Detachment Following Intracapsular Cataract Extraction. Acta Ophthalmol. 68(3):549-553, 1990.

Speaker, M. G., et al.: Role of External Bacterial Flora in the Pathogenesis of Acute Postoperative Endophthalmitis. Ophthalmology 98(4):639-650, 1991.

Stamper, R. L., et al.: Effect of Intraocular Aspiration of Sodium Hyaluronate on Postoperative Intraocular Pressure. Ophthalm. Surg. 21(3):486-491, 1990.

Steinert, R. F., et al.: Cystoid Macular Edema, Retinal Detachment, and Glaucoma After Nd:YAG Laser Posterior Capsulotomy. Am. J. Ophthalmol. 112(3):373-380, 1991a.

Steinert, R. F., et al.: Astigmatism After Small Incision Cataract Surgery. Ophthalmology 98(3):417-424, 1991b.

Tomey, K. F., et al.: The Glaucomas in Aphakia and Pseudophakia. Surv. Ophthalmol. 36(1):79-112, 1991.

van den Berg, T.: On the Relation Between Glare and Stray Light. Documenta Opthalmalogica 78(2):177-121, 1991.

Weatherill, J. R.: The Surgical Management of Age-Related Cataract. In: Douthwaite, W. A. and Hurst, M. A.: Cataract: Detection, Measurement and Management in Optometric Practice. Oxford: Butterworth-Heinemann, 1993.

Weinstein, G. W.: Cataract Surgery. In: Tasman, W. (Ed.): Duane's Clinical Ophthalmology, vol. 5. Philadelphia: Lippincott, 1991.

Wolner, B., et al.: Late Bleb-Related Endophthalmitis After Trabeculectomy with Adjunctive 5-Fluorouracil. Ophthalmology 98(7):1053-1060, 1991.

Young, S. A.: Age-Related and Other Cataract Morphologies. In: Douthwaite, W. A. and Hurst, M. A.: Cataract: Detection, Measurement and Management in Optometric Practice. Oxford: Butterworth-Heinemann, 1993a.

Young, S. A.: The Medical Treatment of Cataract. In: Douthwaite, W. A. and Hurst, M. A.: Cataract: Detection, Measurement and

Management in Optometric Practice. Oxford: Butterworth-Heinemann, 1993b.

Young, R. W.: Age-Related Cataract. New York: Oxford, 1991.

CHAPTER 12

IMPAIRED HEARING IN THE ELDERLY

SCOPE

Hearing impairment is a disability with devastating effects on communication. Although it is disabling at any age, it can be particularly incapacitating in the elderly, who may be losing other important physical and cognitive functions at the same time. Hearing loss in the elderly can contribute to isolation and hasten loss of independence. In addition to the aging process itself, causes of hearing impairment include hereditary factors, drug ototoxicity, infection and trauma. Although most forms of hearing loss cannot be cured, advances in technology can improve hearing capacity and assist in adaptation to impairment. Early diagnosis is especially vital for an older person, so that isolation may be prevented and adaptive processes learned.

SYNOPSIS

12.00 INTRODUCTION

Contemporary society is based to a large degree on auditory communication. Loss of the ability to hear can therefore have a grave impact. The effect can be particularly devastating for an aging person, who is undergoing other physical and social changes that may diminish the sense of competence and independence.

Hearing loss may contribute to a decrease in social interaction and a loss of independence (Appollonio, et al., 1996; Coroni-Huntley, et al., 1992; Gulya, 1992). As hearing acuity diminishes, the individual suffers frustration and tension, a decreasing ability to understand his or her surroundings and a greater sense of vulnerability. This can lead to paranoia and isolation. Feelings of isolation may be exacerbated by failure of family, friends and acquaintances to understand what is happening. Because hearing loss is invisible, even a sympathetic family member may forget such simple adaptive behaviors as facing the hearing-impaired person while speaking slowly (Chen, 1994; Thomsett and Nickerson, 1993). For the older person, this leads to decreases in social interaction and human intimacy at the very stage in life when they are most needed.

Profound hearing loss eliminates feedback about one's own speech and results in unnatural pitch, rhythm and intensity when speaking. This may prove annoying to listeners who do not understand the cause.

13.01 Effects of Late-Onset Hearing Loss

Hearing loss can be particularly devastating in the elderly, contributing to isolation from family and friends and exacerbating the effects of any mental disorders, such as depression or dementia. Studies on the effects of hearing loss have suffered from a lack of consistency in age groups tested and methods of hearing evaluation (Appollonio, et al., 1995); thus they differ in their conclusions about the effects of hearing impairment on quality of life. Recent well-controlled studies suggest, however, that hearing impairment in the elderly not only may contribute to depression and isolation but may affect physical function as well (Appollonio, et al., 1995; Dargent-Molina, et al., 1996).

Elderly persons with hearing impairment report loneliness and lowered self-esteem; the greater the hearing loss, the deeper is the loneliness experienced (Chen, 1994). Hearing loss can lead to a sense of dependence and a reluctance on the part of relatives to permit continuation of independent living. The problem is exacerbated by the frequent reluctance of the elderly to acknowledge hearing impairment because of its association with the aging process. Some studies indicate that more women than men have emotional difficulties as a result of hearing loss (Chen, 1994).

Because hearing loss may lead to inappropriate responses in conversation, an appearance of inattention and a tendency to ask a speaker for repetition, it may be misinterpreted as cognitive dysfunction, such as Alzheimer's disease[1] (Roper, 1995). This situation may be worsened by the fact that the person with hearing loss often does not perceive the deficit to be as serious as family and friends do (Jerger, et al., 1995).

There is an increased mortality among men (but not women) aged 70 to 75 with either a hearing deficit or a combined hearing and vision deficit (Appollonio, et al., 1995). Women aged 75 or older who are living at home have an increased likelihood of becoming physically disabled and dependent if they have a serious hearing impairment (Dargent-Molina, et al., 1996).

Although most forms of hearing impairment cannot be corrected, sensory aids ranging from hearing aids to cochlear implants can preserve social interaction and improve the quality of life. Special considerations apply to the elderly, who may require help in adjusting to these devices. This is particularly true in a health care setting, both office and hospital, where already confusing surroundings may be extremely bewildering to a person who cannot hear (Roper, 1995).

---

[1] *See also* ch. 15 for a discussion of Alzheimer's disease.

Sensorineural hearing loss adversely affects speech perception, particularly in the presence of background noise (Gravel and Ruben, 1996). Cochlear hearing loss acquired in adulthood is characterized by poor frequency resolution and lessened dynamic range. Auditory deprivation in mature individuals with cochlear hearing loss can result in bilaterally symmetric loss.

12.02   Hearing Impairment As a Disability

The American Academy of Otolaryngology and the American Council of Otolaryngology have issued functional definitions of hearing disability: A *permanent impairment* is hearing threshold outside normal limits, caused by a permanent abnormality in anatomy or function; a *permanent handicap* is impairment that interferes with activities of daily living; a *permanent disability* is one that renders a person unable to work full-time (Donaldson, 1996).

12.10   EPIDEMIOLOGY OF HEARING LOSS

Hearing impairment ranks third among chronic conditions in the elderly (Chen, 1994; Rogin, 1996). The hearing threshold generally begins to change between age 40 and 50 and continues to deteriorate throughout life (Staab, 1996).

Statistics on the prevalence of hearing loss vary from study to study, perhaps due in part to its perception as a stigma among many people. It is agreed, however, that its incidence increases dramatically with increasing age (Nadol, 1993).

The elderly constitute more than half of the hearing-impaired population in this country (Winograd, 1995). Studies indicate that at least 50 percent of women over the age of 65 have sufficient hearing loss to make understanding of speech difficult (more than 50 decibels hearing loss at 4000 Hz) (Cohen and Gorlin, 1995). Tinnitus (nearly constant noises in the ears) occurs in nearly 9 percent of persons over the age of 65 (Segal, 1996). The incidence of handicapping hearing loss has been estimated at 36 percent or more among those who are 75 or over (Nadol, 1993).

The rate of hearing loss is two to three times greater among people over the age of 85 than among those between 75 and 84 (Coroni-Huntley, et al., 1992). Nearly half the population aged 80 and over has significant hearing impairment. About 30 percent in this age group are unable to hear and understand normal voices unaided; about 19 percent are unable to do so even when fitted with a hearing aid. The incidence of hearing loss may be as high as 90 percent among nonagenarians (Winograd, 1995).

Men are affected somewhat more frequently than women (33 percent of men, versus 27 percent of women, at age 57) (Staab, 1996). In general, men also suffer more severe impairment (Cherney, et al., 1996).

12.20 AUDITORY ANATOMY AND PHYSIOLOGY

The perception of sound depends on an intricate anatomy that transfers sound vibrations from the air outside to the auditory centers of the brain, where the sound is processed and understood. Sound enters the outer ear as acoustic energy, is converted to mechanical energy at the tympanic membrane barrier to the middle ear, becomes hydraulic energy at the fluid-filled inner ear and stimulates the hair cells within the cochlea. This mechanical stimulus is converted to an electrochemical signal that is sent to the eighth cranial nerve and the brain.

12.21 Anatomy of the Hearing Apparatus

The auditory system consists of the outer ear, the middle ear, the inner ear and auditory nerve and the central auditory pathways (Arts, 1997; Nadol, 1993). *(See Figure 12-1.)* Each plays an important role in conveying sound to the brain. The auditory apparatus is housed within the temporal bone of the skull.

[1] The Outer Ear

The outer (external) ear is comprised of the pinna or auricle, the auditory canal and the outer surface of the tympanic membrane, which separates the outer from the middle ear. The pinna is composed of the skin and cartilage around the external auditory meatus, the opening in the temporal bone that serves as the outer end of the auditory canal. The auditory canal, bounded by the temporal bone and the mastoid process, leads to the tympanic membrane (eardrum). The tympanic membrane is a thin oval approximately 9 to 10 millimeters by 8 to 9 millimeters (Arts, 1997). *(See Figure 12-2.)*

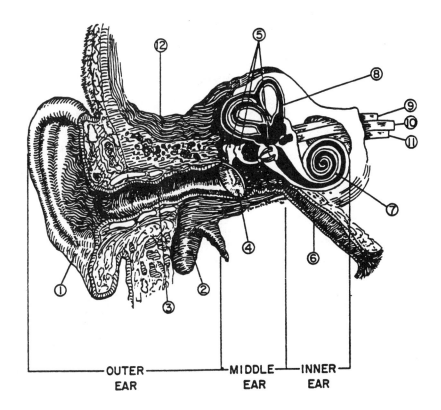

OUTER——————MIDDLE——INNER—
EAR   EAR   EAR

Fig. 12-1. The auditory system and its parts: 1: external ear; 2: mastoid process of the temporal bone; 3: external auditory canal; 4: tympanic membrane (eardrum); 5: auditory ossicles; 6: eustachian tube; 7: cochlea; 8: semicircular canals; 9: facial (seventh cranial) nerve; 10: vestibular nerve (eardrum); 11: cochlear nerve (10 and 11 together constitute the vestibulocochlear or eighth cranial nerve); 12: brain cavity.

[2]   The Middle Ear

Within the air-filled tympanic cavity or middle ear are the auditory ossicles, the eustachian tube extending to the back of the nose and various muscles. The ossicles form a bridge from the tympanic membrane to the oval window of the inner ear and consist of three tiny bones, the malleus (hammer), the incus (anvil) and the stapes (stirrup). *(See Figure 12-3.)* The tip of the manubrium or "handle" of the malleus is attached to the tympanic membrane at its central concavity (umbo) by the connective tissue fibers of its middle layer (lamina propria) (Arts, 1997). The head of the malleus is suspended

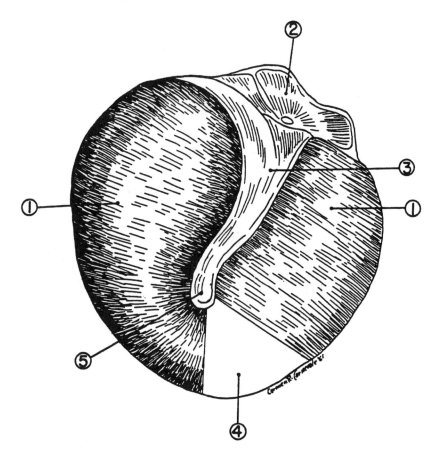

Fig. 12-2. Elements of a normal right tympanic membrane, as seen with an otoscope. 1: pars tensa; 2: pars flaccida; 3: manubrium of the malleus (handle of the hammer); 4: Politzer's light reflex; 5: umbo (point of attachment of the manubrium).

by ligaments from the walls of the middle ear and articulates (forms a joint) with the body of the incus. The incus has two processes, the longer of which articulates with the capitulum (head) of the stirrup-shaped stapes. The footplate of the stapes is attached to the rim of the oval window.

[3] The Inner Ear

The oval window separates the middle ear from the inner ear, which consists of a bony labyrinth within the temporal bone and a membranous labyrinth of ducts and sacs within that. The bony labyrinth

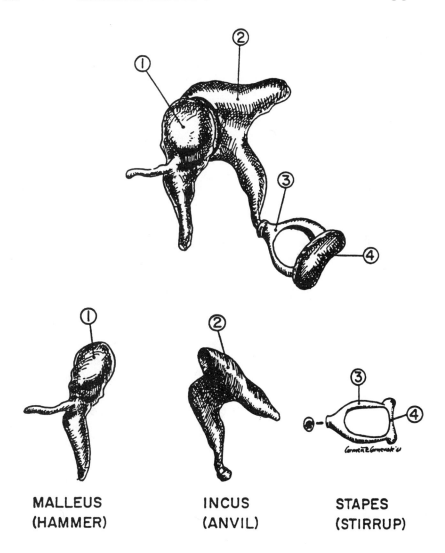

MALLEUS
(HAMMER)

INCUS
(ANVIL)

STAPES
(STIRRUP)

Fig. 12-3. Auditory ossicles as they are joined in the middle ear: 1: malleus (hammer); 2: incus (anvil); 3: stapes (stirrup); 4: footplate of the stapes.

consists of the vestibule, which is connected to the tympanic cavity via the oval window; the cochlea, a spiral-shaped bony tube resembling a snail; the semicircular canals; the vestibular aqueduct and the cochlear aqueduct. The canals and vestibule are the organs of balance.

The cochlea makes 2½ turns about the modiolus, a central cone of spongy bone through which nerves and vessels pass (Arts, 1997). Three parallel cavities, called scala, wind around the modiolus; these are separated from one another by a double plate of bone called the spiral lamina and by the basilar and vestibular (Reissner's) membranes. *(See Figure 12-4.)* The scala vestibuli lies above the spiral lamina and opens into the vestibule through an opening called the fenestra vestibuli. Below the lamina is the scala tympani, connected with the tympanic cavity by the round window. The third cavity, between the other two, is the scala media within the membranous cochlear duct. The duct is formed by the basilar membrane as the floor, the stria vascularis and the vestibular membrane.

Within the scala media is the organ of Corti, the specialized epithelium comprising the acoustic sense organ. This ridge of sensory cells sits on the interior (endolymphatic side) of the basilar membrane. The sensory cells consist of hair cells (cells of Corti), columnar cells with hairlike stereocilia (tubular extensions of the cell surface). There are one row of inner hair cells (about 3500) and three rows of outer hair cells (about 12,000), each row aligned lengthwise within the duct. These auditory receptor cells are connected by nerve fibers running between the two plates of the lamina to 25,000 to 30,000 neurons of the spiral ganglion (Nadol, 1993; Newby and Popelka, 1992). These unite to form the cochlear branch of the eighth cranial nerve (auditory or vestibulocochlear nerve). The organ of Corti is partly overhung by the tectorial membrane, a gelatinous flap within which the stereocilia of the outer hair cells are embedded. *(See Figure 12-5.)*

The auditory nerve proceeds to the pontine brain stem, where all spiral-ganglion fibers form synapses (neural connections) in the cochlear nucleus (collection of specialized cells). From there, nerves project bilaterally (to both sides) to auditory regions of the brain (inferior colliculus, medial geniculate body of the thalamus and auditory cortex of the temporal lobe).

The scala media contains a fluid called endolymph, which differs in composition from the perilymph of the scalae tympanic and vestibuli

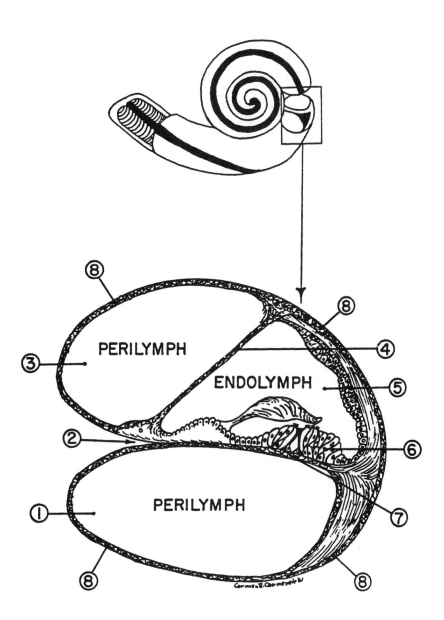

Fig. 12-4. Cross section of the cochlea: 1: scala tympani; 2: spiral lamina; 3: scala vestibuli; 4: Reissner's membrane; 5: scala media (cochlear duct); 6: organ of Corti; 7: basilar membrane; 8: bony cochlea.

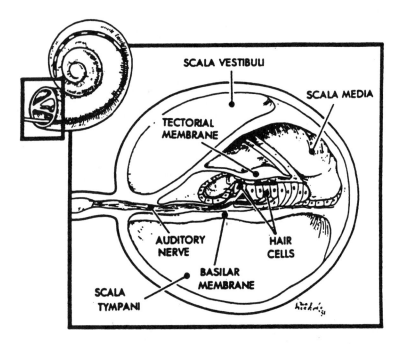

Fig. 12-5. Cross section of the cochlea, showing transduction of sound into hearing. Vibration of the basilar membrane bends hair cell sensory receptors to the acoustic (auditory) nerve, depolarizing them and initiating a chain of electric synaptic events that produce the sensation of sound.

(Salvi and Burkard, 1997). The perilymph has a high sodium concentration and a low potassium concentration. The endolymph, unlike other extracellular fluid in the body, has a high concentration of potassium with low sodium.

12.22   Auditory Physiology

The outer ear acts as a passive sound gatherer and resonator, aiding in detection of the direction of sound. When sound enters the external auditory canal, it sets the tympanic membrane into motion. Because the handle of the malleus is secured to the tympanic membrane, movement of the eardrum sets the ossicular chain into motion.

This movement of the ossicles in the middle ear conveys sound energy from the outer to the inner ear. It matches the low air-based impedance (resistance to being set in motion) of the outer ear to the higher impedance of the fluid within the inner ear.

When the ossicles in the middle ear move, the oval window to the inner ear begins to vibrate, causing displacement of the perilymph of the scala vestibuli. This movement is transmitted to the round window membrane and to the basilar membrane, with a pattern determined by the sound frequency and intensity. Basilar membrane movement causes a shearing between the hair cells and the tectorial membrane. The stereocilia respond by bending, and this deflection initiates nerve action potentials that are transmitted by auditory neurons to the auditory cortex.

About 20 afferent auditory neuron fibers synapse with the basal portion of a single inner hair cell. Other afferent fibers synapse with outer hair cells, about 10 cells per neuron. Thus each hair cell is represented centrally by many nerve processes, whose multiple projections make possible the complex spectrum and quality of hearing. An injury to a few hair cells can therefore make a profound difference centrally (Nadol, 1993).

Normal hearing is binaural: both ears are used, and subtle differences in sound presented to the two ears permit sound localization and filtering out of background noise. The bilateral projections of nerve fibers from the brain stem enables integration of binaural signals.

The auditory system has a tonotopic arrangement: hair cells and their neurons are arranged by the sound frequency to which they respond (Nadol, 1993). Sound is also transmitted to the inner ear by conduction through the temporal bone (Newby and Popelka, 1992). In the person with normal hearing, this component is minor and unnoticed. In the few cases in which air conduction in the outer or middle ear cannot be restored, a hearing aid is used to conduct sound directly to the inner ear.

12.23   Sound Characteristics

A sound wave is vibratory disturbance through air (Staab, 1996). Sound frequency is measured in cycles (number of vibrations) per second, or Hertz (Hz; 1 cycle per second). This is perceived as pitch, measured in mels, in which a simple tone of frequency 1000 Hz results in a pitch of 1000 mels. A doubling in frequency gives a one-octave increase in pitch. The peak frequency of normal human speech is in the 400 to 500 Hz range. Vowels tend to have lower frequency than consonants. Lower frequencies are more audible than higher ones (Donaldson, 1996). The perception of pitch is related to the locus of basilar membrane movement. Studies indicate that higher auditory centers also map in a frequency-specific manner.

Sound intensity (vibration power or pressure) is measured in decibels (dB). Intensity correlates with perceived loudness, measured in sones. Measurement with a hearing instrument is on a logarithmic ratio scale that compares two sound pressure levels (SPL) given in dynes per square centimeter (Donaldson, 1996; Nadol, 1993). In this system, 0 decibels SPL refers to a minimal audible sound of 0.0002 dynes/cm^2. The perception of loudness depends on the number of cochlear nerve cells that are activated (Staab, 1996).

The dynamic range of hearing is the range of frequencies between the softest detectable sounds, about 20 Hz, to the threshold of discomfort, about 20,000 Hz (Staab, 1996). In terms of sound intensity, 0 dB is barely perceptible, 20 dB is a whisper, 65 dB at 3 feet is normal conversation, and discomfort occurs at 100 to 110 dB.

Pure tones consist of a single frequency, and complex tones have multiple frequencies. Noise is defined as sound with irregular frequencies and intensities. Masking—interference by one sound with another—affects hearing acuity. At a given sound intensity, low-pitched tones have a greater masking effect than high-pitched tones. Masking is thought to be related to basilar membrane behavior (Staab, 1996).

Binaural (with both ears) hearing is important for sound localization and for signal processing against a noisy background (Staab, 1996; Sweetow, 1996). Reception of different signals from the two ears, called dichotic listening, improves the brain's ability to cross-correlate input.

12.30   TYPES OF HEARING LOSS

Hearing loss may be conductive, with impairment in conduction of sound from the outside to the inner ear; sensorineural, involving damage to sensory reception or transmission in the inner ear; or mixed. It may also involve central auditory processing. Although hearing impairment in the elderly may be of any type, the most commonly occurring loss—presbycusis—is sensorineural. This may be exacerbated by central hearing deficits (Gravel and Ruben, 1996).

The degree of impairment is described in terms of thresholds for air and bone conduction (Donaldson, 1996). The threshold at which a hearing impairment is considered a handicap to conversation is about

25 to 30 dB (Nadol, 1993). Hearing impairment progression may be rapid or gradual; it may occur in jumps followed by plateaus or declines with a somewhat constant slope.

12.31 Conductive Hearing Loss

Conductive hearing loss affects a mechanism in the outer or middle ear that conducts sound waves to an intact inner hearing organ. It may stem from obstruction of the auditory canal, pathologic changes or structural abnormalities. Such a deficit permits reception of high-intensity and internally produced auditory signals through bone conduction (Gravel and Ruben, 1996). This results in difficulty in hearing low-intensity sounds. Sound is not distorted, and an increase in volume permits normal perception. It is diagnosed when audiometry shows air conduction threshold levels to be poorer than bone conduction levels by 15 dB or more (Donaldson, 1996).[2] Disorders of the outer or middle ear that can lead to conductive hearing loss include blockage by earwax, inflammatory disease leading to accumulation of abnormal tissue in the ear, otosclerosis (growth of abnormal temporal bone), auditory canal collapse and perforation of the tympanic membrane[3] (Nadol, 1993; Newby and Popelka, 1992).

12.32 Sensorineural Hearing Loss (Cochlear Hearing Loss)

Cochlear hearing loss, also called sensorineural loss, involves damage to (or abnormal development of) the inner ear or the eighth cranial nerve (Newby and Popelka, 1992; Roland and Marple, 1997). The most common cause is damage to hair cells. Often the stereocilia are lost. Damage to cochlear neurons may also occur.

[1] Presbycusis

The type of hearing loss most commonly associated with aging is presbycusis, variously defined as inner-ear loss of auditory acuity, bilateral sensorineural loss of high-frequency hearing or progressive hearing loss due to advancing age (Gulya, 1992; Nadol, 1993; Newby and Popelka, 1992). It is found in over ten million elderly persons in the United States, affecting from a third to half of those over the age of 75 years (Cherney, et al., 1996). It typically begins after age 60. Because the loss is sensory, perceived sound is not simply decreased in volume but is distorted as well (Cherney, et al., 1996).

---

[2] See 12.53 *infra.*

[3] See 12.40 *infra.*

Losses occur in the hair cells, peripheral neurons and/or stria vascularis; degeneration of the central auditory pathway is also thought to occur (Gulya, 1992). This age-related degeneration probably results from a combination of factors, including heredity, ototoxicity and noise.[4]

[2] Other Sensorineural Hearing Loss

Other forms of hearing loss due to damage to inner ear structures can occur at any age. Some are more common in the elderly, and it is often difficult to distinguish age-related presbycusis from other types of damage to the inner ear.

Sudden idiopathic (without a known cause) neurosensory hearing loss afflicts about 1 in every 5,000 individuals (Roland and Marple, 1997). Its incidence increases with aging. This can occur within minutes or over the course of a couple of days. It is typically bilateral and is usually associated with tinnitus (ringing in the ears). Most patients begin to recover within a week, but 10 to 40 percent show no recovery. The prognosis is worse when the loss is accompanied by vertigo (sensation of whirling in space). Although the condition is idiopathic, diagnostic evaluation may reveal a tumor, a fistula (abnormal opening) in an inner ear membrane, a viral infection, vascular insufficiency or Meniére's syndrome.[5]

Trauma-induced hearing loss and impairment due to ototoxicity (toxic effect on one or more structures of the auditory system) or infection can occur at any age. However, the accumulation of traumatic influences such as noise may begin to have an effect only in later years. The elderly are more likely to suffer from ototoxic effects of drugs because they take more medications.

12.33 Mixed Hearing Loss

Mixed hearing loss includes components of both conductive and cochlear deficits (Gravel and Ruben, 1996). Many elderly individuals suffer from a combination of conductive hearing loss and presbycusis (Newby and Popelka, 1992).

---

[4] *See* 12.40 *infra.*

[5] *See* 12.40 *infra.*

12.34   Central Auditory Hearing Loss

Perception of the auditory signal is deranged in central auditory loss; this is sometimes termed *auditory processing disorder,* because the problem is with the central processing of the signals (Jerger, et al., 1995). Discrimination and localization of sound and synthesis or fusion of speech may be altered or lost. Many age related changes within the brain can affect perception or interpretation of sound; these include such diverse disorders as tumors and strokes (Newby and Popelka, 1992; Roland and Marple, 1997).

One type of auditory processing disorder specifically affects binaural processing. It is thought that this may result from a decreased efficiency of neural signal transfer from one hemisphere to the other (Jerger, et al., 1995).

12.35   Degrees of Hearing Impairment

Hearing loss varies in degree from none to profound. The degree of impairment is evaluated in terms of decibels of hearing loss: 16 to 25 dB loss is slight, 27 to 40 is mild, 41 to 65 is moderate, 66 to 94 is severe, and more than 95 is profound (Donaldson, 1996).

12.36   Tinnitus

Tinnitus frequently accompanies hearing loss (Segal, 1996). It is the perception of continual sound, usually buzzing, humming or ringing. This condition tends to be more troublesome in the presence of presbycusis. For many, this is one of the most debilitating symptoms accompanying hearing loss (Tyler, 1995). It can occur with either conductive or sensorineural impairment but tends to have a higher pitch in the sensorineural form (Newby and Popelka, 1992).

12.40   ETIOLOGY OF HEARING LOSS

Hearing loss, particularly of high-frequency sound, is a common accompaniment of aging. Thus age itself is a risk factor for hearing impairment. The most common type in the elderly is presbycusis—bilateral sensorineural loss of high-frequency hearing (Cherney, et al., 1996; Nadol, 1993).

Many hereditary and environmental factors act to increase the risk of hearing loss in the elderly. Several commonly administered therapeutic agents have a potential for ototoxicity. The long-term potential damage from noise is a topic of industrial research. Head trauma, tumors, obstruction, infection and radiation are all important causes of hearing impairment.

12.41   Role of Heredity in Hearing Loss

With at least 50 percent of hearing loss having a genetic etiology, hereditary factors are probably the single most common cause of this condition (Nadol, 1993; Ruben, 1996). A major proportion of late-onset hearing loss has a hereditary component. Genetic predisposition plays a significant role in presbycusis and other late-onset hearing loss in adults (as well as in congenital/childhood deafness) (Steel and Kimberling, 1996).

Several genes have been identified in late-onset hearing loss. Such hearing loss may be syndromic (having signs and symptoms that occur together and characterize the disorder) or nonsyndromic (not associated with other detectable abnormalities) (Grundfast and Josephson, 1997). Most hereditary hearing impairment is nonsyndromic autosomal (on a chromosome other than a sex chromosome) recessive (expressed only if a copy is inherited from both parents). Genetically nonsyndromic sensorineural hearing loss most commonly affects hearing in the mid-to high-frequency range and is usually bilateral (Nadol, 1993). Asymmetric or unilateral hearing loss has been found as well. It may be progressive or nonprogressive. Among at least 50 hereditary syndromes associated with conductive hearing loss, the most common is otosclerosis— a progressive replacement of normal hard bone with spongy, vascularized bone (Nadol, 1993).

12.42   Hearing Impairment Due to Ototoxic Substances

A variety of substances have been found to have a toxic effect on the auditory or vestibular system, or both (Nadol, 1993). In many cases, such effects are transient or mild, or they cause only high-frequency impairment that is not detectable without special testing. However, permanent deafness, often sensorineural in type, or vertigo can result from exposure to some chemicals. Most ototoxic substances act by damaging auditory or vestibular hair cells or secretory tissues.

Ototoxic substances include medicines and industrial chemicals. Continual occupational exposure to such chemicals as organic solvents, carbon monoxide and certain metals places the user at risk for hearing impairment (NIOSH, 1996). The most common ototoxicity, however, stems from medications whose lifesaving benefits constantly pose a set of risk-benefit decisions.

Careful monitoring of patients on ototoxic drugs, especially if they are receiving multiple drugs or have compromised renal or hepatic function, may prevent permanent hearing loss. Depending on degree of risk, tests might include serum drug levels, audiometry and vestibular testing, as well as alerting the patient to watch for signs of diminished acuity, tinnitus or vestibular symptoms. Unfortunately, some ototoxic substances may concentrate within the inner ear and lead to continued progressive sensorineural loss after drug discontinuation (Nadol, 1993). Disuse atrophy of neural structures may occur long after damage to the cochlear structures has ceased.

The elderly may have an enhanced susceptibility to ototoxic damage (Garetz and Schacht, 1996). Age alone seems to increase susceptibility, which is further enhanced by malnutrition.

Conditions more commonly found among the elderly, such as diseases that lower hepatic or renal function, can increase the serum concentration of ototoxic agents, exacerbating the risk. Thus a somewhat isolated older person who may take multiple medications and not eat well may enter a downward spiral, in which hearing loss is exacerbated, in turn leading to greater isolation.

Many important clinical drugs are known to have a harmful effect on hearing. These drugs include aminoglycoside antibacterials, antineoplastic (anticancer) agents such as cisplatin (a platinum-based drug) and vinblastine, salicylates, diuretics such as furosemide, quinine (an antimalarial), erythromycin and polypeptide antibiotics. In general, use of medications is more common among the elderly, who use more medications and more types of drugs.[6]

Drug-induced auditory impairment can consist of tinnitus or hearing loss that may be temporary or permanent, may be a mild threshold shift or a profound deafness (Garetz and Schacht, 1996). Vestibular deficits may also result; these may involve mild ataxia (inability to coordinate voluntary muscular movements) or severe vertigo.

Little or no correlation has been found between ototoxicity of various drugs and their molecular structure. Many ototoxic drugs are also nephrotoxic (injurious to the renal system).

---

[6] *See also* ch. 16 for a discussion of drug treatment in the elderly.

[1]   Aminoglycoside Antibiotics

The aminoglycoside antibiotics include gentamicin, amikacin, tobramycin and related medications. Although they are important in the treatment of many serious infections, these drugs can cause permanent hearing loss and vestibular dysfunction. High-frequency perception is usually affected first, but loss then progresses to affect the speech range (Garetz and Schacht, 1996). Prompt cessation of therapy upon detection of early auditory symptoms may reverse some impairment, but in many cases, loss continues after drug administration is stopped. The aminoglycosides vary in their incidence of ototoxicity and in their effects on hearing versus vestibular function.

It is thought that the aminoglycoside toxicity is complex, possibly occurring at multiple sites in the auditory and vestibular systems (Garetz and Schacht, 1996). Early damage occurs at the outer hair cells of the organ of Corti; the nerve processes may suffer if the drug is continued.

Because these drugs have a greater effect on hair cells of the vestibule than on those of the cochlea, they have been used to lessen responsiveness of the vestibular system in Meniére's syndrome (episodes of vertigo, tinnitus and hearing loss) (Garetz and Schacht, 1996; Monsell, et al., 1993). Administration is usually through the tympanic membrane.

[2]   Antineoplastic Agents

Ototoxic antineoplastic agents include nitrogen mustards, vinblastine and other vinca alkaloids and the platinum-containing drugs cisplatin and carboplatin (Garetz and Schacht, 1996). Cisplatin acts against a variety of tumors by suppressing cell growth. Its efficacy makes it an important anticancer drug despite its side effects (Grau, et al., 1996). The most common ototoxic effects are loss of high-frequency hearing and tinnitus. Such hearing loss is dose related, cumulative and permanent (Schweitzer, 1993).

[3]   Salicylates

Salicylates, especially aspirin, are widely used for their anti-inflammatory and analgesic effects. At high doses, which are generally used only for rheumatoid arthritis, they can produce transient hearing loss and tinnitus (Jung, et al., 1993). Such loss is generally mild and bilateral. Hearing typically returns to normal within a few days of ceasing therapy.

[4] Diuretics

Loop diuretics such as furosemide, so called because they inhibit salt and water reabsorption in the loop of Henle of the renal tubules, can cause transient hearing loss and tinnitus (Rybak, 1993). Permanent deficits do occur infrequently.

[5] Other Drugs

Tinnitus and a transient shift in hearing threshold are documented side effects of the antimalarial agents quinine and chloroquine and the antibiotic erythromycin. Medications whose ototoxicity is less frequently seen or less well documented include the antibiotic vancomycin and the antiprotozoal, antitumor agent difluoromethylornithine (Garetz and Schacht, 1996).

[6] Drug-Drug Interactions

Drug-drug interactions are always of particular concern in the elderly, both because multiple medications are more likely to be required and because older persons are more likely to have compromised renal or hepatic function. As with many types of side effects, ototoxic side effects of medications may be more than additive when two or more drugs are given. Some combinations can have profound effects on the auditory system, leading to rapid irreversible damage (Garetz and Schacht, 1996).

The most common kind of potentiation of ototoxic effects occurs when loop diuretic therapy is combined with aminoglycoside antibiotic treatment. This combination can lead to complete deafness. Either class of drugs may also potentiate the ototoxic effects of cisplatin, vancomycin or polymixin B. Noise has also been found to potentiate ototoxicity of drugs, particularly aspirin and aminoglycosides.

Conversely, some therapeutic combinations lessen ototoxicity. Cisplatin effects may be ameliorated by fosfomycin or some sulfur containing compounds.

12.43 Hearing Loss Stemming from Infection

Infections can occur in the outer, middle or inner ear. Many resolve without permanent damage. However, untreated infection can lead to hearing impairment through inflammation or damage to auditory structures. Infection can be viral or bacterial.

[1]   Viral Infections

It has been estimated that viral infections of the inner ear lead to more than 40,000 cases of hearing loss and vestibular dysfunction each year (Woolf, 1996). Up to 33 percent of idiopathic sudden loss of hearing may be due to a preceding or concurrent upper respiratory viral infection. Such impairment is often conductive in type (Donaldson, 1996). Among the effects of infection are tympanic membrane thickening (Nadol, 1993).

Other viruses shown to be associated with hearing loss and vertigo are mumps, chicken pox and measles, which have been implicated in the development of otosclerosis (Nadol, 1993). Many other viruses, including influenza, have been implicated in hearing impairment, although without proof.

[2]   Bacterial Infections

Bacterial infections can cause either conductive or sensorineural damage. Bacterial meningitis results in sensorineural hearing impairment in 5 to 35 percent of disease survivors. Syphilis can cause unilateral or bilateral sensorineural damage. Tuberculosis of the temporal bone, a possible complication of pulmonary tuberculosis, can cause conductive or sensorineural damage.

12.44   Autoimmune Disorders Leading to Hearing Loss

Some progressive hearing loss is thought to have an immunologic basis. Such autoimmune diseases as systemic lupus erythematosus (SLE) and polyarteritis nodosa can cause sensorineural impairment (Nadol, 1993). An immune-mediated hearing loss known as autoimmune inner ear disease (AIED) is poorly understood (Woolf, 1996). Demyelination (a type of nerve damage involving destruction of the sheath that coats nerves) in multiple sclerosis can also lead to sensorineural hearing loss.

12.45   Hearing Impairment Due to Noise or Trauma

Trauma from impact or noise can lead to hearing loss.

[1]   Noise

The Occupational Safety and Health Administration (OSHA) recognizes noise as an occupational hazard of increasing importance

(NIOSH, 1996). Studies indicate that noise of sufficient intensity to cause pain, a sensation of blockage or tinnitus may damage the hair cells, resulting in sensorineural impairment experienced as a shift in hearing threshold. Most individuals recover their hearing after temporary, short-term exposure, but repeated or prolonged exposure to high noise levels results in permanent damage.

Most continual noise exposure is occupational, but such recreational activities as listening to loud music, especially with headphones, can also cause sensorineural damage. Impact (impulsive, sudden, discontinuous) noise may be more deleterious than continuous noise of equivalent energy (NIOSH, 1996). The effects of combined impact and continuous noise appear to be synergistic rather than additive.

Some drugs and chemical agents appear to have a synergistic effect with noise in causing damage to hearing.

[2] Impact Trauma

Skull injuries can lead to either conductive or sensorineural hearing impairment (Nadol, 1993). Conductive loss can result from temporal bone fractures that result in tympanic membrane perforation or damage to the external auditory canal or ossicles. Sensorineural hearing loss is a less common outcome of fractures but may result from concussion.

Blunt or penetrating head injury can perforate the tympanic membrane (Meyerhoff, et al., 1997). Fracture or dislocation of the ossicular chain can occur at the same time. In most instances, the result is a surgically treatable conductive hearing loss.[7]

Impact can cause fistula formation between the middle ear and inner ear by rupture of the membrane between them. Resulting fluid loss from the inner ear can affect hearing or balance. Surgical repair may stabilize hearing and restore balance (Nadol, 1993).

12.46 Hearing Impairment Caused by Obstruction

Perhaps the simplest cause of conductive hearing loss is obstruction of the external auditory canal by accumulation of cerumen (earwax) or collapse of the canal (Nadol, 1993; Wayner, 1996). Cerumen impaction—buildup of earwax to the point that it obstructs the external auditory canal—has an increased frequency in the geriatric population (Marple and Roland, 1997; Parisier, et al., 1997). This can be due to

---

[7] *See* 12.71 *infra.*

proliferation and coarsening of lateral hairs, and tendency of the cerumen to become drier and denser. Unfortunately, an individual's attempts to remove hardened cerumen may introduce bacteria or push the cerumen farther into the canal, increasing the impaction and possibly perforating the tympanic membrane. Hearing loss may be sudden because impairment is minor until obstruction is complete.

Obstruction of the eustachian tube can affect hearing by filling the middle ear with fluid instead of air.

12.47   Other Causes of Hearing Impairment

A variety of other causes can produce hearing impairment. Most of these are more common among the elderly. Therapeutic irradiation to the head or neck may cause conductive or sensorineural damage (Nadol, 1993). Hearing loss is common in patients with chronic renal failure who are on dialysis (Bazzi, et al., 1995). In most cases, the impairment is sensorineural. There does not seem to be a correlation between severity of loss and duration of dialysis. Functional middle ear damage has been found in patients with long-term nasogastric feeding (Vento, et al., 1995).

Acoustic neuroma and other primary tumors of the temporal area can lead to hearing loss. Metastases from tumors elsewhere in the body can also impair hearing and balance.

12.50   DIAGNOSIS OF HEARING LOSS

Hearing evaluation typically begins with the outer ear and progresses inward. The primary care physician can easily screen elderly patients for hearing impairment on a routine basis (Jerger, et al., 1995). Tests for such assessment include a pure tone assessment, involving response to pure tones at set frequencies (typically 500, 1000, 2000 and 4000 Hz at 40 dB), and a questionnaire such as the Hearing Handicap Inventory for the Elderly. If indicated by this test, the patient should be referred to an otolaryngologist or audiologist.

A person may also be prompted by awareness of slowly progressing hearing loss or by family concern to consult a physician, an audiologist or a hearing aid specialist. Although a competent audiologist can determine whether the deficit is a simple impairment requiring a hearing aid or other assistive devices or a disease process requiring an otolaryngologist's services, a medical examination is particularly important for an elderly person who may have multiple problems.

12.51   History and Physical Examination

As with any disorder, an accurate history of onset and progression is the first item of hearing evaluation. Sudden or recent onset or rapid progression indicates the possibility of an acute process and the need for a thorough medical examination, including neurologic evaluation (Donaldson, 1996). Other symptoms requiring referral to a physician include hearing loss accompanied by acute or chronic dizziness, recent or current ear drainage, ear or head pain or discomfort, history or signs of recent trauma, presence of visible cerumen (earwax) or a foreign body within the ear canal. Asymmetric hearing or balance impairment indicate the possibility of a tumor. The examiner should elicit a history of any predisposing factors, such as family tendency or exposure to ototoxic agents, infection or noise (Nadol, 1993).

12.52   Otoscopic Examination

Otoscopy shows abnormalities of the outer ear or tympanic membrane (Donaldson, 1996). Any blockage must be resolved before auditory tests continue. The auditory canal may also collapse in the very old; this requires a special speculum (instrument for enlarging an opening for viewing) or tubing for hearing evaluation.

12.53   Audiometric Evaluation

When hearing loss is detected, specialized audiologic tests are used to determine the person's function and potential for improvement. The American Speech Language Hearing Association and the American National Standard Institute have standards for auditory evaluation procedures and instrumentation (Donaldson, 1996).

Audiometric tests, which are best performed in a sound-isolated room, measure the relation between the hearing threshold for air conduction versus bone conduction, assess the level of hearing loss, determine the levels of hearing comfort and evaluate the degree of sound distortion. Such tests have both prescriptive and fitting value in the process of hearing aid selection.

Tuning fork testing may be used in screening or confirmation (Donaldson, 1996). The Weber test for lateralization and the Rinne test, in which the fork stem is placed on the frontal bone of the skull or the mastoid process of the jaw, respectively, are able to indicate whether hearing loss is sensorineural or conductive. *(See Figure 12-6 and Figure 12-7.)* These tests also indicate whether impairment is unilateral or bilateral.

Pure tone audiometry tests reception of pure tones at a variety of frequencies, commonly at octaves from 250 Hz to 8,000 Hz (Donaldson, 1996). Testing begins with the better ear, using either the ascending method, which begins with inaudible tones, or the descending method.

Air conduction pathways are tested using earphones. Testing each ear separately, audiometry assesses frequency range as well as intensity of sound heard. Sound presented to one ear also reaches the other via air and bone conduction; this can confound test results (Newby and Popelka, 1992). Bone conduction audiometry tests cochlear competence by presenting sound energy directly to the cochlea (Donaldson, 1996).

Speech audiometry presents a live or recorded voice, usually with spondaic (Spondee) words to determine level of word understanding. These are words having two syllables with equal stress on each. The speech threshold and the pure tone audiogram should be within a few decibels of each other (Donaldson, 1996).

Impedance audiometry, or tympanometry, assesses tympanic membrane compliance and movement and the contraction of the stapedius muscle (Donaldson, 1996). As an objective measurement of middle ear function, it is usable with cognitively impaired persons.

Auditory evoked brain-stem response (ABR) uses electroencephalography to determine neural responses to auditory stimuli (Nadol, 1993; Newby and Popelka, 1992). It is measured by using broadband clicks and recording from the surface of the head; measurements of intervals between wave peaks gives information about neural activity through the brain stem pathway. This test can indicate the presence of central neural lesions. It is useful in cognitively impaired or uncooperative patients.

12.54   Imaging Techniques

When symptoms or audiometric tests indicate that the impairment may not be a simple conductive or sensorineural hearing loss, imaging studies may be necessary. Magnetic resonance imaging (MRI) or computed tomography is useful to identify lesions of the brain, brain stem, temporal bone or mastoid process (Nadol, 1993). MRI is also

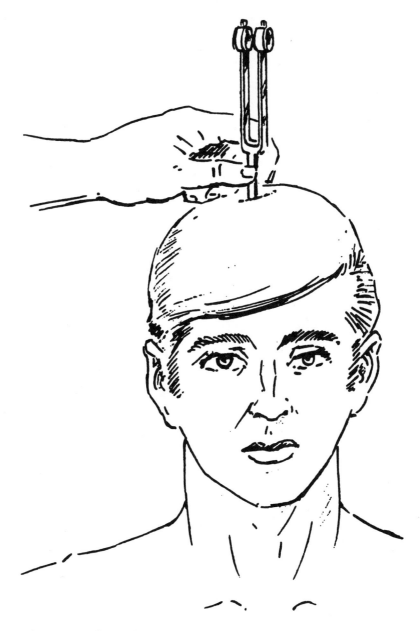

Fig. 12-6. The Weber test is performed when pathology of the middle ear or auditory nerve is suspected. A tuning fork is struck and placed on the top of the skull, and the patient is asked to report in which ear the sound is heard better.

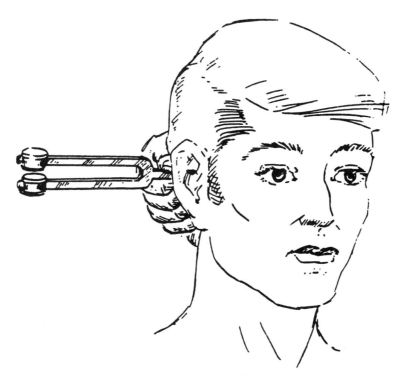

Fig. 12-7. In the first part of the Rinne test, a tuning fork is struck a moderate blow, and the base is held firmly against the mastoid bone. When the person can no longer hear the sound through bone conduction, the tuning fork is held near the opening of the ear, and air conduction is measured.

an important component of assessment prior to cochlear implantation (Ketten, 1995).[8]

12.60   NON-SURGICAL MANAGEMENT OF HEARING IMPAIRMENT

Most hearing impairment is managed by assistive devices, such as hearing aids, with training in adaptive behavior. Management of hearing impairment ideally involves a team consisting of the family physician, who screens and detects hearing loss; an otolaryngologist or otologist, who determines the nature of the deficit; an audiologist, who tests hearing and prescribes a hearing aid type; and a hearing

---

[8] *See* 12.72[1] *infra.*

aid specialist, who fits and tests the device. It is thought that the increase in the number of hearing impaired people as the population ages, changes in health care financing and advances in hearing aid technology will result in a larger role for hearing instrument specialists (Hambley and Cole, 1996).

12.61   Use of Hearing Aids

The most common approach to hearing impairment uses a hearing aid. Hearing aids electronically amplify sound (Mynders, 1996). They are thus most useful for conductive hearing loss, in which the impairment affects sound level rather than clarity. Advances in hearing aid technology in recent years include improvements in both amplification and sound processing as well as impressive miniaturization (House, 1996). In addition, greater emphasis is placed on early detection of hearing impairment and customized fitting of assistive devices so that the patient may begin the adjustment process while the impairment is still mild.

Nevertheless, many persons resist admitting to having hearing loss and perceive the use of an aid as a stigma to be avoided (Sweetow, 1996). Even the best assistive device is of no value to a patient who lacks motivation to be fitted properly and to be trained in its use.

[1]   Hearing Aid Candidates

Hearing aids amplify sound and are most useful when the hearing deficit is a decrease in audibility (Sweetow, 1996). When speech discrimination is decreased because of cochlear distortion or abnormal central processing, a hearing aid may be of little value.

Hearing loss in the elderly is often sensorineural and is less likely to benefit from a hearing aid than is conductive hearing loss (Segal, 1996). However, newer devices that filter and process sound may prove more useful for people with sensorineural loss.

A hearing aid may be prescribed by a physician, typically an otologist or otolaryngologist, or an audiologist. It may be fitted by either or by a hearing aid specialist.

[2]   Hearing Aid Technology

A great many hearing aid styles and technologies have been developed in the effort to improve their utility. A hearing aid may work by air conduction, amplifying sound that passes from the outer to the inner ear, or by bone conduction (Roland and Marple, 1997). Air conduction amplification is generally preferred (Johnson, 1996). Bone conduction is used mainly in cases of uncorrectable ear drainage or ear canal stenosis.

Components include sound input microphones, telecoils to transduce the sound to an electric current, amplifiers to increase its energy and receivers to transduce current back to sound. Batteries provide power. Additional components may include preamplifiers, circuit limiters, signal processors, filtering devices and programming circuits. Patient controls include volume, tone, directional microphones and telephone switches, as well as on/off.

The several styles include in-the-ear (ITE), behind-the-ear (BTE), in-the-canal (ITC) and completely-in-the-canal (CIC) (Johnson, 1996; Sweetow, 1996). The ITE is the most commonly used, comprising at least 60 percent of those now worn. The choice of style may be dictated in part by ear anatomy. Comfort is important to continued wearing. Ears that produce excessive cerumen (earwax) or are draining may need bone conduction systems that do not enter the ear.

Because a hearing aid in the canal is nearer to the eardrum than one behind or in the ear, less amplification is needed to produce adequate sound pressure at the tympanic membrane, and feedback and distortion are lessened (Sweetow, 1996). A CIC hearing aid may reduce feedback problems when the hearing loss is the high-frequency sensorineural type. These devices require greater manual dexterity and are more likely to be uncomfortable.

Various hearing aid technologies have been developed (Mynders, 1996). A linear circuit simply amplifies sound, which is changed only in loudness (Sweetow, 1996). Because loud sounds may be uncomfortable if they are amplified to the same degree as soft sounds, compression circuits soften or compress selected sounds, so that faint sounds are amplified more than are loud ones (Mynders, 1996). Adaptive compression circuits differentiate among incoming signals. Automatic signal processor (ASP) circuits electronically monitor and modify incoming sounds with respect to frequency, intensity or time. Soft sounds are amplified and loud sounds are softened. The new digital programmable circuits allow the patient and the instrument vendor to program several different circuits, which may then be selected for different environments, such as television watching or business conferences. These are often the best solution for hard-to-fit patients, but cost and complexity may make them unsuitable for many of the elderly (Johnson, 1996).

[3] Advantages and Limitations of Hearing Aids

Hearing aids amplify sounds, which must still be processed by the inner ear. Thus they are helpful only when the hearing impairment is peripheral in origin (Sweetow, 1996).

Persons with high-frequency sensorineural hearing impairment lose the ability to hear high-pitched sounds but may retain hearing in the lower pitches. It is difficult to fit them with hearing aids because they may find annoying overamplification in the low-pitch range, discomfort at moderately elevated intensity, feedback (squealing or whistling) and perception of unnatural voice quality.

Hearing assisted by a hearing aid lacks the normal ear's ability to compensate for background noise and to select a voice from background babble (Roland and Marple, 1997). The aid may also distort sound so that desired sounds are less prominent than some background ones. Optimum use of hearing aids may require attention to the problem of background noise, which hinders speech perception in cochlear hearing loss (Gravel and Ruben, 1996).

Background noise is a particular problem when the listener is a distance from the sound source, as in an auditorium (Sweetow, 1996). The speech intensity decreases with distance, while background noise surrounding the listener remains. To some degree, the individual can compensate by choosing environments, such as restaurants, with a quiet atmosphere and without background music. Use of infrared sound transmission is increasingly available in theaters and concert halls. [9]

Hearing aid wearers may find that their own voices sound peculiar. This is partly due to ear occlusion, which results in hearing one's own voice by bone conduction rather than air conduction, and partly due to elimination of resonance provided by the ear canal (Sweetow, 1996).

Although much progress has been made in speech processing by hearing aids, inner ear or central nervous system distortion is not corrected.

---

[9] *See* 12.62 *infra.*

[4]   Binaural Versus Monaural Hearing Aid Use

More than 60 percent of hearing aids in use in the United States are binaural (one in each ear) (Sweetow, 1996). Despite cosmetic and financial considerations, most audiologists recommend two aids, even when one ear is nearly normal. For most individuals, this approach improves sound localization and filtering of background noise (Donaldson, 1996). It also permits use of a lower volume because of summation of sound. Although some people find the input from binaural aids confusing, most adjust well.

In the elderly, however, binaural amplification is not always the best approach. Deleterious effects of binaural amplification have been found in some elderly individuals, who experience interference with speech perception, particularly following use of a monaural hearing aid (Gravel and Ruben, 1996).

For some, the best course may be to use an aid that transmits the signal arriving at the poor ear to the opposite ear. This may be done through a wire or an FM signal and is called contralateral routing of signal (Johnson, 1996; Sweetow, 1996).

[5]   Selection and Use of a Hearing Aid

It is important that a person experiencing hearing loss consult an otolaryngologist (ear, nose and throat specialist) prior to trying a hearing aid. Proper diagnosis of the impairment and its cause are prerequisites to the decision to use a hearing aid.

An otolaryngologist or audiologist should consider occupation and living arrangements in determining the best course of action for a hearing-impaired individual (Sweetow, 1996). Psychosocial factors that may influence an individual's hearing ability or response to sound include intelligence, education, cognitive impairment, motivation and age (Donaldson, 1996).

An audiologist who will work closely with the patient in fitting and fine-tuning the instrument is of great importance for an elderly person. The process of adaptation requires cooperation and communication (Hambley and Cole, 1996).

Testing of a new device should be conducted in high-demand conditions rather than in a quiet room (Sweetow, 1996). It is important to establish that the instrument delivers a comfortable listening level (Donaldson, 1996). The ideal instrument should make speech audible while avoiding uncomfortable loudness. Computer-aided real-ear measurements use a probe microphone in the ear canal to assess the functional gain (difference between aided and unaided thresholds) resulting from a hearing aid (Hambley and Cole, 1996).

Counseling to establish realistic expectations is an important aspect of the fitting procedure. Hearing does not become loud and clear as soon as the device is inserted. The patient has also become accustomed to impaired hearing, so that the brain has forgotten how to process some sounds, which now seem new and unfamiliar (Hambley and Cole, 1996). Orientation to a hearing aid involves gradual increases in wearing time, practice in use and maintenance, and patient adjustment to a new way of hearing in a variety of settings (Wayner, 1996). Hearing aid use should be combined with such forms of rehabilitation as speech reading.

An understanding of other possible age-related infirmities is also important. The elderly may be particularly resistant to using a hearing aid because they view it as another sign of diminishing ability. Such disorders as arthritis can aggravate difficulties with hearing aid use, making it harder to change batteries or insert the ear mold. Diminished visual acuity can interfere with maintaining and adjusting the device.

12.62   Assistive Devices for the Hearing Impaired

A variety of assistive devices to enhance the hearing-impaired person's understanding of speech or awareness of the environment are available to promote a person's continued independence (Roland and Marple, 1997). Assistive technology may be used alone or in combination with a hearing aid or cochlear implant and may provide auditory, visual or tactile information. Alerting devices include telephone amplifying receivers and flashing lights on telephones, doorbells, timers and clocks, or tactile stimulators.

Use of infrared listening systems in theaters and auditoriums is increasing. In this method, microphones pick up the speech, and infrared rays transmit the sound to the listener's receivers. This has the advantage of eliminating background noise (Johnson, 1996). Another method—frequency modulating (FM) transmission—uses radio waves to transmit sound.

Devices to improve use of the telephone may amplify sound, providing auditory enhancement, or enable the person to communicate using a keyboard via the phone lines. Use of a computer with a modem is a recent aid to telecommunications.

An answering service with an operator who is trained to relay information to a hearing-impaired person is particularly helpful for a person who continues to work. The answering service might relay information from incoming calls by use of e-mail.

12.63   Aural Rehabilitation

Aural rehabilitation to enhance the communication functions of a hearing-impaired individual encompasses psychological support and training in compensatory techniques as well as facilitating the use of assistive devices (Nodar, 1996). Unlike much rehabilitation, aural rehabilitation does not restore lost function. It does, however, train the person with hearing loss to use her or his remaining functions and available technology.

[1]   Speechreading

In speechreading (the term preferred over "lipreading"), the hearing-impaired individual watches the speaker and synthesizes context, environment, gestures, facial expressions and body language with lip movements and sound in order to understand conversation (Nodar, 1996). Some individuals have a natural facility for this, but it can be learned.

Although speechreading may not be necessary in the early stages of hearing impairment, instruction in its use before it is required will ease the transition from hearing to impairment. An additional consideration is that the aging process may slow the learning process and diminish visual acuity. In many cases, speechreading is needed the most when eyesight is also failing (Roland and Marple, 1997). However, many individuals resist such training when hearing impairment is mild.

[2]   Psychosocial Skills

It is difficult for many hearing-impaired persons to admit their disability, yet doing so enlists the help of family, friends and colleagues (Wayner, 1996). Acknowledgment of the problem opens the door to asking others to speak slowly and clearly, while facing the hearing-impaired person. Many simple adjustments can be made to the environment in terms of seat placement and lighting if requested.

Lighting that illuminates the speaker's face will help the hearing-impaired person read lips and body gestures.

[3] Sign Language

Use of sign language is seldom an option, because the person who loses hearing late in life still lives in a world of hearing people, who do not know it (Roland and Marple, 1997). Modifications in its use may be needed as the person ages. The older person who may have previously been skilled in its use may, for example, be losing visual acuity, so that extra attention must be given to environmental factors.

12.70 SURGICAL APPROACHES TO HEARING IMPAIRMENT

A surgical approach is used when there is a clear need for an anatomic correction or when a profound hearing deficit cannot be improved by hearing aid use.

Surgical implantation of electronic devices to deliver sound directly to the proximal (nearer the center of the body) auditory nerve elements offers hearing to many persons with severe to profound sensorineural hearing loss. These cochlear implants partially replace the function of the cochlea, bypassing the outer and middle ear and the hair cells that are most often the dysfunctional components in sensorineural deafness (Balkany, 1993).

12.71 Surgical Correction of Conductive Hearing Loss

Conductive hearing loss due to mechanical defects can often be restored (Hall and Grose, 1993; Nadol, 1993). Perhaps the easiest method is removal of cerumen (earwax). This may be done to restore hearing after complete obstruction or as a regular prophylactic measure for patients who experience increased secretion (Parisier, et al., 1997).

Surgery may be helpful when hearing loss is due to chronic ear disease (Glasscock, et al., 1997). The location of such surgery presents unusual risks. The most common complication is facial nerve injury, which can happen with even the most skilled surgeon performing the operation. Knowledge of facial nerve location coupled with intraoperative facial nerve monitoring should minimize this complication. Other potential complications are injury to the dura (outer membrane) covering the brain, corda tympani nerve or vestibule.

[1] Tympanoplasty

Tympanoplasty (myringoplasty) repairs a perforated tympanic membrane, with or without grafting (Glasscock, et al., 1997). Grafts may use autogenous (from the patient) cartilage to provide greater support for the membrane or autogenous fascia to close large perforations (Perkins and Bui, 1996). Tympanoplasty with mastoidectomy (hollowing out of the mastoid process) may be necessary to eradicate middle ear disease such as chronic suppurative otitis media (middle ear infection) or cholesteatoma (aggressive but noncancerous proliferation of keratinizing epithelial tissue, which forms fingernails and hair, in the middle ear) (Cook, et al., 1996; Meyerhoff, et al., 1997).

[2] Ossicular Reconstruction

Ossicular reconstruction repairs or replaces a member of the ossicular chain, usually the stapes, which may have been damaged or destroyed by a disease process (Glasscock, et al., 1997). Today's prostheses are comprised of biocompatible materials, such as hydroxyapatite.

[3] Surgical Treatment of Otosclerosis

Although otosclerosis usually has its onset prior to age 40, recent improvements in surgical treatment enable restoration of hearing to both young and old who suffer from this disorder (House, 1997; Newby and Popelka, 1992). Otosclerosis initially affects the stapes, often resulting in fixation. In stapedectomy, the ankylosed (stiffened by a disease process, with fibrous or bony union across the joint) stapes is replaced with a prosthesis.

12.72 Cochlear Implants

Cochlear implants bypass the outer and middle ear and deliver processed sound directly to spiral ganglion cells in the cochlea or the axons of the auditory nerve. They are suitable for adults with profound binaural sensorineural hearing loss from damage to inner ear structures who no longer benefit from conventional hearing aids (Roland and Marple, 1997). Although the sound perceived through an implant is very different from normal hearing, most patients find that this technology improves their quality of life (Maillet, et al., 1995; Thomsett and Nickerson, 1993). The technology has been called "the most significant advance in the surgical management of profound deafness in history" (Black, 1995).

[1] Eligibility for Cochlear Implantation

Only patients with profound sensorineural deafness who have been shown to derive little or no benefit from hearing aids are eligible for cochlear implantation. Generally the guideline for consideration of an implant is an ability to understand less than 30 percent of speech. An individual who has not tried a powerful hearing aid must attempt to use one before being accepted for surgery (Balkany, 1993; Miyamoto, 1996).

[2] Cochlear Implant Components and Variations in Technology

The components of a cochlear implant are a microphone worn over the ear, a speech processor worn on a belt or in a pocket, a transmitter/receiver that transmits an electric signal across the skin by an electromagnet-coil combination and electrodes in the cochlea (Roland and Marple, 1997). The microphone receives sounds as acoustic waves and sends them to the speech processor, which transduces sound signals into electric signals (encodes the sound). The electric impulses are sent via the transmitter/receiver to the electrodes, which stimulate the auditory nerve endings.

Implants vary in a number of technologic features, including the encoded speech features and the filters applied to the sound (Miyamoto, 1996; Roland and Marple, 1997). The newest speech processors can separate speech and other meaningful sounds from background sounds by analyzing incoming sounds by amplitude.

From 1 to 22 electrodes may be implanted into the inner ear. Stimulation by several electrodes at more than one site gives a wider variety of sound, including variation in pitch, and gives better speech recognition, than does use of a single-electrode device (Cohen, et al., 1993).

[3] Implantation and Adaptation

Preimplantation testing includes audiologic assessment to determine degree and type of hearing loss, and radiologic evaluation of the cochlea by magnetic resonance imaging or computed tomography to assure the presence of the intact auditory neural elements that are essential to success (Miyamoto, 1996). No tests have been developed, however, to evaluate the functional status of the auditory nerve. The ear must be infection free, and the tympanic membrane must be intact.

Outcomes research has shown that it is impossible to predict implant benefit reliably.

Surgery to open the cochlea and insert the electrode in the scala tympani is done under general anesthesia, usually with overnight hospitalization. Mastoidectomy (removal of the mastoid bone) is required to gain access to the cochlea. Surgical complications are rare but include necrosis of the skin flap covering the implant and temporary facial nerve paresis (incomplete paralysis) (Balkany, 1993).

Programming of the external components to communicate with the implanted components is done by an audiologist four to six weeks after implantation (Roland and Marple, 1997). Most patients report immediate improvement upon implant activation, and this increases over time (Cohen, et al., 1993).

Benefits from cochlear implants range from improved ability to speechread through better cue perception to understanding of speech without looking directly at the speaker (Cohen, et al., 1993). Up to 90 percent of recipients show some improvement. Decreased tinnitus has been reported by 28 to 55 percent of individuals in whom it had been bothersome prior to surgery (Tyler, 1995).

In addition to the practical adjustment to sounds received via cochlear implants, there are important psychological adaptations. Despite preoperative counseling, many patients expect miracles that do not occur. The brain must learn to interpret the nerve impulses from the implant as recognizable sounds. Such adaptation to processed sounds takes time and work. Despite initially unfulfilled expectations and the amount of work required, most implant recipients find the results worthwhile. Patient motivation is a strong determinant of implant success.

[4]   Cochlear Implants in the Elderly

There is no upper age limit for cochlear implantation as long as the individual's health permits the surgery (Miyamoto, 1996). Persons as old as 87 years have received implants. Some studies have found that younger adults do better with cochlear implants than the elderly (Cohen, et al., 1993). However, most studies show that elderly patients experience increased self-confidence, greater social interaction and improved quality of life after implantation (Facer, et al., 1995; Kelsall, et al., 1995).

12.73   Tumor Removal

When hearing impairment is due to a tumor, such as an acoustic neuroma, excision of the tumor may halt the progression of the loss. Early detection with new scanning instrumentation, coupled with stereotactic surgical procedures, has made it possible to preserve hearing in many cases. With improved surgical approaches, significant restoration of hearing may result (Nadol, 1993; Weber and Gantz, 1996). However, some experts caution that the risk of removal of an acoustic neuroma is so great that a conservative approach of watching is preferable to immediate surgery (Jorgensen and Pedersen, 1994).

12.80   PROGNOSIS

Technology to serve the hearing impaired population has progressed rapidly, and many older persons can now be assisted by it. Because it has been shown that the elderly can benefit from sensory aids, it is important that these be made available to them (Appollonio, et al., 1995; Appollonio, et al., 1996; Jerger, et al., 1995; Kelsall, et al., 1995).

Early detection and assistance are important for any hearing-impaired person, because a longer period of deafness impedes adjustment to assistive devices. Early detection and assistance are particularly vital for the elderly because other aspects of the aging process, such as decreasing manipulative dexterity and visual acuity, may exacerbate the difficulties of learning to use hearing aids and other devices. The correlation between hearing impairment and decreased physical mobility also supports the need for early detection in order to sustain general health and function (Dargent-Molina, et al., 1996). Early detection and rehabilitation may prevent the loneliness, loss of self-esteem and decreased independence that are frequent accompaniments of hearing impairment (Chen, 1994).

Screening for hearing impairment is simple, and the equipment is relatively inexpensive.[10] Thus it may be feasible for nurses and social workers, as well as primary care physicians, to assess hearing in the elderly (Chen, 1994).

---

[10] See 12.50 supra.

12.100   BIBLIOGRAPHY

Text References

Appollonio, I., et al.: Effects of Sensory Aids on the Quality of Life and Mortality of Elderly People: A Multivariate Analysis. Age Ageing 25:89-96, 1996.

Appollonio, I., et al.: Sensory Impairments and Mortality in an Elderly Community Population: A Six-Year Follow-Up Study. Age Ageing 24:30-36, 1995.

Arts, H. A.: Anatomy of the Ear. In: Roland, P. S., et al.: Hearing Loss. New York: Thieme, 1997.

Balkany, T.: A Brief Perspective on Cochlear Implants. N. Engl. J. Med. 328::281-282, 1993.

Bazzi, C., et al.: Hearing Loss in Short-and Long-Term Haemodialysed Patients. Nephrol. Dial. Transplant. 10:1865-1868, 1995.

Black, F. O.: Forward: Multicenter Comparative Study of Cochlear Implants: Final Reports of the Department of Veterans Affairs Cooperative Study Program. Ann. Otol. Rhinol. Laryngol. Suppl. 16S:4-5, 1995.

Chen, H. L.: Hearing in the Elderly. Relation of Hearing Loss, Loneliness, and Self-Esteem. J. Gerontol. Nurs. 20:22-28, 1994.

Cherney, L. R., et al.: Effects of Aging on Communication. In: Lewis, C. B. (Ed.): Aging: The Health Care Challenge, 3rd ed. Philadelphia: Davis, 1996.

Cohen, M. M. and Gorlin, R. J.: Epidemiology, Etiology, and Genetic Patterns. In: Gorlin, R. J., et al. (Ed.): Hereditary Hearing Loss and Its Syndromes. New York: Oxford University Press, 1995.

Cohen, N. L., et al.: A Prospective, Randomized Study of Cochlear Implants. N. Engl. J. Med. 328:233-237, 1993.

Cook, J. A., et al.: Hearing Results Following Modified Radical Versus Canal-Up Mastoidectomy. Ann. Otol. Rhinol. Laryngol. 105:379-383, 1996.

Coroni-Huntley, J. C., et al.: Epidemiology of Disability in the Oldest Old. In: Suzman, R. M., et al.: The Oldest Old. New York: Oxford University Press, 1992.

Dargent-Molina, P., et al.: Sensory Impairments and Physical Disability in Aged Women Living at Home. Int. J. Epidemiol. 25:621-629, 1996.

Donaldson, L. L.: Evaluating the Patient. In: Goldenberg, R. A. (Ed.): Hearing Aids: A Manual for Clinicians. Philadelphia: Lippincott-Raven, 1996.

Facer, G. W., et al.: Cochlear Implantation in the Senior Citizen Age Group Using the Nucleus 22-Channel Device. Ann. Otol. Rhinol. Laryngol. Suppl. 166:187-190, 1995.

Garetz, S. L. and Schacht, J: Ototoxicity: Of Mice and Men. In: Van De Water, T. R., et al.: Clinical Aspects of Hearing. New York: Springer-Verlag, 1996.

Glasscock, M. E., et al.: Surgery for Chronic Ear Disease. In: Hughes, G. B., et al. (Eds.): Clinical Otology, 2nd ed. New York: Thieme, 1997.

Grau, J. J., et al.: Calcium Supplementation and Ototoxicity in Patients Receiving Cisplatin. Br. J. Clin. Pharmacol. 42:233-235, 1996.

Gravel, J. S. and Ruben, R. J.: Auditory Deprivation and Its Consequences: From Animal Models to Humans. In: Van De Water, T. R., et al.: Clinical Aspects of Hearing. New York: Springer-Verlag, 1996.

Grundfast, K. M. and Josephson, G. D.: Hereditary Hearing Loss. In: Hughes, G. B., et al. (Eds.): Clinical Otology, 2nd ed. New York: Thieme, 1997.

Gulya, A. J.: Disorders of Hearing. In: Evans, J. G. and Williams, T. F.: Oxford Textbook of Geriatric Medicine. New York: Oxford University Press, 1992.

Hall, J. W. and Grose, J. H.: Short-Term and Long-Term Effects on the Masking Level Difference Following Middle Ear Surgery. J. Am. Acad. Audiol. 4:307-312, 1993.

Hambley, C. M. and Cole, R. E.: Fitting the Hearing Aid. In: Goldenberg, R. A. (Ed.): Hearing Aids: A Manual for Clinicians. Philadelphia: Lippincott-Raven, 1996.

House, J. W.: Otosclerosis. In: Hughes, G. B., et al. (Eds.): Clinical Otology, 2nd ed. New York: Thieme, 1997.

House, J. W.: Preface I. In: Goldenberg, R. A. (Ed.): Hearing Aids: A Manual for Clinicians. Philadelphia: Lippincott-Raven, 1996.

Jerger, J., et al.: Hearing Impairment in Older Adults: New Concepts. J. Am. Geriatr. Soc. 43:928-935, 1995.

Johnson, E. W.: Selecting a Hearing Aid. In: Goldenberg, R. A. Hearing Aids: A Manual for Clinicians. Philadelphia: Lippincott-Raven, 1996.

Jorgensen, B. G. and Pedersen, C. B.: Acoustic Neuroma. Follow-Up of 78 Patients. Clin. Otolaryngol. 19:478-484, 1994.

Jung, T. T. K., et al.: Ototoxicity of Salicylate, Nonsteroidal Anti-Inflammatory Drugs, and Quinine. Otolaryngol. Clin. N. Am. 26:791-810, 1993.

Kelsall, D. C., et al.: Cochlear Implantation in the Elderly. Am. J. Otol. 16:609-615, 1995.

Ketten, D. R.: Radiologic Assessment. In: NIH Consensus Development Conference: Cochlear Implants in Adults and Children. Bethesda: National Institutes of Health, 1995.

Maillet, C. J., et al.: Change in the Quality of Life of Adult Cochlear Implant Patients. Ann. Otol. Rhinol. Laryngol. Suppl. 16S:31-48, 1995.

Marple, B. F. and Roland, P. S.: External Auditory Canal. In: Roland, P. S., et al. (Eds.): Hearing Loss. New York: Thieme, 1997.

Meyerhoff, W. L., et al.: Tympanic Membrane, Middle Ear, and Mastoid. In: Roland, P. S., et al. (Eds.): Hearing Loss. New York: Thieme, 1997.

Miyamoto, R. T.: Cochlear Implants. In: Goldenberg, R. A. (Ed.): Hearing Aids: A Manual for Clinicians. Philadelphia: Lippincott-Raven, 1996.

Monsell, E. M., et al.: Therapeutic Use of Aminoglycosides in Meniére's Disease. Otolaryngol. Clin. N. Am. 26:737-746, 1993.

Mynders, J. M.: How Hearing Aids Work. In: Goldenberg, R. A. (Ed.): Hearing Aids: A Manual for Clinicians. Philadelphia: Lippincott-Raven, 1996.

Nadol, J. B., Jr.: Hearing Loss. N. Engl. J. Med. 329:1092-1102, 1993.

NIOSH (National Institute for Occupational Safety and Health), Education and Information Division, Division of Biomedical and Behavioral Science: Criteria for a Recommended Standard: Occupational Noise Exposure, Revised Criteria, 1996.

Newby, H. A. and Popelka, G. R.: Audiology, 6th ed. Englewood Cliffs, N.J.: Prentice Hall, 1992.

Nodar, R. H.: Effective Listening. In: Goldenberg, R. A. (Ed.): Hearing Aids: A Manual for Clinicians. Philadelphia: Lippincott-Raven, 1996.

Parisier, S. C., et al.: Diseases of the External Auditory Canal. In: Hughes, G. B., et al. (Eds.): Clinical Otology, 2nd ed. New York: Thieme, 1997.

Perkins, R. and Bui, H. T.: Tympanic Membrane Reconstruction Using Formaldehyde-Formed Autogenous Temporalis Fascia: Twenty Years' Experience. Otolaryngol. Head Neck Surg. 114:366-379, 1996.

Rogin, C. M.: Preface 3. In: Goldenberg, R. A. (Ed.): Hearing Aids: A Manual for Clinicians. Philadelphia: Lippincott-Raven, 1996.

Roland, P. S. and Marple, B. F.: Disorders of Inner Ear, Eighth Nerve, and CNS. In: Roland, P. S., et al. (Eds.): Hearing Loss. New York: Thieme, 1997.

Roper, T, A.: The Use of Deaf-Aid Communicators in a Salford Hospital: A Failure of Communication? Age Ageing 24:160-162, 1995.

Ruben, Robert J.: Introduction. In: Van De Water, T. R., et al.: Clinical Aspects of Hearing. New York: Springer-Verlag, 1996.

Rybak, L. P.: Ototoxicity of Loop Diuretics. Otolaryngol. Clin. N. Am. 26:829-844, 1993.

Salvi, R. and Burkard, R.: Auditory Physiology. In: Roland, P. S., et al. (Eds.): Hearing Loss. New York: Thieme, 1997.

Schweitzer, V. G.: Ototoxicity of Chemotherapeutic Agents. Otolaryngol. Clin. N. Am. 26:759-789, 1993.

Segal, E. S.: Common Medical Problems in Geriatric Patients. In: Cartensen,Check spelling L. L., et al. (Ed.): Practical Handbook of Clinical Gerontology. Thousand Oaks, Calif.: SAGE Publications-Check: Publications or Publishers, 1996.

Staab, W. J.: The Perception of Sound by Normal Listeners. In: Goldenberg, R. A. (Ed.): Hearing Aids: A Manual for Clinicians. Philadelphia: Lippincott-Raven, 1996.

Steel, K. P. and Kimberling, W.: Approaches to Understanding the Molecular Genetics and Hearing and Deafness. In: Van De Water,

T. R., et al.: Clinical Aspects of Hearing. New York: Springer-Verlag, 1996.

Sweetow, R. W.: Advising a New Hearing Aid Candidate. In: Goldenberg, R. A. (Ed.): Hearing Aids: A Manual for Clinicians. Philadelphia: Lippincott-Raven, 1996.

Thomsett, K. and Nickerson, E.: Missing Words: The Family Handbook on Adult Hearing Loss. Washington: Gallaudet University Press, 1993.

Tyler, R. S.: Tinnitus in the Profoundly Hearing-Impaired and the Effects of Cochlear Implants. Ann. Otol. Rhinol. Laryngol. Suppl 165:25-30, 1995.

Vento, B. A., et al.: Middle Ear Effects Secondary to Nasogastric Intubation. Am. J. Otol. 16:820-822, 1995.

Wayner, D. S.: Using the Hearing Aid. In: Goldenberg, R. A. (Ed.): Hearing Aids: A Manual for Clinicians. Philadelphia: Lippincott-Raven, 1996.

Weber, P.C. and Gantz, B. J.: Results and Complications from Acoustic Neuroma Excision via Middle Cranial Fossa Approach. Am. J. Otol. 17:669-675, 1996.

Winograd, C. H.: Common Clinical Disorders in Geriatric Patients. In: Federman, D. D. (Ed.): Scientific American Medicine. New York: Scientific American, 1995.

Woolf, N. K.: The Role of Viral Infection in the Development of Otopathology: Labyrinthitis and Autoimmune Disease. In: Van De Water, T. R., et al.: Clinical Aspects of Hearing. New York: Springer-Verlag, 1996.

CHAPTER 13

URINARY INCONTINENCE

SCOPE

Urinary incontinence is not a disease in and of itself but rather a symptom of a variety of conditions. About half of these conditions are transient and relatively easy to correct, while the other half are chronic and more difficult to resolve. Although advanced age is a predisposing factor, incontinence is not a direct consequence of aging. The five basic types of incontinence are often intermixed: stress, urge, reflex, overflow and total. Incontinence is diagnosed by a medical history, a physical and neurologic examination, laboratory tests and urodynamic tests. Treatment ranges from simple noninvasive therapy to drugs and surgery.

SYNOPSIS

13.00   INTRODUCTION

Urinary incontinence is the involuntary loss of urine. Whether the condition is mild, moderate or severe, it may be one of the most devastating of all medical conditions (Norton, 1982).

Incontinence has psychological as well as physiologic consequences. If the condition is left untreated, the patient's quality of life can be dramatically diminished. He or she may shun social and family obligations, curtail exercise and other leisure pursuits, avoid sexual activity and pass up career opportunities. In extreme cases, the sufferer may become a virtual recluse. Fortunately, with better diagnostic criteria and heightened physician awareness of the problem, most incontinent patients now can be completely cured, achieve significant improvement or at least be made more comfortable.

13.01   Definition

According to the International Continence Society, incontinence is "the loss of urine at inappropriate times, which presents a social or hygienic problem and is objectively demonstrable" (Bates, et al., 1979). Although this definition, formulated in 1972, is widely accepted, it is somewhat controversial. Questions have been raised as to when urine loss actually becomes a social or hygienic "problem," and whether current tests are sensitive enough to produce "objective" results. Indeed, specifying that leakage must be "objectively demonstrable" implicitly assumes a certain degree of severity (Herzog, 1988). In addition, the emotional consequences of urine loss vary substantially among individuals, with minor leakage being upsetting to some and greater leakage being well tolerated by others. Some experts suggest that *any* urine loss that creates a problem for an individual, or for his or her family or caretakers, should be taken seriously by physicians (Jeter, 1985).

13.02   Myths

Social taboos associated with the physiologic functions of elimination have made it difficult for society to discuss incontinence as openly as many other medical conditions. As a result, incontinence has become clouded by myth and misapprehension. One widespread myth is that incontinence is a relatively rare phenomenon. Another is that it is an expected consequence of aging. Yet another holds that few effective treatments are available. These myths present significant barriers to care. People wait an average of nine years before seeking treatment (Jeter, 1988), and they are often told by physicians that nothing can be done.

13.03   Epidemiology

Urinary incontinence is a pervasive condition that is not limited to the elderly and the infirm. According to the National Institutes of Health, at least 10 million Americans are afflicted, 85 percent of whom are women. Nearly 40 percent of women over 60 suffer from incontinence (Fantl, 1991).

13.04   Anatomy and Physiology

The urinary bladder is a muscular sac that stores and evacuates urine. It is supported by ligaments attached to the pubic bone and by pelvic floor muscles (extending between the pubic bone and the lowest part of the spine). These muscles are an integral part of the continence mechanism.

The bladder wall consists of three layers of tissue: the fatty outer covering, the central muscular layer (the detrusor muscle) and the inner mucous membrane (lining). The detrusor muscle is separated from the mucous membrane by the lamina propria, a thin, loose layer of connective tissue. The trigone is an inverted triangular area in the wall of the bladder, with the apex ending near the bladder neck.

The ureters are tubes that conduct urine from the kidney to the bladder. They enter the bladder near the corners of the trigone base and release small amounts of urine every 10 to 15 seconds. The normal or functional capacity of the bladder is about 12 to 16 ounces (360 to 480 mL) of urine. When distended (enlarged) under anesthesia, the true capacity is often more than double that amount—about 25 to 30 ounces (750 to 900 mL).

The urethra is the channel through which urine is carried from the bladder to the outside of the body. (*See Figure 13–1.*)

[1] Normal Urination

Adults urinate between four and eight times a day. The elderly may retain excess fluid during the day, causing them to produce more urine in the evening and making voiding (bladder emptying) once or twice nightly a normal occurrence.

Urination (micturition) is controlled from an area near the base of the brain called the pons. (*See Figure 13–2.*) As the bladder fills, parasympathetic (involuntary) nerves are inhibited, causing the detrusor to relax, and sympathetic (involuntary) nerves cause the internal sphincter muscles (ringlike muscles that control the bladder's opening and closing) to contract. As filling of the bladder approaches its functional capacity, a frank urge to urinate is created. When a decision to void is made, the parasympathetic nerves are stimulated by a chemical substance called acetylcholine, which causes the detrusor to contract, and the sympathetic impulses are inhibited by a hormone called norepinephrine. At this point, the external sphincter muscles can be relaxed consciously, effecting urination.

[2] Abnormal Urination

Symptoms of urinary dysfunction can generally be divided into two categories: irritative and obstructive. Irritative symptoms include frequent, urgent and/or painful urination; meager urine output; and nocturia (excessive or frequent urination at night). Obstructive symptoms include nocturia as well as difficulties in initiating urination or in emptying the bladder, decreased urinary stream and bladder pain that is relieved by voiding.

13.10 CLASSIFICATION OF DYSFUNCTION

Over the years, a number of systems have been developed for describing voiding dysfunction. The most prominent classifications are the Bors-Comarr system, the Bradley "loop" system, the Lapides system and the functional system.

The *Bors-Comarr* system describes incontinence in spinal-cord-injured patients, noting the location of the injury and the amount of

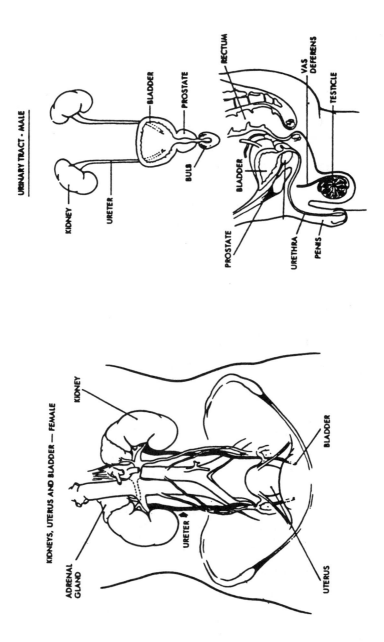

Fig. 13–1. The bladder and related structures in the female (left) and the male (right).

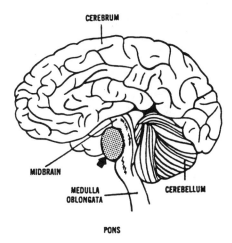

Fig. 13–2. The pons (at arrow) in relation to other parts of the brain. This nerve structure controls urination, among other things.

incontinence (Bors and Comarr, 1971). The *Bradley "loop"* system, applicable only to spinal cord injuries, describes dysfunction in terms of neurologic loops that may be interrupted or broken by spinal trauma (Bradley, 1986). The *Lapides* system, which is widely used by urologists for all types of voiding dysfunction, focuses on disruptions of the motor and/or sensory functions of the bladder (Lapides, 1970). The *functional* system views incontinence as either a failure to store urine properly or a failure to empty the bladder completely (Wein, 1987). Because of its simplicity and clarity, the functional system is gradually coming into widespread use.

Wein (1981) points out that none of these systems is perfect and that patients should be referred for further evaluation before irreversible treatment is contemplated.

13.20   TYPES OF INCONTINENCE

According to the functional view of incontinence, the failure to store urine results from either an overactive bladder muscle or a displaced bladder neck and urethra. An overactive bladder muscle is variously characterized as *detrusor hyperreflexia, uninhibited bladder contractions* or *unstable bladder.* The condition of displaced bladder neck and urethra has been called *vesicourethral prolapse* and *dysfunctional (damaged) urethra.*

Failure to empty urine properly can result from an underactive detrusor muscle, referred to as "detrusor areflexia," or a blocked urethra. If the activity of the detrusor, the sphincters or both is uncoordinated, this failure is referred to as "dyssynergia."

There are five basic types of incontinence: stress, urge, reflex, overflow and total. Frequently patients experience more than one type. For example, older women tend to exhibit both stress and urge incontinence, while older men often suffer from urge and overflow incontinence.

13.21   Stress Incontinence

Stress incontinence occurs when pelvic floor muscles are weakened or damaged, most often by childbirth, surgery, disease or injury. It is the most common type of incontinence in women under the age of 60 (Yarnell, et al., 1981). Contrary to popular belief, it is not caused by emotional stress.

When the bladder is in its normal position, intravesical (within the bladder) pressure is applied equally to the detrusor, the bladder neck and the proximal (internal) urethral sphincter muscle. In this way, continence is maintained. However, when the bladder slips, the sphincter assumes an inferior position. A sudden movement, such as that produced by a sneeze or a cough, causes pressure to be applied unequally. The sphincter is overwhelmed, and leakage results.

In women, muscular damage may cause conditions in which portions of urogenital (pertaining to the urinary tract and the genital organs) structures prolapse (herniate) into the vagina. Among such conditions are cystocele (herniation of the bladder), urethrocele (herniation of the urethra), cystourethrocele (herniation of the bladder and the urethra), enterocoele (herniation of the small intestine), rectocele (herniation of the rectum) and uterine prolapse (herniation of the uterus). (*See Figure 13–3.*)

Stress incontinence can be classified according to the following types (Blaivas, 1987):

> Type 0: No urinary leakage is demonstrated urodynamically (by the forces that move urine along the urinary tract).[1] The bladder neck is closed and in normal position.

---

[1] *See* 13.44 *infra.*

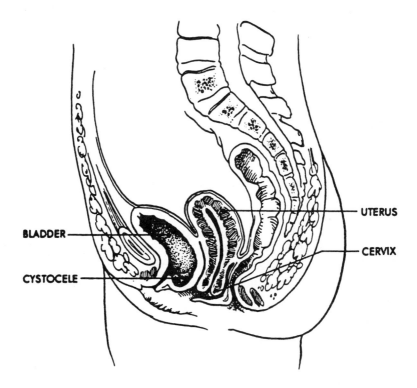

Fig. 13–3. Cystocele is a type of hernia in which the bladder protrudes into the vagina. It is among the conditions that can cause stress incontinence.

Type I: Leakage is caused by sudden movement but no cystocele is present.

Type IIA: Leakage occurs upon sudden movement and cystourethrocele is present.

Type IIB: The bladder neck descends, the urethra opens and incontinence occurs.

Type III: The bladder neck and urethra are open at rest and total incontinence occurs.

13.22   Urge Incontinence

Urge incontinence is characterized by a strong urge to urinate, followed quickly by involuntary urination. It is the most common type of incontinence in the elderly, occurring both day and night and often resulting in moderate to severe urine loss. Urge incontinence is most often caused by a hyperactive or unstable detrusor muscle, a degenerative disease or irritation of the bladder lining.

13.23   Reflex Incontinence

Reflex incontinence is actually a variation of urge incontinence in which the bladder contracts involuntarily without a warning. It typically occurs in patients who have suffered a stroke or a spinal cord injury.

13.24   Overflow Incontinence

If the bladder muscle is weak or underactive because of neurologic disease, the bladder may not empty completely. Subsequently it fills beyond its normal functional capacity. At some point, the sphincter is overwhelmed, and leakage results, manifesting as a continual dribble of urine or as a gush without warning. This condition is called overflow incontinence.

Overflow incontinence is commonly caused by neurologic degeneration or diabetes. In men, it is often seen in association with benign prostatic hypertrophy (abnormal enlargement of the prostate gland).

13.25   Total Incontinence

Total incontinence is a rare condition caused by severe urethral damage or degeneration, or by urinary fistulas (abnormal channels that allow urine to escape) that bypass the sphincter muscles. It results in an uncontrollable flow of urine.

13.30   ETIOLOGY

Incontinence is not a disease in and of itself; rather, it is a symptom of many underlying conditions resulting from physiologic or neurologic dysfunction. These conditions fall into two categories: transient and chronic.

13.31 Transient Incontinence

Transient conditions usually have an acute onset and are relatively easy to treat. They are the most common cause of incontinence in the elderly (Resnick, 1986).

[1] Drugs

A number of drugs may cause bladder irritability or sphincteric relaxation, and result in incontinence. They include anticholinergics, alpha agonists, alpha antagonists and diuretics.

Anticholinergics, which block the action of the parasympathetic nervous system,[2] are a major component of prescription and over-the-counter varieties of antihistamines and antidepressants. They can interfere with the bladder's ability to contract, causing overflow incontinence. *Alpha agonists,* which are found in many over-the-counter decongestants and cold medications, can cause urinary retention and result in overflow incontinence. *Alpha antagonists,* frequently found in antihypertensive (high blood pressure–reducing) medication, block nerve impulses to the urethra and may cause stress incontinence. *Diuretics,* which stimulate the kidney to produce more urine, can stimulate the bladder through filling, causing or exacerbating stress and urge incontinence.

[2] Mental Impairment

Depression, disorientation and frank dementia (mental deterioration) may result in a lack of awareness of the need to urinate or a lack of motivation to use the toilet.

[3] Estrogen Deficiency

Estrogen is a female sex hormone that stimulates the activity of the sex organs and the development of secondary sex characteristics. All the functional parts of the female urethra are estrogen-sensitive (Tapp and Cardozo, 1986). When estrogen levels decrease due to surgical or natural menopause, some urethral atrophy (wasting) may occur. This may result in a failure of urethral edges to coapt (fit together) or provide a tight seal, thereby causing incontinence.

---

[2] *See* 13.04 *supra.*

[4] Restricted Mobility

When a patient is confined to bed or a wheelchair because of an illness, an accident or surgery, the ability to reach a toilet in time may be restricted.

[5] Catheters

Urinary catheters (tubes placed in the urethra to withdraw urine from the bladder) can cause urinary tract infection, leading to bladder irritation and, consequently, stress or urge incontinence. (*See Figure 13–4.*) They can also cause significant morbidity and mortality (Platt, et al., 1982).

[6] Alcohol

Alcohol is a classic bladder irritant as well as a diuretic. In susceptible individuals, even small amounts of alcohol may precipitate

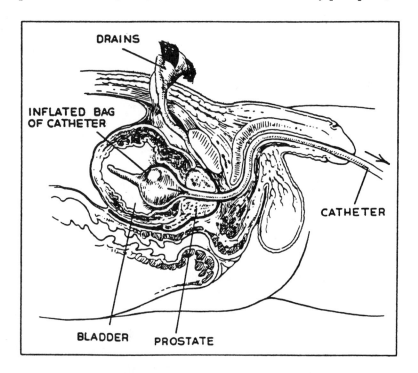

Fig. 13–4. Catherization of the urethra in a male patient. This procedure can cause urinary tract infection, resulting in incontinence.

or exacerbate all types of incontinence. Excessive consumption can impair both cognitive function and mobility, and interfere with the motivation or ability to reach a toilet.

[7] Impacted Stool

Stool impaction, which commonly occurs in the elderly, can press on nerves or on the bladder itself, resulting in urge or overflow incontinence.

13.32 Chronic Incontinence

Chronic incontinence is more difficult to resolve than transient incontinence.

[1] Obstetric Injuries

During vaginal childbirth, the pelvic floor muscles may be stretched or torn, resulting in stress incontinence. The support mechanisms of the bladder neck may be damaged if the symphysis pubis (soft-tissue joint formed by the pubic bones) is stretched, broken or separated surgically (in a procedure known as symphysiotomy) during delivery. (*See Figure 13–5.*)

[2] Abdominal or Pelvic Surgery

Stress incontinence, and sometimes total incontinence, can result from hysterectomy (surgical removal of the uterus); surgery for colon cancer, prostate enlargement or cancer, cervical or ovarian cancer; or abdominal procedures impairing neurologic function or damaging the urinary sphincter mechanism.

[3] Urethral Obstruction

Prostate enlargement, bladder stones, cystocele,[3] scarring from surgical procedures (especially previous incontinence surgery) or from infections such as gonorrhea may narrow the urethra, causing stress or overflow incontinence.

[4] Diseases with Neuropathic Complications

Alzheimer's disease, Parkinson's disease, diabetes mellitus, multiple sclerosis and advanced syphilis are among the diseases with neuropathic complications that may cause incontinence.

---

[3] *See* 13.21 *supra.*

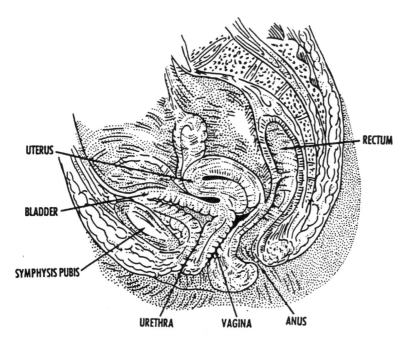

Fig. 13–5. The symphysis pubis and related structures in the female. Stress incontinence may occur if the symphysis pubis is damaged during childbirth.

- *Alzheimer's disease,* which affects the frontal and occipital areas of the brain, causes central nervous system (brain and spinal cord) degeneration.[4] In the bladder, it may manifest as detrusor hyperreflexia (overactivity) and result in urge incontinence.

- *Parkinson's disease,* a degenerative disorder of the brain, interferes with neurologic function, also causing urge incontinence.

- *Diabetes mellitus,* a metabolic disorder causing, among other things, degeneration of nerve fibers, can eventually interfere with the ability to sense the need to urinate.[5] The detrusor

---

[4] *See also* ch. 15.

[5] *See also* ch. 9.

decompensates, becoming flaccid (weak) and inefficient, and resulting in overflow incontinence.

- *Multiple sclerosis* gradually demyelinates (destroys the protective sheaths of) nerve fibers in the spinal cord. This can cause detrusor hyperreflexia and/or sphincter dyssynergia (disturbance in muscular coordination) and, hence, urge incontinence. The incontinence is occasionally complicated by urinary retention.

- *Advanced syphilis* affecting the posterior spinal cord can diminish neurologic sensation and result in overflow incontinence.

[5] Spinal Cord Injuries or Degeneration

Spinal trauma, especially compression fractures of the pelvis, disrupts the functioning of the central nervous system and can diminish the bladder's neurologic functioning, resulting in all types of incontinence.

[6] Cerebrovascular Accidents and Tumors

Strokes[6] and tumors, especially those located in the spine or the frontal lobe of the brain, may diminish neurologic function, causing urge incontinence.

[7] Chronic Urinary Tract Infections

Urge incontinence may be caused by chronic urinary tract infections or inflammation due to indwelling catheters; radiographic therapy in the pelvic region; chemotherapy for bladder, prostate or uterine cancer; or bladder stones.

[8] Obesity

Large internal fat deposits found in obese patients can displace the bladder neck and urethra, causing stress incontinence.

[9] Alcohol Abuse

Over the long term, excessive alcohol ingestion can damage neurologic function, causing stress or overflow incontinence.

---

[6] *See also* ch. 8.

[10] Congenital Birth Defects

Spina bifida (herniation of the spinal cord though the walls of the spinal canal) can result in incomplete urination. In severe cases, it can cause a total inability to urinate, requiring intermittent self-catheterization. Exstrophy (a turning inside out of the bladder) and some cases of epispadias (malformation of the bladder neck and urethra) can result in lifelong total incontinence, unless the condition is corrected surgically.

13.40 DIAGNOSIS

The diagnosis of incontinence requires careful and sometimes persistent investigation. The condition has various manifestations and a substantial array of potential etiologies, all of which may co-exist.

The diagnosis is based on a medical history, including a voiding diary; a physical and neurologic examination; blood, urine and renal (kidney) function tests; and urodynamic tests. Often, enough information for a presumptive diagnosis can be gleaned from the medical history and the routine office procedures. In many cases, noninvasive therapy[7] can be initiated without resorting to more elaborate, invasive tests, which should be used with great caution in the elderly.

13.41 Medical History

A thorough medical history should ascertain the following:

- family history of incontinence;
- first experience of incontinence;
- urinary habits and symptoms associated with voiding, including frequency and amount of leakage, difficulties in emptying bladder and whether a warning occurs before leakage;
- physical activity associated with urine loss;
- type and number of absorbent pads used per 24-hour period;
- previous treatments for incontinence;
- current prescription and over-the-counter medications being taken;
- other medical conditions;

---

[7] See 13.51 infra.

- surgical history;
- if female, births;
- if male, prostate problems and recent changes in sexual function;
- bowel habits;
- previous neurologic problems; and
- pelvic radiation therapy or chemotherapy for cancer.

An associated part of the medical history is a voiding diary. For two or more days, the patient or the caretaker should record the following: time of day, type and amount of fluid intake, amount of urine loss, activity engaged in at time of urine loss and whether a perceptible urge was present just before an accident. The diary often reveals a pattern of incontinence tied to medication, fluid intake or food allergy.

The medical history and voiding diary should illuminate potential etiologies and areas for further examination. If no obvious clues arise, a neurologic workup is appropriate.

13.42 Physical and Neurologic Examination

A thorough physical examination should focus on the pelvic and urogenital areas. In women, the physician should check for cystocele, urethrocele, rectocele, enterocele or uterine prolapse.[8] In men, the physician should perform a rectal examination to check for prostatic hypertrophy (abnormal enlargement of the prostate gland) or nodules (small lumps).

The examiner should also rule out neurologic deficiencies and assess mental and motor function, coordination, and sacral (situated at the lower end of the spine) and perineal (pertaining to the region at the underside of the trunk) reflexes.

13.43 Laboratory Tests

Laboratory tests should include a urinalysis and a urine culture if pyuria (pus in the urine) is present. If the patient is experiencing irritative bladder symptoms, a urine cytology (cell) test should be performed to rule out bladder cancer. If there is blood in the urine, an intravenous pyelogram (kidney x-ray in which the contrast medium

---

[8] *See* 13.21 *supra.*

is injected into a vein) should be taken to rule out kidney tumors, stones or other abnormalities. Tests to measure kidney function include routine blood urea nitrogen tests (which determine the amount of nitrogen present in the blood in the form of urea, a component of urine) and serum creatinine tests (which determine how well the kidney eliminates creatinine, a substance found in muscles, urine and blood).

13.44 Urodynamic Tests

Urodynamic tests seek to duplicate and quantitate urine loss. The techniques vary from "eyeball urodynamics," which can be performed during a regular office visit, to procedures employing multichannel video equipment (Blaivas, 1987). In general, 90 percent of the information needed to diagnose incontinence can be gleaned from routine office procedures (Resnick and Yalla, 1988). However, if irreversible therapy (i.e., surgery) is contemplated and a conclusive diagnosis has not been achieved, then more sophisticated procedures should be performed.

The tests are invaluable in pinpointing the etiology of incontinence. However, specialists warn that there may be a poor correlation between urodynamic findings and a patient's symptoms. In addition, the tests may elicit urinary symptoms of which the patient was hitherto unaware. Most typically, urge incontinence may manifest after testing for what appeared to be uncomplicated stress incontinence.

Urodynamic tests include cystometry, uroflowmetry, residual urine volume measurement, electromyography and urethral pressure profile.

[1] Cystometry

Cystometry provides a graphic record, called a cystometrogram, of intravesical pressure (pressure inside the bladder) and the efficiency of bladder function. Pressure is recorded as the bladder is filled and emptied, either voluntarily or involuntarily.

The cystometrogram provides information on bladder compliance (how the bladder responds to pressure changes), contractility (involuntary bladder contractions) and sensation (at what point a patient experiences initial sensations of bladder filling, a strong desire to void and extreme discomfort). Maneuvers designed to provoke leakage, such as coughing, standing or brief exercise, should be performed when the patient experiences a strong desire to void.

[2]   Uroflowmetry

Uroflowmetry assesses the quality of urine flow with regard to the rate, volume and strength of the stream. An erratic pattern may reveal bladder-sphincter dyssynergia (uncoordinated muscle activity), while a consistently low rate of flow may indicate urinary obstruction.

[3]   Residual Urine Volume

After the uroflow exam is completed, a catheter is inserted into the bladder, and any residual urine is drained and measured. A significant amount of residual urine can indicate outlet or urethral obstruction, or poor detrusor tone.

[4]   Electromyography

An electromyogram (EMG) is a graphic or an electronic recording of muscle activity. In a urodynamic EMG, patch electrodes are placed on the perineum. Under normal circumstances, EMG activity increases as the bladder fills. It stops suddenly upon urination and resumes at a lower level when urination is complete. An abnormal EMG can reveal bladder-sphincter dyssynergia.

[5]   Urethral Pressure Profile

Continence is maintained when intravesical pressure is less than the resistance of the urethral sphincter muscle. To obtain a urethral pressure profile (UPP), a catheter with holes along its side and a sensor on its tip is drawn through the urethra. Fluid is emitted through the holes, and the sensor transmits information about the response of the urethral wall to the escaping fluid. The UPP is not as valuable as other tests for stress incontinence, but it can be useful in assessing the effectiveness of surgery, the efficiency of an artificial sphincter and the function of the external sphincter.

13.50   TREATMENT

The key to effective treatment is a correct diagnosis. In patients with multiple etiologies or mixed incontinence, a combination of approaches may be used. If the condition is traced to a transient cause, it may be cured simply by identifying the precipitating factor and eliminating it.

13.51   Noninvasive Measures

The National Institutes of Health Consensus Development Conference on Incontinence recommends that as a general rule, the least invasive or dangerous procedures should be tried first, before undertaking riskier and perhaps irreversible therapy. Noninvasive treatment may be the only option for elderly patients who are not candidates for surgery.

[1]   Dietary Changes

In cases of urge or mixed incontinence, detrusor activity can be reduced or eliminated by identifying bladder irritants and removing them from the diet. The most common irritants include alcohol, caffeine, acidic or spicy foods, and milk products. The patient may be able to identify offending substances by keeping a food diary for several days.

[2]   Prompted Voiding

Reflex and overflow incontinence precipitated by involuntary bladder contractions can be managed simply and effectively by emptying the bladder before a voiding accident is likely to occur. A patient's "safe period" can be determined by maintaining a voiding chart for several days. He or she is then instructed to urinate before this period expires. Prompted voiding is the treatment of choice for elderly patients who have difficulty with independent toileting or who may be unaware of the need to void (Schnelle, et al., 1983).

[3]   Bladder Training

Bladder training, also called bladder retraining or bladder drill, is an effective, noninvasive treatment option for patients with urge, reflex or overflow incontinence. It is designed to lengthen the interval between voiding.

The technique is based on the precepts of childhood toilet training, in which urination is brought under voluntary control by repetitive efforts to inhibit micturition (urination), coupled with suggestive voiding at appropriate times. A voiding chart kept for several days is used to establish the minimum interval of continence, and the patient is instructed to urinate on a strict schedule within that interval. When continence is maintained for three days, the interval is increased by up to 30 minutes at a time, until a reasonable voiding schedule, usually every three to four hours, can be achieved. In a recent study, bladder training reduced by 57 percent the number of voiding accidents suffered by 60 incontinent women over the age of 54 (Fantl, 1991).

Bladder training can be combined with tranquilizers or anticholinergic drugs[9] to suppress involuntary bladder contractions while the interval is lengthened, or with pelvic floor exercises to help maintain continence when an urge to urinate occurs.

[4] Kegel's (Pelvic Floor) Exercises

In the late 1940s, Dr. Arnold Kegel popularized an exercise for women to strengthen the pelvic floor muscles supporting the bladder and the urethra (Kegel, 1948). These muscles can be easily identified by stopping the flow of urine, by tightening the muscles around a finger inserted into the vagina or by using an electronic sensor attached to a biofeedback device. Then they are contracted, or squeezed, in sets several times a day.

Although Kegel's exercises have been shown to be highly effective in treating stress incontinence, they are somewhat controversial. At the present time, there is little consensus on how many times a day the exercises should be done or how long each contraction should be held. As a result, their effectiveness has been spotty, and the exercises have fallen into general disrepute among physicians. It has been suggested that the exercises are generally more effective when combined with biofeedback techniques (Burgio, et al., 1986).

[5] Biofeedback

Grounded in the principles of behavioral medicine, biofeedback training is the process of making involuntary and unconscious bodily functions perceptible to the senses so they can be controlled by a conscious mental effort. To treat stress or urge incontinence, pelvic floor muscle contractions can be monitored by patch electrodes placed on the perineum or by an electronic probe in the vagina or rectum (in women or men). Monitoring systems provide a visual, audio or graphic assessment of pelvic floor muscle activity and, thereafter, a record of progress in a training program designed to strengthen this critical muscle group. Most patients begin to see changes within three to six weeks, although a sustained program of several months is usually necessary for significant improvement.

---

[9] *See* 13.31[1] *supra.*

Low-grade electrical stimulation of the pelvic floor muscles, delivered with a vaginal or an anal probe, can be combined with biofeedback to contract the muscles passively. This technique, sometimes referred to as "interferental therapy," has been widely used in Europe over the past decade. Electrical stimulation can be especially useful for people with severely atrophic (wasted or withered) pelvic muscles.

13.52   Pharmacologic Therapy

Pharmacologic therapy for urinary incontinence is designed to (1) improve the storage of urine by decreasing detrusor hyperactivity or increasing outlet resistance; or (2) improve bladder emptying by stimulating more efficient bladder contractions or relaxing the sphincter muscles.

The advantages of drug treatment are that it is fast acting and quickly reversible and does not require great effort on the part of the patient. The side effects, however, often weigh heavily against long-term use, and incontinence generally returns or worsens when drugs are discontinued. Therefore, drug treatment might best be looked at as a management tool for incontinence rather than as a "magic bullet." The drugs noted in this section are used to facilitate urinary function, not to address the plethora of underlying etiologies of urinary incontinence.

[1]   Drugs to Improve Urine Storage

Among the drugs used to improve urine storage are propantheline bromide, oxybutynin chloride, imipramine hydrochloride, flavoxate hydrochloride, phenylpropanolamine hydrochloride and estrogens.

[a]   Propantheline Bromide

Propantheline bromide blocks receptors of acetylcholine (a nerve impulse transmitter) in the bladder wall and thereby inhibits involuntary bladder contractions. It is one of the most widely used drugs in treating urge and reflex incontinence. Side effects include dry mouth, blurred vision, urinary retention, increased heart rate, nervousness, drowsiness, nausea, vomiting and constipation.

[b]   Oxybutynin Chloride

Oxybutynin chloride is a smooth muscle relaxant that has a strong anticholinergic effect (blocks the effects of acetylcholine). It is frequently employed to decrease involuntary bladder contractions in urge and reflex incontinence, and it may decrease symptoms of frequency and urgency as well. It is also one of the few drugs found to be effective in managing childhood enuresis (bedwetting).[10] Side effects include dry mouth, tachycardia (increased heart rate), blurred vision, drowsiness, bloating, nausea, vomiting, insomnia and impotence. Glycopyrollate, which is used to relax the gastrointestinal tract, is similar in indications and action.

[c]   Imipramine Hydrochloride

Imipramine hydrochloride is a tricyclic (containing three fused rings in its chemical structure) antidepressant that inhibits involuntary bladder contractions and increases outlet resistance. It is used to treat urge and reflex incontinence. At present, the mechanism of action is unclear. The side effects are numerous, including dry mouth, blurred vision, urinary retention, cardiovascular effects, psychiatric aberrations, neurologic disturbances, allergic reactions, hematologic (blood) problems (such as bone marrow depression), gastrointestinal symptoms (such as nausea, vomiting and diarrhea), endocrine (hormonal) disruptions and general systemic problems (such as jaundice and fatigue).

[d]   Flavoxate Hydrochloride

Flavoxate hydrochloride, a smooth muscle relaxant, has both antispasmodic (spasm-relieving) and anesthetic (numbing) properties. It is useful in the treatment of urge and reflex incontinence. Side effects include nausea, vomiting, blurred vision and mental confusion.

[e]   Phenylpropanolamine Hydrochloride

Phenylpropanolamine hydrochloride is a decongestant that stimulates alpha-adrenergic receptors (sites that are innervated by fibers of the sympathetic nervous system and react to norepinephrine and certain blocking agents) in the bladder neck (outlet) urethral smooth muscle, causing contraction of the internal urinary sphincter and increasing urethral closure. It is useful in the treatment of stress, urge and reflex incontinence. Side effects include nervousness, dizziness and sleeplessness.

---

[10] *See* 13.62 *infra.*

[f] Estrogens

Hormone replacement therapy is often prescribed for postmenopausal stress incontinence, although this remains a matter of controversy. There are numerous anecdotal reports of subjective symptomatic improvement, but only a few studies have been able to confirm such improvement urodynamically. Nonetheless, the use of conjugated (mixed) estrogens in pill or cream form, or the new transdermal (through the skin) patch, is often considered when other treatments fail. Long-term use of hormone replacement therapy, with its attendant known and suspected risks, should be weighed carefully. As with other drugs, the effects last only as long as the medication is taken.

The side effects of conjugated estrogens range from minor discomfort to serious medical disorders. They include changes in the menstrual cycle, breast tenderness, nausea, bloating, chloasma (spotty discoloration of the facial skin, which may be permanent), dizziness migraine headaches, depression and weight gain.

[2] Drugs to Improve Bladder Emptying

Prazosin hydrochloride, phenoxybenzamine and diazepam are amomg the drugs used to improve bladder emptying.

[a] Prazosin Hydrochloride

Prazosin hydrochloride is an antihypertensive drug that blocks alpha-adrenergic receptors in the smooth muscle of the bladder neck and the urethra. It is useful in treating overflow incontinence by improving urinary flow. Side effects include vomiting, diarrhea, constipation, nervousness, skin rashes and urinary frequency. Ironically, it may also cause or exacerbate stress and urge incontinence. Terazosin hydrochloride is another drug in this category with similar indications and actions.

[b] Phenoxybenzamine

Phenoxybenzamine is a potent drug that also blocks alpha-adrenergic receptors in smooth muscles. It was formerly the drug of choice for relaxing the bladder outlet and the urethra in order to decrease overflow incontinence, as well as for decreasing symptoms of frequency and urgency. However, it has been found to cause stomach and bowel cancer in laboratory animals. Now, prazosin hydrochloride is preferred, especially for long-term use. Side effects include nasal congestion, orthostatic hypotension (low blood pressure upon standing) and tachycardia (rapid heartbeat).

[c] Diazepam

Diazepam, a potent central nervous system depressant, has been employed in the treatment of overflow incontinence to relax the striated (striped and voluntary) muscles of the urinary sphincters. Common side effects include drowsiness, fatigue and ataxia (lack or loss of muscular coordination). Paradoxically, in a few cases, the drug may cause urinary retention. Because of problems with habituation and dependence, diazepam should be used with caution, especially in the elderly, and withdrawal should be gradual. Buspirone hydrochloride is a newer drug of this class that is less habit-forming.

13.53 Surgery

Surgery may be used to treat stress incontinence, mixed stress and urge incontinence, and total incontinence. It is not effective for other types of the condition. In most cases, the primary goal of surgery is to return the bladder neck as close as possible to its normal position within the abdominal cavity. If the bladder is placed too high, urinary retention may result. If significant vaginal prolapse (slippage) occurs, it must be corrected at the same time to assure continence.

Because of the possibility of failure or of exacerbating existing incontinence, surgery should be the remedy of last resort. Effectiveness rates for incontinence surgery are often overstated, partly because the follow-up time for many studies is less than 1 year (Stanton, 1988). To determine longer term results, Leach re-evaluated patients up to 4.5 years after surgery and found that 50 percent were symptom-free, 25 percent were improved and 25 percent were worse. Of the 25 percent who were worse, some had to self-catheterize. In addition, urge incontinence, which had been nonexistent previously, occurred in some patients, and stress incontinence recurred in others up to 2 years postoperatively (Kelly, et al., 1991).

Surgery for incontinence may involve bladder neck suspension procedures, the pubovaginal sling procedure, artificial urinary sphincter implants or urinary diversion. The complications of these procedures include infection, blood loss, urinary retention with the potential for long-term self-catheterization, bladder perforation and possible precipitation of urge incontinence.

[1]   Bladder Neck Suspension Procedures

The Marshall-Marchetti-Krantz (MMK) procedure was first used in the 1940s. Employing an abdominal approach, the surgeon uses sutures (surgical strings) to attach fascia (connective tissue) surrounding the bladder neck and the urethra to fascia covering the pubic bone (Marshall, et al., 1949). Unfortunately, in addition to normal postoperative complications, about 5 percent of patients develop osteitis pubis (infection of the pubic bone) (Stanton, 1988). To avoid the possibility of this infection, Burch modified the MMK procedure by attaching the sutures to Cooper's ligament, which runs along the pectineal line (on the back surface of the thigh) of the pubic bone (Burch, 1961).

In 1959, A. J. Pereyra performed the first transvaginal bladder neck suspension operation, using a primary vaginal incision and a minor suprapubic (above the pubic bones) incision. The procedure, in its various modifications, is now the most widely used operation for stress incontinence.

In the Raz modification, an incision is made in the vagina and a suture is placed on each side of the urethra at the bladder neck. Forming a loop under the bladder neck, the two ends of the suture are then pulled up through the suprapubic incision, adjusted and tied over the abdominal muscles (Hadley, et al., 1985). The Cobb and Radge variation (1978) utilizes two suprapubic incisions, and the Stamey procedure (1973) buttresses the periurethral fascia with two Dacron® (synthetic polyester) arterial grafts.

Compared with the abdominal approach, the vaginal approach produces less damage to abdominal wall fascia and less postoperative discomfort, and requires a shorter hospital stay.

[2]   Pubovaginal Sling Procedure

The pubovaginal (pertaining to the pubic bone and the vagina) sling procedure is used in cases of intractable incontinence when the urethra is nonfunctional, or when a patient has had several unsuccessful surgical procedures. A sling made of the patient's own fascial tissue or of synthetic material (polypropylene mesh, nylon or silicone) is tunneled beneath the bladder neck and attached to the fascia of the rectus abdominus muscles (in the front part of the abdomen).

In addition to normal surgical complications, this procedure carries a significant risk of precipitating or exacerbating urge incontinence or urinary retention, which may require permanent self-catheterization. The sling materials, with the exception of silicone, have a tendency to fuse with adjacent tissue and may be difficult to remove if voiding difficulties occur postsurgically.

[3] Artificial Urinary Sphincter

An artificial urinary sphincter can be used to treat total incontinence caused by prostate surgery, pelvic trauma or unsuccessful surgery for stress incontinence (in women only). The device consists of an inflatable cuff that surrounds the urethra, a balloonlike reservoir and a pump-release mechanism. During bladder filling, the cuff remains inflated with fluid and holds the urethra in a closed position. When the patient desires to empty the bladder, he or she presses the pump, thereby allowing the fluid to transfer from the urethral cuff to the reservoir. After urination is completed, the cuff slowly refills, again closing the urethra.

Complications include mechanical breakdown of the device, tissue erosion and precipitation of urge incontinence. The artificial sphincter has been used less widely and less successfully in women than men. In part, this is because the pump must be imbedded underneath the labia (folds of skin surrounding the opening of the vagina), which may cause pain or discomfort during sexual activity.

[4] Urinary Diversion

A urinary diversion may be considered as treatment for total incontinence. In a "regular" urinary diversion, the ureters are detached from the bladder and attached to a bowel segment that has been isolated and brought to the skin surface as a stoma (surgically created opening in the abdominal wall). Urine drains continuously into a collecting bag, which must be emptied once or twice a day. Immediate postoperative complications include excessive bleeding and infection of the bladder, kidneys or abdominal cavity. The primary long-term complication is chronic kidney infection.

In a continent urinary diversion, urine is diverted from the bladder and channeled into a surgically constructed reservoir. The reservoir is fashioned from a piece of bowel and housed within the abdominal cavity. A stoma provides an outlet, and the patient self-catheterizes four to six times a day. Immediate postsurgical complications include bowel obstruction; bleeding; urinary or fecal leakage from the suture line; and kidney, bladder or abdominal infections. Long-term complications include leakage of the reservoir, kidney infection and stoma breakdown.

13.54   Other Methods of Treatment

Other methods of treatment include pessaries, vaginal weights and periurethral injections.

[1]   Pessaries

A pessary is a device that is inserted into the upper part of the vagina to hold the uterus in place. It is indicated for women who want to avoid surgery for stress incontinence accompanied by uterine descensus (abnormal slipping of the uterus). Pessaries come in a number of sizes and shapes. After fitting by a physician, the device may be used for several months, although some types must be removed for coitus, and all must be removed and cleaned periodically to avoid infection.

[2]   Vaginal Weights

Vaginal weights are small, graduated, tamponlike weights that are inserted into the vagina. To hold them in place, the user is forced to isolate and constrict the pelvic floor muscles. They represent a relatively new and highly effective treatment for stress incontinence (Peattie and Plevnik, 1988). The weights, which are employed twice daily for 15 minutes at a time during normal activity, can be especially helpful for women who have trouble isolating the pelvic floor muscles or holding contractions long enough.

[3]   Periurethral Injections

Periurethral (around the urethra) injections of synthetic polytef (an artificial resin) or collagen (a fibrous material) can be used to facilitate urethral closure after unsuccessful surgery, chronic infection or damage from radiation therapy for cancer in the pelvic region. Repeat injections may be necessary to achieve optimal results. The advantages of the procedure are that it is less invasive than surgery and can be done when there is considerable tissue destruction. Unfortunately, the collagen may be entirely absorbed by the body, necessitating repeat injections, and the polytef particles may separate and migrate to the lymph nodes or more distant sites, potentially causing adverse reactions or the development of tumors.

13.100   BIBLIOGRAPHY

Text References

Bates, P., et al.: The Atandardization of Terminology of Lower Urinary Tract Function. J. Urol. 121:551, 1979.

Bors, E. and Comarr, A. E.: Neurological Urology. Baltimore: University Park Press, 1971.

Blaivas, J. G.: Sphincteric Incontinence in the Female: Pathophysiology, Classification and Choice of Corrective Surgical Procedure. Am. Urolog. Assoc. Update Series 4(25):4–5, 1987.

Bradley, W. E.: Physiology of the Urinary Bladder. In: Walsh, P., et al. (Eds.): Campbell's Urology. Philadelphia: Saunders, 1986.

Burch, J. C.: Urethrovaginal Fixation to Cooper's Ligament for Correction of Stress Incontinence, Cystocele and Prolapse. Am. J. Obstet. Gynecol. 81:281, 1961.

Burgio, K. L., et al.: The Role of Biofeedback in Kegel Exercise Training for Stress Urinary Incontinence. Am. J. Obstet. Gynecol. 154:58–64, 1986.

Cobb, O. E. and Radge, H.: Correction of Female Stress Incontinence. J. Urol. 20:418, 1978.

Fantl, J. A., et al.: Efficacy of Bladder Training in Older Women with Urinary Incontinence. J.A.M.A. 265(5):609–613, Feb. 6, 1991.

Garrett, R. A.: Enuresis. Am. Urolog. Assoc. Update Series 2(34):2–3, 1983.

Hadley, R. H., et al.: Transvaginal Needle Bladder Neck Suspension. Urol. Clin. North Am. 23(2):294, May 1985.

Herzog, R.: Urinary Incontinence in Adults: Prevalence and Incidence in a Community-Dwelling Population. Bethesda, Md.: Proceedings of the NIH Consensus Development Conference, Oct. 3–5, 1988.

Jeter, K. J.: Incontinence in the American Home: A Survey of 36,500 Incontinent People. Bethesda, Md.: Proceedings of the NIH Consensus Development Conference, Oct. 3–5, 1988.

Jeter, K. J.: Living with the Problems of Bladder Control. In: Gartley, C. B. (Ed.): Managing Incontinence. Ottawa, Ill.: Jameson Books, 1985.

Kegel, A. H.: Progressive Resistance Exercise in the Functional Restoration of the Perineal Muscles. Am. J. Obstet. Gynecol. 56:238–248, 1948.

Kelly, M., et al.: Symptomatic Analysis of Patients Undergoing Modified Pereyra Bladder Neck Suspensions for Stress Incontinence: Pre-and Post-Op Findings. Urology 37(3):213, March 1991.

Lapides, J.: Neuromuscular, Vesical and Ureteral Dysfunction. In: Campbell, M. F. and Harrison, J. H. (Eds.): Urology, pp. 1343–1379. Philadelphia: Saunders, 1970.

Marshall, V. F., et al.: The Correction of Stress Incontinence by Simple Vesicourethral Suspension. Surg. Gynecol. Obstet. 88:509, 1949.

Mikkelsen, E. J. and Rapoport, J. L.: Enuresis: Psychopathology, Sleep Stage and Drug Response. Urol. Clin. North Am. 7:361, 1980.

Norton, C.: The Effects of Urinary Incontinence in Women. Int. Rehabil. Med. 4:9–13, 1982.

Peattie, A. B. and Plevnik, S.: Cones Versus Physiotherapy As Conservative Management of Genuine Stress Incontinence. J. Neurourol. Urodyn. 7(3):265, 1988.

Platt, R., et al.: Mortality Associated with Nosocomial Urinary Tract Infections. N. Engl. J. Med. 307:637, 1982.

Resnick, N. R.: Urinary Incontinence in the Elderly. Hosp. Pract. 21(11):80C, Nov. 15, 1986.

Resnick, N. R. and Yalla, S. V.: Proceedings of the 18th Annual Meeting of the International Incontinence Society, 1988.

Scharf, M.: Waking Up Dry. Cincinnati: Writer's Digest Books, 1986.

Schnelle, J. F., et al.: Management of Geriatric Incontinence in Nursing Homes. J. Appl. Behav. Anal. 16:235–241, 1983.

Stamey, T. A.: Cystoscopic Suspension of the Vesical Neck for Urinary Incontinence. Surg. Gynecol. Obstet. 136:547, 1973.

Stanton, S. L.: Urinary Incontinence in Adults: Suprapubic Approaches for Stress and Urge Incontinence in Women. Bethesda, Md.: Proceedings of the NIH Consensus Development Conference, Oct. 3–5, 1988.

Tapp, A. J. S. and Carodozo, L. D.: The Post-Menopausal Bladder. Brit. J. Hosp. Med. 35:20, 1986.

Wein, A. J.: Classification of Voiding Dysfunction. Amer. Urolog. Assoc. Update Series 6(4), 1987.

Wein, A. J.: Lower Urinary Tract Function and Pharmacologic Management of Lower Urinary Tract Dysfunction. Urol. Clin. N. Am. 12(2):67, 1985.

Wein, A. J.: Classification of Neurogenic Voiding Dysfunction. J. Urol. 125:605, 1981.

Yarnell, J. W. G., et al.: The Prevalence and Severity of Urinary Incontinence in Women. J. Epidemiol. Community Health 35:71, 1981.

CHAPTER 14

DISORDERS OF THE PROSTATE

SCOPE

Benign prostatic hypertrophy (BPH) and prostate cancer are independent disease entities that may, however, co-exist in the same patient. The primary risk factor for BPH is age. Other possible risk factors have been identified, but more and larger studies are needed to confirm them. Risk factors for prostate cancer include advancing age, black race, family history of the disease, smoking, vasectomy (excision of a segment of the sperm duct to produce sterility) and high dietary fat intake. Diagnosis includes urinalysis, measurement of serum creatinine level and serum prostate-specific antigen (PSA) concentration, uroflowmetry, postvoid residual volume, imaging of the urinary tract and cystourethroscopy. Treatment ranges from watchful waiting to surgery.

SYNOPSIS

14.00   INTRODUCTION

The prostate gland can be affected by both benign and malignant disease processes. A common benign disorder of the prostate is called benign prostatic hyperplasia (BPH), sometimes referred to as benign prostatic hypertrophy. The latter term is a misnomer, however, because the condition is characterized by an increase in the number of cells in the prostate (hyperplasia) rather than an enlargement of prostatic cells (hypertrophy) (Narayan, 1995). The term "benign" is used because BPH does not involve cancerous cells and is rarely life threatening.

Unlike BPH, prostate cancer is a malignant disease; that is, it is characterized by the uncontrolled reproduction of abnormal cells that, if unchecked, results in death. BPH and prostate cancer are independent disease entities, and BPH is not thought to predispose to prostate cancer (Sagalowsky and Wilson, 1994). The two diseases can occur together, however, in the same organ (Moul, 1993).

14.10   BENIGN PROSTATIC HYPERPLASIA

The prostate, which is shaped like a small walnut, is located between the urinary bladder and the base of the penis. *(See Figure 14-1.)* The prostate of a boy weighs only a few grams. Starting at puberty, the prostate undergoes a period of growth that lasts for about eight years and ends when the organ weighs about 20 grams. The prostate remains at this weight for 15 to 25 years but then starts to grow again by a process of cell proliferation in the area closest to the urethra. This growth may eventually compress the normal parts of the organ and the urethra, thereby obstructing the outflow of urine from the bladder (Villers, 1994). This obstruction is responsible for the urinary symptoms associated with BPH,[1] which are referred to collectively as prostatism. About 50 percent of men with BPH eventually develop prostatism (McConnell, 1995).

14.11   Epidemiology

BPH increases in prevalence with age (Chute, et al., 1993). More than 90 percent of men aged 80 years have BPH to at least some degree, and 75 percent of these men have clinical symptoms. The average age for the development of symptoms of BPH is about 60 years in blacks and about 65 in whites. About 50 percent of men aged 60 to 69 have symptoms of BPH. Each year in the United States, more than one million men seek medical care for the symptoms of BPH, and BPH is responsible for more than 300,000 surgical procedures (O'Leary, 1995a).

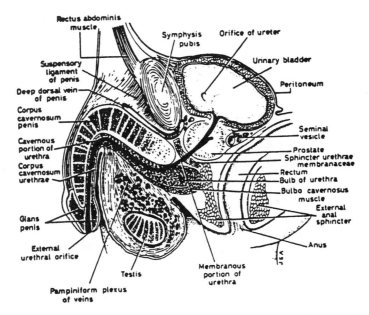

Fig. 14-1. The prostate in relation to surrounding structures of the male urogenital system.

---

[1] See 14.16[1] *infra.*

BPH probably does not have environmental origins. In addition, the prevalence of BPH increases with age in all countries, suggesting that all men will develop the disease if they live long enough (Isaacs and Coffey, 1989).

14.12   Risk Factors

The primary risk factor for BPH is age. Other possible risk factors have been identified, but more and larger studies are needed to confirm them. A study of 910 men who had undergone surgery for BPH found that the risk for surgery to treat BPH was greater in Jews than in Christians, in blacks than in whites, in never-married men than in ever-married men, in poorly educated men than in educated men, in men with a small body habitus (build) than in men with a large body habitus and in non-beer-drinking men than in beer-drinking men (Morrison, 1992). A family history of BPH may also be a risk factor for the development of clinical symptoms of the disease (Sanda, et al., 1994)

14.13   Etiology

The etiology of BPH is not well understood, but two factors are known to be necessary for it to occur: the presence of the hormone dihydrotestosterone, which mediates prostatic growth at all ages, and aging. Dihydrotestosterone is produced in the prostate from testosterone, the primary male hormone produced by the testes. As men age, their blood estrogen levels increase and their testosterone levels decrease. In laboratory animals, estrogen enhances the effect of dihydrotestosterone on the prostate, and if this occurs in humans, it may explain the role of aging in the development of BPH. It has also been hypothesized that with age, the number of stem cells (cells whose daughter cells differentiate into other cell types) in the prostate increases and the rate of cell death decreases.

14.14   Pathogenesis

The cell proliferation of BPH does not occur throughout the organ but only in the area near the urethra. The hyperplastic tissue that is formed is nodular and composed of varying amounts of stroma (supporting framework), glandular epithelium and muscle. The first changes of BPH are seen as microscopic stromal nodules around the periurethral glands. These changes are followed by acinar (glandular) hyperplasia that begins around the nodules. Over a period of years, the nodules reach diameters that range from a few millimeters to several centimeters. Hyperplastic glands are often large, with infoldings of the acini (the small, saclike secretory portions of the glands).

14.15 Adverse Effects on the Urinary System

Because BPH develops over a long period, the adverse effects that it causes in the urinary system are insidious. The changes are a result of complex interactions among the resistance to urinary flow in the urethra (produced by both spastic and mechanical effects of BPH), the pressure generated in the bladder by the muscle of the bladder as it tries to expel urine, and the general health of the individual. Paradoxically, there is no straightforward relationship between urethral obstruction and the size of the prostate; severe obstruction can occur even when the organ still is of normal size.

Initially the bladder muscle becomes hypertrophic to compensate for increased resistance in the urethra. Later, however, the muscle loses tone, and the bladder develops diverticula (outpocketings). There is also some degeneration of the nerve cells that supply the muscle. Eventually poor contractility (weakness) of the bladder muscle and a high volume of residual urine (urine not expelled during urination) in the bladder can lead to vesicoureteral reflux (backward flow of urine from the bladder into the ureters), hydronephrosis (dilation of the pelvis and calices of the kidneys) and kidney failure.

14.16 Symptoms

Persons with BPH may have urinary symptoms, systemic symptoms related to the urinary tract, symptoms unrelated to the urinary tract and symptoms related to complications. Up to a third of men with urinary symptoms of BPH show spontaneous improvement or stabilization of their symptoms with time (Narayan, 1995). It is not clear, however, whether this improvement is objective (due to regression of the BPH) or subjective (due to the man adapting to his symptoms). The urinary symptoms of BPH fall into two categories: obstructive and irritative.

[1] Obstructive Urinary Symptoms

An early and universal obstructive symptom of BPH is a weak urinary stream (reduction in the force or caliber of the urinary stream due to urethral compression). Hesitancy (involuntary delay in starting the urinary stream) occurs because the bladder muscle takes longer to overcome urethral resistance. Intermittency (stopping and starting of the urinary stream several times during voiding), postvoid dribbling and incomplete bladder emptying are caused by failure of the bladder muscle to sustain the required pressure until the end of voiding. The latter two symptoms may also be a result of a "ball-valve" effect caused by obstructive prostate tissue at the neck of the bladder.

[2] Irritative Urinary Symptoms

The irritative symptoms of BPH are nocturia (urinating at night), urinary frequency (urination at short intervals), urinary urgency (strong desire to void) and dysuria (difficulty or pain on urination). Nocturia and urinary frequency can be due to several factors:

- incomplete emptying of the bladder may result in shorter periods between voidings;

- enlargement of the prostate, especially if it extends into the bladder, can result in an abnormally frequent triggering of the voiding response; and

- hypertrophic bladder muscle may be sensitive to minimal changes in urine volume.

Urinary urgency and dysuria are less common than nocturia and urinary frequency. These symptoms may be due to an inability to empty the bladder, caused by inadequate relaxation of the sphincter in the neck of the bladder or by bladder instability in which the muscular contractions are not coordinated with sphincteral relaxation.

[3] Systemic Symptoms Related to the Urinary Tract

Long-term obstruction of the outflow of urine from the bladder usually leads to hydronephrosis (dilation of the pelvis and calyces of the kidneys), which can cause abdominal discomfort and flank pain. Renal failure may lead to the symptoms of uremia (excessive urea and other nitrogenous waste in the blood), which include chronic fatigue, weakness, loss of appetite and sleepiness.

[4] Symptoms Unrelated to the Urinary Tract

Increased abdominal pressure and straining during voiding can cause hernia (protrusion of a structure through the tissues normally containing it) and hemorrhoids (dilation of the external hemorrhoidal veins that causes painful swellings at the anus). An extremely enlarged prostate can interfere with bowel movements.

[5] Symptoms Related to Complications

Persons with late-stage BPH may have flank pain, fever and pain on urination (dysuria) due to inflammation of the bladder (cystitis) or kidneys (pyelonephritis). The inflammation may be due to infection or calculi (stones, usually composed of salts of inorganic or organic acids) caused by urinary stasis. The presence of infection or calculi may cause the prostate to bleed, causing hematuria (blood in the urine).

14.17 Signs

Patients with advanced BPH may show signs of renal failure, including high blood pressure, rapid heart rate, pericarditis (inflammation of the covering of the heart), pallor of the nail beds and peripheral nerve disease. Examination with the hands may reveal flank tenderness, a palpable kidney or a distended bladder.

Digital rectal examination (examination by inserting a gloved, lubricated finger into the rectum) may reveal enlargement of the prostate. BPH commonly produces a smooth, firm, elastic enlargement. Nodularity of the prostate due to BPH often is not palpable because the nodules are covered by a smooth, compressed peripheral zone. The furrow between the two lateral lobes of the prostate usually is lost in BPH and cannot be palpated, but this loss can occur in prostate cancer as well. The presence of firm nodules and irregularities suggests prostate cancer rather than BPH (Denis, 1995).[2]

14.18 Diagnosis

Because of the high prevalence of BPH in the aging male population, the high cost of treatment and the increasing number of new treatments under investigation and entering the marketplace, the Agency for Health Care Policy and Research (AHCPR), a division of the United States Department of Health and Human Services, commissioned a panel of experts to review the medical literature on BPH and develop guidelines for its diagnosis and treatment. The guidelines drafted by the panel were reviewed by other experts in the fields of urology, internal medicine and family practice, and opinions and suggestions were obtained from men with BPH. The final report was published in February 1994 (McConnell, et al., 1994). Similar guidelines have been issued by the International Consultation on

---

[2] *See* 14.29[1] *infra.*

Benign Prostatic Hyperplasia, which met under the auspices of the World Health Organization (Cockett, et al., 1993).

[1] Medical History

The AHCPR guidelines recommend that the clinical evaluation of a man with symptoms of BPH begin with the taking of a detailed medical history that focuses on past disorders of the urinary tract and a physical examination. When taking the medical history, the physician should specifically ask whether the patient has a history of hematuria (blood in the urine), urinary tract infection, nervous system disease or urethral stricture (reduction of the caliber of the urethra). In addition, the patient should be questioned about current medication to determine whether he is taking drugs that impair bladder contractility (e.g., anticholinergics) or that increase resistance to urinary outflow (e.g., sympathomimetics). The patient should also be queried about his general health and asked about surgical procedures that he has undergone.

[2] Physical Examination

The recommended physical examination of a man with symptoms of BPH includes a neurologic examination and a digital rectal examination. These examinations help differentiate BPH from prostate or rectal cancer, evaluate sphincter tone and rule out any neurologic problems that may be causing the symptoms. Digital rectal examination also helps determine the size of the prostate, knowledge of which is important in selecting the most appropriate treatment (but not in determining whether treatment is required). As mentioned, prostate size does not correlate with the presence or severity of symptoms.

[3] American Urological Association Symptom Score

The American Urological Association has developed a questionnaire for use in discriminating between men with and without BPH and between men with BPH who need therapy and those who do not (Barry, et al., 1992; O'Leary, 1992). (*See Table 14-1.*) The AHCPR guidelines recommend use of this questionnaire in the initial evaluation of patients with prostatism and in assessing response to treatment and disease progression.

Each of the seven questions on the questionnaire is answered on a scale of 1 to 5, so the highest score possible is 35. Scores of less than 7, 8 to 19, and 20 to 35 are considered indicative of mild, moderate and severe BPH, respectively. Other sections of the questionnaire rate the degree to which the man has problems with or is bothered by his symptoms and the degree to which his symptoms reduce the quality of his life.

[4]   Urinalysis

A urinalysis is recommended to detect bacteria and/or blood in the urine (hematuria). The presence of bacteria indicates urinary tract infection, and hematuria is the most frequent presenting symptom of bladder cancer. Urinary tract infection and bladder cancer can produce symptoms (e.g., urinary frequency and urgency) that mimic the symptoms of BPH.

[5]   Measurement of Serum Creatinine Level

Serum creatinine level is an indicator of kidney function. Measurement of this variable in men with symptoms of BPH is recommended for several reasons. One is that on average, about 14 percent of patients with BPH have renal insufficiency. Another is that patients with BPH and renal insufficiency have an increased risk of postsurgical complications (Mebust, et al., 1989). A third reason is that surgically treated BPH patients with renal insufficiency have a mortality rate that is up to six times greater than that of patients with normal kidney function.

[6]   Measurement of Serum Prostate-Specific Antigen (PSA) Concentration

In the AHCPR guidelines, measurement of serum levels of prostate-specific antigen (PSA)[3] is an optional test for ruling out impalpable prostate cancer in patients with BPH. The test is not considered mandatory because there is significant overlap in the PSA values between men with BPH and men with clinically localized (organ-confined) prostate cancer (Wolff, et al., 1995); there is no consensus on the significance of minimally elevated serum PSA levels; and at present, data do not show that PSA testing leads to a reduction in the morbidity or mortality of men with prostate cancer.

---

[3] *See* 14.29[2] *infra.*

Table 14-1

Questionnaire for Deriving the American Urological Association BPH
Symptom Score

Urinary Symptoms	Not at all	Less than 1 time in 5	Less than half the time	About half the time	More than half the time	Almost always
Over the past month or so, how often have you had a sensation of not emptying your bladder completely after you finished urinating?	0	1	2	3	4	5
Over the past month or so, how often have you had to urinate again less than 2 hours after you finished urinating?	0	1	2	3	4	5
Over the past month or so, how often have you found you stopped and started again several times when you urinated?	0	1	2	3	4	5
Over the past month or so, how often have you found it difficult to postpone urination?	0	1	2	3	4	5
Over the past month or so, how often have you had a weak urinary stream?	0	1	2	3	4	5
Over the past month, how often have you had to push or strain to begin urination?	0	1	2	3	4	5
Over the past month, how many times did you most typically get up to urinate from the time you went to bed at night until you got up in the morning?	0	1	2	3	4	5

[7] Uroflowmetry

A uroflowmeter is an instrument that makes a continuous recording of urine flow rate (expressed in milliliters per second) throughout the course of urination. Uroflowmetry is commonly used in the evaluation of patients with symptoms of bladder outlet obstruction. In the AHCPR guidelines, uroflowmetry is an optional test in the evaluation of men with prostatism.

An abnormally low urine flow rate can be caused by obstruction or by weakness of the bladder muscle, and uroflowmetry cannot distinguish between the two causes. The method also cannot reveal the cause of lower urinary tract obstruction, but uroflowmetric determination of peak flow rate can be useful in distinguishing between normal men and men with BPH, urethral stricture or prostatitis (inflammation of the prostate).

At very low urine volumes, the bladder cannot create enough pressure for uroflowmetry to record a representative urine flow. Therefore, for the test to be accurate, the patient must void at least 125 to 150 milliliters (mL). At this volume, normal men have an average flow rate of about 12 mL per second and a peak flow rate of about 20 mL per second. Mild bladder outlet obstruction reduces average flow to 6 to 8 mL per second and peak flow to 11 to 15 mL per second. Severe obstruction reduces the rates to even lower levels.

[8] Postvoid Residual Volume

The postvoid residual volume is the amount of urine remaining in the bladder immediately after the completion of urination. Residual volume normally ranges from 0.09 to 2.25 mL, but there is substantial variability among individuals. There is no absolute cutoff point for abnormal residual volume, but a volume greater than 150 mL generally is considered significant (i.e., indicative of severely abnormal bladder function or severe obstruction) because it represents about a third of the volume of the normal bladder.

Postvoid residual volume can be measured noninvasively by ultrasonography (delineation of deep structures by measuring the reflection or transmission of ultrasonic waves) or invasively by catheterization (passage of a tubular instrument through the urethra into the bladder to drain it of urine). Dedicated small bladder scanners have recently become available for the measurement of residual volume.

In the AHCPR guidelines, determination of postvoid residual volume is an optional test in the evaluation of men with prostatism.

[9] Imaging of the Urinary Tract

Imaging of the upper urinary tract of a man with prostatism is not recommended unless he has hematuria, renal insufficiency, urinary tract infection, a history of urolithiasis (stones in the urinary system) and/or a history of urinary tract surgery. The urinary tract can be imaged by intravenous urography (x-ray examination of kidneys, ureters and bladder by means of a contrast agent injected into a vein) or ultrasonography (Geboers, et al., 1994). Ultrasonography is preferred by some urologists because it is noninvasive, relatively inexpensive and has no known side effects. It is considered more specific in determining the nature of a mass lesion in the kidney, whereas intravenous urography has been found to be more sensitive in determining the cause of hematuria.

Ultrasonography also can be used to estimate the size of the prostate, knowledge of which may be useful in choosing an appropriate treatment for BPH. Ultrasonography to measure prostate volume can be performed either suprapubically (from above the pubic bone) or transrectally (from inside the rectum). To assess the volume of the prostate accurately, measurements of the organ must be made in three planes: the anterior-posterior, the sagittal (parallel to the midline) and the coronal (a vertical plane at right angles to a sagittal plane, dividing the body into anterior and posterior portions). Prostate weight can be easily estimated from prostate volume, because the specific gravity of the prostate is between 1 and 1.05.

[10] Cystourethroscopy

Cystourethroscopy is the examination of the inside of the urethra and bladder through an endoscope (a slender tube equipped with a lens and a light that allows visualization of the interior of a canal or hollow organ). The procedure is performed with the aid of local or general anesthesia, or both. The AHCPR guidelines do not recommend this procedure as a means of determining the need for treatment, but it may be useful in selecting or excluding specific invasive therapies.

Cystourethroscopy to exclude unrelated bladder and urethral conditions is recommended for men with prostatism who have a history of hematuria, urethral stricture disease, bladder cancer or lower urinary tract surgery. Cystourethroscopy can be used to detect enlargement of the prostate and obstruction of the urethra and bladder neck, as well as to identify bladder tumors, bladder stones, diverticula and specific anatomic abnormalities that may affect clinical decisions. In addition, residual urine can be removed through the endoscope for determination of postvoid residual volume.[4]

Cystourethroscopy is associated with risks, including discomfort to the patient, adverse effects of the sedative or anesthetic used in the procedure, urinary tract infection, bleeding and urinary retention. Except for discomfort, these effects occur infrequently.

14.19   Treatment

The AHCPR guideline panel reviewed the published data on treatments for BPH and decided that enough information was available to estimate the outcomes of seven treatments and that these treatments therefore could be presented to patients as options (McConnell, 1995). (*See Table 14-2.*) All other therapeutic modalities were classified as experimental. Since the publication of the AHCPR guidelines, a device for the delivery of microwave energy for the treatment of BPH has been approved by the United States Food and Drug Administration (FDA).[5]

[1]   Treatment Outcomes

Treatment outcomes can be indirect or direct. The indirect outcomes most commonly used in research to measure the effectiveness of a treatment for BPH are peak urinary flow rate[6] and postvoid residual volume.[7] Direct outcomes of treatment for BPH include degree of improvement of symptoms due to treatment, risk of complications or side effects of treatment, duration of hospital stay and loss of days of work.

[2]   Treatments with Estimatable Outcomes

Among the treatments for BPH the outcomes of which can be estimated are watchful waiting, alpha blockers, finasteride and others.

---

[4] *See* 14.18[8] *supra.*

[5] *See* 14.19[2][h] *infra.*

[6] *See* 14.18[7] *supra.*

[7] *See* 14.18[8] *supra.*

[a] Watchful Waiting

In watchful waiting (also called expectant management or surveillance), no active therapy is undertaken, but symptoms and clinical course are periodically monitored to determine whether the disease has progressed (Barry, et al., 1988).

[b] Alpha Blockers

Alpha blockers are drugs such as alfuzosin, doxazosin, prazosin and terazosin that inhibit the contraction of smooth muscle. Use of these drugs in the treatment of BPH is based on the theory that bladder outlet obstruction secondary to BPH is due not only to compression of the urethra by hyperplastic prostate tissue but also by contraction of the smooth muscle of the prostate (Lepor, et al., 1996).

[Please see Table 14–2 on following page.]

Table 14-2

Direct Outcomes of BPH Treatments

Outcome	BD	TUIP	OS	TURP	WW	AB	F
Chance (%) for improvement of symptoms*	37-76	78-83	94-99.8	75-96	31-55	59-86	54-78
Reduction (%) in AUA symptom score	51	73	79	85	?	51	31
Chance (%) of complications (about 20% are significant)*	1.78-9.86	2.2-33.3	6.98-4.27	5.2-30.7	1-5†	2.9-43.3	13.6-18.8
Chance (%) of dying within 30-90 days of treatment*	0.72-9.78‡	0.2-1.5	0.99-4.56	0.53-3.31	0.8		
Chance (%) of total urinary incontinence*	?	0.06-1.1	0.34-0.74	0.68-1.4	?		
Chance (%) of need for operative treatment of surgical complications in the future*	?	1.34-2.65	0.6-14.1	0.65-10.1	0		
Chance (%) of impotence*	§	3.9-24.5	4.7-39.2	3.3-34.8	§	2.5-5.3	

Patients (%) with retrograde ejaculation	?	6-55	36-95	25-99	0	4-11	0
Loss of work time (days)	4	7-21	21-28	7-21	1	3.5	1.5
Hospital stay (days)	1	1-3	5-10	3-5	0	0	0

*90% confidence interval (90% probability that value will fall within the range given).
†Complications from progression of BPH. ‡Patients treated in study were high-risk or elderly. §About 2% of men aged 67 years become impotent per year. BD = balloon dilation; TUIP = transurethral incision of the prostate; OS = open surgery; TURP = transurethral resection of the prostate; WW = watchful waiting; AB = alpha blocker therapy; F = finasteride therapy.

[c]   Finasteride

Finasteride is a drug that lowers serum levels of dihydrotestosterone[8] and thereby, over a period of months, reduces the size of the prostate and relieves symptoms (Pascual, et al., 1994).

[d]   Balloon Dilatation

Balloon dilatation is a procedure in which a catheter with a balloon at one end is inserted into the prostatic urethra and inflated with the aim of stretching the urethra where it is narrowed by pressure from the prostate (McLoughlin and Williams, 1990; Reddy, 1990).

[e]   Transurethral Incision

Transurethral incision is a surgical procedure performed through an endoscope in which one or two cuts are made in the prostate to reduce constriction of the urethra. The operation is performed only in patients with bladder outlet obstruction whose prostate weighs an estimated 30 grams or less (Riehmann, et al., 1995).

[f]   Transurethral Resection

Transurethral resection is the surgical removal of the inner portion of the prostate through an endoscope. The procedure usually requires a hospital stay. Transurethral resection is considered the treatment of choice for BPH when the prostate weighs between 30 and 80 grams (Hartung, 1995).

[g]   Open Prostatectomy

Open prostatectomy is the surgical removal of the inner portion of the prostate via an incision made through the skin above or posterior to the pubic bone. The operation requires a hospital stay and is used for prostates weighing more than 80 grams (Murphy, et al., 1994).

[h]   Microwave Hyperthermia

Microwave hyperthermia involves the transrectal or transurethral delivery of microwaves to the prostate via a catheter containing a microwave antenna and a cooling system for the purpose of thermally destroying prostate tissue without damaging surrounding structures (Blute, et al., 1994; Venn, et al., 1995).

---

[8] *See* 14.13 *supra.*

[3]   Experimental Treatments

A number of experimental treatments are under investigation for BPH. In *laser ablation,* a laser beam, usually delivered through optical fibers contained in an endoscope, is used to thermally destroy prostate tissue that is compressing the urethra (Anson, et al., 1995a, 1995b; Strauss, 1995). Another treatment involves the placement of *prostatic urethral stents* (expandable metallic devices) in the prostatic urethra to maintain the patency of the urethra. With time, epithelial tissue grows over and covers the stent (Kletscher, et al., 1995).

Antiandrogen therapy is the selective blockade of the activity of androgens (male hormones) at the prostate level, using drugs known as antiandgrogens (e.g., flutamide). *Transurethral needle ablation* is the use of high-frequency radio waves to thermally destroy prostate tissue. The waves are delivered through a urethral catheter equipped with adjustable needles that are placed in selected areas of prostate tissue (Issa, 1996).

High-intensity focused ultrasound involves the delivery of ultrasound energy through a computer-controlled transrectal probe to create thermal injury of prostate tissue (Bihrle, et al., 1994; Foster, et al., 1994).

[4]   AHCPR Treatment Recommendations

If the patient's American Urological Association symptom score is 7 or lower[9] and he has no complications, watchful waiting is recommended. If the man's symptoms progress to moderate or severe levels (American Urological Association symptom score greater than 7), it is recommended that his physician discuss the symptoms with him again and, if his BPH has become bothersome or detrimental to his health, offer him other treatment options.

Patients with moderate or severe symptoms should be given information in an unbiased manner on the benefits and risks of watchful waiting, alpha blocker therapy, finasteride therapy, balloon dilation, microwave hypothermia and surgery. Risks of surgery include urinary incontinence (inability to prevent the discharge of urine), impotence (inability to have an erection) and retrograde ejaculation (semen travels toward the bladder instead of to the outside of the body).

---

[9] *See* 14.18[3] *supra.*

Actual treatment outcome data should be given to the patient to allow him to choose the treatment that he considers best for himself. When informing the patient about his treatment options, the physician should be wary of using educational materials developed by groups or manufacturers with an economic or other interest in a particular treatment.

If a man chooses watchful waiting or a treatment other than surgery and later experiences a worsening of symptoms, surgery can be discussed again as an option. Failure to respond to nonsurgical therapy does not mean, however, that the patient must undergo surgery. The patient may well choose watchful waiting over the risks of surgery.

According to the AHCPR guidelines, the following groups should receive surgical treatment for BPH: (a) patients with refractory urinary retention who have failed at least one attempt at catheter removal of retained urine, (b) men with recurrent urinary tract infections or recurrent gross hematuria, (c) patients with bladder stones and (d) patients with renal insufficiency clearly caused by BPH.

14.20   ADENOCARCINOMA OF THE PROSTATE

Adenocarcinoma accounts for the vast majority of tumors of the prostate. Because of this, the term *prostate cancer* has become essentially synonymous with prostate adenocarcinoma, both in medical terminology and in common speech.[10]

Prostate cancer poses a particular challenge to physicians for a number of reasons: its natural progression is not known and appears to vary among individuals (Dearnaley, et al., 1993), there is no consensus on the advisability and efficacy of routine screening for the disease (Chodak, 1993; Krahn, et al., 1994; Schröder, 1995), and considerable controversy exists regarding the most appropriate methods of staging, diagnosis and treatment (Schröder, 1990), especially for patients whose cancer has not spread beyond the prostate (Whitmore, 1994). Studies designed to resolve some of these issues are in progress (Catalona, 1994; Wilt and Brawer, 1995), but final results are not expected until about 2005 (Begg, 1994).

---

[10] *See* 14.30 *infra* for a brief discussion of other cancers of the prostate.

14.21   Epidemiology

In the United States, prostate cancer has overtaken lung cancer and colorectal cancer as the most commonly diagnosed cancer in men. Between 1980 and 1990, the incidence of prostate cancer increased by 50 percent, primarily because of improved detection but also because of the increasing number of men who are over the age of 50. A further increase in incidence is expected as screening tests continue to improve and to be more widely used. The incidence of prostate cancer in black men is about 37 percent greater than it is in white men (Morton, 1994). In fact, black Americans have the highest incidence of prostate cancer in the world (American Cancer Society, 1996).

Incidences and death rates of clinically evident prostate cancer vary greatly among countries, even when differences in the availability and efficacy of screening programs are taken into consideration. In 1988, for example, the age-adjusted death rates per 100,000 persons in the population were 15.7 for men in the United States but only 3.5 for men in Japan (Boring, et al., 1992a). On the other hand, autopsy data from many nations show that between 15 and 30 percent of men over the age of 50 years have microscopic evidence of prostate cancer. By age 80 years, 60 to 70 percent of men have evidence of prostate cancer at autopsy (Pienta and Esper, 1993).

It is estimated that a 50-year-old American man has a 40 percent chance of developing microscopic prostate cancer during his lifetime, a 10 percent chance of being diagnosed with the disease and a 2 to 3 percent chance of dying of prostate cancer (Garnick, 1993). Eighty percent of prostate cancers are diagnosed in men over the age of 65 years.

14.22   Risk Factors and Etiology

Risk factors for prostate cancer include advancing age, black race, family history of the disease, smoking, vasectomy (excision of a segment of the sperm duct to produce sterility) and high dietary fat intake. Socioeconomic class, infectious agents, sexual behavior, smoking and BPH (benign prostatic hyperplasia) do not appear to increase the risk. Some reports indicate an increased risk of prostate cancer among men in certain occupations, including mechanics, printers, plumbers, farmers and factory workers, but these reports have not been confirmed by large-scale studies (Pienta and Esper, 1993).

[1]   Age

The prevalence of both clinically apparent and microscopic prostate cancer increases with age. Prostate cancer increases more rapidly with age than any other major cancer, although the reasons that it does are unclear. The development of a cancer cell is thought to be a multistep process that requires genetic events to initiate the transformation of normal cells to cancerous cells and other events that promote the transformation process. The presence of microscopic cancer appears to be related to age, but other risk factors probably are responsible for the promotion aspects of transformation (Pienta and Esper, 1993).

[2]   Family History

The results of several studies suggest that the incidence of prostate cancer is higher in men who have relatives with the disease than in men who do not (Steinberg, et al., 1990a; Spitz, et al., 1991; Carter, et al., 1992). In one series of analyses, it was found that men whose father or brother had prostate cancer are twice as likely to develop prostate cancer as are men without affected relatives; the risk increases with the number of affected relatives (Carter, et al., 1992). The American Cancer Society (ACS) recommends that screening for prostate cancer in men with a positive family history of the disease begin earlier than that of the rest of the male population (Mettlin, et al., 1993).[11]

[3]   Race

The incidence of prostate cancer varies greatly among races. Both incidence and mortality data indicate that the incidence of clinical prostate cancer is low in Asian men and high in Scandinavian men (Boring, et al., 1992a). Research shows that men tend to take on the risk of the country to which they emigrate (Meikle and Smith, 1990). Both research and census data show that in the United States, black men have a higher incidence of clinical prostate cancer at all ages than do white men and that the racial difference does not correlate statistically with education or socioeconomic class (Baquet, et al., 1991).

---

[11] *See* 14.29 *infra.*

[4] Vasectomy

Studies have revealed a small increase in the risk for prostate cancer in men who have undergone vasectomy (Mettlin, et al., 1990). The risk appears to increase with the number of years since the operation was performed (Giovannucci, et al., 1992a and 1992b).

[5] Dietary Fat

Epidemiologic and migrant studies have found a positive association between prostate cancer and dietary fat (especially animal fat), and this may explain why the risk of microscopic prostate cancer is similar among countries but the risk of clinically evident disease is higher in Western nations (Morton, et al., 1996). Inasmuch as a low-fat, high-fiber diet is known to affect male sex hormone metabolism, it has been postulated that the effect of dietary fat in the development of prostate cancer may be mediated through endogenous (produced by the body) hormones.

It is thought that both genetic and environmental factors are involved in the etiology of prostate cancer, with male hormones possibly playing an essential role as tumor promoters. The etiologic role of male hormones on prostate cancer is suggested by several observations:

- prostate cancer does not occur in men deprived of testicular function;
- castration results in regression of prostate tumor growth; and
- isolated prostate cancer cells grow rapidly in the presence of male hormones.

Studies also have shown an association between the presence of male hormones and the expression of oncogenes (genes capable of causing the conversion of normal cells into cancer cells).

14.23 Pathology

The vast majority of cancers of the prostate are adenocarcinomas arising from the epithelial lining of the prostate glands. About 70 percent of prostate adenocarcinomas arise in the peripheral zone, 10 to 20 percent originate in the central zone, and 10 to 15 percent arise in the transition zone. In up to 85 percent of cases, the disease is polycentric (has multiple sites of origin). Transitional cell carcinomas that arise in the prostatic ducts, squamous cell carcinomas, adenosquamous carcinomas, mucinous carcinomas, small cell carcinomas and sarcomas (connective tissue cancers) also occur in the prostate but are rare.

14.24   Tumor Grade and Stage

The grade of a prostate tumor is determined by the microscopic examination of tissue removed from the tumor during a diagnostic biopsy or from a resected organ. Several systems have been devised for grading prostate adenocarcinoma. The most widely used is the Gleason system, which is based on the degree of differentiation of the glandular tissue of the organ (Spires, et al., 1994). The five grades of prostate cancer in the Gleason system are defined as follows:

> Grade 1: Well-differentiated carcinoma with uniform gland pattern.
>
> Grade 2: Well-differentiated carcinoma with glands varying in size and shape.
>
> Grade 3: Moderately differentiated carcinoma with either irregular acini (the saclike secretory portions of glands) that are often widely separated or well-defined papillary (fingerlike) or cribriform (sievelike) structures.
>
> Grade 4: Poorly differentiated carcinoma with fused glands widely infiltrating the stroma. Malignant cells may grow in cords or sheets.
>
> Grade 5: Very poorly differentiated carcinoma with no or minimal gland formation. Tumor cell masses may have central necrosis (cell death).

About 50 percent of prostate tumors have more than one pattern of differentiation. The most common pattern is called the primary, and the second most common pattern is called the secondary. The two patterns are often added and averaged to produce what is known as a Gleason score. Tumor grade and stage are useful prognostic indicators. Patients with low-grade/low-stage tumors generally do well; those with high-grade/high-stage cancers usually do poorly, regardless of treatment.

Stage is a designation used to describe the extent of spread of a cancer. Two systems are widely used for the staging of prostate cancer:

the tumor-node-metastasis (TNM) system, developed by the International Union Against Cancer, and the American Urological Association system (Catalona and Whitmore, 1989). (*See Table 14-3* for comparison of the two staging systems.)

T1a, T1b and T1c tumors (roughly equivalent to A1 and A2 tumors) are not palpable on digital rectal examination. They usually are found at the time of transurethral or open prostatectomy for BPH and therefore are referred to as occult (hidden) or incidental. T2a and T2b (exactly equivalent to B1 and B2) describe tumors that are identifiable on digital rectal examination, appear to be confined to the prostate and have a diameter of less than or more than 1.5 centimeters, respectively. Stage T3 (corresponding to stage C) denotes disease that has extended through the capsule of the prostate. Prostate cancer in stages T1, T2 and T3 usually is asymptomatic. The designations "N" and "M" are used to denote metastasis (dissemination of tumor cells by the lymphatic or blood vessels) to regional lymph nodes or distant sites, respectively.

14.25   Natural Progression

The natural progression of prostate cancer is unknown. Some prostatic carcinomas are slow growing and may exist for long periods without causing significant symptoms, whereas others are more aggressive. It is not known whether tumors can become more malignant with time.

One hypothesis is that prostate cancers are small in the beginning and then progress to a larger volume. Tumor grade may change during the process, due to genetic instability and mutation. According to this hypothesis, the natural progression of prostate cancer is to eventually spread beyond the organ and metastasize to distant sites (Narayan, 1995).

Prostate cancer can spread by three routes: direct extension, the lymphatic system and the bloodstream. The prostatic capsule is a natural barrier against the growth of a tumor into surrounding structures, but tumors often grow by direct extension into the seminal vesicles, urethra and bladder because the capsule is weak at these points. Prostate cancer cells spread by the blood most often cause secondary tumors (in decreasing order of frequency) in bone, lung, liver and adrenal glands.

Table 14-3

American Urological Association (AUA) and TNM Staging Systems for Prostate Cancer

AUA		TNM	
A	Occult carcinoma (not palpable on digital rectal examination)	T1	Incidental (not palpable on digital rectal examination)
		T1a	Three foci or less
A1	One lobe	T1b	More than three foci
A2	Multifocal or diffuse	T1c	Detected by biopsy because of an elevated serum PSA level
B	Confined to prostate	T2b	Greater than 1.5 cm/more than one lobe
B1	One lobe	T2a	Less than or equal to 1.5 cm
B2	Diffuse	T2	Clinically or grossly limited to prostate
C	Extracapsular extension	T3	Invades prostatic apex/beyond capsule/bladder neck/seminal vesicle/not fixed
		T4	Fixed or invades other adjacent structures
D1	Pelvic lymph node metastasis	N1	Single less than or equal to 2 cm
		N2	Single greater than 2 cm but less than or equal to 5 cm; multiple less than or equal to 5 cm
		N3	Greater than 5 cm
D2	Distant metastasis	M1	Distant metastasis

14.26 Symptoms and Signs

In most patients, prostate cancer develops slowly (tumor volume doubling time is about two years) (Stamey and McNeal, 1992), and most tumors develop in the periphery of the organ rather than in the area around the urethra. Early prostate cancer, therefore, rarely causes symptoms of urethral obstruction. When such symptoms do occur, they are identical to those of BPH.[12] The most frequent presenting symptom of prostate cancer is hematuria (bloody urine). Symptoms and signs of advanced disease may include neurologic symptoms due to spinal cord compression, myelophthisis (wasting or atrophy of the spinal cord), deep venous thrombosis, pulmonary emboli and bone pain.

14.27 Diagnosis

Tools used in the diagnosis of prostate cancer include digital rectal examination, transrectal ultrasonography, measurement of serum PSA concentration and biopsy of the prostate. The accuracy of the commonly used combination of digital rectal examination, PSA test and transrectal ultrasonography is about 85 percent (Akdas, et al., 1995).

[1] Digital Rectal Examination

Clinical trials have shown digital rectal examination to have an accuracy of only 30 to 45 percent (Lee, et al., 1988). Because of the minimal time, expense and discomfort involved in the procedure, however, the American Cancer Society recommends that it be performed as part of the routine physical examination of all men over the age of 40 (American Cancer Society, 1996).

The posterior surfaces of the lateral lobes, where prostate cancer commonly begins, are readily palpable on digital rectal examination. Prostate cancer typically is felt as hard, nodular and irregular. Hardness of the organ, however, can also be due to BPH or calculi (stones), and the furrow between the lateral lobes can be obscured by both BPH and cancer. Extension of a tumor into the seminal vesicles may also be detectable by digital rectal examination.

[2] Measurement of Serum PSA Concentration

PSA is a protease (an enzyme that breaks down protein) that is thought to function normally to liquefy the semen. PSA is secreted by the epithelial cells of the normal prostate, and small amounts pass into the blood if the blood-prostate barrier is broken in any way by cell destruction. Thus, PSA is prostate specific and not prostate cancer specific.

BPH is thought to elevate serum PSA levels in direct proportion to the size of the prostate, whereas the degree of PSA production by

---

[12] *See* 14.16[1] *supra.*

malignant prostate glands is variable and depends on the degree of glandular differentiation in the tumor. Glands that are well differentiated produce more PSA than do glands that are poorly differentiated.

It is estimated that 25 to 30 percent of men with serum PSA levels greater than 4 nanograms per mL have prostate cancer. The sensitivity of PSA testing for detecting prostate cancer can be enhanced by applying age-specific criteria (Oesterling, et al., 1993). The upper limits of normal PSA concentrations for white men aged 40 to 49 years, 50 to 59 years, 60 to 69 years, and 70 to 79 years are 2.5, 3.5, 4.9 and 5.8 nanograms per mL, respectively (Garnick and Fair, 1996). Black men tend to have higher PSA levels, and their levels vary more with increasing age. Therefore, the recommended upper limits of normal concentrations for black men in their 40s, 50s, 60s and 70s are 2, 4, 4 and 5.5 nanograms per mL, respectively (Morgan, et al., 1996).

In August 1994, the United States Food and Drug Administration approved the use of PSA testing in association with digital rectal examination for the early detection of prostate cancer. The use of serum PSA for the detection of prostate cancer has significantly changed the profile of clinical stage at diagnosis. In the era before PSA testing (before 1980), up to a third of men diagnosed with prostate cancer had metastatic disease at diagnosis (Murphy, et al., 1982). Now, because of the widespread use of the PSA test, about 95 percent of patients have clinically localized disease (stages T1c and T2) at diagnosis (Boring, et al., 1994; Catalona, et al., 1993).

In the diagnosis of prostate cancer, PSA is used in a variety of ways. Measurement of PSA can detect cancer not discernible on digital rectal examination. In patients with elevated PSA levels and negative biopsy findings, the need for follow-up biopsies can be ascertained by determining PSA velocity (rate of increase in PSA serum level over time) and PSA density (serum PSA concentration divided by prostate volume). PSA levels that rise at a rate of 0.75 nanograms per mL per year or greater are considered indicative of prostate cancer. Thus, if three PSA values obtained at 6–or 12–month intervals show a rise of 0.75 nanograms per mL or more, a repeat biopsy should be performed (Carter, et al., 1992).

Because prostate cancer tissue produces more PSA per gram of tissue than does normal prostate tissue or BPH tissue, an elevated PSA density may indicate the presence of prostate cancer. A PSA density of more than 0.15 nanograms per mL has been found to be associated with an approximately 50 percent chance of finding prostate cancer on biopsy (Benson, et al., 1992). PSA density may be especially useful for patients whose prostate is large and whose elevated PSA levels, therefore, may be due to BPH, and for patients whose initial biopsy was negative and whose follow-up tests show a rising trend in PSA levels. Problems in the use of PSA density in determining the likelihood of prostate cancer include the potential for errors in measuring the prostate volume by transrectal ultrasonography and a variation of up to 15 percent in repeated examinations in the same patient (Brawer, et al., 1993).

Research indicates that men with a high ratio of bound PSA (PSA that is bound to serum protein) to free PSA are more likely to have prostate cancer detected by biopsy, regardless of total (bound and free) PSA level, although confirmatory studies are needed to establish the usefulness of the bound-to-free PSA ratio in the diagnosis of prostate cancer (Oesterling, et al., 1995).

New methods are being developed that combine measurement of PSA level with other modalities to aid in the staging of prostate cancer. In one such method, PSA concentration is combined with Gleason score[13] and biopsy data to predict whether a patient's disease is still confined to the prostate. Another method exploits the fact that aggressive prostate tumors are highly vascular. By combining PSA level, Gleason score and the density of small vessels in the tumor (vessel count per unit area of tissue, determined microscopically), the clinician is able to calculate the probability that a patient's cancer has extended beyond the prostate (Brawer, et al., 1994; Furusato, et al., 1994).

PSA level may be valuable in the detection of residual cancer in patients who have undergone radical prostatectomy (surgical removal of the prostate). After removal of the prostate, the PSA level should fall to zero (or to less than 0.1 nanogram per mL in the measurements of most commercially available test kits). If it does not, residual disease is suspected. Rising PSA after a drop to zero indicates either microscopic recurrence of cancer in the prostatic bed or metastasis (Garnick and Fair, 1996).

---

[13] *See* 14.25 *supra.*

[3]   Transrectal Ultrasonography

Transrectal ultrasonography can detect up to 60 percent of prostate cancers, even if they are nonpalpable. This accuracy is thought to be a result of the compact, highly cellular nature of prostate tumors, which causes them to be hypoechogenic (poorly reflective of high frequency sound waves). Ultrasonography is also useful in directing needle biopsy and for determining the degree of extension of the tumor into the bladder and seminal vesicles. Transrectal ultrasonography is recommended if either the digital rectal examination is positive or the PSA level is elevated.

[4]   Computed Tomography (CT)

Computed tomography (CT; a modality in which an x-ray tube moves around the patient, creating an image of a cross section of the body) is used in the diagnosis and staging of prostate cancer only when metastasis to the lymph nodes is suspected on the basis of high PSA or Gleason scores. The computed tomographic criterion for nodal involvement is nodal size, which means that false-negative and false-positive findings are not uncommon.

[5]   Magnetic Resonance Imaging (MRI)

Magnetic resonance imaging (MRI; a procedure in which the patient's body is placed in the field of a powerful magnet and then subjected to radiofrequency pulses to produce detailed images of soft tissues) is not used in the diagnosis of prostate cancer because of its high cost and the overlap in the appearance of BPH and cancerous processes. Magnetic resonance imaging appears to be somewhat more accurate than transrectal ultrasonography in assessing the extension of a prostate tumor to structures outside the prostatic capsule (Schiebler, et al., 1993; Tempany, et al., 1994). For most patients, however, cost, time and duplication of information preclude the use of both transrectal ultrasonography and MRI.

[6]   Pelvic Lymphadenectomy

Pelvic lymphadenectomy is a surgical procedure in which lymph nodes are removed from the pelvic region and examined for cancer. The surgery often is performed with a laparoscope (a tube equipped with a lens and a light that allows the physician to see inside the body) inserted through a small incision in the abdominal wall (Schuessler, et al., 1991). Pelvic lymphadenectomy is considered the most accurate technique for detecting metastasis to the lymph nodes in patients with prostate cancer.

[7] Bone Scanning

Bone scanning is the most common and reliable way to determine whether prostate cancer has metastasized to bone in distant sites. In this procedure, the patient swallows or is injected with a small amount of a radioisotope (e.g., technetium-99m-labeled methylene diphosphonate) that binds to bone cells. A camera displays an image of the gamma rays emitted by the radioisotope on a screen. The way the material is absorbed by the cells of the bones can indicate the presence of cancer. The diagnosis is confirmed by a plain radiograph of the area. Less than 2 percent of bone scans produce false-positive results. Common causes of false-positive scans are degenerative arthritis, Paget's disease[14] and prior injury of the bone in any area.

[8] Biopsy

A definitive diagnosis of prostate cancer can be provided only by a pathology examination of a tissue specimen taken from the tumor. The prostate is biopsied when an abnormality is detected on digital rectal examination, by an elevated PSA level, by imaging or when a man has obstructive urinary tract symptoms that have no known cause.

Several biopsy procedures are used in the diagnosis of prostate cancer. In fine-needle biopsy (also called aspiration biopsy), tissue is removed by drawing it through a needle that pierces the skin of the area between the thighs (transperineal biopsy) or the rectum (transrectal biopsy) and the capsule of the prostate. Fine-needle biopsy carries a lower risk of infection, and transrectal biopsy provides more precise sampling. The most accurate sampling is obtained with a spring-loaded needle that is operated under ultrasonographic guidance. Open perineal biopsy (removal of prostate tissue through an incision in the skin between the thighs) is rarely used, both because it is a more extensive procedure and because it can cause at least temporary impotence. Transurethral biopsy is also infrequently used because most early cancers are located in the peripheral regions of the prostate. Tissue specimens for staging can be obtained from the tumor itself at the time of tumor resection.

---

14 *See also* ch. 5.

14.28   Screening

Numerous studies have assessed the efficacy of digital rectal examination, serum PSA testing and transrectal ultrasonography as screening tools for prostate cancer. On the basis of the results, the American Urological Association and the American Cancer Society have recommended that prostate cancer screening with digital rectal examination and PSA testing begin at age 50 years for white men without a family history of prostate cancer and at age 40 years for black men and men with one or more first-degree relatives with prostate cancer (Andriole and Catalona, 1994). A study involving more than 6,000 men found that screening with digital rectal examination and PSA testing doubled the detection rate of tumors that were organ confined (and thus highly curable) from about 35 percent (when traditional indications for biopsy were used) to about 70 percent (Richie, et al., 1993). The specificity of transrectal ultrasonography is considered too low for it to be useful in screening programs.

Not all advisory groups endorse routine screening of men for prostate cancer. Consensus conferences held in Canada, France and Sweden, and statements by the International Union against Cancer and the United States Public Health Service Task Force have not endorsed routine screening (Garnick, 1993). Critics of PSA testing of all men over the age of 50 point out that a large proportion of screening-detected cancers are incidental tumors that have little clinical significance. These groups argue that there is a lack of evidence showing that PSA testing leads to a reduction in the morbidity or mortality of men with prostate cancer, and that routine PSA testing may lead to overdiagnosis and, therefore, to unnecessary treatment-related morbidity and mortality (Kantoff and Talcott, 1994). Trials are underway to determine whether screening programs can reduce the number of deaths due to prostate cancer, but definitive results are not expected until about 2005.

14.29   Treatment

Prostate cancer may be treated by watchful waiting, curative treatment or palliation. Valid comparisons of the various treatment strategies are lacking in the medical literature. For this reason, there are no absolute recommendations for the treatment of individual patients (Catalona, 1994). In making decisions about treatment, physicians are advised to give less weight to information about the value of various treatments than to the patient's age and general health, the stage and grade of the cancer (Catalona and Whitmore, 1989), and factors concerning quality of life, such as the risks and complications of treatment versus the risks of advanced cancer (Emberton, et al., 1996).

[1]   Clinically Localized Disease

In 1996, the five-year relative (adjusted for normal life expectancy) survival rate of men with clinically localized prostate cancer was 98 percent (American Cancer Society, 1996). The Prostate Cancer Clinical Guidelines Panel of the American Urological Association has published recommendations for treatment of clinically localized prostate cancer (Middleton, 1996). The panel based its recommendations on treatment outcome data from all available published reports on clinically localized prostate cancer. The panel found the data inadequate for valid comparisons of the following four types of treatment commonly used for stage T1c and T2 prostate cancer: radical prostatectomy (removal of the entire prostate and the seminal vesicles), external beam radiotherapy (exposure of the tumor to cancer-killing rays produced by a machine outside the body), brachytherapy (radiotherapy in which the source of radiation is placed within the body; also called interstitial radiotherapy) and watchful waiting.

The panel's report states that differences were too great among treatment series regarding such significant characteristics as age, tumor grade and pelvic lymph node status for one of the four treatments to be considered superior to another. The panel recommended the following standards:

- Assessment of the patient's life expectancy, overall health status and tumor characteristics is necessary before any treatment decision can be made.

- A patient with clinically localized prostate cancer should be informed about the commonly accepted initial interventions, including, at a minimum, radical prostatectomy, radiation therapy and watchful waiting. A discussion of the estimates of the benefits and harms of each intervention should be offered to the patient.

- The patient's preference, based on his attitude toward the course of the disease and the benefits and risks of the different interventions, should be considered in determining his treatment.

The panel made the following treatment recommendations:

- In general, the patient who is most likely to benefit from a radical prostatectomy is a healthy man with a relatively long life expectancy, no significant surgical risk factors and a preference to undergo surgery.

- Radiation therapy is appropriate for a man with a relatively long life expectancy, no significant risk factors for radiation toxicity and a preference to undergo radiation therapy.

- Surveillance is probably most suited to the patient with a shorter projected life span and/or a low-grade tumor.

The most common risks of radical prostatectomy are impotence and incontinence. Improvements in surgical technique now allow preservation of the nerve and vascular supply of the penis (and thus preservation of potency) in most patients below the age of 60. The most common complications of radiation therapy are cystitis (inflammation of the urinary bladder) and proctitis (inflammation of the mucous membrane of the rectum).

Adjuvant hormonal therapy has been used in the treatment of stage T2 prostate cancer, with the aim of reducing the size of the tumor before surgery and lowering the incidence of positive surgical margins (cancer found at the margins of tissue removed with the tumor) (Fair, et al., 1993). In hormonal therapy, a drug that reduces circulating levels of male hormones is administered for three to six months prior to surgery. The effectiveness of adjuvant hormonal therapy has not yet been adequately tested.

Cryoablation of the prostate (destruction of the prostate by freezing it with liquid nitrogen) is under investigation as a way of controlling clinically localized prostate cancer. At present, insufficient data are available for recommendation of the technique as an alternative to radical prostatectomy.

[2]   Locally Advanced Disease

Currently there is no efficient therapy for locally advanced prostate cancer (disease that has spread beyond the prostate capsule; stages T3 and T4). The treatments described herein all are associated with survival rates that are about 25 to 50 percent lower than the rate in the general population (Catalona, 1994). The five-year relative survival rate for patients with locally advanced prostate cancer is 92 percent (American Cancer Society, 1996).

Surgery generally is not recommended for men with stage T3 and T4 disease because most have occult distant metastases and because complete removal of the tumor is seldom achieved, even with a wide excision. In some patients, low-grade stage T3 tumors have been managed with transurethral resection with acceptable results. In about 20 percent of men diagnosed with stage T3 prostate cancer, the stage is really lower and the tumor is amenable to radical prostatectomy (Morgan, et al., 1993). Adjuvant hormonal therapy may improve the results of radical prostatectomy in men with T3 disease.

Radiation therapy for stage T3 and T4 tumors is associated with a 15-year survival rate that is about half that of the normal population (Epstein and Hanks, 1992). Adjuvant hormonal therapy has been used with the goal of improving survival after radiation therapy (Pilepich, et al., 1990), but the long-term efficacy of such treatment is not known.

[3] Lymph Node Metastases

Less than 15 percent of patients with lymph node metastases (stages N1 through N3) are cured by any treatment (Epstein and Hanks, 1992). For this reason, a pelvic lymphadenectomy (surgical removal of the lymph nodes) to determine whether there has been metastasis to the lymph nodes is usually performed before radical prostatectomy and sometimes before radiotherapy. Lymphadenectomy itself is not therapeutic.

Treatments used in patients with nodal metastases include hormonal therapy, radical prostatectomy and radiation therapy. Hormonal therapy may delay progression of the cancer and provide local control of the primary tumor (Steinberg, et al., 1990b). Transurethral resection usually is effective in relieving obstruction of the bladder outlet caused by the tumor. Some clinicians do not perform radical prostatectomy in patients with nodal metastases, whereas others do so as a means of providing local control. In a study comparing radical prostatectomy, radiation therapy and watchful waiting in patients with pelvic node metastases, the men treated with prostatectomy fared the best (Steinberg, et al., 1990b). Encouraging results have been obtained with radical prostatectomy and postoperative hormonal therapy (Zincke, et al., 1992), but equivalent results may be obtainable with hormonal therapy alone (Myers, et al., 1992). There is little evidence that radiation therapy is effective in treating men with nodal metastases of prostate cancer (Catalona, 1994).

[4]   Metastases to Distant Sites

The primary treatment used for patients with disseminated prostate cancer is androgen-deprivation therapy (the elimination, by either medical or surgical means, of androgens). With this treatment, most patients show an objectively measurable response, but evidence of a survival benefit is lacking. The five-year relative survival rate of patients with distant metastases is 30 percent (American Cancer Society, 1996).

Methods of reducing serum levels of male hormones include orchiectomy (surgical castration), administration of luteinizing hormone-releasing hormone agonists (e.g., goserelin acetate, megestrol acetate, and leuprolide acetate) and the administration of antiandrogens (substances that prevent full expression of the biological effects of androgenic hormones on tissue; e.g., flutamide and estrogens such as diethylstilbestrol). Orchiectomy is a simple outpatient operation that reduces serum androgen concentrations without the problems of compliance with medical regimens. This procedure, understandably, is not acceptable to all patients.

The timing of hormonal therapy is a matter of controversy, both because patients with metastatic prostate cancer who are not treated sometimes live for long periods without symptoms and because the side effects of androgen deprivation (hot flashes; breast enlargement; diminished muscle mass; fatigue; decreased stamina, libido and sexual potency; and psychological changes) are not unimportant to asymptomatic, sexually active men (Garnick and Fair, 1996). There is only equivocal evidence that early hormonal therapy is more effective than delayed therapy (Kozlowski, et al., 1991). Symptomatic men with disseminated disease should be treated immediately, however.

A controversial area is the use of combined treatments for the achievement of maximal androgen deprivation (McLeod, et al., 1995). Combination therapy may provide no more than a 6-month increase in survival (Beland, et al., 1991) or, in patients with early metastatic disease, survival may be increased by up to 20 months (Crawford, et al., 1989). In a study comparing orchiectomy with a combination of flutamide and goserelin acetate, the combination resulted in a

10-month delay in the progression of disease and a 10-month survival advantage (Denis, et al., 1993).

An agent under investigation for the treatment of metastatic prostate cancer in patients who do not respond to hormonal treatment is suramin, an anti-growth-factor drug that also has antiandrogenic activity. There have been no reports of complete response to suramin, but some studies have shown responses in about a third of patients that last for more than a year (Meyers, et al., 1995). Chemotherapy has not been shown to be useful in the treatment of metastatic prostate cancer.

Patients with spinal cord compression due to the metastasis of prostate cancer to the dura mater (the fibrous membrane forming the outer envelope of the brain and the spinal cord) should be treated with a high-dose corticosteroid such as dexamethasone (Garnick, 1993), usually followed by radiation therapy. If such patients have not previously received hormonal therapy, androgen suppression is best initiated with orchiectomy or the administration of the antifungal drug ketoconazole, because these treatments rapidly lower testosterone secretion (Catalona, 1994). Surgical decompression of the spinal cord is indicated for patients with severe or rapidly progressing lesions and those with spinal instability.

Patients with metastatic prostate cancer often suffer excruciating bone pain that can be controlled with localized palliative radiation therapy and narcotic analgesics. Patients commonly require increasing doses of morphine or another narcotic to control their bone pain while they are receiving radiation therapy.

14.30 OTHER CANCERS OF THE PROSTATE

Although adenocarcinoma is by far the most common type of cancer affecting the prostate, other types may be seen as well.

14.31 Transitional Cell Carcinoma

Transitional cell carcinoma is derived from transitional epithelium and occurs chiefly in the urinary bladder, ureter or renal pelvis. Transitional cell carcinoma of the prostate is usually secondary to primary disease in one of these structures. Primary transitional cell carcinoma of the prostate is very rare. Patients who develop it are usually in the sixth decade and seek medical care because of obstructive urinary symptoms and hematuria.

14.32 Squamous Cell Carcinoma

Squamous cell carcinoma accounts for less than 1 percent of prostate cancers. It is associated with both transitional cell carcinoma and treated prostatic adenocarcinoma. Patients come to their physicians complaining of prostatism.

14.33 Carcinoid and Small Cell Carcinoma

Carcinoid is a small, slow-growing neoplasm that sometimes occurs in a bronchus. It is composed of islands of rounded or spindle-shaped cells of medium size and covered by intact mucosa. Small cell carcinoma is a highly malignant cancer that occurs primarily in the wall of a bronchus. In the prostate, it is uncertain whether these two cancers are distinct. As it does in the bronchus, the tumor may respond to chemotherapy.

14.34 Sarcoma

Sarcomas make up about 0.1 percent of prostate cancers and are either rhabdomyosarcoma (a tumor derived from striated muscle) or leiomyosarcoma (a tumor derived from smooth muscle). The former occurs in young patients. The latter occasionally occurs in children, but the main incidence is in men in the 40-to 70-year-old age group.

14.100 BIBLIOGRAPHY

Text References

Akdas, A., et al.: The Diagnostic Accuracy of Digital Rectal Examination, Transrectal Ultrasonography, Prostate-Specific Antigen (PSA) and PSA Density in Prostate Carcinoma. Br. J. Urol. 76:54-56, 1995.

American Cancer Society. Cancer Facts & Figures 1996. Atlanta: American Cancer Society, 1996.

Andriole, G. L. and Catalona, W. J.: Prostate Carcinoma. Annu. Rev. Med. 45:351-359, 1994.

Anson, K., et al.: A Multicenter, Randomized, Prospective Study of Endoscopic Laser Ablation Versus Transurethral Resection of the Prostate. Urology 46:305-310, 1995a.

Anson, K., et al.: The Current Status of the Use of Lasers in the Treatment of Benign Prostatic Hyperplasia. Br. J. Urol. 75(Suppl. 1):34-41, 1995b.

Baquet, C. R., et al.: Socioeconomic Factors and Cancer Incidence among Blacks and Whites. J. Natl. Cancer Inst. 83:551-557, 1991.

Barry, M. J., et al.: Watchful Waiting vs. Immediate Transurethral Resection for Symptomatic Prostatism: The Importance of Patients' Preferences. J.A.M.A. 259:3010-3017, 1988.

Barry, M. J., et al.: The American Urological Association Symptom Index for Benign Prostatic Hyperplasia. J. Urol. 148:1549-1557, 1992.

Begg, C. B.: Methodological Issues in Studies of the Treatment, Diagnosis, and Etiology of Prostate Cancer. Semin. Oncol. 21:569-579, 1994.

Beland, G., et al.: Total Androgen Ablation: Canadian Experience. Urol. Clin. North Am. 18:75-82, 1991.

Benson, M. C., et al.: The Use of Prostate Specific Antigen Density to Enhance the Predictive Value of Intermediate Levels of Serum Prostate Specific Antigen. J. Urol. 147:817-821, 1992.

Bihrle, R., et al.: High-Intensity Focused Ultrasound for the Treatment of Benign Prostatic Hyperplasia: Early United States Clinical Experience. J. Urol. 151:1271-1275, 1994.

Blute, M. L.: Microwave Thermotherapy for the Treatment of Benign Prostatic Hyperplasia. Semin. Urol. 12:181-192, 1994.

Boring, C. C., et al.: Cancer Statistics, 1994. CA Cancer J. Clin. 44:7-26, 1994.

Boring, C. C., et al.: Cancer Statistics, 1992. CA Cancer J. Clin. 42:19-39, 1992a.

Boring, C. C., et al.: Cancer Statistics for African Americans. CA Cancer J. Clin. 42:7-18, 1992b.

Brawer, M. K., et al.: Predictors of Pathologic Stage in Prostatic Carcinoma. The Role of Neovascularity. Cancer 73:678-687, 1994.

Brawer, M. K.: The Role of Alpha 1-Blockade in Benign Prostatic Hyperplasia. J. Clin. Pharmacol. 33:891-895, 1993.

Carter, B. S., et al.: Mendelian Inheritance of Familial Prostate Cancer. Proc. Natl. Acad. Sci. U.S.A. 89:3367-3371, 1992.

Carter, H. B., et al.: Longitudinal Evaluation of Prostate Specific Antigen Levels in Men with and without Prostate Cancer. J.A.M.A. 257:2215-2221, 1992.

Catalona, W. J.: Management of Cancer of the Prostate. N. Engl. J. Med. 331:996-1004, 1994.

Catalona, W. J. and Whitmore, W. F., Jr.: New Staging Systems for Prostate Cancer. J. Urol. 142:115-1304, 1989.

Catalona, W. J., et al.: Comparison of Digital Rectal Examination and Serum Prostate Specific Antigen in the Early Detection of Prostate Cancer: Results of a Multicenter Clinical Trial of 6630 Men. J. Urol. 151:1283-1290, 1994.

Catalona, W. J., et al.: Detection of Organ-Confined Prostate Cancer Is Increased Through Prostate-Specific Antigen-Based Screening. J.A.M.A. 270:948-954, 1993.

Chodak, G. W.: Questioning the Value of Screening for Prostate Cancer in Asymptomatic Men. Urology 42:116-118, 1993.

Chute, C., et al.: The Prevalence of Prostatism: A Population-Based Survey of Urinary Symptoms. J. Urol. 150:85-89, 1993.

Cockett, A. T. K., et al.: Proceedings of the Second International Consultation on BPH, Jersey: Scientific Communication International, 1993.

Crawford, E. D., et al.: A Controlled Trial of Leuprolide with and without Flutamide in Prostatic Carcinoma. N. Engl. J. Med. 321:419-424, 1989.

Dearnaley, D. P., et al.: Prostate Cancer (Grand Round). Lancet 342:901-905, 1993.

Denis, L. J.: Diagnosing Benign Prostatic Hyperplasia Versus Prostate Cancer. Br. J. Urol. 76(Suppl. 1):17-23, 1995.

Denis, L. J., et al.: Goseriln Acetate and Flutamide Versus Bilateral Orchiectomy: A Phase III EORTC Trial (30853). Urology 1993; 42:119-130.

Emberton, M., et al.: The Effect of Prostatectomy on Symptom Severity and Quality of Life. Br. J. Urol. 77:233-247, 1996.

Epstein, B. E. and Hanks, G. E.: Prostate Cancer: Evaluation and Radiotherapeutic Management. CA Cancer J. Clin. 42:223-240, 1992.

Fair, W. R., et al.: Use of Neoadjuvant Androgen Deprivation Therapy in Clinically Localized Prostate Cancer. Clin. Invest. Med. 16:516-522, 1993.

Foster, R. S., et al. High-Intensity Focused Ultrasound for the Treatment of Benign Prostatic Hypertrophy. Semin. Urol. 12:200-204, 1994.

Furusato, M., et al.: Tumour Angiogenesis in Latent Prostatic Carcinoma. Br. J. Cancer 70:1244-1246, 1994.

Garnick, M. B.: Prostate Cancer: Screening, Diagnosis, and Management. Ann. Intern. Med. 118:804-818, 1993.

Garnick, M. B. and Fair, W. R.: Prostate Cancer: Emerging Concepts. Ann. Intern. Med. 125:118-124, 1996.

Geboers, A. D., et al.: Imaging in BPH Patients. Arch. Esp. Urol. 47:857-864, 1994.

Giovannucci, E., et al.: A Retrospective Cohort Study of Vasectomy and Prostate Cancer in U.S. Men. J.A.M.A. 269:878-882, 1992b.

Giovannucci, E., et al.: A Prospective Cohort Study of Vasectomy and Prostate Cancer in U.S. Men. J.A.M.A. 269:873-877, 1992a.

Hartung, R.: Transurethral Prostatectomy (TURP): Still the Gold Standard? J. Urol. (Paris) 101:18-21, 1995.

Isaacs, J. T. and Coffey, D. S.: Etiology and Disease Process of Benign Prostatic Hyperplasia. Prostate 2(Suppl.):33-50, 1989.

Issa, M. M.: Transurethral Needle Ablation of the Prostate: Report of Initial United States Clinical Trial. J. Urol. 156:413-419, 1996.

Kantoff, P. W. and Talcott, J. A.: The Prostate Specific Antigen: Its Use as a Tumor Marker for Prostate Cancer. Hematol. Oncol. Clin. North Am. 8:555-572, 1994.

Kletscher, B. A., et al.: Prostatic Stents: Current Perspectives for the Management of Benign Prostatic Hyperplasia. Urol. Clin. North Am. 22:423-430, 1995.

Kozlowski, J. M., et al.: Advanced Prostatic Carcinoma: Early Versus Late Endocrine Therapy. Urol. Clin. North Am. 18:15-24, 1991.

Krahn, M. D., et al.: Screening for Prostate Cancer. A Decision Analytic View. J.A.M.A. 272:773-780, 1994.

Lee, R., et al.: Prostate Cancer: Comparison of Transrectal Ultrasound and Digital Rectal Examination for Screening. Radiology 168:389-394, 1988.

Lepor, H. and Rigaud, G.: The Efficacy of Transurethral Resection of the Prostate in Men with Moderate Symptoms of Prostatism. J. Urol. 143:533-537, 1990.

McConnell, J. D.: Benign Prostatic Hyperplasia: Treatment Guidelines and Patient Classification. Br. J. Urol. 76(Suppl. 1):29-46, 1995.

McConnell, J. D., et al.: Benign Prostatic Hyperplasia: Diagnosis and Treatment. Clinical Practice Guideline No. 8. AHCPR Publication No. 94-0582. Rockville, MD: Agency for Health Care Policy and Research, Public Health Service, U.S. Department of Health and Human Services, 1994.

McLeod, D. G., et al.: Controversies in the Treatment of Prostate Cancer with Maximal Androgen Deprivation. Surg. Oncol. Clin. N. Am. 4:345-359, 1995.

McLoughlin, J. and Williams, G.: Prostatic Stents and Balloon Dilatation. Br. J. Hosp. Med. 43:422-426, 1990.

Mebust, W. K., et al.: Transurethral Prostatectomy: Immediate and Postoperative Complications. A Cooperative Study of 13 Participating Institutions Evaluating 3,885 Patients. J. Urol. 141:243-247, 1989.

Meikle, A. W. and Smith, J. A.: Epidemiology of Prostate Cancer. Urol. Clin. North Am. 17:709-718, 1990.

Mettlin, C., et al.: Defining and Updating the American Cancer Society Guidelines for the Cancer-Related Check-up: Prostate and Endometrial Cancers. CA Cancer J. Clin. 43:42-46, 1993.

Mettlin, C., et al.: Vasectomy and Prostate Cancer Risk. Am. J. Epidemiol. 132:1056-1061, 1990.

Meyers, G. P., et al.: Suramin: A Novel Growth Factor Antagonist with Activity in Hormone-Refractory Metastatic Prostate Cancer. J. Clin. Oncol. 10:881-889, 1992.

Middleton, R. G., et al.: Prostate Cancer Clinical Guidelines Panel Summary Report on the Management of Clinically Localized Prostate Cancer. J. Urol. 154:2144-2148, 1995.

Morgan, W. R., et al.: Long-Term Evaluation of Radical Prostatectomy as Treatment of Clinical Stage C (T3) Prostate Cancer. Urology 41:113-120, 1993.

Morgan, W. R., et al.: Age-Specific Reference Ranges for Serum Prostate-Specific Antigen in Black Men. N. Engl. J. Med. 335:304-310, 1996.

Morrison, A. S.: Risk Factors for Surgery for Prostatic Hypertrophy. Am. J. Epidemiol. 135:974-980, 1992.

Morton, M. S., et al.: The Preventive Role of Diet in Prostatic Disease. Br. J. Urol. 77:481-493, 1996.

Morton, R. A., Jr.: Racial Differences in Adenocarcinoma of the Prostate in North American Men. Urology 44:637-645, 1994.

Moul, J. W.: Benign Prostatic Hyperplasia. New Concepts in the 1990s. Postgrad. Med. 94(6):141-146, 151, 152, 1993.

Murphy, G. P., et al.: National Patterns of Prostate Cancer Treatment by Radical Prostatectomy: Results of a Survey by the American College of Surgeons Commission on Cancer. J. Urol. 152:1817-1819, 1994.

Murphy, G. P., et al.: The National Survey of Prostate Cancer in the United States by the American College of Surgeons. J. Urol. 127:928-934, 1982.

Myers, R. P., et al.: Hormonal Treatment at Time of Radical Retropubic Prostatectomy for Stage D1 Prostate Cancer: Results of Long-Term Follow-up. J. Urol. 147:910-915, 1992.

Narayan, P.: Neoplasms of the Prostate Gland. In: Tanagho, E. A. and McAninch, J. W. (Eds.): Smith's General Urology, 14th ed.. Norwalk, Conn.: Appleton & Lange, 1995.

O'Leary, M. P.: Evaluating Symptoms and Functional Status in Benign Prostate Hyperplasia. Br. J. Urol 76:25-28, 1995.

O'Leary, M. P., et al.: Hard Measures of Subjective Outcomes: Validating Symptom Indexes in Urology. J. Urol. 148:1546-1564, 1992.

Oesterling, J. E., et al.: Serum Prostate-Specific Antigen in a Community-Based Population of Healthy Men: Establishment of Age-Specific Reference Ranges. J.A.M.A. 270:860-864, 1993.

Oesterling, J. E., et al.: Free, Complexed and Total Serum Prostate Specific Antigen: the Establishment of Appropriate References Ranges for Their Concentrations and Ratios. J. Urol. 154:1090-1095, 1995.

Pascual, J., et al.: Pharmacological Treatment of Benign Prostatic Hyperplasia. Br. J. Clin. Pract. 48:137-138, 1994.

Pienta, K. J. and Esper, P. S.: Risk Factors for Prostate Cancer. Ann. Intern. Med. 118:793-803, 1993.

Pilepich, M. V., et al.: Phase II Radiation Therapy Oncology Group Study of Hormonal Cytoreduction with Flutamide and Zoladex in

Locally Advanced Carcinoma of the Prostate Treated with Definitive Radiotherapy. Am. J. Clin. Oncol. 13:461-464, 1990.

Richie, J. P., et al.: Effect of Patient Age on Early Detection of Prostate Cancer with Serum Prostate Specific Antigen (PSA) and Digital Rectal Examination. Urology 42:365-374, 1993.

Riehmann, M., et al.: Transurethral Resection Versus Incision of the Prostate: A Randomized, Prospective Study. Urology 45:768-775, 1995.

Sagalowsky, A. I. and Wilson, J. D.: Hyperplasia and Carcinoma of the Prostate. In: Isselbacher, K. J., et al. (Eds.): Harrison's Principles of Internal Medicine, 13th ed. New York: McGraw-Hill, 1994.

Sanda, M. G., et al.: Genetic Susceptibility of Benign Prostatic Hyperplasia. J. Urol. 152:115-119, 1994.

Schiebler, M. L., et al.: Current Role of MR Imaging in the Staging of Adenocarcinoma of the Prostate. Radiology 189:339-352, 1993.

Schröder, F. H.: Screening, Early Detection, and Treatment of Prostate Cancer: A European View. Urology 46(3 Suppl. A):62-70, 1995.

Schröder, F. H. (Ed.): EORTC Genitourinary Group Monograph 8. Treatment of Prostatic Cancer: Facts and Controversies. New York: Wiley-Liss, 1990.

Schuessler, W. W., et al.: Transperitoneal Endosurgical Lymphadenectomy in Patients with Localized Prostate Cancer. J. Urol. 145:988-991, 1991.

Spires, S. E., et al.: Gleason Histologic Grading in Prostatic Carcinoma. Arch. Pathol. Lab. Med. 118:705-708, 1994.

Spitz, M. R., et al.: Familial Patterns of Prostate Cancer: A Case-Control Analysis. J. Urol. 146:1305-1307, 1991.

Stamey, T. A. and McNeal, J. E.: Adenocarcinoma of the Prostate. In: Walsh, P. C., et al. (Eds.): Campbell's Urology, 6th ed. Philadelphia: Saunders, 1992.

Steinberg, G. D., et al.: Family History and the Risk of Prostate Cancer. Prostate 17:337-347, 1990a.

Steinberg, G. D., et al.: Management of Stage D1 Adenocarcinoma of the Prostate. The Johns Hopkins Experience 1974 to 1987. J. Urol. 144:1425-1432, 1990b.

Strauss, B. S.: Laser Ablation of Prostatic Hypertrophy. N.J. Med. 92:455-458, 1995.

Tempany, C. M., et al.: Staging of Prostate Cancer: Results of Radiology Diagnostic Oncology Group Project Comparison of three MR Imaging Techniques. Radiology 192:47-54, 1994.

Venn, S. N., et al.: Microwave Hyperthermia in Benign Prostatic Hypertrophy: A Controlled Clinical Trial. Br. J. Urol. 76(Suppl. 1):73-76, 1995.

Villers, A.: Anatomy of the Prostate: Insight into Benign Prostatic Hyperplasia Anatomy and Pathogenesis. Prog. Clin. Biol. Res. 386:21-30, 1994.

Whitmore, W. F., Jr.: Localized Prostatic Cancer: Management and Detection Issues. Lancet 343:1263-1267, 1994.

Wilt, T. J. and Brawer, M. K.: Early Intervention or Expectant Management for Prostate Cancer. The Prostate Cancer Intervention Versus Observation Trial (PIVOT): A Randomized Trial Comparing Radical Prostatectomy with Expectant Management for the Treatment of Clinically Localized Prostate Cancer. Semin. Urol. 13:130-136, 1995.

Wolff, J. M., et al.: Evaluation of Patients with Diseases of the Prostate Using Prostate-Specific Density. Br. J. Urol. 76:41-46, 1995.

Yachia, D., et al.: Self-Retaining Intraurethral Stent: An Alternative to Long-Term Indwelling Catheters or Surgery in the Treatment of Prostatism. Am. J. Roentgenol. 154:111-113, 1990.

Zincke, H., et al.: Stage D1 Prostate Cancer Treated by Radical Prostatectomy and Adjuvant Hormonal Treatment. Cancer 70:311-323, 1992.

CHAPTER 15

ALZHEIMER'S DISEASE

SCOPE

Alzheimer's disease is an organic disorder affecting the brain. It usually begins with deficits in memory and progresses slowly. Increasing deficits in cognition and intellect are often accompanied by changes in behavior and personality. Eventually the patient loses the skills needed in the activities of daily life, and finally there is total loss of intellect and complete inability to function. Alzheimer's disease is irreversible and essentially fatal, with no known treatment. Diagnosis can be confirmed only with postmortem evidence of damage to the brain. As the population ages, large numbers of new cases are expected in coming decades. Despite extensive investigations, the etiology remains obscure, except for the understanding that the disease is probably multifactorial.

15.00   INTRODUCTION

Alzheimer's disease is a progressive, degenerative disorder affecting the brain. Its presentation is multifaceted, involving deficits in memory and impaired cognition and, eventually, total loss of intellect and ability to function. Although it may be accompanied by changes in personality, Alzheimer's disease is classified as an organic mental disorder, that is, the symptoms noted reflect measurable physical damage to the brain.

Loss of intellectual function with an organic cause marks this as a dementia, and Alzheimer's disease is usually considered the most common of the more than 60 conditions that have been associated with dementia. It has become a particular focus of concern because it is strongly linked to age and, with the portion of the population over age 65 growing rapidly, many millions of new cases can be expected in the years to come.

Alzheimer's disease is irreversible, as there is no known effective drug treatment, and considered fatal, though it is very often not the direct cause of death.

15.01 Alzheimer's Disease and Aging

Accounts connecting age with fading intellect appear throughout history. Plato, for example, thought extreme old age excused certain crimes; the second century physician Galen wrote of *morosis,* a condition in which "the knowledge of letters and other arts are totally obliterated, indeed those so afflicted cannot even remember their own names."

For centuries, dementia was considered a normal and an inevitable part of aging. In modern times, this was explained as a product of age-connected narrowing of the blood vessels—"hardening of the arteries"—reducing the supply of oxygen to the brain. But although the aging process itself does involve neurologic changes that are often manifested as memory loss, dementia of Alzheimer's type is a distinct disease. It bears the name of Alois Alzheimer, a psychiatrist and neuropathologist who in 1907 reported on a "singular sickness of the cerebral cortex" of a female patient, age 51. She exhibited rapidly progressive memory failure, restlessness, spatial disorientation and many other symptoms that are now recognized as characteristic of this disorder. She died, bedridden and incontinent, less than five years later.

Until quite recently, Alzheimer's disease was considered synonymous with "presenile dementia," that is, a dementia appearing in someone younger than 65 and distinct from the problems connected with aging. However, it is now generally agreed that one pathology correlates with the clinical findings that mark Alzheimer's disease, whether it appears before age 65 ("early onset"), which is rare, or after ("late onset"). The term "senility" is generally avoided.

15.02 Epidemiology

Any statement concerning the prevalence (occurrence in a given population) of Alzheimer's disease must be treated with great caution.

An estimate of 4 million people in the United States is often given, but the number of all those with the disease who never receive medical attention is unknown and may be quite large.

Inconsistencies in the types of populations that have been studied and in the criteria used to identify the disease, as well as the difficulty of correlating clinical symptoms with the postmortem findings required for a definitive diagnosis, mean that variations of severalfold between studies are not unusual. For example, a study published in 1989 showed a prevalence of 47 percent in East Boston, Massachusetts, and another study the same year in Rochester, Minnesota, showed a prevalence of 12.6 percent (Larson, 1993).

These and most similar disparities can be explained, to a considerable extent, by methodologic differences. But all accounts do show a firm relationship with age. Thus several metastudies (involving many different published results and attempting to combine comparable findings) show prevalence nearly doubling approximately every five years among people age 60 to age 95. The data include an assessment of 22 surveys of general populations (Henderson, 1990) and a review of 47 studies (Jorm, 1987). Most investigations show prevalence of from 2 to 4 percent for all those over age 65, rising to 20 percent or more among individuals who are 85 years of age and over.

Most (but not all) studies also find that the incidence of Alzheimer's disease is about equal in males and females, whites and nonwhites at a given age. Some regional differences do appear, notably in the proportion of all dementias attributed to Alzheimer's disease as opposed to some sort of vascular dementia.[1]

The link with age means that the absolute number of cases will grow quite rapidly in the years to come: in the United States, the over–85 age group is the most rapidly growing age cohort.

[1]   Mortality

Although Alzheimer's disease is a fatal disease and is considered the fourth leading cause of death among those over 65 in the United States, inconsistent diagnostic criteria make it difficult to speak with certainty about relative or absolute mortality. An additional problem facing researchers is that death certificates often do not note the presence of Alzheimer's disease; indeed, the majority of Alzheimer's

---

[1] See 15.20 infra.

patients die of something else, most often bronchial pneumonia (Burns, 1990).

Changes over time are also difficult to analyze. For example, the death rate from Alzheimer's disease in the United States reportedly increased more than tenfold in the years from 1979 to 1987: from 0.4 cases per 100,000 persons to 4.2 per 100,000 persons (Centers for Disease Control, 1990). This may reflect a real increase, heightened awareness or a change in the way physicians diagnose (for example, the number of deaths attributed to "senility" has gone down), though similar increases have been reported from other countries.

In discussing relative mortality, one problem is that most studies involve individuals in clinical settings rather than in the community, which seems likely to overstate the risk of death. A sampling of all residents over the age of 65 in a defined urban community indicated that overall, those with Alzheimer's disease had a relative risk of death 1.44 times that of unaffected persons. However, both the severity of the disease and cachexia (the state of being visibly very ill) played a strong independent role: Those with relatively slight impairment had death rates comparable to the unaffected population; the most severe cases had a risk of death 4.6 times the norm (Evans, et al., 1991).

A report that surveyed some 90 published studies describing populations in both community and institutional settings in several countries found few accounts of how long patients survive after onset of the disease and little examination of whether deaths attributed to Alzheimer's disease could be traced to deficits in cognition, memory or performance; to the disease itself; and/or to some other coexisting illness. Nevertheless, all comparable studies showed some excess mortality for people with dementia, and this excess increases with age, although it is not certain whether the difference reflects Alzheimer's disease in particular or other age-dependent difficulties (van Dijk, et al., 1991).

In general, most studies show a more favorable prognosis among female than male patients. This may simply reflect the fact that women live longer, but a number of theories have been proposed based on role differences. Also, some investigators have found that early onset, poor cognition and psychotic symptoms are associated with higher death rates (Burns, et al., 1991).

[2]   Risk Factors

The one significant risk factor that has been consistently associated with Alzheimer's disease is age. An extraordinary amount of investigation has been devoted to the attempt to identify other risks, but no body of work as yet points convincingly to any one causal or marking factor. Indeed, published results can be characterized as inconclusive at best and are often contradictory. For example, of ten published studies of a possible link between Alzheimer's disease and head injury, three find evidence of some connection, six find no such evidence and one finds a negative correlation (Henderson, 1990).

Most of the factors that have been investigated are, like head injury, known to be related to dementia of one sort or another.[2] Some elements now generally dismissed include birth order, age of mother at birth, use of therapeutic radiation and stress. The one risk factor other than age that does seem significant is a history of dementia in the family, particularly among first-degree relatives, i.e., a parent, child or sibling.[3]

Screening large populations is not now considered feasible for a number of reasons (Canadian Task Force, 1991):

- All known procedures leave uncertainties about diagnosis.

- Many of these procedures are costly.

- Identifying an individual as being impaired can have a number of negative consequences.

15.10   PATHOLOGY AND CLINICAL COURSE

Dementia of Alzheimer's type usually starts insidiously and develops slowly. Some deterioration of memory is one of the earliest and most notable signs, followed by progressive loss of intellectual function. It is possible to speak of a "usual" pattern, but there are many significant individual variations in both the nature and the severity of symptoms and in the course of the disease.

For these reasons, estimates of duration of the disease—in each stage and overall—must be considered approximations at best. In addition, the disorder may not be recognized for a considerable time after it is well established, and, again, there are contradictory findings.

---

[2] *See* 15.20 *infra* for a discussion of the most significant of these factors.

[3] *See* 15.23 *infra.*

Some studies show that on average, clinical manifestations last longer in patients with early-onset Alzheimer's disease than in those who first develop symptoms after age 65; others show that the course is longer in those over 65. Down's syndrome patients who live until the age of 40 invariably develop Alzheimer's disease, and the course in these patients is about 5 years. However, it is difficult to speak of an actual date of onset among these patients.

15.11   The Three Stages of Alzheimer's Disease

Many discussions of Alzheimer's disease posit a progression involving three stages of severity: mild (some researchers suggest an even earlier "very mild" phase), moderate and severe. Note that these are broad categories, and the borders between them are somewhat blurred. Many scales are in use to measure the characteristics considered in categorizing patients, and the progression varies markedly from case to case and rarely moves at a constant rate; indeed, plateaus are one hallmark of Alzheimer's disease. It should also be noted that these stages may be more valid for describing averages for groups of patients than for describing any one individual.

[1]   Mild

The mild, or initial, stage typically lasts two to four years. Those close to the patient usually notice signs of short-term memory loss affecting both verbal and spatial memory; the patient is likely to be more troubled by flaws in long-term memory. These changes in memory are subtle but consistent; they are followed, sooner or later, by signs of deficiency in other cognitive functions, including orientation, judgment and problem solving. This interactive combination gradually makes it more and more difficult to conduct the activities of daily life.

At this early stage, many symptoms are somewhat vague and subjective. The patient may use a variety of strategies to conceal any disability but will often complain of fatigue and difficulty concentrating, and become noticeably less active socially. Signs of severe anxiety, hypochondria, depression and paranoia (as with Dr. Alzheimer's first patient) can appear but are relatively uncommon at this stage.

[2]   Moderate

In this second phase, which lasts two to four years or more, memory difficulties become more pronounced, and other symptoms of deterioration begin to manifest themselves as well, including impaired speech (aphasia), some loss of physical coordination (apraxia) and increasing inability to recognize familiar sights or sounds (agnosia). There are also indications of further disturbances of intellectual function and spatial orientation. A general fading of emotional affect and lack of vitality are often noted, but in some patients, personality and social behavior may be relatively intact.

[3]   Severe

Generally the severe stage continues for no less than a year. Mental deterioration of patients in this stage of Alzheimer's disease affects all cognitive functions, verbal and nonverbal. Speech may become nearly incomprehensible, and visual perception may continue to degrade. Apathy becomes more general; however, even at this stage, patients may make short coherent comments and have reactions that resemble problem-solving behavior.

Movement symptoms like involuntary tremor, which are often an early sign of neurologic disorder, are relatively late to appear. In advanced cases, there is a marked increase in muscle tension, and myoclonic seizures (spasms involving alternate contraction and relaxation of a muscle) are fairly common. These shocklike contractions of a muscle or group of muscles in one or several areas of the body are apparently more common with early-onset Alzheimer's disease. Some authors describe epileptic seizures as well.

15.12   Psychopathology

The term *psychopathology* refers to the medical study of the causes and nature of mental disorders. In Alzheimer's disease, these causes are by definition organic, but the symptoms often involve some behaviors that are not usually in the realm of physical medicine. One way to consider these is to discuss cognitive difficulties and behavioral difficulties as separate entities, but it should be kept in mind that there is no firm border between the two.

[1]   Symptoms of Cognitive Deterioration

Although difficulties with short-term memory are usually considered a first indication of Alzheimer's disease, it is important to note that minor memory complaints, such as inability to recall a name, are quite common in healthy elderly individuals and are neither a sign nor a predictor of dementia. However, consistent deficits in memory that interfere with everyday functioning, such as forgetting important messages and conversations or failing to recall major public events, may be a sign of very mild dementia. Among individuals who are in fact in the early stage of Alzheimer's, prompting may elicit a recollection, but even then, details are likely to be sketchy.

Other symptoms that are usually early to appear include difficulties with orientation, that is, confusion with respect to time and, less often, location: the amount of spatial disorientation varies considerably from one individual to another.

Aphasia (deficiency in or loss of the ability to produce or comprehend spoken or written language) appears in approximately a third of patients at the mild stage, with deficits in reading comprehension and written expression usually becoming detectable before errors in naming, auditory comprehension and speaking. This difficulty becomes more common and more pronounced as time goes on, with some 80 percent of all patients showing signs of aphasia at the moderate stage (Morris and Rubin, 1991). As degeneration continues, speech may deteriorate and become fragmented, with repetitions of the end syllables of words (logoclonia); eventually patients can become mute and unable to communicate.

Writing disturbances—agraphia—are also common in Alzheimer's disease and seem to become more severe as the disease progresses. These probably reflect the combined burden of linguistic difficulties (aphasia), apraxia (loss of physical coordination), difficulty paying attention and visuoperceptual disturbances—all of which are commonly seen in these patients (Henderson, et al., 1992). The ability to perceive odors—to discriminate, recognize and recall them—is diminished later in life for everyone, but the decline is more pronounced in those with Alzheimer's disease and is often a very early sign (Doty, 1991).

Visual agnosia can reach a level of confusion (called misrecognition or misidentification) in which patients fail to recognize not only familiar faces but their own reflections in a mirror. They may also think images on television are human beings actually present in a room.

Social skills may stay intact for a time, but changes in psychomotor activity, lack of energy and reduced ability to concentrate, together with diminished cognitive function, mean that patients gradually lose the ability to perform the myriad tasks of everyday life. This first appears with complex and unfamiliar demands but eventually reaches routines: handling a checkbook or bank account, regular work or hobbies may become difficult. Eventually the patient loses the ability to feed himself or herself, dress, use a toilet and so forth.

A set of bizarre behaviors called Kluver-Bucy syndrome is sometimes described at this final stage, although it is thought to reflect damage to regions of the brain not directly affected in Alzheimer's disease: these include severe amnesia, a tendency to examine objects orally, bulimia (abnormal hunger) and, less often, an uninhibited hypersexuality.

[2]   Symptoms of Behavioral Changes

A galaxy of symptoms usually considered under the rubric of personality changes or behavioral changes commonly accompany Alzheimer's disease. These range from slight alterations in temperament, such as increased passivity, to full psychotic syndromes.

Depression is the single most frequently reported difficulty, with studies typically finding depression or depressed mood in 20 to 50 percent of all patients; a review of 30 studies finds it present in an average of 41 percent (Wragg and Jeste, 1989). Put another way, the proportion of depressed persons among Alzheimer's disease patients is at least ten times higher than in the general population, but it is not clear if this is more true of this than any other illness (Alexopolous and Abrams, 1991). Depression may or may not be correlated with the severity of the disease; it is far more likely to be reported by patients themselves than by relatives and to be reported more often by relatives than by professional interviewers.

Depression may be mostly a matter of mood (major depressive disorders are rare in Alzheimer's patients with no prior history of depression), but increasing passivity and insecurity, and a less cheerful affect, are usually consistent and lasting. Persons asked to describe a patient's personality in the most advanced stages commonly say there isn't any (Morris and Rubin, 1991).

Delusions are also quite common among Alzheimer's patients, with several studies showing an incidence of from 31 to 47 percent (Burns and Levy, 1992). The problems seems to become more common as the disease progresses. These delusions usually take the particular form of paranoia, and a number of themes appear with great regularity: patients are convinced that items have been stolen, that they are dealing with impostors, that they are being abandoned and so forth. These syndromes can become quite elaborate, involving accusations of infidelity and a general level of suspicion that can be very trying for caregivers.

Hallucinations (visual more often than auditory) are reported in some 20 to 30 percent of patients (Deutsch and Rovner, 1991). These may represent in part the misidentification that is symptomatic of the condition; when these elements combine, the effect is sometimes bizarre. For example, one study tells of a patient who believed his wife was a man and refused to sleep in the same bed with her (Deutsch and Rovner, 1991).

Some behavioral manifestations of Alzheimer's disease present possibilities of real danger to both patients and caregivers, including physical aggression. These agitated behaviors, which appear in about 25 percent of all patients, tend to increase as the disease continues.

Patients with a tendency to wander or get lost are a special source of concern. They need constant supervision, as a momentary lapse could lead to disaster. Not surprisingly, many Alzheimer's disease patients who experience hip fracture have wandered. It is not clear whether this tendency to wander reflects discrete pathologic damage or is simply a combination of the difficulties associated with the disease; efforts to find a marker for this specific symptom have not been successful.

15.13 Neuropathology

The existence of three distinct pathologic changes in brain tissue is essential to confirm the presence of Alzheimer's disease: senile plaques, neurofibrillary tangles and granulovacuolar neurons, which are degenerated nerve cells with spherical holes containing granules seen mainly in the hippocampus (an elevated portion of one of the chambers of the brain). Note that these changes can be found only at autopsy (or with a brain biopsy) and therefore cannot be part of routine clinical diagnosis.

Other signs of Alzheimer's disease can be discerned, to some extent, in living patients, including reduced brain weight, atrophy of the cerebral cortex and enlargement of the ventricles, cavities within the brain that are filled with cerebrospinal fluid. But although these indicators of gross pathology are relatively easy to see, there is so much overlap between diseased and healthy individuals of the same age that they are of little use in establishing a diagnosis.

The changes noted in the brains of those who have had Alzheimer's disease are diffuse rather than focal, but there is a consistent pattern of accentuation in certain areas of the brain. These are most marked in the posterior temporal and parietal associational cortex, that is, in the area of the cerebral cortex responsible for higher mental and emotional processes, including memory, learning and so forth. (*See Figure 15–1.*) Similar losses in other regions are also assumed to have direct and discernible effects, for example, on the hippocampus, which is involved in new learning, and the amygdala, hypothalamus and olfactory cortex, which are involved in emotions and behavior. The precentral areas of the cortex, which are more involved with sensation and muscle movement, are relatively spared, although they can become more involved after the disease has continued for some time. As a rule, these changes are symmetric; if not, the localization correlates with clinical abnormalities: aphasia if the left side is not functioning properly, apraxia if there is diminished activity on the right.

There may also be lesions in white matter, which comprises the nerve fibers covered with an insulating sheath of myelin that act as conductors in the brain; the source and significance of these changes, however, is a matter of some controversy.

Technologic advances in recent years have considerably enhanced the ability to analyze tissue at the cellular level, and this has led many investigators to try correlating the clinical signs of Alzheimer's disease precisely with discrete pathologic changes, in the hope of discovering (and perhaps correcting) just what causes dementia in these patients. Much of this work has focused on the constituents and role of the plaques and tangles that are characteristic of this disorder.

[1] Neuritic Plaques

Neuritic plaques (sometimes termed senile plaques) are focal collections of degenerating nerve terminals that surround a core of abnormal fibrillar protein, called amyloid beta protein (ABP). The word *amyloid* means starchlike and refers principally to the staining properties of this material. These plaques, which were noted by Alzheimer, have been a subject of intense investigation principally designed to determine if they play a significant causal role in the process of degeneration or if they are a product of that degeneration.

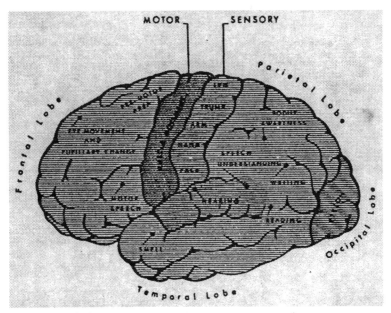

Fig. 15-1. The lobes of the brain. Alzheimer's disease generally affects the frontal and temporal lobes, and therefore their respective motor and sensory functions.

Amyloid beta protein is a fragment of another protein called amyloid precursor protein (APP). The two are normally split by the actions of certain enzymes; in Alzheimer's disease, it is supposed that something has gone wrong with this process, so that ABP builds up in excessive amounts between cells, forming plaques that damage the nerve cells; the damage, in turn, may lead to the formation of more amyloid beta protein.

Most recently this research has focused on a genetic defect linked with APP protein. As a result, early-onset Alzheimer's disease is now considered a genetically heterogeneous disease, as genes on two separate chromosome have both been associated with this subtype of the disease (Marx, 1992). Most recently a third gene, on yet another chromosome, has appeared to show a possible relationship with the far more common late-onset Alzheimer's disease.

Amyloid deposits are also seen in the walls of cerebral blood vessels in some Alzheimer's disease patients.

[2] Neurofibrillary Tangles

Neurofibrils are the delicate, interlaced threads that pass through the cytoplasm of the body of a neuron (nerve cell) and extend from one dendrite to another or into the axon. (Dendrites are nerve cell extensions that pass electrical impulses toward the nerve cell; axons extend from the neuron and function to direct the impulses to other neurons.) (*See Figure 15–2.*) The neurofibrillary tangles seen within nerve cells in Alzheimer's disease are bundles of paired helical filaments (PHF) that are morphologically unlike normal neurofibrils. PHFs also accumulate in affected areas as threads and plaques, often surrounding the amyloid core.

Postmortem examinations of patients with Alzheimer's disease usually reveal neurofibrillary tangles in the cerebral cortex, especially in the hippocampus and in small pyramidal neurons in outer laminae of the fronto-temporal cortex. They are not seen in the cerebellar cortex, spinal cord, peripheral nervous system or extraneuronal tissue: in contrast, amyloid deposits are seen in both the cerebrum and cerebellum in Alzheimer's disease. (*See Figure 15–3.*)

The question of whether amyloid deposits precede the development of neurofibrillary tangles, or vice versa, has been vigorously discussed. Some have argued that the ABP is first to appear and is in effect the causative agent in Alzheimer's disease, with all other damage following from these deposits. It is not known if plaques or tangles appear as part of the normal aging process. It is possible that many clinically normal individuals with these signs may actually have very mild, unrecognized Alzheimer's disease.

15.14   Neurochemical Abnormalities

Chemicals called neurotransmitters are essential to the passage of impulses between nerve cells. As an impulse goes along the nerve to the synapse (the site of apposition between nerve cells), these chemical "messengers," which are stored in the nerve ending, are released. The neurotransmitter diffuses across the cleft between synapses from the stimulated (presynaptic) cell, to bind with a receptor (a highly specialized protein) on the outside of the receiving (postsynaptic) cell.

In Alzheimer's disease, postmortem studies show that levels of one kind of neurotransmitter, acetylcholine, are below normal. This is thought to reflect the fact that in these individuals, an enzyme called acetylcholinesterase, which regulates acetylcholine levels, does not function properly. Partly because therapy based on this finding was not successful, it is now understood that other neurotransmitter systems are also deficient. (*See Figure 15–4.*)

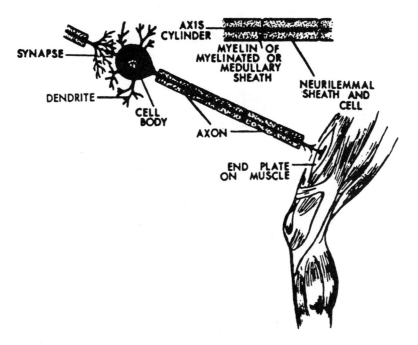

Fig. 15-2. Nerve cells. Communication between nerve cells occurs across the synapse separating the dendrites. Note the long axon, which makes it possible for damage to the nerve to have an effect on distant structures.

15.20 ETIOLOGY

Many apparently well founded theories on the cause of Alzheimer's disease have not withstood the test of time. At this point, there is some consensus that the condition may be multifactorial, that is, involving genetic predisposition as well as one or more exogenous or environmental elements, including exposure to substances with known neurotoxic effects. The strong and consistent relationship with age suggests that some time-dependent decline in neural function could also play a part.

Among the plausible etiologic factors that have been studied but are now generally discounted are the following:

- history of Down's syndrome in relatives;
- alcohol abuse; and

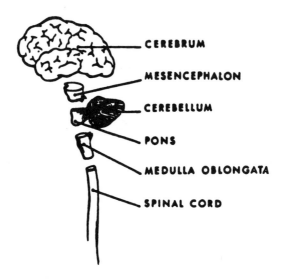

CEREBRUM

MESENCEPHALON

CEREBELLUM

PONS

MEDULLA OBLONGATA

SPINAL CORD

Fig. 15-3. The major divisions of the brain, including the cerebrum and cerebellum.

- stress.

Studies continue on exposure to chemical factors, cerebrovascular difficulties, genetic predisposition and infectious disease, and these are briefly discussed here.

15.21   Chemical Imbalances and Toxic Factors

Many exogenous chemical factors are known to trigger neuronal changes, as demonstrated by longitudinal study of a number of disorders, but none so far has shown any unique relationship to Alzheimer's disease. For example, the activity of monoamine oxidase, an enzyme that plays a key role in the degradation of monamine neurotransmitters, increases with age, but this increase is more marked in Alzheimer's patients. However, above-average increases are also seen in patients with Huntington's disease and Parkinson's disease.

Aluminum is found in neurofibrillary tangles and plaques in Alzheimer's patients, but it is also found in the brains of individuals with no reported signs of dementia. And though aluminum is neuro-toxic, it is also very common, so it is difficult to associate tissue concentrations with diet or the environment. Some studies of particular populations (e.g., miners who inhaled aluminum powder and people living in areas with high levels of aluminum in drinking water) have

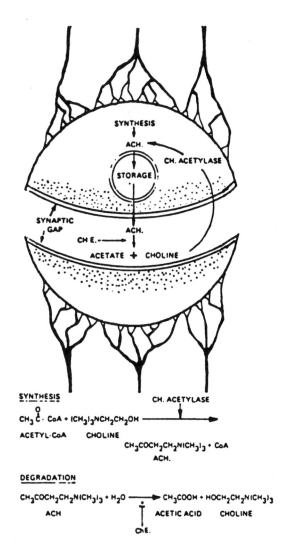

Fig. 15-4. A cholinergic synapse. Note the cycle of ACh synthesis and storage in presynaptic bodies.

suggested a correlation between Alzheimer's disease and environmental exposure to aluminum, but the evidence is considered suggestive rather than certain.

These findings have been put in question by an investigation involving a highly sensitive technique called nuclear microscopy. In this study, plaque cores from people who were known to have suffered from Alzheimer's disease revealed no aluminum at all, suggesting that earlier results were a product of contamination from the ubiquitous substance (Landsberg, et al., 1992).

15.22   Vascular Impairment

The important question of whether many dementias now attributed to Alzheimer's disease are in fact a result of some sort of vascular pathology is a matter of considerable controversy. As vascular dementias are both preventable to a degree and somewhat amenable to treatment, a shift of even a few percentage points would make a major difference in public health terms.

Vascular dementias follow from some ischemic episode (interruption in blood flow) that cuts the supply of blood-borne oxygen and glucose to the brain, popularly called a stroke.[4] Stroke is often accompanied by sudden memory disturbance, and the idea that blood flow was reduced in older people seemed to make dementia an inevitable consequence of aging: a view that proved "logical, compelling, and wrong" (Hachinski, 1992). Establishing the fact that dementia is not an unavoidable aspect of normal aging, some argue, has led to an underemphasis on the role of vascular damage.

The exact relationship between vascular interruption and dementia is not clear. No universally accepted criteria exist for establishing vascular dementia, so considerable variations in reports of their comparative prevalence are common. However, some consistent differences appear in populations from different regions. Incidence of Alzheimer's disease is thought to exceed that of vascular dementias in western Europe, for example, but the situation is reversed in Japan and Russia. If this is in fact the case, epidemiologic investigations of differences between the populations might reveal some helpful information.

Most surveys of dementia patients are conducted not among members of populations but in hospital settings, where it is possible to check the reliability of clinical diagnoses. These generally show that 50 to 70 percent of dementias are attributable to Alzheimer's disease. However, one detailed study of all citizens age 85 and over in a Swedish town found Alzheimer's dementia accounted for a smaller proportion of cases than vascular dementia (Skoog, et al., 1992).

---

[4] *See also* ch. 8.

15.23   Genetic Factors

Of all possible etiologic factors besides age, perhaps the most consistent relationship has involved family history, or some genetic link. Many studies since the early 1950s have found a pattern of Alzheimer's disease appearing within particular families that strongly suggests the disease is inherited as an autosomal dominant factor, that is, the gene can produce the disorder in either parent, and the children have, on average, a 50 percent chance of having the disease. This has appeared particularly with the early-onset subtype of Alzheimer's disease, as occurred in one Italian family in which over eight generations since 1850 demonstrated evidence of the disease (Bergamini, et al., 1991).

All such investigations have certain difficulties in common: One is the problem associated with establishing a diagnosis; another is the high proportion of older individuals overall who are affected by the disorder, which makes it difficult to trace family patterns with confidence.

Another suggestion comes from a link between Alzheimer's disease and Down's syndrome, which is hereditary. People with Down's syndrome who live to age 40 invariably show the plaques and tangles of Alzheimer's disease at autopsy. However, studies of twins have generally been unconvincing: Variations in both age of onset and severity indicate that nongenetic factors play a major role.

A review of seven published case-control studies finds accounts showing a relative risk to family members of Alzheimer's disease patients ranging from 1.0 to 7.7, with a mean of about 4.0. The review also notes a possible bias: Those who have seen the disease in their own families are more likely to recognize and report it (Larson, et al., 1992).

15.24   Transmissible Agents

A clinical picture resembling that seen in Alzheimer's disease can be found in patients who have acquired one of several virus-borne degenerative diseases of the brain (encephalopathies) called spongiform because they lead to the formation of small spaces (vacuoles) in the cerebral cortex. But postmortem examinations of Alzheimer patients' brain tissue show no consistent pattern of viral involvement. Assays of cerebrospinal fluid and blood designed to note exceptional levels of many other common viruses have also shown no correlation with Alzheimer's disease (Renvoize, et al., 1987). If an infectious agent is involved in Alzheimer's disease, it has not been detected.

15.25   Head Injury

The plaques characteristic of Alzheimer's disease can develop very quickly after head injury and are often found in long-term survivors of such injury. Their rapid appearance suggests that they could be a normal response to injury and, conversely, that it is possible that those who survive such trauma should be watched more carefully for signs of Alzheimer's disease. A number of studies suggest that Alzheimer's patients are more likely than those with no dementia to have recovered from head trauma, but the correlation is not a strong one. Also, the fact that the source is usually someone other than the patient could mean that the degree of injury is overestimated (Larson, et al., 1992).

Continuing insult to the head leads to a syndrome called dementia pugilistica (being "punch-drunk"), and autopsy evidence indicates a loss of neurons in these cases. It is possible that Alzheimer's disease and dementia pugilistica share some common pathogenetic mechanisms that lead to tangle and plaque formation.

15.30   DIAGNOSIS

Since the diagnosis of Alzheimer's disease is not complete without a postmortem examination of brain tissue, the task of the clinician who suspects the presence of this disorder is largely a matter of excluding other possible causes of dementia. This is evidently not a simple task: attempts to match diagnoses with postmortem evidence show that 20 percent or more of these cases are misdiagnosed even in the setting of a teaching hospital (Nielsen, et al., 1991).

Correct early diagnosis can be important for several reasons. Some treatment approaches that are appropriate for dementia may actually do damage to a patient with certain conditions, for example, a depressive episode. Also, patients with Alzheimer's disease may deteriorate if they are treated with medications designed for those with Parkinson's disease. Moreover, there is some chance of noticeable improvement in the very earliest phases of Alzheimer's disease, and prompt care can avoid irreversible damage in some other kinds of dementia. Finally, patients with unrecognized dementia are at risk of victimization and abuse, more likely to suffer falls and other injuries, and exposed to a particular kind of medical risk: If medication is unsatisfactory, the demented patient may not be able to report problems that are normally easily detected.

For these reasons, there has been an intense search for reliable "markers," signs of biochemical or other pathologic changes that can be obtained in a living subject. But despite improvements in imaging techniques, novel ways to discover the existence of protein abnormalities in skin and other peripheral areas, and advances in our understanding of genetics, no specific tests can confirm the diagnosis with absolute accuracy.

In 1984, in direct response to findings that a noticeable percentage of patients with diagnosed Alzheimer's disease showed no sign of the disease at autopsy, the National Institute of Neurological and Communicative Disorders and Stroke (NINCDS) and the Alzheimer's Disease and Related Disorders Association (ADRDA) published a set of suggested criteria for clinicians (McKhann, et al., 1984). These much-cited standards, which have shown generally good agreement with postmortem findings, describe three categories: *probable, possible* and *definite*.

Very briefly, the *probable* category requires:

- dementia as established by clinical examination and neuropsychological testing;
- evidence of a deficit in two or more areas of cognition;
- progressive worsening of memory and other cognitive functions; and
- age between 40 and 90 at onset.

In addition, to fit into this category, the individual should have no sign of disturbance of consciousness or of any other disorder that might account for the noted deficits.

The diagnosis is supported by progressive deterioration of cognitive function, impaired ability to carry out activities of daily living, altered behavior, a family history of similar disorders and an uneven course of progression. The diagnosis is made less likely by sudden onset, focal neurologic findings and seizures or disturbances of gait early in the course of the illness.

Possible Alzheimer's disease involves similar but somewhat fewer and less rigorously detailed symptoms; *definite* involves the "probable" criteria as well as pathologic evidence from a biopsy or an autopsy. In many studies of the disease, this distinction is reflected in the use of the term "dementia of Alzheimer's type" or "senile dementia of Alzheimer's type" for conditions that meet the probable standard, with "Alzheimer's disease" reserved for the histologically verified disorder.

The one other diagnostic standard most often invoked (and often used in tandem with NINCDS-ADRDA) is that of the American Psychiatric Association's *Diagnostic and Statistical Manual* (DSM) (1994). This book defines Alzheimer's disease as a primary degenerative dementia and sets as diagnostic signs both evidence of short- and long-term memory impairment and one of the following:

- impairment in abstract thinking;
- impairment in judgment;
- evidence of aphasia, apraxia, agnosia or personality change.[5]

These must be severe enough to interfere with performance of everyday activities. Also, the DSM criteria specifically exclude delirium and nonorganic mental disorders.

15.31 The Diagnostic Workup

As the focus of diagnosis in these cases is to exclude, insofar as that is possible, any treatable cause of dementia, the recommended workup is quite thorough, involving a history, physical and neurologic examination, considerable laboratory work, electrophysiologic measures, chest x-ray and, often, computed tomography (CT).

15.32 History

Typically those close to the patient are first to notice the consistent deficiencies in memory that are the hallmark of Alzheimer's disease. Other common early signs, such as difficulties with language, change in handwriting and, less often, impaired sense of locality, can be and often are concealed by the patient.

The most important part of the history involves change over time. It is important to remember that there is considerable overlap between healthy elderly individuals and those with Alzheimer's disease, especially in the early stages, in terms of almost every available diagnostic measure. Thus to a great extent, detection of the disease

---

[5] *See* 15.12 *supra.*

must be based on decline from previous levels as reported by someone close to the patient or recorded by a clinician after a series of visits.

In talking with the patient or informants, the examiner should try to elicit information that will help establish baseline measures of cognitive function. History of stroke or any ischemic episode (interruption of blood flow), use of alcohol or medications of any sort and past diagnosis of mental disorders all may be suggestive of another pathology; a family history of dementing disorders may suggest Alzheimer's disease.

15.33 Physical and Neurologic Examination

In the majority of physical and neurologic examinations, the key finding is that the Alzheimer's patient is unexceptional by most measures. Thus the clinician's task consists largely of looking for signs of other disorders that are connected with dementia. The most common of these involve cerebrovascular difficulties or other neurologic pathologies, including Parkinson's disease, Huntington's disease, Pick's disease, frontotemporal dementia and progressive supranuclear palsy. Outside the brain proper, other not uncommon organic causes of dementia include metabolic hypothyroidism, renal dialysis, chronic pulmonary disease, tuberculosis, meningitis, some forms of syphilis and human immunodeficiency virus (HIV; the virus that causes AIDS), severe malnutrition, alcohol abuse and some drugs, especially psychoactive medications. Major depressive disorders and other psychiatric disorders can also produce symptoms like those seen in organic dementias ("pseudodementia"); the NINCDS-ADRDA standards recommend a complete psychiatric examination to exclude these.

The order in which symptoms appear can be telling. Gait disturbances usually come some time after signs of cognitive deficit in Alzheimer's disease, but that progression is reversed in hydrocephalus (enlargement of the cerebral ventricles and accumulation of cerebrospinal fluid in the skull) and in Creutzfeldt-Jakob disease, a viral disease that leads to dementia.

Some differentiations are subtle and require detailed somatic and psychological examination. For example, frontotemporal degeneration and Pick's disease are also slowly progressive dementias, but patients with either of these conditions are usually more likely than those with Alzheimer's disease to show early personality changes, such as lack of insight and disinhibition, but less likely to exhibit impaired memory or spatial disorientation, although their speech and motor responses may be slow.

Separating the symptoms of dementia from those of depressive syndromes can also be challenging, especially as depression is likely to occur in a large number of Alzheimer's disease patients. In these cases, the patient's own overall behavior is important, and attention should be paid to the possibility that apathy, withdrawal and the like may be a product of long-term use of certain medications.

Perhaps the most difficult differentiation is among Alzheimer's disease, vascular or multi-infarct dementia and situations in which both are present. The most accepted tool for diagnosis involves a standard measure of ischemia (Hachinski, 1983). Some symptoms suggesting ischemic brain disorder, including severe headache and dizziness, are not uncommon with mild Alzheimer's disease. Multi-infarct dementia tends to be marked by abrupt onset, a variable and stepwise or episodic progress, and focal neurologic signs and symptoms.

Another type of vascular dementia is Binswanger's disease, in which the white matter cells lose their myelinated covering because of an interruption in the blood supply, although the diagnosis is difficult to establish, as changes to white matter appear in over 40 percent of Alzheimer's patients and over 80 percent of those with multi-infarct dementia (Hachinski, 1992). Binswanger's disease, too, is slowly progressive, with gradual accumulation of mental and neurologic deficits, but unlike Alzheimer's, it is often episodic and remitting. Personality changes, psychotic reactions, memory failure and emotional incontinence are reported and are thought to be connected with damage to white matter in the frontal lobes. Speech difficulties are common, but not the apraxia or agnosia (loss of physical coordination and increasing inability to recognize familiar sights or sounds, respectively) often seen with Alzheimer's disease. Hypertension (high blood pressure) and cardiac arrhythmias (conditions involving irregular heartbeat) are common in Binswanger's disease, while Alzheimer's patients often have low blood pressure.

15.34   Laboratory Tests

Analysis of cerebrospinal fluid has long been used as a way to discover signs of neurologic disorders, but none is specific for Alzheimer's disease. The cholinergic deficit found consistently in postmortem assessments is not necessarily found in cerebrospinal fluid. Other (noncholinergic) neurotransmitter abnormalities may appear, but these are neither consistent nor in agreement with autopsy evidence.

Thus the principal value of laboratory tests in these cases is as an aid in identifying other causes of dementia, including infections and immunologic disorders, thyroid deficiency and so forth.

15.35 Electrophysiologic Tests

Patients with Alzheimer's disease generally have some slowing of dominant alpha wave activity that is visible on an electroencephalogram (EEG), and there is some correlation between EEG pathology and cognitive deterioration (Gustafson, 1991). (*See Figure 15–5.*) These measurements can help distinguish conditions such as epilepsy and frontotemporal degeneration, in which the EEG is relatively normal, from vascular dementias, which can produce a distinct pattern. However, in general, this and more sophisticated devices designed to map electrical activity in the brain have not been helpful in diagnosing Alzheimer's disease.

15.36 Imaging Devices

The development of new and extremely sophisticated imaging devices has changed—and continues to change—the understanding of Alzheimer's disease. Indeed, at present, as more than one observer has commented, the ability to see has outpaced the ability to understand.

[1] Computed Tomography (CT)

Computed tomography is a noninvasive, relatively rapid technique that provides accurate views of the neuronal anatomy of the brain with digital reproductions of radiographic images. At times, the device is connected directly with a computer that is programmed to provide an analysis of the image as well. For example, technicians can use a "light pen" to outline an area of interest, and the computer will provide a reading on density in that area. This provides a measurement of the amount of atrophy, as the cell loss that is part of Alzheimer's disease means that the brain appears to shrink.

In fact, computed tomography may provide the most sensitive indication of gross changes in brain pathology that is available, as autopsy measures are subject to technical and fixation artifacts when

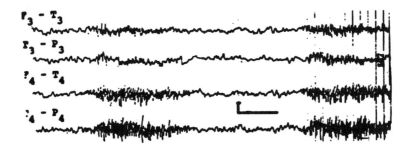

Fig. 15-5. A normal electroencephalogram (EEG) tracing of an adult. The time interval from the beginning to the end of the tracing is 10 seconds.

matter is being prepared for examination and cannot, of course, determine changes over time.

Computed tomography can also give indications of ventricular dilation, but its principal value is as a way to exclude difficulties that may mimic Alzheimer's disease, such as neoplasm (brain tumor), subdural hematoma (accumulation of blood below the membrane surrounding the brain), cerebrovascular disorders and hydrocephalus (accumulation of fluid on the brain). It cannot show plaques and neurofibrillary tangles, and has been of questionable value as a tool for early diagnosis.

For the most part, computed tomography exams performed early in the course of Alzheimer's disease reveal nothing abnormal. Again, there is considerable overlap between demented and nondemented individuals, and it is hard to distinguish those changes that do appear from age-related anatomic changes of the brain. For example, autopsy studies show that brain weight falls by 2 percent per decade from about age 40, with a similar reduction in the amount of gray and white matter. Ventricular enlargements also tend to be correlated with age, though in a more dramatic and less linear fashion. Thus just finding evidence of atrophy and ventricular enlargement is not very helpful (deCarli, et al., 1990).

Use of computed tomography as a diagnostic tool involves making some choice between sensitivity and specificity: If one uses highly sensitive criteria, many normal subjects will be mislabeled as having Alzheimer's disease; if highly specific criteria are employed, many will be missed. This effect is demonstrated in attempts to correlate premortem computed tomography with postmortem evidence

(Mendez, et al., 1992) or with results of neuropsychological tests (Albert and Lafleche, 1991). Considerable work is now directed at establishing parameters.

[2]   Magnetic Resonance Imaging (MRI)

Like computed tomography, magnetic resonance imaging is more useful in excluding other dementias than in diagnosing Alzheimer's disease itself. It can distinguish gray and white matter, and is particularly helpful for showing changes in white matter. Used in conjunction with computed tomography, it may help exclude frontotemporal dementia by revealing the anterior-posterior gradient of changes.

[3]   Positron Emission Tomography (PET) and Single
Photon Emission Computed Tomography (SPECT)

Positron emission tomography (PET) or single-photon emission computed tomography (SPECT) should show regional abnormalities in blood flow and metabolism. These techniques involve scintigraphy, i.e., "tagging" with a radioactive material (a radionuclide) by injection (or, recently, inhalation) and tracking the flow of material with a scintillation camera.

In an aging patient with a clinical diagnosis of Alzheimer's disease, this method has revealed a decline in cortical metabolism (the physical and chemical processes in the brain) that is thought to parallel the severity of the dementia. In milder stages, the posterior temporal and parietal regions are most markedly affected, and occipital and motor sensory areas are relatively spared; in more severe cases, these areas also show a marked decline, and metabolic rates become as low as those in the associational cortex.

However, although this technique is valuable for revealing bilateral insufficiency, it does not show unilateral or exclusively frontal defects, which are seen in some 20 percent of Alzheimer's disease patients. In addition, many of the defects noted in Alzheimer's disease may also appear in other conditions, like Parkinson's disease (Holman, et al., 1992).

15.37   Antemortem Examination

Many factors, including cause of death and delay before the procedure can begin, may change the state of tissue in the brain and cloud the results of postmortem examination. In particular,

Alzheimer's disease patients often die after protracted bronchial pneumonia, which can affect a number of neurochemical traits. Some investigators believe antemortem examinations will allow more solid conclusions about early change in the disease and help relate neurochemical measures to specific behavioral changes. Such studies so far show a sizable minority of patients (30 to 35 percent) with no specific neuropathologic changes (Palmer and Bowen, 1991).

15.38   Neuropsychological Examination

Neuropsychological assessment of dementia involves subjective rating by a clinician using one or more of many available scales, designed to measure such characteristics as concentration, recent and remote memory, orientation and ability to function in the world. Some of these scales are supposed to parallel characteristic Alzheimer's disease syndromes as they change over time, so that a deviation from the scale may be taken to suggest the presence of some other disorder. In addition, one or more formal psychometric tests are usually administered, with attention paid to language function, praxis (performance of action), visual perception, abstract thinking and decision making.

As cognitive decline is both an early and a prominent symptom of Alzheimer's disease, there is hope that careful examination, involving both quantitative results and assessments of quality and attitude, will provide early recognition of the disease. A great deal of effort has been devoted to defining differences from aging itself and from other dementias. For example, considerable work has been devoted to developing paradigms to measure impairment in recent memory, often seen as the most important early manifestation of the disorder. But these are difficult to devise: memory involves idiosyncratic individual experience, emotion and imagination as well as perception, and longitudinal studies show that many available measures are not sensitive or, if they are sensitive, not helpful in staging (Welsh, et al., 1992).

One problem is the so-called *floor effect,* that is, the fact that severe mental impairment may be present even in early stages. It is difficult, especially with aged patients, to establish a baseline without considerable life history data, yet it may well be necessary to consider premorbid individual differences if any standardized tests are to be effective in detecting very mild Alzheimer's disease.

A few cognitive tests or subtests concern specific debilities. For example, apraxia might be gauged by asking the patient to draw complex objects and then work downward to a cube, from a cube to a rectangle to a circle inside a circle and finally a straight line.

One novel (and patented) proposal suggests that the decline seen in Alzheimer's disease is more or less literally a trip backward through time. Proponents of this theory point to step-by-step regressions along the stages of the illness that are homologous to a child's acquisition of skills. The authors concede that there are important differences (for example, Alzheimer's patients never crawl or cry like infants) but suggest that using psychometric tests designed for children might demonstrate progression of the disease (Reisberg, et al., 1991).

Some scales are called global, as they have both cognitive and noncognitive components, the latter noting such dimensions as mood, behavior, agitation, delusions and hallucinations. One often-cited measure is the Clinical Dementia Rating scale, which is based on a 90-minute semi-structured interview with the subject and/or a knowledgeable collateral source, in which the clinician notes five degrees of impairment on each of six categories of cognitive function: memory, orientation, judgment and problem solving, community affairs, home and hobbies, and personal care. These resolve into a three-point scale paralleling the NINCDS-ADRDA mild (1), moderate (2), and severe (3), with a 0.5 rating for very mild Alzheimer's disease. Over time, this measure has shown some relationship to the progression of Alzheimer's disease.

A number of scales are also available for noncognitive assessments, particularly for gauging depression. Some of these are especially geared to geriatric patients or those with cognitive impairment.

Active Daily Living scales concern concrete physical tasks, such as the ability to feed oneself, get in and out of bed, use a toilet and the like, and more complex instrumental tasks, such as the ability to handle personal finances, plan and prepare meals, use a phone and travel. There are more than 40 published versions of these indexes, including some that are supposed to closely parallel the progression of Alzheimer's disease (Kluger and Ferris, 1991).

Another device that is widely used for screening and for assessing any change in cognitive abilities over time is the Mini Mental State Examination (MMSE). This simplified examination, which is designed to deal especially with elderly and/or demented patients, involves 11 questions and takes five to ten minutes. It measures orientation (knowledge of time and place), registration (ability to name familiar objects), short-term and delayed recall, attention and calculation (asking the patient to count backward from 100 by sevens for a few seconds or to spell "world" backward), command of simple language and ability to copy a design (Folstein, et al., 1975).

Criticisms of the MMSE include the fact that it "bottoms out" relatively early in the evolution of Alzheimer's disease, so that it is of little use in the later stages. Like many similar measures, it tends to overdiagnose cognitive deficits in those with less than eight years of schooling or with cultural differences (Escobar, et al., 1986). In fact, age itself may be an element: when all residents over 65 in a given community were given a brief test of memory, attention and orientation, the results showed a strong inverse correlation between age and performance (Scherr, 1988). These distortions may be balanced by the fact that in making their diagnoses, physicians are more strongly influenced by their own judgment of a patient's state than by test results (Pittman, et al., 1992).

One other reason for caution is that depressed patients with no signs of dementia perform about the same on formal psychometric examinations as those with very mild Alzheimer's disease. Therefore, a careful psychiatric evaluation is advisable before interpreting poor test performance as a sign of Alzheimer's disease (Rubin, et al., 1991).

15.40   TREATMENT AND MANAGEMENT

Most existing medical treatments of Alzheimer's disease must be described as palliative. The striking individual variations in presentation and course, as well as the generally bleak prognosis, suggest that treatment efforts should deal with each patient in every aspect of his or her life. As a result, major efforts are directed at social service, counseling and the like for both patient and family.

Broadly speaking, attempts to cure or even slow the disease have apparently not succeeded, although it is difficult to gauge the effectiveness (or lack of effectiveness) of treatment approaches for several reasons. By the time the disease is diagnosed, the patient is typically in the moderate stage, which means it is difficult to measure any subtle response or to follow up for any considerable period of time. In addition, with so many variables to be considered—both cognitive and behavioral symptoms—there is the problem of deciding just what the target is for the therapy in question. Once that is decided, the question remains of what test or test battery is best able to gauge the improvements, if any, that are effected by a particular remedy. Note that the usual goal of these efforts is not to reverse the disease process or even stop it but to slow the decline: even a small delay or slight improvement in intellectual capacity allowing self-care for a bit longer would be considered worthwhile.

Over the years, therapeutic approaches have followed current understandings of etiology in relatively straightforward fashion. Thus some early attempts to medicate patients with Alzheimer's disease involved vasodilators (drugs that expand blood vessels), based on the idea that lack of blood in the brain was the cause of dementia. Other attempts have been more directed toward behavior. For example, central nervous system stimulants were chosen to counter the usual lethargy, but (although some are still in use) the problem is not in fact one of generalized lack of arousal but of specific deficits. Psychotropic drugs found to have some effects in nonorganic disorders, such as schizophrenia, proved ineffective and sometimes exacerbated cognitive deficits.

A class of drugs called *nootropic* (a coinage suggesting "toward the mind"), which are supposed to interact directly with neurotransmitters, was developed specifically to improve cognitive function in neurologically damaged patients, but these have proved disappointing in tests with human subjects.

The discovery that cholinergic activity was below normal in the brain of Alzheimer's disease patients, and that this played a role in memory loss and problems of cognition, suggested that a single neurotransmitter was largely responsible for the disorder (as dopamine is for Parkinson's disease). There followed attempts to produce medications that would restore or enhance cholinergic function, first with chemicals known to act as precursors in the synthesis of acetylcholine (choline and lecithin), then with agents known to block the action of acetylcholinesterase, the enzyme that breaks down acetylcholine.

One of these blocking agents, tacrine, has had some modest success in a few trials. One investigator found a slowing of deterioration by the equivalent of some 6 to 12 months, but the effects were quite discrete, generally involving more improvement on simple tasks than on complex ones, and attention and judgment more than memory. The clinical relevance of these gains was a "matter of individual judgment," the authors concluded, but the drug had no effect on the basic disease process and presented a real risk of liver toxicity (Eagger, et al., 1991).

A much larger multicenter study involving only patients who responded to tacrine in a preliminary trial also found less decline in cognitive function in treated patients than in those receiving a placebo, though again results were discrete; indeed, physicians did not notice any difference (but caregivers noted less decline in activities of daily living). The authors concluded that some patients might benefit from treatment with tacrine (Davis, et al., 1992).

In line with a more recent view of Alzheimer's disease as a heterogeneous disorder involving multiple neurotransmitter systems in particular anatomic sites, rather than particular neurotransmitters, therapies have been designed to replace or enhance the efficacy of other active elements. Some have shown promise in animal experiments, but results in humans have been disappointing.

Investigations of one class of drugs are considered promising. These drugs are designed to reduce or retard the progress of Alzheimer's disease based on certain endogenous (already in the body) polypeptides (proteins) that are called neurotrophic, meaning relating to nutrition and metabolism of nerve tissue. There is some controversy over a theory that overactivity of these elements may be responsible for Alzheimer's disease. Most prominent among these substances is nerve growth factor (NGF), which is essential for neurons. To date, most work on these has been done in the laboratory. Work also continues on drugs that might modify the abnormal amyloid protein found in brain plaques.[6]

Trials of a chelator (a chemical that combines with metal) that removes aluminum from the system showed a significant reduction in the rate of decline of daily living skills, but investigators called for caution in interpreting these results (Crapper-McLachlan, et al., 1991). One other possible avenue of treatment being explored involves grafting tissue into the brain (Gage, et al., 1989).

15.41 Behavioral Medications

Some therapeutic work with Alzheimer's disease patients is directed at specific behavioral aspects of the disorder, particularly the agitation,

---

[6] *See* 15.13 *supra.*

irritability, aggression and wandering that often appear as symptoms of the illness. Behavioral medications (drugs designed to modify psychotic behaviors), such as neuroleptics, antianxiety and antidepressive preparations, and sedatives, hypnotics and antihypertensives (medications used to treat high blood pressure) have all been studied.

Use of these drugs has been justified partly on the grounds that deteriorating behavior puts a great burden on caregivers and may be more likely than cognitive problems to precipitate institutionalization. Neuroleptics especially have been of some modest assistance in dealing with delusions and hallucinations and with aggressive and agitated behavior, and patients on these medications tend to be more cooperative. However, many of these drugs have side effects that interfere with the cholinergic system and may thereby effectively promote dementia. When their use is discontinued, patients show major gains in cognitive abilities. Other neurologic side effects include seizures and tardive dyskinesia.

Using minor tranquilizers avoids these effects, and benzodiazepines, such as Valium®, are often employed. But here, too, there are real problems. Often, cognitive impairment appears as a late sign in a patient who has taken these drugs for many years. Also, these drugs have a longer half-life and stronger per-dose effect in elderly people. Indeed, a review of published work on the use of these medications among elderly patients suggests that any benefits may be outweighed by risks, including an increase in hip fractures, oversedation and faster deterioration of cognitive abilities (Stern, et al., 1991). If they are used, a short-acting formulation is indicated, with dosage adjusted for each patient's age and health status, and with a careful check of any other drug use, since drug interactions can also create major problems.

15.42 Psychosocial Management

With Alzheimer's disease, it is certainly valid to think in terms of management, as many patients live a number of years in need of full-time care. These efforts require a consistent, stable environment with few changes in routine for the patient and considerable counseling and support for the family.

Those who treat Alzheimer's disease patients face some unique problems. For example, although it is generally agreed that patients with terminal disease should be told their diagnosis, there can be reason for hesitation with Alzheimer's disease, including the facts that no existing method allows an unquestioned diagnosis and that the course is so variable that prognosis and life expectancy are uncertain. It is also agreed that patients should have the best possible information about their condition before deciding on any course of treatment, but in these cases, the patients's ability to make decisions will inevitably diminish, so there is the issue of determining when the patient becomes too demented to understand (Drickhamer and Lachs, 1991).

15.43   Physical Management

Care of Alzheimer's patients begins with attention to the immediate living environment, especially if orientation is impaired. Lighting should be relatively intense during the daytime but decreased in the evening, with low nightlights in the bedroom and bathroom. Colors and graphic symbols to signal particular locations, and oversize clocks and calendars can all help. For those with visual impairment, it is important to keep heavy-base lamps and cords out of the usual line of traffic. For the physically impaired, round edges, sturdy furniture and a bed on the floor may make life less dangerous and more easeful.

Aphasia is a condition in which both comprehension and production of language are disrupted, and loss of speech is perhaps the most distressing of the typical symptoms. This can occur fairly early in the course of the disease, though that is unusual. In these cases, the caregiver must guard against the assumption that trouble vocalizing indicates impaired understanding, and vice versa—some patients can repeat instructions verbatim or read written instructions, yet have no understanding.

Hearing and vision should be checked, and the family should be aware that the patient may seem uncooperative when, in fact, there is a problem of comprehension. With these individuals, it is best to speak slowly, look for nonverbal cues and ask questions that can be answered with yes or no.

Patients with agnosia (inability to recognize familiar objects and faces) reaching the point of misrecognition benefit from a simple environment: soft colors, good lighting, nonabstract and nonthreatening wall hangings. Television sets can be threatening, especially if they issue disturbing noises (such as explosions or a baby crying), and mirrors and even reflecting window glass should be removed.

With apraxia (loss of ability to perform familiar motor acts), it is helpful to have large utensils or large handles on much-used objects.

Elderly patients have less need for calories, but adequate nutrition is extremely important, and caregivers must pay attention to food intake. When eating becomes difficult, it may be helpful to allow the patient to eat (or be fed) in private. Regular exercise demonstrably reduces restlessness and agitation.

A number of techniques are employed in the hope of enhancing memory, but they should take into account the special situation of these patients. For example, cognitive retraining, usually employed with victims of closed head injuries, is based on the assumption that cortical function is intact, but this is not the case for Alzheimer's disease patients, who will need constant prompting.

Reality orientation involves continually repeated reminders from caregivers to keep the patient stimulated. This requires not simply conversation but also the use of props, such as a blackboard with information about place and time and a written daily schedule of activities, photo albums, flash cards, maps, globes, etc., in everyday interactions. In addition, this kind of program involves regular, structured sessions during which the caregiver has a chance to reinforce accurate statements. Although quantitative research on this approach shows mixed results, care providers tend to find it useful, even though it is a very demanding system (Dippel and Hutton, 1992).

All such efforts must be varied to reflect the stage of the disorder. A patient who can at first read newspaper headlines and do crossword puzzles, then perhaps only read recipes or sports news, play checkers or cards, in the last stages may only be able to repeat his or her name, address and telephone number. The caregiver's goal throughout is to rebuild self-confidence and dignity.

With severe cases, in general, caregivers are advised to keep eye contact when speaking and to use a calm tone, gestures and exaggerated facial expressions to reinforce meaning. Avoiding talking when there is competing noise will also aid understanding. Other techniques are to use short words, sentences containing one thought, repeatedly mention the patient's name (and avoid pronouns) and ask one question at a time. Even in these situations, it is best never to assume incomprehension and to be sensitive to the individual's attitude: Some patients do not like having a word supplied while they are "reaching" for it; some do.

Other particular problems can have particular solutions. For patients who tend to wander, inside locks, doorknob covers that must be gripped tightly to turn and painted grid patterns can be helpful preventive devices. Some studies indicate that walking with these patients and paying some attention to their emotional needs also reduces their tendency to wander away.

When dealing with delusion, caregivers are advised to reassure, not argue; similarly with agitated patients, they can benefit from one of the few advantages the disease offers: a simple distraction may help, as patients often forget quickly.

15.44   Family and Caregivers

More than a million Alzheimer's patients are cared for at home by a spouse or family members; 72 percent of the caregivers are women. This is about 80 percent of the total of Alzheimer's patients; only 20 percent are in institutions. This care often takes more than 40 hours a week (Levine and Lawlor, 1991).

Thus an important part of therapy for Alzheimer's disease involves considering the burdens placed on the patient's family, who are likely to experience an extraordinary range of disturbing emotions:

- anger with the patient for being stubborn or abusive;
- resentment at the load of responsibilities—and guilt about feeling resentful;
- frustration at the patient's lack of response;
- embarrassment at the patient's behavior;
- love for the person the patient used to be and dislike for the person the patient now is;
- isolation and yet denial of the need for assistance; and
- trying to decide if and when a nursing home might be a good idea.

One important element in dealing with the patient's behavioral problems, then, is to educate the family. Those who know that Alzheimer's disease patients lose items, repeat themselves, wander, get lost, might accuse caregivers of stealing, say they have not eaten and so forth will often be less hostile. In some cases, individual or family therapy can be helpful in dealing with such feelings as confusion at reversal of the parent-child relationship.

Caregivers should also be made aware that a patient's needs will change as the disease progresses. Early on, little care is needed, but planning for the future is very important; in more severe cases, it will be necessary to supervise finances and the like. At this stage, "denial" by caregivers can pose a problem. As the burden escalates, there is a need for more formal kinds of support, such as respite and home care, and still later, help with placing the patient in an institution. The stress is relentless, so those providing health care should be well informed about community support services and agencies like the Alzheimer's Association.

Within families, the physical, mental, social and financial impact can be devastating. As well, there can be disagreement about the advisability of different kinds of treatment and when to tell outsiders, anger at those who do not share the chores of care and disruption when the patient can no longer fill his or her role.

15.45 Institutional Care

As the aged—especially the very old—population grows, more and more attention is being paid to the question of long-term care. This is especially true regarding individuals who are victims of Alzheimer's disease, which accounts for about half of nursing home admissions in the United States.

In recent years, segregated "special care units" for demented patients have been created within some nursing homes. There are as yet few studies of these facilities, but an investigation of a representative sample of such units across the country found a considerable range of quality, from ideal to execrable. The ideal facility, the investigation found, had the following attributes:

- clean and carefully maintained physical plant;
- cheerful staff;
- allowances for both privacy and planned activities;
- low patient-staff ratios, with pleasant interactions; and
- trained administrators who believe in the value of segregated units.

Investigators also noted that appearances could be deceptive: Some facilities that looked unappealing had well-trained staff members, and some quite handsome homes had staffs with little training or interest in caring.

Toward the bottom of the scale, investigators found noise, crowding and lack of cleanliness. The worst institutions were genuinely detrimental to the well-being of patients, with staff ratios often lower than 1 to 12 and free use of chemical and physical restraints. Patients in these institutional settings tend to have neither family nor friends, and administrators are usually charged with keeping the facility full (Gold, et al., 1991).

15.100   BIBLIOGRAPHY

Text References

Albert, M. S. and Lafleche, G.: Neuroimaging in Alzheimer's Disease. Psychiatr. Clin. N. Am. 14:433–457, June 1991.

Alexopoulos, G. S. and Abrams, R. C.: Depression in Alzheimer's Disease. Psychiatr. Clin. N. Am. 14:327–340, June 1991.

American Psychiatric Association: Diagnostic and Statistical Manual of the Mental Disorders, 4th ed. (DSM-IV). Washington, D.C.: American Psychiatric Association, 1994.

Bergamini, L., et al.: Familial Alzheimer's Disease: Evidences for Clinical and Genetic Heterogeneity. Acta Neurol. 534–538, Dec. 1991.

Burns, A. and Levy, R.: Clinical Diversity in Late Onset Alzheimer's Disease. Oxford: Oxford University Press, 1992.

Burns, A., et al.: Factors Affecting Survival in Alzheimer's Disease. Psychol. Med. 21:363–370, 1991.

Burns, A., et al.: Cause of Death in Alzheimer's Disease. Age Ageing 19:341–344, Sept. 1990.

Canadian Task Force on the Periodic Health Examination. Periodic Health Examination: 1991 Update. 1. Screening for Cognitive Impairment of the Elderly. Can. Med. Assn. J. 144:425–431, Jan. 15, 1991.

Centers for Disease Control: Mortality from Alzheimer Disease— United States, 1979–1987. M.M.W.R. 39:785–788, 1990.

Crapper-McLachlan, D. R., et al.: Intramuscular Desferrioxamine in Patients with Alzheimer's Disease. Lancet 336:1304–1308, June 1, 1991.

Davis, K. L., et al.: A Double-Blind, Placebo-Controlled Multicenter Study of Tacrine for Alzheimer's Disease. N. Engl. J. Med. 327:1253–1259, Oct. 29, 1992.

DeCarli, C., et al.: Critical Analysis of the Use of Computer-assisted Transverse Axial Tomography to Study Human Brain in Aging and Dementia of the Alzheimer Type. Neurology 40:872–883, June 1990.

Deutsch, L. H. and Rovner, B. W.: Agitation and Other Noncognitive Abnormalities in Alzheimer's Disease. Psychiatr. Clin. N. Am. 14:341–350, June 1991.

Dippel, R. L. and Hutton, J. T.: Caring for the Alzheimer's Patient, 2nd ed. Buffalo: Prometheus Books, 1992.

Doty, R. L.: Olfactory Capacities in Aging and Alzheimer's Disease: Psychophysical and Anatomic Considerations. In: Growdon, J. H., et al. (Eds.): Aging and Alzheimer's Disease. New York: Annals N.Y. Academy of Science, 1991.

Drickhamer, M. A. and Lachs, M. S.: Should Patients with Alzheimer's Disease Be Told Their Diagnosis? N. Engl. J. Med. 325:947–951, Apr. 7, 1991.

Eagger, S. A., et al.: Tacrine in Alzheimer's Disease. Lancet 37:989–992, Apr. 27, 1991.

Escobar, J. I., et al.: Use of the Mini-Mental State Examination (MMSE) in a Community Population of Mixed Ethnicity: Cultural and Linguistic Artifacts. J. Nerv. Ment. Dis. 174:607–614, 1986.

Evans, D. A., et al.: Risk of Death from Alzheimer's Disease in a Community Population of Older Persons. Am. J. Epidemiol. 134:403–412, Aug. 15, 1991.

Folstein, M., et al.: "Mini-Mental State": A Practical Method for Grading the Cognitive State of Patients for the Clinician. J. Psychiatr. Res. 12:189–198, 1975.

Gage, F., et al.: Neuronal Grafting and Alzheimer's Disease. Berlin: Springer-Verlag, 1989.

Gold, D. T., et al.: Special Care Units: A Typology of Care Settings for Memory-Impaired Older Adults. Gerontologist 31:467–475, Aug. 1991.

Gustafson, L.: The Clinical Diagnosis of Dementia of Alzheimer Type: Prospects and Limitations. In: Fowler, C. J., et al. (Eds.): Biological Markers in Dementia of Alzheimer Type. London: Smith-Gordon, 1991.

Hachinski, V.: Preventable Senility: A Call for Action Against the Vascular Dementias. Lancet 340:645–647, Sept. 12, 1992.

Hachinski, V.: Differential Diagnosis of Alzheimer's Dementia: Multi-Infarct Dementia. In: Riseberg, B. (Ed.): Alzheimer's Disease. New York: Free Press, 1983.

Henderson A. S.: Epidemiology of Dementing Diseases. In: Wurtman, R. J., et al. (Eds.): Alzheimer's Disease. Advances in Neurology, vol. 51. New York: Raven Press, 1990.

Henderson, V. W., et al.: The Agraphia of Alzheimer's Disease. Neurology 42:776–784, Apr. 1992.

Holman, B. L., et al.: The Scintigraphic Appearance of Alzheimer's Disease: A Prospective Study Using Technetium–99m-HMPAO SPECT. J. Nucl. Med. 33:181–185, Feb. 1992.

Jorm, A. F., et al.: The Prevalence of Dementia; A Quantitative Integration of the LIterature. Acta Psychiatr. Scand. 76:465–479, Nov. 1987.

Kluger, A. and Ferris, S. H.: Scales for the Assessment of Alzheimer's Disease. Psychiatr. Clin. N. Am. 14:309–326, June 1991.

Landsberg, J. P., et al.: Absence of Aluminium in Neuritic Plaque Cores in Alzheimer's Disease. Nature 360:65–68, Nov. 5, 1992.

Larson, E. B.: Illnesses Causing Dementia in the Very Elderly [Editorial]. N. Eng. J. Med. 328:203–205, Jan. 21, 1993.

Larson, E. B., et al.: Cognitive Impairment: Dementia and Alzheimer's Disease. Ann. Rev. Pub. Health 13:431–439, 1992.

Levine, J. and Lawlor, B. A.: Family Counseling and Legal Issues in Alzheimer's Disease. Psychiatr. Clin. N. Am. 14:385–396, June 1991.

Marx, J.: Familial ALzheimer's Linked to Chromosome 14 Gene. Science 258:550, Oct. 23, 1992.

McKhann, G., et al.: Clinical Diagnosis of Alzheimer's Disease: Report of the NINCDS-ARDRA Work Group under the Auspices of Department of Health and Human Services Task Force on Alzheimer's Disease. Neurology 34:939–944, July 1984.

Mendez, M. F., et al.: Risk Factors in Alzheimer's Disease: A Clinicopathologic Study. Neurology 42:770–775, Apr. 1992.

Morris, J. C. and Rubin, E. H.: Clinical Diagnosis and Course of Alzheimer's Disease. Psychiatr. Clin. N. Am. 14:223–236, June 1991.

Nielsen, H., et al.: The Accuracy of Early Diagnosis and Predictors of Death in Alzheimer's Disease and Vascular Dementia—a Follow-up Study. Acta Pscyhiatr. Scand. 84:277–282, Sept. 1991.

Palmer, A. M. and Bowen, D. M.: Neurochemical Basis of Dementia of the Alzheimer Type: Contribution of Postmortem and Antemortem Studies. In: Fowler, C. J., et al. (Eds.): Biological Markers in Dementia of Alzheimer Type. London: Smith-Gordon, 1991.

Pittman, J., et al.: Diagnosis of Dementia in a Heterogeneous Population. A Comparison of Paradigm-Based Diagnosis and Physician's Diagnosis. Arch. Neurol. 49:461–476, May 1992.

Reisberg, B., et al.: Dementia of the Alzheimer Type Recapitulates Ontogeny Inversely on Specific Ordinal and Temporal Parameters. In: Fowler, C. J., et al. (Eds.): Biological Markers in Dementia of Alzheimer Type. London: Smith-Gordon, 1991.

Renvoize, E. B, et al.: A Sera-epidemiological Study of Conventional Infections. Age Aging 16:311–314, Sept. 1987.

Rubin, E. H., et al.: The Influence of Major Depression on Clinical and Psychometric Assessment of Senile Dementia of the Alzheimer Type. Am. J. Psychiatry148:1164–1171, Sept. 1991.

Scherr, E., et al.: Correlates of Cognitive Function in an Elderly Community Population. Am. J. Epidemiol. 128:1084–1101, Nov. 1988.

Skoog, I., et al.: A Population-Based Study of Dementia in 85–Year-Olds. N. Engl. J. Med. 328:153–158, Jan. 21, 1993.

Stern, R. G., et al.: The Use of Benzodiazepines in the Management of Behavioral Symptoms in Demented Patients. Psychiatr. Clin. N. Am. 14:375–384, June 1991.

van Dijk, P. T. M., et al.: Survival of Patients with Dementia. J. Amer. Geriatr. Soc. 39:603–610, June 1991.

Welsh, K. A., et al.: Detection and Staging of Dementia in Alzheimer's Disease. Use of the Neuropsychological Measures Developed for the Consortium to Establish a Registry for Alzheimer's Disease. Arch. Neurol. 49:448–452, May 1992.

Wragg, R. E. and Jeste, D. V.: Overview of Depression and Psychosis in Alzheimer's Disease. Am. J. Psychiatry 146:577–587, May 1989.

CHAPTER 16

DRUG TREATMENT IN THE ELDERLY

SCOPE

Compared to younger patients, persons over 65 years of age are twice as likely to require medication on a long-term basis and at least three times as likely to take multiple medications. The physiologic changes associated with aging alter the body's ability to absorb and metabolize drugs, and they may alter the effects drugs have on the various organ systems. In order to properly manage the medical therapy of an elderly patient, the physician must consider the effects aging has on the ability to absorb and metabolize drugs, the presence of various diseases and the possible interactions that could occur among medications. Although the demands of managing medications in elderly patients are complex, when this is done properly, elderly patients are no more likely to have adverse medication reactions than are younger patients.

SYNOPSIS

725

16.00 INTRODUCTION

The likelihood of a person having a chronic disease begins to increase after age 60 and increases markedly after age 70 (Troncale, 1996). Because of the frequency of disease in this age group, persons over age 65 consume over 30 percent of all prescription drugs used in the United States, although they account for only 13 percent of the population (Carlson, 1996).

New medications treat many diseases effectively and with few side effects, allowing many people to continue living productive and healthy lives into their eighth and ninth decades, despite the presence of significant diseases. Medications are now used to treat diseases that once would have required surgery or for which no treatment was available as recently as a decade ago (Lonergan, 1996).

Unfortunately no medication is free of adverse effects and side effects. As the number of persons over age 65 increases—and each patient is prescribed more medications—the incidence of drug-related complications has skyrocketed. Currently one of every six Americans over age 65 can expect to suffer an adverse drug reaction severe enough to require hospitalization (Steiner, 1996).

16.10 SPECIAL CONSIDERATIONS IN THE ELDERLY

Adverse reactions to medication are more likely to occur in elderly than in younger patients, for several reasons. The physiologic changes of aging are likely to affect two major aspects of drug therapy: the pharmacokinetics (the absorption, distribution within the body and metabolism or excretion of drugs) and the pharmacodynamics (the effects the drug will have upon the body's organs). As a result of these changes, the dosage of most drugs must be reduced by varying degrees. In addition, various diseases cause additional physiologic changes that further alter the effects of medication. Since the average elderly (over age 65) person suffers from four to six chronic diseases (Troncale, 1996), drug therapy must be further modified to take disease states into account.

In addition, elderly patients are often poorly compliant with their prescribed drug regimen (Doucet, et al., 1996). Side effects, the cost of medication and patient confusion all contribute to this poor compliance rate (Borchelt, 1995). Elderly patients are also more likely to receive prescriptions from several different physicians than are younger patients (Carlson, 1996). Often, physicians depend on the patient to inform them of medications other physicians have prescribed. Since both hearing impairment and a mild degree of cognitive dysfunction are common in the geriatric population, this practice is likely to result in miscommunication and the potential for two (or more) physicians to prescribe similar medications.

All these factors contribute to the high potential for adverse drug reactions (ADRs) in elderly patients. It is not surprising that between 10 percent and 30 percent of all geriatric hospitalizations are associated with an adverse drug reaction, a drug-drug interaction (DDI) or an accidental drug overdose (Doucet, et al., 1996; Lonergan, 1996). The problem is not limited to outpatients; ADRs are involved in 10 percent of the complications experienced by hospitalized elderly patients (Lonergan, 1996).

In order to safely prescribe medications for elderly persons, proper precautions and vigilant monitoring are required to assure that the patient receives the maximum possible benefit, with minimal adverse effects. Only about 15 percent of physicians have received formalized training in prescribing for geriatric patients, however (Semla, et al., 1997), and there is no evidence to suggest that adverse drug reactions are becoming less frequent in the elderly population.

16.20   CHANGES IN PHARMACOKINETICS ASSOCIATED WITH AGING

The pharmacokinetics of a drug include the following factors:

- rate and quantity of absorption;
- distribution of the absorbed drug to the various tissues of the body; and
- metabolism or excretion of the drug to end its effects.

In general, all these aspects of drug pharmacokinetics are altered to some degree by the aging process and by the various disease states that are likely to occur in older patients.

Older patients often require a lower dose or a longer interval between doses than do younger patients. However, the various physiologic changes that accompany aging have different effects on each of the different classes of drugs. For this reason, the prescribing physician must be aware of the type and degree of physiologic change present and the effect these changes are expected to have on the specific type of medication being prescribed.

16.21   Changes Affecting Gastrointestinal Absorption of Drugs

Older patients are likely to have diminished function of the gastrointestinal tract, including decreased saliva production, decreased motility (ability to move food) of the esophagus, slowed gastric emptying and decreased absorption from the intestines (Lonergan, 1996). Congestive heart failure and vascular disease are also likely to slow the initial absorption of drugs because of diminished circulation to the stomach and intestines. In most elderly persons, these changes are mild and result in only a slight delay between taking oral medication and the actual absorption of the medication into the body.

Because of delayed gastric emptying (food remains in the stomach longer), interactions between drugs and food are more pronounced in the elderly. The absorption of most medications, especially antibiotics, is likely to be delayed and reduced by the presence of food. A few medications, especially beta-blocking medications and diuretics taken by patients with heart disease and high blood pressure, actually have an increased absorption in the presence of food, which could result in a drug overdose. The nutritional supplements often taken by elderly patients are particularly likely to interfere with drug absorption and may require special precautions.

For this reason, elderly patients should take their medication at least one hour before or two hours after eating. Elderly patients should take oral medications with a full glass of water in order to speed passage through the esophagus and stomach.

16.22   Changes of Drug Distribution in the Body

Once a drug has been absorbed into the bloodstream, it will spread through all the tissues of the body. Drugs are not all distributed evenly throughout the body, however, but will tend to accumulate in different tissues, depending on their biochemical composition. Changes that occur with aging in the proportion of different body tissues can affect the distribution of certain drugs.

[1]   Changes of Body Tissue Composition

Depending upon its biochemical composition, an individual drug is either more soluble in water or in lipids (fats and oils). Once a drug has been absorbed into the body, most of the drug molecules will enter either the watery fluids of the body or the fatty tissues. These drug molecules will remain as a "drug reservoir" in the tissues, staying in balanced equilibrium with the portion of the drug that remains in the bloodstream. As the drug supply in the bloodstream is continuously metabolized by the body, the remaining drug is slowly released from this tissue reservoir.

In old age, the composition of the various tissues in the body changes. Muscle mass (which is largely water) decreases by at least 30 percent compared to that of young adults, and as a result, the water content of the body decreases by about 15 percent. The portion of the body that is composed of lipid increases by at least 25 percent in old age, even in individuals whose weight does not change. Persons who gain weight as they age will often have doubled the lipid proportion of their bodies compared to that expected for young adults (Lonergan, 1996).

The dosage of drugs is routinely determined according to a certain number of milligrams of drug per kilogram of body weight, using data obtained in studies on young adults. Using these standard formulas to prescribe drugs for elderly patients will tend to result in an overdose for water-soluble drugs (*see Table 16-1*) and an underdose for lipid-soluble drugs (*see Table 16-2*).

Table 16-1
Commonly Prescribed Water-Soluble Drugs

---

aspirin
aminoglycoside antibiotics, except Tobramycin®
cimetidine (Tagamet®) and similar drugs
digoxin (Lanoxin®)
loazepam (Ativan®), oxazepam (Serax) and most short acting
  benzodiazepines
methyldopa (Aldomet®)
procainamide (Procan®)

A second effect that occurs only in the case of lipid-soluble drugs is the "increased reservoir" effect. Since elderly persons have a higher proportion of fatty tissue, a larger portion of lipid-soluble drugs will enter the "tissue reservoir," and less will be in the bloodstream. Since more of the drug remains in the reservoir to replenish that which is metabolized, the interval between doses can often be increased without a loss of drug effectiveness.

In general, water-soluble drugs should be prescribed at a lower dose for elderly patients than they would be for younger patients. Lipid-soluble drugs may be prescribed at a similar dose as that recommended for younger persons, but since the duration of action may be prolonged by the reservoir effect, the interval between doses can be prolonged. With either type of drug, careful follow-up should be performed to evaluate for potential overdose.

Table 16-2
Commonly Prescribed Lipid-Soluble Drugs

---

amiodarone (Cordarone®)
barbiturates
diazepam* (Valium®) and some long acting benzodiazepines
digitoxin (Crystodigin®)
ethylchlorvynol (Placidyl®)
propranolol (Inderal®) and other beta-blockers

---

*NOTE: Diazepam has an extremely prolonged duration of action in elderly patients. A single dose may have an effect for as long as 100 hours (Semla, et al., 1997).

[2] Changes in Serum Proteins

The blood plasma (the liquid portion of blood, in which cells and particles are suspended) contains many different protein molecules in solution. Many drugs bind tightly to these proteins in the plasma. The net effect of this "protein binding" is that only a fraction of the drug is available to give a clinical effect, while the majority of drug molecules remain bound to plasma proteins. As with lipid binding, this provides a reservoir of drug, prolonging its duration of action. When a highly protein bound drug is given to a person with reduced plasma protein levels, more of the drug than expected is available to cause its clinical effect. (*See Table 16-3.*) This results in an apparent overdose of drug in the body, even though the dosage may have been calculated correctly.

The normal aging process does not markedly alter plasma proteins, but chronic disease, which occurs in 25 percent of elderly persons, can dramatically reduce the amount of plasma protein (Roe, 1994). Malnutrition, which affects about 20 percent of elderly persons, can also reduce plasma protein levels (Nikolaus, et al., 1995). Concentrations of plasma albumin (the plasma protein present in highest quantity) should be measured in patients at risk for having low plasma protein levels.

A second effect of protein binding is a drug-drug interaction (DDI) occurring when a patient takes two different drugs that are both highly protein bound. If the two drugs compete for the same protein binding sites, an increased free concentration of one or both drugs occurs, effectively causing a drug overdose. Many cardiac medications, anti-inflammatory medications and antidepressant medications are highly protein bound. Because elderly patients are especially likely to take these types of medication, a protein binding DDI is one of the most common adverse drug reactions among these individuals (Lonergan, 1996).

Table 16-3
Highly Protein Bound Drugs

Anti-inflammatories	
aspirin	mefenamic acid
fenoprofen	oxaprozin
ibuprofen	naproxyn
indomethacin	piroxicam
Cardiac Medications	
amiodarone	nimodipine
clofibrate	prazosin
diltiazem	propranolol
felodipine	quinidine
nicardipine	warfarin
nifedipine	verapamil
Psychoactive Medications	
amitriptyline	haloperidol
buprenorphene	nefazodone
chlordiazepoxide	nortriptyline
chlorpromazine	oxazepam
desipramine	quazepam
fluoxetene	sertraline
flurazepam	temazepam
Other	
diphenhydramine	phenytoin
doxycycline	spironolactone
glyburide	tolbutamide

16.23   Changes in Metabolism of Drugs

The ability of the body to remove drugs once they have been absorbed is only slightly affected by aging itself. However, many of the disease states associated with old age can have a dramatic effect on the body's ability to metabolize drugs. Patients with renal disease, heart failure or liver disease are very likely to have altered drug metabolism.

[1] Changes in Renal Function

Most drugs are eliminated by the kidneys and excreted into the urine. With regard to drug elimination, the most important aspect of kidney function is the glomerular filtration rate (GFR), which is a direct measure of blood flow to the kidney. The clearance of most drugs is directly proportional to the glomerular filtration rate.

The GFR declines steadily with age after the third decade. By the age of 70, an otherwise healthy person will have a 30 percent reduction in glomerular filtration rate, even if she or he has never had kidney disease (Lonergan, 1996). In individuals with a past history of kidney disease (including recurrent kidney infections or kidney stones), with current kidney problems or with significant cardiovascular disease, the GFR will be reduced even further.

In younger patients, the GFR can be estimated by checking the patient's serum creatinine level, since creatinine is constantly produced by muscle cells and removed by the kidneys. In elderly patients, this method of estimation is much less accurate because of the decreased muscle mass that occurs with age. In order to accurately assess kidney function and GFR in an elderly patient, a 12–or 24–hour creatinine clearance test must be performed. This test involves collecting both urine and blood samples, and calculating the percentage of creatinine that is being removed by the kidneys.

The dosage of drugs that are primarily cleared by the kidney should routinely be reduced slightly, or the interval between doses increased, in elderly patients. (*See Table 16-4.*) If the patient's history suggests impaired kidney function, a creatinine clearance test should be performed, and the medication dosage reduced according to the results of the test. For example, if the GFR is reduced to 25 percent of normal or less, the dose of drugs should be reduced to about a third of the standard dose (Greenblatt, 1993).

The kidneys can also be damaged by certain medications, especially if an overdose occurs. The two groups of drugs most commonly associated with renal damage are the aminoglycoside antibiotics and the nonsteroidal anti-inflammatory drugs (NSAIDs). When these drugs are used in elderly patients, kidney function should be monitored regularly.

Table 16-4
Drugs Excreted Primarily by the Kidneys

acyclovir	cimetidine
amantadine	clonidine
amiloride	digoxin
aminoglycoside antibiotics	ethambutol
atenolol	lisinopril
carteolol	metoclopramide
cephalosporin antibiotics	nadolol
chlorpropamide	thiazide diuretics

[2]   Changes in Liver Function

The liver is involved in drug metabolism in two ways. The cyto-chrome metabolic pathways in the liver chemically break down and inactivate many drugs as they pass through the liver (also known as Phase I drug metabolism). This is a rapid chemical process that is sometimes referred to as *first-pass elimination,* since a large portion of drugs metabolized by this route are eliminated the first time they pass through the liver. Phase II metabolism in the liver involves the attachment of chemicals to the drug molecule so that they can be easily excreted. This process is slower than first-pass metabolism but is necessary for excretion of some types of drugs.

Even though liver function decreases up to 30 percent during old age, the liver has sufficient reserves that the effects of aging on drug metabolism are minimal. If a geriatric patient also has liver disease, however, he or she may have enough deterioration of liver function to interfere with the metabolism of some drugs. (*See Table 16-5.*) Additionally, some medications, such as cimetidine, can interfere with the Phase I metabolism of other drugs by the liver.

16.30   CHANGES IN PHARMACODYNAMICS ASSOCIATED WITH AGING

As the body ages, a general deterioration in the function of the individual organ systems occurs. This can alter the overall effects a drug has on the organ that it is targeted to help, and it can also alter the frequency and severity of side effects. These changes in pharmaco-dynamics are generally specific to the drug category involved. How-ever, side effects involving the cardiovascular and nervous systems are much more likely to occur in elderly patients than in younger patients.

Table 16-5
Drugs Metabolized Primarily by the Liver

acebutolol	metoprolol
acetaminophen	morphine
amoxapine	naproxen
buprenorphine	nifedipine
chlorpromazine	nitroglycerin
codeine	pentaerythritol tetranitrate
diazepam	phenylzine
diltiazem	propranololranitidine
enalapril	rifampin
felodipine	timolol
flurazepam	verapamil
isosorbide dinitrate	warfarin
labetalol	
lorazepam	

16.31 Cardiovascular System

Unlike the liver and kidney, the cardiovascular system generally has very limited reserves in elderly patients. Because of this, elderly patients are very sensitive to any medication that either decreases the contracting ability of the heart or causes dilation of the blood vessels. They also have decreased sensitivity to medications that stimulate the sympathetic nervous system, so medications that stimulate the heart or contract the blood vessels may be less effective.

[1] Postural Hypotension

Postural hypotension is a decrease in blood pressure that occurs when a person changes position from sitting or lying down to standing. It is caused by blood pooling in dilated blood vessels of the abdomen and legs, resulting in less blood returning to the heart. Postural hypotension of some degree occurs in 5 percent to 15 percent of persons over 75 years of age (Lonergan, 1996).

Any medication that causes vasodilation or interferes with the contracting ability of the heart can cause postural hypotension in elderly patients. In most cases, these effects aren't severe and will resolve as the patient adjusts to the medication. However, postural hypotension is a common cause of falls and injury among elderly patients (Borchelt, 1995). Elderly patients should be made aware of the potential for postural hypotension whenever they begin a new medication.

[2] Volume Depletion

The impaired kidney function that occurs in old age can interfere with the ability of the body to maintain an adequate level of fluid and salt. Because of impaired cardiac function, elderly patients cannot tolerate significant loss of fluid without suffering hypotension (low blood pressure). Medications that either have a diuretic (salt- and water-losing) effect or that interfere with kidney function can cause volume depletion in elderly patients.

Volume depletion results in decreased blood pressure. In elderly patients, a significant decrease in blood pressure often causes alterations of mental function, such as confusion or agitation. It may also result in muscle weakness or falls, and may impair the function of other organs, especially the kidneys. Elderly patients taking cardiac medications or diuretics are especially at risk of volume depletion during mid-summer heat waves. Over 80 percent of all heat stroke and other heat-related illnesses occur in persons over age 65 who are taking medications of this type (Faunt, et al., 1995).

[3] Heart Failure

The diminished cardiac reserves of elderly patients make them more likely to suffer symptoms of heart failure when taking any medication that interferes with heart function. At the same time, elderly patients are more likely than younger patients to require such medications. Usually medication-induced heart failure will progress gradually over several days. Symptoms include weakness, shortness of breath and swelling of the ankles and hands. Severe cases will involve hypotension, altered mental status and decreased urine output.

Beta-blocking and calcium-channel-blocking drugs, antihypertensive medications and some forms of chemotherapy for cancer are most likely to cause symptoms of heart failure. In most cases, the symptoms are entirely reversible once the offending medications are removed, but severe cases will require hospitalization.

16.32   Nervous System

Elderly patients are much more sensitive to the effects of central nervous system drugs than are younger patients. Benzodiazepines, sedatives and antidepressant medications are the drugs most likely to result in a deterioration of mental function in elderly patients, even when their dosage has been reduced (Greenblatt, 1993). Confusion, agitation and a decreased level of consciousness are all commonly reported in elderly patients taking these medications. Some drugs, such as cimetidine, that have no central nervous system effects in younger patients can cause a significant change in mental status in older patients (Semla, et al., 1997).

Drug-induced changes in mental status are much more likely to occur in patients who have some pre-existing alteration of their mental function. Since 28 percent of elderly patients are reported to have mental alterations (Ames and Tuckwell, 1994), the proportion of patients at high risk is quite large. In particular, patients with both Alzheimer's disease[1] and Parkinson's disease may suffer catastrophic deterioration of mental function when they are exposed to medications that affect the central nervous system (Greenblatt, 1993).

16.40   COMMON ADVERSE DRUG REACTIONS IN THE ELDERLY

Some adverse drug reactions, such as gastrointestinal upset and allergic reaction, are no more likely to occur in elderly patients than in young patients. However, elderly patients are much more likely to suffer certain types of adverse drug reactions than are younger patients (Lonergan, 1996; Naranjo, et al., 1995). In some cases, these side effects develop after taking medications that are not associated with such effects in younger persons. (*See Table 16-6.*)

16.41   Falls

Elderly patients are likely to have several medical conditions that could contribute to a fall: impaired muscle strength and vision, neurologic disease that affects gait or balance, and cardiovascular problems that result in hypotension (low blood pressure) or fainting. Almost a third of community-dwelling persons over age 75 will require hospitalization each year as a direct result of a fall. Falls in elderly

---

[1] *See also* ch. 15.

persons account for 250,00 fractured hips each year in the United States alone, and accidents (two thirds of which are falls) are the sixth most common cause of death in elderly persons worldwide (Sagar, 1996).

Table 16-6
Specific Adverse Drug Effects in the Elderly

Drug	Side Effect
amitriptyline (Elavil®)	confusion, hypotension, cardiac dysrhythmia, urinary retention
cimetidine (Tagamet®)	sedation, confusion, alteration of hepatic metabolism
diazepam (Valium®)	prolonged sedation (lasting for days)
digitalis (Lanoxin®)	high potassium levels
imipramine (Tofranil®)	hypotension, cardiac dysrhythmia
methyldopa (Aldomet®)	sedation, confusion
prazosin (Minipress®)	severe hypotension
verapamil (Calan®, Isoptin®)	constipation

Adverse medication reactions have been reported to cause or contribute to between 20 percent and 40 percent of all falls in the elderly (Liu, et al., 1995; Davies and Kenny, 1996), and falls are most likely to occur within 28 days of starting a new medication (Neutel, et al., 1996). An additional 5 percent of all falls in elderly patients are associated with the use of alcohol while taking a prescription medication (Sagar, 1997). The adverse medication reactions most likely to result in a fall are hypotension or postural hypotension, confusion and sedation, and cardiac dysrhythmia. Specifically the benzodiazepines, diuretics, antidepressants, beta-blocking drugs and calcium channel blocking drugs are most likely to be associated with such reactions and are the medications most commonly reported to be associated with falls (Neutel, 1996; Liu, 1995).

16.42   Hypotension

The cardiovascular system of young persons has large reserves and can compensate easily for changes in blood volume, blood vessel dilation or the contraction strength of the heart. With age, blood vessels loose some of their ability to contract, while at the same time, the heart is less able to increase the amount of blood it pumps. Because of these changes, elderly persons are very sensitive to any medications that interfere with the heart's contraction or that dilate the blood vessels.

If either of these changes occurs, the cardiovascular system cannot compensate, and hypotension (lowered blood pressure) results. When the major effect is dilation of the blood vessels, lowered blood pressure may only be apparent when the patient stands (postural hypotension). If the heart's contracting ability is affected, hypotension may occur even when the patient lies flat. Postural hypotension is one of the most frequent side effect of medication among elderly patients, although generalized hypotension also occurs regularly (Nikolaus, 1995).

Postural hypotension usually causes fainting or dizziness when a person rises from a sitting position. Blood flow to the brain is dramatically reduced when an elderly person develops generalized hypotension, and the individual may have symptoms of confusion, fainting or increased dementia (severe impairment of cognitive function), loss of consciousness, rapid pulse and a drop in urine output. Severe or long-lasting hypotensive episodes in elderly patients can result in stroke or heart attack. Less severe episodes are strongly associated with falls and may contribute to renal failure.

Numerous drugs are known to frequently cause hypotension in elderly patients. Cardiovascular medications such as beta-blockers, calcium-channel blockers, antihypertensive medications and diuretics are all common causes of hypotension. Antidepressants, benzodiazepines and other medications that are not associated with hypotension in younger patients may cause it in the elderly (Preskorn, 1993). In fact, hypotension resulting from the combination of an antidepressant medication with a cardiac medication is one of the most common adverse drug-drug interactions (Borchelt, 1995).

16.43   Confusion and Dementia

A mild degree of mental impairment is not uncommon in elderly patients. Between 15 percent and 20 percent of patients over 65 years of age, and more than 40 percent of those over 75, have some form of organic mental impairment (Greenberg, 1997). Additionally, over 25 percent of persons 65 or older suffer depression or significant anxiety (Ames and Tuckwell, 1994). Many of these patients have only mild symptoms, however, and are able to compensate well and live independently.

Medication can significantly worsen the symptoms of mental dysfunction in elderly patients. As many as 10 percent of all cases of confusion and sudden dementia (severe impairment of cognitive function) are caused by adverse reactions to drugs (Greenberg, 1996). Such reactions may originate from direct effects of the drugs on the central nervous system or from secondary effects, such as decreased blood circulation to the brain.

In addition to sudden deterioration of mental function occurring soon after a new drug therapy is begun, drug treatment can be associated with a slow deterioration of mental function that can be mistaken for the mental changes of aging (Doucet, et al., 1996). When the designers of one study reviewed the medication regimens of elderly patients, over 60 percent were taking some medication that could interfere with mental function (Borchelt, 1995). Simply reducing the number of medications taken has been reported to improve mental function in a significant fraction of elderly patients (Doucet, et al., 1996; Schrader, et al., 1996).

Drugs frequently associated with a deterioration of mental function in elderly persons are listed in *Table 16-7.*

16.44   Kidney Damage

The decrease in kidney function that occurs with age can alter the excretion of many different drugs.[2] Conversely, many medications can also interfere with renal function. The most common adverse effect of medications on the kidneys is to reduce glomerular filtration.[3] This decreases the amount of blood flow to the kidney, which further reduces renal function. A few drugs can also have a direct toxic effect on the kidney, especially if they are given in high doses.

Many drugs, including the nonsteroidal anti-inflammatory medications and diuretics, reduce glomerular filtration rate. The effect is usually temporary, and function will return to normal when the drugs are discontinued. The drugs most commonly associated with actual kidney damage are the aminoglycoside antibiotics, especially if they are used in high doses. Whenever these drugs are used, the patient's creatinine clearance should be assessed at the beginning of therapy,[4]

---

[2] *See* 16.23[1] *supra.*

[3] *See* 16.23[1] *supra.*

[4] *See* 16.23[1] *supra.*

and regularly while the treatment continues. Additionally, serum concentrations of the aminoglycoside should be measured for both peak and trough levels, and the dosage adjusted accordingly (Semla, et al., 1997).

Table 16-7
Drugs Causing Altered Mental Status in the Elderly

---

alpha methyldopa
analgesics (all, including nonsteroidal anti-inflammatory agents)
antiarrhythmics: lidocaine, procainamide, quinidine, mexilitine, disopyramide
antibiotics: penicillin, methicillin, ciprofloxacin, gentamycin, isoniazid, chloroquin
anticholinergics: benztropine, dicyclomine, oxybutinin, propantheline, scopalamine
anticonvulsants: carbamazepine, phenytoin, valproic acid
antidepressants (all)
antihistamines: diphenhydramine, chlorpheniramine, hydroxyzine, promethazine
antispasmodics (all)
benzodiazepines (all)
beta-blockers: propranolol, metoprolol
calcium channel blockers: verapamil, nifedipine
decongestants: ephedrine, pseudoephedrine
digitalis
disulfiram
gastrointestinal drugs: cimetidine, ranitidine, metoclopramide, misoprostolol

---

16.50   COMMON DRUG-DRUG INTERACTIONS IN THE ELDERLY

When any patient takes more than one medication, the potential for an adverse drug-drug interaction (DDI) exists. Such adverse interactions can take place whenever one drug alters the pharmacokinetics of another drug, or if the two drugs have similar and additive effects on the same organ system.

The average elderly person takes between three and five prescription medications on a regular basis. About 10 percent of all elderly persons—and over 30 percent of all nursing home residents—take eight or more different medications every day (Lonergan, 1996; Banys, 1996). Since the possibility of adverse drug-drug interactions is proportional to the number of different medications taken, these patients are at particularly high risk.

16.51   Alteration of Pharmacokinetics

Because many medications are chemically similar, they may interfere with some aspect of the pharmacokinetics of another medication. Such interactions have been reported between literally thousands of different medication combinations, but most occur when one drug either interferes with the absorption or metabolism of another drug, or when two drugs compete for protein binding sites.

[1]   Interference with Absorption

The presence of food is more likely to interfere with a drug's absorption than is the presence of another drug. However, many over-the-counter antacids and laxatives can decrease the absorption of a number of drugs. Although this usually happens in an unpredictable fashion, a few generalizations can be made. Digoxin, benzodiazepines, tetracycline antibiotics, corticosteroids and supplemental iron are all likely to have decreased absorption in the presence of antacids. Any drug that lowers the acid content of the stomach is likely to interfere with the absorption of ketoconazole, an antifungal medication (Semla, et al., 1997).

[2]   Interference with Liver Metabolism

Drugs that are extensively metabolized by the liver may have a prolonged duration of action and reach toxic levels if another drug interferes with their metabolism.[5] The liver generally has large reserves and can metabolize many drugs simultaneously, but elderly patients with pre-existing liver disease often have limited reserves of hepatic function. Cimetidine (Tagamet®), an H2-blocking drug (used to prevent histamine from stimulating receptors that work to cause the stomach to secrete more acid) commonly used to treat gastric acidity, can reduce the metabolizing capability of the liver significantly. Many authors recommend avoiding this drug when treating patients taking other medications that depend on liver metabolism for removal (Lonergan, 1996).

---

[5] *See* 16.23[2] *supra.*

[3] Interference with Renal Excretion

The dose of drugs excreted by the kidney must be reduced in patients who have renal disease.[6] The addition of other drugs that decrease renal blood flow may further reduce the clearance of such drugs by the kidney. Diuretics, nonsteroidal anti-inflammatory medications and aminoglycoside antibiotics can all reduce renal blood flow and cause such changes. Antihypertensive medications, beta-blocking agents and calcium channel blocking drugs can also reduce renal excretion of other drugs by reducing blood flow to the kidneys.

[4] Interference with Protein Binding

Whenever highly protein bound drugs are absorbed, only a small fraction of the drug is actually free in the body. The majority of the drug is bound to albumin and other proteins in the blood plasma, where it is not available to cause any effect on the target organs. If the amount of protein in the plasma is reduced, then a larger amount of the drug will be free in the plasma, resulting in an unexpectedly high concentration of free drug and a potential for drug toxicity. This can occur in elderly patients who are malnourished or become chronically ill (Lonergan, 1996).

If two different drugs that each are highly protein bound are given to a patient, the drugs may compete for protein-binding sites.[7] This results in the displacement of molecules of one drug from the protein, raising the serum level of free (active) drug, possibly to toxic levels. Even if toxicity does not occur, the protein-bound drug will serve as a reservoir of drug, prolonging its duration of action. Displacing the drug from protein-binding sites therefore shortens the duration of the effect of the drug. Displacement of one drug from its protein-binding sites by another drug is one of the most common DDIs (Borchelt, 1995; Carlson, 1996).

16.52 Alterations of Pharmacodynamics

Because the reserves of the body's various organ systems diminish with age, the elderly are more likely than younger patients to suffer symptoms when two or more drugs have actions on the same organ system. Such DDIs may occur when two drugs have an unexpectedly large additive actions on their target organ system. For example, the

---

[6] *See* 16.23[1] *supra.*

[7] *See* 16.22[2] *supra.*

addition of a second antihypertensive drug rarely causes problems in patients under age 55 but sometimes causes severe hypotension in elderly patients.

Similarly, elderly patients are particularly prone to suffering from the additive side effects of two or more drugs (Kruse, 1995). These interactions are often dramatically more severe in elderly patients and may cause side effects almost never reported in younger patients (Naranjo, et al., 1995). For example, the addition of a nonsteroidal anti-inflammatory drug (NSAID) to a beta-blocker rarely causes significant side effects in a young person. However, it is not uncommon for the combination of mild fluid retention (from the NSAID) with decreased cardiac contraction (from the beta-blocker) to cause congestive heart failure in an elderly patient with diminished cardiovascular and renal function.

16.60   FACTORS AFFECTING MEDICATION COMPLIANCE IN THE ELDERLY

Between a third and half of all elderly patients are not compliant with their medication therapy (Lonergan, 1996). Many factors affect patient compliance, including poor physician-patient communication, medication costs, impaired mental status of patients, the presence of unpleasant side effects and complex medication schedules. Some of these factors are present in persons of any age, but most occur more commonly in elderly patients.

16.61   Altered Physical and Mental Status

It has been documented that as many as 25 percent of patients over age 65 have a decreased ability to learn and remember new tasks (Fitten, et al., 1995). When this is coupled with the fact that as many as 40 percent of chronically ill elderly patients will have a medication change during any three-month period (Nikolaus, et al., 1996), it is not surprising that many elderly patients become confused about their medication schedules.

In addition, many elderly persons have physical limitations that further affect their ability to manage a complex medical schedule. Hearing difficulties often interfere with the patient's ability to understand their doctor's instructions. As many as 40 percent of elderly patients have cataracts[8] or other visual difficulties that interfere with

---

[8] *See also* ch. 11.

reading the print on medication bottles or medication instructions (Atkin, et al., 1994). Arthritis and generalized weakness may also interfere with an elderly person's ability to take medication. For example, between 10 percent (Nikolaus, et al., 1996) and 40 percent (Atkin, et al., 1994) of elderly patients cannot open "childproof" medicine bottles, while as many as 70 percent (Atkin, et al., 1994) cannot break a pill in half.

Studies have shown that ability to accurately follow a medication schedule decreases with age after age 65 (Atkin, et al., 1994; Fitten, et al., 1995). The worse the patient's overall health, the less likely the patient is to take medication as prescribed, yet the more likely the patient is to have a complex medical regimen (Ruscin and Semla, 1996). Females are reported to have more difficulty following medication regimens than males (Fitten, et al., 1995; Ruscin and Semla, 1996), but this may be related to the greater number of females living past their eighth decade.

Although the difficulty elderly patients have in taking medication as prescribed is well documented in the literature, many physicians continue to simply assume that their patients are accurately following the medical regimen. Most authors recommend that elderly patients should be assessed for their ability to follow a medical regimen using a few simple techniques (Fitten, et al., 1995; Ruscin and Semla, 1996):

1. Patients should demonstrate an ability to open prescription bottles, read medication labels and differentiate various pills.

2. All patient directions should be given in writing, as well as verbally.

3. Brief tests of cognitive abilities, such as the Mini-Mental State Examination (MMSE), should be administered to identify patients who are most likely to be unable follow prescription directions.

Patients at high risk for inadvertent noncompliance may benefit from home health visits on a regular basis. It has also been shown that frequent, repeated patient counseling by a nurse or pharmacist can increase compliance in such cases (Kruse, 1995). When possible, a spouse or other relative can take charge of the patient's medications, but in many cases, the spouse has similar physical or mental deficits. In addition, when serum blood analysis of medication levels are available, blood levels should be checked frequently to assure that the medication is being taken in proper quantities.

16.62   Polypharmacy and Complex Medication Regimens

The ability of elderly patients to follow their medical regimen decreases as the number of different medications involved increases (Ruscin and Semla, 1996). Additionally, the likelihood of drug-drug interactions increases proportionally with the number of different medications prescribed (Sternon and Gilles, 1996). Unfortunately, elderly patients are quite likely to be taking multiple medications. In fact, half of all outpatients over age 65 take three or more different medications simultaneously, 40 percent take five or more drugs, and 15 percent take eight or more different medications (Lonergan, 1996; Borchelt, 1995).

Several factors contribute to the high incidence of polypharmacy in older patients. Separate specialists treating different conditions often prescribe medications simultaneously for the patient. Individual physicians also have a tendency to prescribe more medications more frequently for older patients than for younger patients with similar symptoms, although the reasons for this are not clear (Kruse, 1995; Carlson, 1996).

Current estimates are that as many as 25 percent of all geriatric patients are receiving some form of inappropriate or unnecessary medication (Lonergan, 1996; Borchelt, 1995). This could include selection of an inappropriate medication, improper dosage of an appropriate medication, or receiving a combination of medications that are likely to result in a drug-drug interaction. Studies have shown that careful review of the medication regimen of elderly patients, combined with patient education, results in a reduction of the number of medications being prescribed (Schrader, et al., 1996). Other studies have demonstrated that when the medical regimens of elderly patients are reviewed by independent practitioners, the reviewer can find no indication for as many as 30 percent of the medications that are prescribed (Sheehan, et al., 1996). When the number of medications is reduced, elderly patients report an improvement in their mental status and perceived health (Schrader, et al., 1996; Carlson, 1996).

Reduction in the number of medications prescribed also directly reduces the potential number of drug-drug interactions. An analysis of patients taking an average of four different drugs showed that 85 percent of patients had at least one potential drug-drug interaction (DDI) that could lead to overdose, while 52 percent had at least one

DDI in which some drugs actually interfered with the action of others (Borchelt, 1995).

16.63 Other Factors Affecting Medication Usage

In addition to the medical factors involved in compliance, other factors can play a significant role in the overuse and underuse of medications.

[1] Cost of Medications

Most elderly persons live on a fixed income, and the cost of medication can become a large monthly expense. The cost of a single nongeneric medication can be several hundred dollars a month. In many cases, physicians prescribe medication without actual awareness of its cost or of their patient's ability to pay for it. When patients cannot afford their medication, they may reduce their dose of medication, miss taking the medication for days or weeks, or stop taking the medication entirely. Often they will not inform the prescribing physician of this because of embarrassment. In many cases, a generic alternative could be prescribed, resulting in a significant cost saving for the patient.

For patients participating in Medicaid or many types of managed care, medications are often available at a nominal cost or for free. Often, however, the formulary of drugs available under such programs is strictly limited. This may result in a physician using a less acceptable drug because it is the only one available through the program. In a few programs, physicians' prescriptions may automatically be changed to a formulary drug of the same classification. In some instances, this may result in the substitution of a drug that has an entirely different pharmacokinetic or side effect profile.

[2] Habituation and Substance Abuse

Although most physicians consider alcoholism and substance abuse to be diseases of the young, there is increasing evidence that substance abuse is also a significant problem in geriatric patients (King, et al., 1994; Szwabo, 1993). Although persons over 60 are less than half as likely to abuse alcohol as younger patients, those elderly people who drink are much more likely to be hospitalized and have chronic medical illness than those who don't (Banys, 1996).

While older patients are very unlikely to use illicit or illegal drugs, it has been estimated that as many as 13 percent of elderly patients misuse or abuse prescription medications (Banys, 1996). The drugs most commonly abused by patients in this age group are narcotic analgesics and sedative-hypnotics. Most commonly, elderly patients who overuse narcotics have underlying chronic pain. Anxiety and sleep problems are the underlying complaints in many elderly patients who overuse benzodiazepines and other sedative-hypnotics. In the vast majority of cases, elderly patients who overuse medications obtain them by prescriptions from more than one physician (Szwabo, 1993).

Patients who abuse alcohol are likely to have chronic liver damage that can interfere with the metabolism of other drugs (Lonergan, 1996). Alcohol also interacts with several types of medication in elderly patients, increasing the incidence of postural hypotension and falls (Sagar, 1997). Chronic narcotic and benzodiazepine use can result in depression, decreased mental function and insomnia (King, et al., 1994). All these medications can also result in drug-drug interactions, especially the benzodiazepines.

Because prescription medications account for the majority of drugs that are abused by elderly patients, physicians must consider the appropriateness of medications they prescribe and the possibility that other physicians are prescribing similar medications. Often, centralized pharmacy records can reveal a pattern of multiple prescriptions when a patient denies or "forgets" such activity.

Even when clear records are kept, however, it is sometimes difficult to decide what amount of medication is appropriate for elderly patients. Although opinions concerning the appropriate use of narcotic analgesics vary widely, the Health Care Financing Administration has published guidelines for the use of sedative-hypnotics in elderly patients. Summarized, the guidelines are as follows (Semla, et al., 1997):

1. Long-acting benzodiazepines should only be used when a shorter-acting drug has failed. Long-acting benzodiazepines include chlordiazepoxide (Librium®), clonazepam (Klonopin®), diazepam (Valium®), flurazepam (Dalmane®) and quazepam (Doral®).

2. Short-acting benzodiazepines should only be used when other causes of the patient's distress have been eliminated. Use should not exceed four months without an attempt at dose reduction and withdrawal.

3. Drugs for sleep induction should only be used when all reasons for insomnia have been investigated. The use of the drug must result in improvement of the patient's symptoms. Use should not exceed 10 consecutive days.

4. Barbiturates, ethchlorovynol (Placidyl®), meprobamate (Equanil®, Miltown®), paraldehyde and glutethimide (Doriden®) should not be used to treat elderly patients.

Although these guidelines have the force of regulations only in nursing home patients in the United States, they are excellent guidelines for prescribing sedative-hypnotics for all elderly patients. It has been reported that alprazolam (Xanax®) and clonazepam (Klonopin®) tend to have higher abuse potential in the elderly, and there use should therefore be avoided (Banys, 1996).

16.64 Steps to Improve Patient Compliance with Medication

In summary, three basic steps seem to effectively improve compliance with a medical regimen in elderly patients. The first—and perhaps most important—is to simplify the medical regimen of elderly patients whenever possible. Studies have demonstrated that up to a third of medications the elderly take can be safely removed from the regimen, resulting in a significant decrease in the likelihood of drug-drug interactions and adverse drug effects (Kruse, 1995; Borchelt, 1995).

The second step is to evaluate the patient to determine if compliance is possible. Such an evaluation must consider hearing and visual impairment as well as manual strength and dexterity. A brief evaluation of mental and cognitive function is appropriate in patients with significant illness. When patients are obviously unable to comply with therapy recommendations because of physical or mental limitations, another individual must be found who is willing to take charge of the medication, or appropriate home or institutional care should be arranged.

The final step is continued and repeated patient education and follow-up. Such programs can be administered by physicians, nurses or pharmacists. In all cases, education programs have been shown to increase compliance, reduce complications and minimize expense to the patient (Sorrento, et al., 1996; Sheehan, et al., 1996).

16.70   COMMON PROBLEMS ASSOCIATED WITH SPECIFIC MEDICATION GROUPS

With thousands of prescription drugs currently on the market, it is impossible to identify even a significant fraction of the potential adverse drug reactions, drug-drug interactions and side effects that can occur in elderly patients. Most pharmacies have computer programs that will perform this function and routinely check their patients' medication list for such events. However, certain groups of medications are commonly associated with adverse effects in elderly patients, and these deserve special mention.

16.71   Antidepressants

More than 25 percent of persons over 65 years of age show clinical evidence of depression (Johnson, 1996). At least 10 percent of elderly persons (Ames and Tuckwell, 1994) and at least 15 percent of elderly females (Szwabo, 1993) are known to take antidepressant medication, although the actual number may be higher. Unfortunately, antidepressant medications have a very high incidence of causing side effects and adverse reactions in the elderly.

The tricyclic antidepressants (TCAs), including amitriptyline, imipramine, doxepin and nortriptyline, have been available since the 1950s. Although they remain in common use today, they are associated with several side effects in the elderly. Trazodone, although it is chemically different from the tricyclics, has similar effects and side effects. All these drugs can cause significant sedation and impairment of mental function in elderly patients. They also can result in dry mouth and urinary retention. Amitriptyline in particular has been reported to cause severe sedation in elderly patients, while desipramine is less likely to cause dry mouth and urinary retention (Semla, et al., 1997; Skerritt, et al., 1997).

All the tricyclic antidepressants are also associated with postural hypotension when used by elderly patients. Postural hypotension may occur as an adverse drug reaction when these are the only medication prescribed, but it is more commonly reported in patients who are also taking antihypertensive or cardiac medications. The tricyclics also are reported to result in cardiac dysrhythmias when used in combination with any of several different medications (Naranjo, et al., 1995; Skerritt, et al., 1997).

The selective serotonin reuptake inhibitors (SSRIs), such as fluoxetine, sertraline and paroxetine, are a newer class of antidepressants. When compared to the tricyclics, the SSRIs have a much lower incidence of postural hypotension and cardiac disturbances in elderly patients (Skerritt, et al., 1997). They also appear less likely to cause sedation or to have adverse effects on mental function (Preskorn, 1993). However, these drugs are likely to interfere with hepatic (pertaining to the liver) clearance of other drugs (Preskorn, 1993), and care must be taken when they are prescribed to elderly patients taking hepatically metabolized medications.

When TCAs are used in elderly patients, the dose must be significantly reduced in order to avoid toxic effects. However, individual patients metabolize these drugs at different rates, and it is quite possible for a reduced dose to result in inadequate concentrations of the drug in the body. Serum concentrations of all the tricyclic drugs can be determined by laboratory analysis, and this is recommended when this class of drugs is used to treat elderly patients (Eilers, 1995; Semla, et al., 1997). The SSRI antidepressants require only a slight reduction in dosage when used in elderly patients, and sertraline requires no dosage reduction at all (Preskorn, 1993).

16.72 Other Psychotropic Medications

Although the use of benzodiazepines is controversial, many elderly patients do take them for their tranquilizing or sedating effects. Benzodiazepine use is strongly associated with falls in elderly patients (Neutel, et al., 1996), and they are the most common causes of drug-overdose hospitalization in the elderly (Kruse, 1990). Benzodiazepines cause daytime sedation or deterioration of mental function in many, if not most, of the elderly patients who take them (Kruse, 1990).

As a general rule, the dose of benzodiazepines should be no more than half that used for young adults. Long-acting benzodiazepines, particularly diazepam, chlorazepate, flurazepam and quazepam, should not be used to treat elderly patients (Semla, et al., 1997). Oxazepam has a more predictable duration of action in elderly patients and is recommended by some authors (Johnson, 1997; Naranjo, et al., 1995). Buspirone, a nonbenzodiazepine tranquilizer, is also recommended (Naranjo, et al., 1995).

The antipsychotic tranquilizers are sometimes used to treat elderly patients who suffer from dementia or psychosis (Colenda, et al., 1996).

Elderly patients are extremely sensitive to the hypotensive and other side effects of these drugs, however, and only physicians who have broad experience with these drugs should prescribe them for elderly patients (Naranjo, et al., 1995). Carbamazepine has been reported to be an effective alternative to the neuroleptics and is not associated with hypotension. It does cause severe depression of white blood cell production in a few elderly patients, however (Lemke, 1995). Newer antipsychotic medications, such as clozapine and risperidone, may prove superior to the older agents, but their use has not been studied in the elderly (Colenda, et al., 1996).

16.73   Digitalis Preparations

The digitalis drugs are invaluable as inotropes—drugs that improve the contracting ability of the heart. They are used frequently to treat elderly patients with congestive heart failure and certain cardiac dysrhythmias, particularly atrial fibrillation or flutter. However, the absorption and metabolism of digitalis is notoriously unpredictable in elderly patients, and the drug has a very narrow range between effective dose and toxic dose. For this reason, serum concentrations of digitalis should be measured regularly until the dosage of medication is properly adjusted.

Elderly patients are much more likely to experience the toxic effects of digitalis than are younger patients, even when the dosage is regulated properly. Loss of appetite or nausea, visual changes, confusion and depression are commonly reported by elderly patients taking digitalis, although these effects may improve over time. Headache, muscular weakness and irregular heartbeat can also occur.

A number of other drugs interfere with digitalis absorption and metabolism. All antacids, most antidiarrhea preparations and many cholesterol binding drugs decrease the absorption of digitalis compounds, and patients should avoid taking these for several hours after taking digitalis. A number of drugs interfere with the metabolism of digitalis, and digitalis dosage should be reduced if any of these drugs are added to the patient's drug regimen. (*See Table 16-8.*) A few medications, including the hydantoins, increase the metabolism of digitalis, while diuretic medication can enhance digitalis toxicity by altering serum potassium levels (Semla, et al., 1997).

Table 16-8
Drugs Reducing Metabolism and Clearance of Digitalis

amiodarone	quinidine
captopril	quinine
diltiazem	spironolactone
erythromycin	tetracycline
ibuprofen	tolbutamide
indomethacin	verapamil
nifedipine	

16.74   Cimetidine

Cimetidine (Tagamet®) was the first H2 blocking agent introduced and the first to be available without a prescription. It is used to treat peptic ulcer disease and excess gastric acid. Cimetidine interferes with the hepatic metabolism of a number of drugs, including digitalis, benzodiazepines and beta-blockers. Although its effects are unpredictable, cimetidine can cause a marked elevated in the blood levels of these drugs. It also has been reported to cause sedation and confusion in elderly patients. For this reason, most authors recommend the use of a different H2 antagonist in elderly patients. Because the medication is available without prescription, however, elderly patients are likely to take cimetidine without their doctor's knowledge (Semla, et al., 1997).

16.100   BIBLIOGRAPHY

Text References

Ames, D. and Tuckwell, V.: Psychiatric Disorders Among Elderly Patients in a General Hospital. Med. J. Aust. 160:671-675, 1994.

Atkin, P. A., et al.: Functional Ability of Patients to Manage Medication Packaging: A Survey of Geriatric Inpatients. Age Ageing 23:113-116, 1994.

Banys, P.: Substance Abuse. In: Lonergan, E. T. (Ed.): Geriatrics. Stamford, Conn.: Appleton and Lang, 1996.

Borchelt, M.: Potential Side-Effects and Interactions of Multiple Medication in Elderly Patients: Methodology and Results of the Berlin Study of Aging. Z. Gerontol. Geriatr. 28:420-428, 1995.

Carlson, J. E.: Perils of Polypharmacy: 10 Steps to Prudent Prescribing. Geriatrics 51:26-35, 1996.

Colenda, C. C., et al.: Clinical Variables Influencing Treatment Decisions for Agitated Dementia Patients: Survey of Physician Judgments. J. Am. Geriatr. Soc. 44:1375-1379, 1996.

Davies, A. J. and Kenny, R. A.: Falls Presenting to the Accident and Emergency Department: Types of Presentation and Risk Factor Profile. Age Ageing 25:362-366, 1996.

Doucet, J., et al.: Drug-Drug Interactions Related to Hospital Admissions In Older Adults: A Prospective Study of 1000 Patients. J. Am. Geriatr. Soc. 44:944-948, 1996.

Eilers, R.: Therapeutic Drug Monitoring for the Treatment of Psychiatric Disorders:Clinical Use and Cost Effectiveness. Clin. Pharmacokinet. 29:442-450, 1995.

aunt, J. D., et al.: The Effete in the Heat: Heat-Related Hospital Presentations During a Ten Day Heat Wave. Aust. N.Z. J. Med. 25:117-121, 1995.

en, L. J., et al.: Assessment of Capacity to Comply with Medication egimens In Older Patients. J. Am. Geriatr. Soc. 43:361-367, 1995.

nberg, D. A.: Dementia. In: Lonergan, E. T. (Ed.): Geriatrics. mford, Conn.: Appleton and Lang, 1996.

blatt, D. J.: Basic Pharmacokinetic Principles and Their Applica- to Psychotropic Drugs. J. Clin. Psychiatry. 54:8-13, 1993.

n, F.: Psychiatric Disorders. In: Lonergan, E. T. (Ed.): Geriat- Stamford, Conn.: Appleton and Lang, 1996.

. J., et al.: Diagnosis and Assessment of Substance Abuse In Adults: Current Strategies and Issues. Addict. Behav. 55, 1994.

. H.: Problems and Pitfalls in the Use of Benzodiazepines lderly. Drug Saf. 5:328-344, 1990.

H.: Comprehensive Geriatric Assessment and Medication ce. Z. Gerontol. Geriatr.28:54-61, 1995.

R.: EffeConn. of Carbamazepine on Agitation in Al- Inpatients Refractory to Neuroleptics. J. Clin. Psychiatry. 7, 1995.

Liu, B. A., et al.: Falls Among Older People: Relationship to Medication Use and Orthostatic Hypotension. J. Am. Geriatr. Soc. 43:1141-1145, 1995.

Lonergan, E. T.: Medications. In Lonergan, E. T. (Ed.): Geriatrics. Stamford, Conn.: Appleton and Lang, 1996.

Naranjo, C. A.: Recent Advances in Geriatric Psychopharmacology. Drugs Ageing 7:184-202, 1995.

Neutel, C. I., et al.: New Evidence On Benzodiazepine Use and Falls: The Time Factor. Age Ageing 25:273-278, 1996.

Nikolaus, T., et al.: Assessment of Nutritional Risk in the Elderly. Ann. Nutr. Metab. 39:340-345, 1995.

Nikolaus, T., et al.: Elderly Patients' Problems With Medication. An In-Hospital and Follow-Up Study. Eur. J. Clin. Pharmacol. 49:255-259, 1996.

Preskorn, S. H.: Recent Pharmacologic Advances in Antidepressant Therapy for the Elderly. Am. J. Med. 94:2S-12S, 1993.

Roe, D. A.: Medications and Nutrition in the Elderly. Prim. Care 21:135-147, 1994.

Ruscin, J. M. and Semla, T. P.: Assessment of Medication Management Skills In Older Outpatients. Ann. Pharmacother. 30:1083-1088, 1996.

Sagar, S. M.: Gait Instability and Falls. In: Lonergan, E. T. (Ed.): Geriatrics. Stamford, Conn.: Appleton and Lang, 1996.

Schrader, S. L., et al.: The Medication Reduction Project: Combating Polypharmacy in South Dakota Elders Through Community-Based Interventions. S.D. J. Med. 49:441-448, 1996.

Semla, T. P., et al.: Geriatric Dosage Handbook. Cleveland: Lexi-Comp, 1997.

Sheehan, J., et al.: The Effects of Hospital Admission on Drug Prescribing in an Elderly Population. Ir. Med. J. 89:115-116, 1996.

Skerritt, U., et al.: Selective Serotonin Reuptake Inhibitors in Older Patients. A Tolerability Perspective. Drugs Aging 10:209-218, 1997.

Sorrento, T. A., et al.: Pharmaceutical Services in a Capitated Geriatric Care Program. Am. J. Health Syst. Pharm. 53:2848-2852, 1996.

Steiner, J. F.: Pharmacotherapy Problems in the Elderly. J. Am. Pharm. Assoc. 36:431-437, 1996.

Sternon, J. and Gilles, C.: Poly-medication and Drug Interactioni In Geriatrics. Rev. Med. Brux. 17:389-396, 1996.

Szwabo, P. A.: Substance Abuse in Older Women. Clin. Geriatr. Med. 9:197-208, 1993.

Troncale, J. A.: The Aging Process: Physiologic Changes and Pharmacologic Implications. Postgrad. Med. 99:11-114, 1996.

CHAPTER 17

PSYCHOLOGICAL ADAPTATION TO LONG-TERM CARE

> **SCOPE**
> Toward the end of the life cycle, a person normally has to cope with issues of endings and losses, as well as the natural waning of faculties. The superimposition of chronic illnesses (e.g., Alzheimer's disease, hip fractures) and the need for long-term care—common features of later life for the majority of people—accentuate the sense of decline and place further demands on the aging individual's coping resources. The nature and severity of a person's psychological reactions, as well as his or her ways of coping with them and adjusting to changed life circumstances, vary according to intrapersonal, environmental and other factors. Various models have been developed to describe and facilitate the process of adaptation to both chronic illness and long-term care. In the elderly, the relationship between physical health and mental health is particularly acute. The promotion of maximum adaptation to old age, chronic illness and long-term care should thus be given a high priority in the care of the elderly.

SYNOPSIS

17.100 BIBLIOGRAPHY

17.00   INTRODUCTION: THE ELDERLY

As do individuals in other stages of the life cycle, the elderly face unique challenges in adapting to chronic illness and its care. The added prominence of this group in contemporary health care discussions is due to its increasing numbers.

17.01   The Nature of the Adaptive Challenge

Toward the end of the life cycle, issues of endings and losses and the natural waning of faculties are the predominant realities and normal developmental tasks a person has to cope with and adapt to. In addition, approximately 8 in 10 elderly individuals have at least one chronic condition. The superimposition of chronic illness, which is often age-related (e.g., Alzheimer's disease, osteoporosis), and the need for long-term care place further demands on the aged individual's adaptive resources (Mockenhaupt, 1993).

The relation between physical health and mental health is particularly strong among the elderly (Kaufman, 1996). Any downswings in the course of a chronic physical illness will have significant adverse effects on the person's mental health. The promotion of maximum adaptation to old age, chronic illness and long-term care should thus be given a high priority in the care of the elderly.

17.02   Scope and Current Status of Long-term Care Among the Elderly

Approximately 35 percent of the elderly population require care in a long-term-care facility (e.g., nursing home) at some point during their lives, though only about 5 percent of the aged population is institutionalized at any given time (Kaplan and Sadock, 1994c). The nursing home population consists mainly of widowed women, about half of whom are past age 85 (Kaplan and Sadock, 1994c).

The family caregiver is usually a daughter or daughter-in-law. Within the health care system, the primary caregiver is the nurse. As with the chronic care situation in general, the need remains to refocus health care for the elderly on chronic care and away from acute care (Estes, et al., 1993). In recent years, rising health care costs and limited resources have sparked a somewhat negative attitude regarding the type and amount of health care that should be provided to the elderly (Walters, 1996).[1]

17.10 PSYCHOLOGICAL CHALLENGES OF NORMAL AGING

Normal aging brings with it various physical, psychological and social losses and declines with which the person must cope. All these age-related changes will be exaggerated by illness or distress. However, the need to be aware of individual differences is particularly important for accurate assessment and care of the elderly. In general, it appears that those with the best psychological functioning in youth end to show less decline in function with age (Twining, 1996). Thus lderly individuals with the best psychological functioning may inction as well as the average young person. This is also generally ie, within narrower limits, of physical functioning.

17.11 Cognitive Changes

'ognitive changes include changes in mental functioning, thinking language. Memory is perhaps the change most often thought of lation to the elderly, but a great amount of misunderstanding exists tactly what those changes are.

1] Memory

1ory changes are typically thought of as the most characteristic change in old age. In fact, although there is a decline in function the elderly as a group, the perceived extent of decline is ' due to confusion of observers concerning dementias. With ɔ short-term memory (the ability to remember events of the seconds or minutes), a person in her or his late 70s might) remember only six to eight items, for example, whereas n young adulthood might be able to recall seven to nine ining, 1996). The decline in short-term memory has little laily functioning, and any effect can easily be compensated nting information in a way that is within the older person's of these compensations have already been made at the , such as the "chunking" of telephone numbers into small an be easily remembered by people of any age. Similar

fra.

compensations should be made, if necessary, in providing medical and treatment information.

Long-term memory also shows a decline with aging, but the extent of the decline depends on the task. Recognition (prompted) memory is much less affected than unprompted memory. This suggests that the ability to retrieve information, not the ability to store it, is what is primarily affected by aging.

How new information is asked for and processed also has an effect on memory function. Older people tend to use less effective strategies in this regard; their memory can be improved by helping them learn and use effective strategies for acquiring and storing new information. Since older people expect to have worse memories, the self-fulfilling prophecy of perception can also be a factor in apparent memory impairment. Training in memory skills can help eliminate this source of memory problems.

Finally, the quality of memory may also be affected with age. In particular, older people tend to be less accurate in remembering, often confusing what they actually did with what they thought they did. Obviously, thinking that one took medication instead of actually taking it, for example, can have serious adverse effects on a treatment plan. The discrepancy between remembering things as being done rather than thought about or discussed can also create conflicts between the patient and the caregiver.

[2] Thinking and Language

The most prominent changes in thinking and language abilities involve declines in speed of information processing. Thus slowing down the presentation of information aids in the acquisition of it. This is true of people of all ages, but it is particularly important in presenting medical and treatment information to the elderly patient. Failure to understand staff prescriptions and instructions is a major reason for failure to adhere to them.

17.12 Personality and Emotional Changes

Although some small personality changes may occur with aging, notably increased emotional sensitivity and extroversion, continuity is the overwhelmingly predominant feature of personality at all ages. Marked changes in personality, with no obvious cause other than aging, may therefore be a sign of illness or distress.

Factors that may strongly influence a person's contentment and morale during older age are health, income and interpersonal relationships (Twining, 1996). Discontent, depression and loneliness in later life are generally related to poor health, poverty and/or family or other interpersonal difficulties. These areas are thus prime focal points for intervention. The emphasis, it is generally believed, should be on quality—not quantity—and this can be provided by even a small amount of contact with one trusted person the patient can confide in and communicate with.

Whether the older person should be active or "disengaged" on his or her rocking chair is a matter of individual variability. Either approach can represent healthy psychological adjustment in later life, depending on the personality of the individual.

Events that present the most serious challenges to adjustment in later life are long-term health problems, retirement, loss of spouse or close friends, and having to change one's home and living arrangements. Several of these may occur at once, as when a person's spouse dies and poor health forces him or her to move to a nursing home. At any rate stressful life events are better coped with one at a time. In the situation just cited, for example, family and friends should not pressure the person into moving out of his or her home immediately but should allow the individual some time to adjust. Rapid change, such as sudden illness or unexpected spousal death, is also more difficult to adjust to than slower, anticipated change for which the individual has time to prepare.

PSYCHOLOGICAL CHALLENGES OF CHRONIC ILLNESS

Knowledge of the psychological challenges of normal aging, as described, is essential for assisting the elderly individual in facing chronic illness and long-term care. Specific issues and concerns are described in the following sections.

Grief and Loss

In the elderly, reactions to chronic illness and care are often accompanied by feelings of grief, anxiety and depression; issues of personal loss are also a focus. All these must be managed to assure maximum adaptation to the condition and compliance with care. Although specialists in clinical psychology will play an important role, the primary responsibility for management of the patient's emotional state belongs to the health care team and, under their guidance, the family caregiver.

Grief and loss are not unique to old age, but some features of bereavement in the elderly are more characteristic of later life than of other stages in the life cycle. Moreover, a grief reaction may be precipitated by any type of major loss, including loss of a loved one, loss of bodily or mental function due to a chronic condition and its treatment, loss of hoped-for goals and loss of what is perceived of as a previous self.

[1] Loss of a Loved One

Loss of a loved one may occur at any age, but the cumulative grief of multiple losses of people who have been close to the person for a long time is more characteristic of later life. (A notable exception is the experience of younger people during the HIV/AIDS, epidemic, particularly in the 1980s. Many, in fact, compared their experience of multiple losses of close friends to the experiences of their grandparents.) Loss of adult children is an experience that is, of necessity, virtually unique to later life. It is a major source of distress, and adjustment is typically very difficult.

The grief reaction has been described in terms of phases, which usually include an initial stage of psychic shock or numbing, characterized by disbelief and absence of feeling; acute grief, characterized by painful longings; and integration or assimilation, characterized by gradual acceptance of the loss at an emotional level and adaptation to life without the lost person.

Adjustment and adaptation can be a long process. It does not follow a straightforward path through these phases; anniversaries and other reminders can trigger acute feelings of grief months or years after the lost person's death. Other factors that affect adaptation include the circumstances of the loss, the quality of the relationship and the availability of support. Most people do not need professional grief counseling. However, this should be provided to those at risk for complex grief and impaired adjustment; for example, when the departed person died suddenly while the bereaved was on bad terms with him or her and/or if the bereaved person has little or nothing in the way of a support group in daily life.

[2] Loss of Function

The loss or impairment of function caused by a chronic condition and its treatment can precipitate a grief reaction similar to that caused by the loss of a loved one. This is especially true of conditions with sudden onset, such as stroke (cerebrovascular accident, or CVA)[2] (Hayn and Fisher, 1997). A major difference between the grief reaction to loss of function and that due to loss of a loved one is that in the former case, the loss of function usually follows serious illness, as in stroke. During the acute phase, pain, unconsciousness and threat to life may be present, so that grief and emotional support or counseling are not priorities at this time.

The point at which psychological issues emerge and need to be addressed varies with the individual. Often the person's reaction to treatment is a good guide, with episodes of acute distress or problems of motivation signaling problems with adjustment. In general, patients will not express problems directly to staff they perceive as having high status (that is, the physician) but will rather confide in "lower status" staff members during a bath or treatment session. The home visit, taking place in the more familiar and secure environment of the person's home, is often the best setting for discovering and addressing psychological issues. Often, therefore, the visiting nurse is the member of the health care team who is most likely to be the source of information and intervention.

The family as well as other patients may be important sources of emotional support. They can also be the source of inaccurate information and misleading advice, however. It is thus important for the nurse to keep in touch with the patient's perceptions about his or her condition and progress.[3]

Discharge from the hospital can also be a threatening experience, especially following prolonged rehabilitation. A change in the person's role is being forced on him or her again, and the new life with a chronic condition holds many uncertainties. This can cause psychological problems out of proportion to the actual functional impairment.

[3] Loss of Hoped-for Goals

Lowered expectations for the future are another potential source of loss, grief and mourning. Whether a person will be able to return home

---

[2] See also ch. 8.

[3] See 17.31 infra.

and recover sufficient mobility for independent living are common questions during the early period of chronic illness. All health care professionals need to be versed in the skills necessary to communicate the need for lowered expectations and other "bad news" to the patient.

Fortunately, such skills can be learned. The objective in presenting bad news is to bridge the gap between the reality of the situation and what the patient knows or perceives about it, in order to make these two perspectives as congruent as possible. This can require a very delicate balancing act. The tendency is to err on the side of optimism. This is usually advisable, in fact, in the early stages of treatment, in order to promote motivation and a positive attitude. Sometimes, as with stroke patients, for example, the outcome really is unpredictable, so that excessive pessimism, at any rate, is not justified. On the other hand, excessive optimism in the beginning can create disillusionment and compliance problems later on, if goals have to be lowered. This, and discharge from the hospital itself, can also give rise to feelings of abandonment. Patients may become entrenched in the belief that more therapy and/or different therapists are what is needed in order to realize the original expectations. They may be right or wrong about this.

In general, the approach in communicating with the patient should be positive and focused on skills attained rather than on failures and losses. How much the patient wants to know and how he or she should best be told must also be taken into account.

[4]　Loss of Previous Self

Finally, all the losses just described add up to an overall sense of a loss of the former self. Psychotherapies aimed at helping the person redefine his or her self-concept, sources of self-esteem, body image and so on can be useful in helping the person integrate the losses and adjustments to them into a new sense of self that feels, of necessity, different but not diminished as a person.[4]

[5]　Reminiscence and Life Review

It has been suggested that for the elderly, thinking about the past and telling others about it are both important parts of coming to terms with one's mortality and a potential form of therapy. The role and effects of reminiscence are rather complex, however (Gibson, 1994).

---

[4] *See* 17.44 *infra.*

For one thing, people of all ages engage in reminiscence and life review. Moreover, life review is not necessary for good adjustment to later life. There are maladaptive patterns of reminiscence, in which only the bad and distressing experiences of life are recalled and dwelled on; alternatively, all thought of the past may be avoided. No universal rule can be made, therefore, about the benefits or disadvantages of reminiscence and life review.

The psychological astuteness and skill of the clinician are critical in selecting those patients for whom therapy might be helpful and for facilitating their recollections. The use of the richness of an older person's life stories in person-centered psychotherapy may suggest helpful ways to approach the psychological problems that arise in connection with long-term care and rehabilitation, but few outcome data are available on the efficacy of this (Viney, 1993).

17.22 Anxiety

Although depression and dementia are symptoms more commonly requiring psychiatric intervention in the elderly, from 5 to 10 percent of the aged suffer from anxiety of clinical proportions (Twining, 1996). The anxiety-based disorder of *agoraphobia* (fear of leaving familiar surroundings), for example, most commonly follows a recent trauma, such as a fall, fracture or mugging.

One major manifestation of anxiety related to the accompanying sense of vulnerability is loss of confidence. Thus anxiety can not only keep an older person housebound but can interfere with motivation and the ability to follow a treatment plan.

Anxiety in the elderly is treated in essentially the same way as it is in younger people; that is, with anxiolytic medications and/or psychotherapeutic interventions such as relaxation exercises. One valuable modification for the elderly is the use of taped relaxation programs, which can be adjusted to a comfortable decibel level for the individual patient's hearing capacity. This eliminates the contradictory need for the therapist to shout soothing relaxation instructions and for the patient to strain in order to hear them.

17.23 Depression, Mortality and Suicidal Intent

Depression is relatively common among older persons in poor health and among those who are having difficulty coming to terms with their mortality. Common symptoms of depression include disturbances of appetite and sleep patterns, irritability, loss of interest in activities and interpersonal relationships that were formerly enjoyed, having feelings and making remarks about being worthless, thoughts that life is no longer worth living, and impairments of memory, cognition, concentration and judgment. It is essential that health care personnel as well as family and friends appreciate that depression is a maladaptive response to life events (such as chronic illness) that is now highly treatable.

Depression can lead to suicide. The rate of suicide among the elderly is high (40 per 100,000 people) (Kaplan and Sadock, 1994c), but the rate of attempted suicide is low (Twining, 1996). Based on these facts, it must be concluded that expressions of suicidal wishes or intentions must be taken seriously. On the other hand, many older individuals express the idea that life is no longer worth living and that they will be glad when their time has come but have no suicidal intent. These may be individuals who are in particularly poor health or individuals who have come to terms with their mortality and feel that they have had a satisfying life that should now come to its inevitable end. It is clearly important to distinguish between these different types of individuals.

A number of simple screening tests for depression have been devised. These should be used in combination with clinical skill to assess a person's potential for suicide. One common distinction is that those who express the wish to die but have no real desire to do so typically find satisfaction in what the present and the future have to offer and have undiminished interest and enjoyment in customary activities and social contacts.

17.30   DETERMINANTS OF PSYCHOLOGICAL REACTIONS

The nature and severity of a person's reactions to chronic illness and long-term care will be influenced by a variety of factors beyond the chronic condition and treatment themselves. These factors include personal coping resources and external support networks as well as barriers to adaptation. Intervention is aimed at maximizing adaptation through facilitation and/or bolstering of coping and support resources, and minimizing or eliminating barriers.

17.31 Perceptions, Values and Beliefs About Health and Illness

The effectiveness—indeed, the very acceptance—of health care is related to a person's perceptions, values and beliefs about health and illness (Kaufman, 1996). In other words, a person's health-related behavior is influenced by how he or she views and defines health and illness. This is particularly true of the elderly. When the definition of health used by a health care professional differs in important ways from that of the elderly patient, it is likely that medical advice will be discounted by the patient.

For example, the definition of health subscribed to by most health care professionals is the one offered by the World Health Organization (WHO) in the 1940s; namely, that health is a "state of complete physical, mental, and social well-being, and not merely the absence of disease or infirmity" (Kaufman, 1996). But between 75 percent and 85 percent of elderly patients have at least one chronic condition, so the WHO definition will leave them puzzled and confused, at best. Worse, they may assume that they are unhealthy, when their health status may be normal for their age.

Many studies have found a strong link among the elderly between self-assessment of health status and survival (Idler and Kasl, 1995). Moreover, at a given level of health status, the older the person, the better her or his self-assessed health is likely to be. It is thus crucial to the promotion of adherence and adaptation to long-term care for the clinician to determine the patient's perceptions and definition of health at the very beginning of the doctor-patient relationship. Without this, the relationship and the patient's health care will be off in the wrong direction from the outset.

17.32 Autonomy

The question of patient autonomy is a complex one that involves ethical as well as medical and psychological issues. The central dilemma involves how to safeguard the patient's right to personal control while providing optimum long-term health care, including promotion of risk reduction and a healthier life-style (Rice, et al., 1997).

The concept of personal autonomy has been a central tenet in biomedical ethics for the past two decades (Kane, 1995). It is generally agreed that attempts at coercing (versus encouraging) a person to follow prescribed treatment and a health-promoting life-style are both ethically wrong and psychologically unproductive; in fact, attempts at coercion are usually counterproductive. A new ethic has emerged in the 1990s, however; known as *collectivism,* it asserts the rights of society to expect individual citizens to curb their independence to the extent of forgoing unhealthy behaviors such as smoking and overeating that result in their becoming a burden on society in terms of health care costs and resources consumed in later life (Clark, 1991). Attempts to implement this new ethic by both government and private insurance companies include measures such as health care rationing (denying access to certain procedures, such as organ transplants) (Walters, 1996) and differential pricing policies for healthy as opposed to unhealthy life-style practices (e.g., nonsmoking vs. smoking) (Kelly and Maas, 1994). In general, however, the elderly have not yet been held accountable for past unhealthy behaviors (Gerety, 1994). Neither has the government stopped giving mixed messages, such as advocating smoking cessation and maintenance of healthy weight on the one hand and refusing to allow Medicare or Medicaid reimbursement for smoking cessation or weight loss clinics on the other (Rice, et al., 1997).

Although the collectivist position is certainly not merely academic, the reality of the individual's plight on entering the health care system—and the need for advocacy on behalf of personal control—can be seen quite clearly in the experience of elderly individuals who are institutionalized for long-term care (Estes, 1993). The health care system, which has been described as a "higher power" (Rice, et al., 1997), is sprawling, alien, intimidating, paternalistic and subtly coercive (Gamroth, et al., 1995). Because the current generation of elderly people were socialized to believe in the absolute power of authority figures, they tend to relinquish control more readily than do younger individuals, thus magnifying their vulnerability to the higher power (Rice, et al., 1997). It is essential to the working relationship among health care providers, patients and their families that health care providers begin to teach patients and their families about the system and their options and rights within it.

Providers should encourage elderly patients and their families to become partners in their own health care and to accept services that are offered, but they should not try to coerce them. It must be remembered that what is being promoted is better health care through patient autonomy. Numerous studies have shown a strong positive correlation between a sense of personal control and physical and emotional well-being and quality of life (Barder, et al., 1994). Conversely, when a person is deprived of control or a role in the decision-making process, a phenomenon known as *postdecision dissonance* occurs, which correlates with low morale, poor quality of life and excess mortality (Rodin and Tribo, 1992). Some authors have made a distinction between autonomy and decision making: An individual who elects to designate another person to make health care decisions on his or her behalf, for example, is considered to be exercising autonomy, even though he or she will not take part in the decision-making process beyond this fundamental initial decision.

[1] Cognitive Impairment

The issue of autonomy is further complicated among the elderly by the question of cognitive impairment (CI) and the impending issue of death and dying.[5] Approximately 75 percent of elderly patients in nursing homes are cognitively impaired due to causes such as senile dementia of the Alzheimer type (SDAT) (Beck and Vogelpohl, 1995). Often these individuals have had to be institutionalized to protect both themselves and their families, because their cognitive impairment makes them functionally dependent.

Unfortunately, admission to a custodial setting further exacerbates the cognitive impairment, due to further loss of independence (e.g., loss of decision-making power), loss of privacy, loss of familiar surroundings and routines, and regimentation (Reinhardy, 1995). To date, little data exist as to what constitutes autonomy for cognitively impaired persons or how best to intervene in order to preserve as much autonomy for them as possible (Beck and Vogelpohl, 1995).

[2] Impediments to Autonomy

Several impediments to autonomy have been identified; these are especially prominent with the cognitively impaired, but they are problems all elderly patients face (Vogelpohl, et al., 1996). First, health care providers tend to have low expectations of what an impaired elderly person is capable of; as a result, these patients achieve at the low level expected of them. This is seen in the setting of goals that are too low. Rather than assessing the elderly patient's abilities

---

[5] *See* 17.33 *infra.*

comprehensively and identifying strengths as well as weaknesses, health care workers tend to generalize and conclude that because an elderly person has poor function in one area, he or she must have poor function in all areas.

Codified (generalized) institutional policies and regulations contribute to this lack of individualized, control-enhancing care, as does high rate of staff turnover and poor staff understanding of dementia and other cognitive impairments. Society at large contributes its own adverse effects to the autonomy of elders by valuing dependence over autonomy, compliance over individuality and youth over aging, and by failing to support policies and funding aimed at maintaining autonomy in health care among the elderly. Finally, the elderly themselves present an impediment to their autonomy by being willing, because of their socialization, to go along with these societal values and the attitudes and pronouncements of authorities.

Of course, the question must be answered: When does the degree of cognitive impairment make a substitute decision maker (guardian) necessary? Unfortunately, few good assessment instruments exist for making this determination, and family caregivers, professional health care providers and lawyers frequently have different views as to which areas should be assessed in determining incapacity or disability (Kjervik, et al., 1993). It seems clear, however, that revision of the laws governing guardianship in this area would be beneficial (Coker and Johns, 1992; Rice et al., 1997).

In brief, the court assigns responsibility to a guardian to care for another person whom the court has found incapable of managing his or her own affairs. Guardianship is assigned as limited (partial: e.g., money management) or plenary (full: supervision of all aspects of the person's life). In addition to the problem of monitoring the guardianship, it is very difficult to have the terms changed from more to less restrictive. Thus, the patient becomes trapped in loss of autonomy. Cognitive impairment is changeable over time in many patients, and the law does not reflect this (Gerety, 1994) or the fact that when individuals are able to be autonomous, they should be permitted to be. This would require better monitoring and better assessment methods, however, than are now in use.

17.33 Issues of Death and Dying

The elderly, as well as those with chronic conditions whose status is terminal (e.g., cancer, HIV/AIDS), need to address issues of death and dying in addition to all the other issues involved in having a chronic condition that requires long-term care. The issue of decision making about one's own death and dying is, in fact, an extension of the issue of autonomy in health care just discussed (Husted and Husted, 1995). Current opinion in biomedical ethics is that a competent, independent adult has the right to choose final treatment as well as treatment that will be administered prior to a condition's becoming terminal (Beauchamp and Childress, 1995).

[1]   Advance Directives

A number of mechanisms are available to the individual for making his or her decisions on final treatment known. These may be put into effect in anticipation of future incompetence and dependence and include natural death acts (NDAs), advance directives regarding treatment and proxies (so-called living wills) (Annas, 1991; Winslade, 1991; Rice, et al., 1997).

NDAs were first introduced in Indiana in 1969, in response to the consumer movement for greater patient participation in one's own health care. They consist of broad written specifications of the types of treatment the person does and does not want a physician to administer when he or she is no longer able to make such decisions.

Since 1969, most of the other states have enacted statutes that provide for living wills (advance directives). Approximately 1 in 10 adults in the United States has a living will (Rice, et al, 1997). Two types of living will are generally recognized: patient-specified treatment instructions and designation of a proxy (Winslade, 1991).

Patient-specified treatment instructions specify the types of treatment a person does or does not want a physician to administer in the event that the patient is not competent to participate in the decision. Difficulties with patient-specified advance directives may arise due to differences in laws from state to state. For example, some states recognize living wills only if they have been written after the person has become terminally ill. Other states require living wills to be updated periodically. In some cases, the type of treatment an elderly patient can refuse is limited to "extraordinary" or artificial measures.

Designation of proxy directives involve the appointment, by the patient or the court, of a surrogate individual who is authorized to make treatment decisions for the patient, in light of wishes the patient has previously made known to the surrogate. The surrogate thus serves as a "durable power of attorney" (DPA). To date, the DPA option has been used infrequently by elderly individuals. Two disadvantages of the DPA are the challenge of finding someone willing to take on the responsibilities, and the need for a lawyer to legitimize the arrangement.

Physician compliance with the written directives set out in both types of living will has been problematic. In general, there is a tendency for physicians to give precedence to considerations of what they believe to constitute proper medical care over the patient's autonomous wishes (Rice, et al., 1997). The reasons for this deserve investigation.

The implementation of the Patient Self-Determination Act (PSDA) in 1990 gives all hospitals that receive Medicare and Medicaid funds the following obligations (Mezey, et al., 1994; Pinch and Parsons, 1992):

- to provide all patients with information about their rights to accept or reject treatment and to draw up advance directives;

- to provide staff and community education on the use of advance directives, including the relevant law and hospital policy;

- to assure that the patient's medical record reflects his or her status with respect to advance directives;

- to assure that there is no discrimination against or conditional care practiced with patients who do not have an advance directive; and

- to maintain written policies and procedures for adherence to the Patient Self-Determination Act.

Although the enactment of the PSDA has led to an increase in the number of health care professionals encouraging patients to formulate advance directives, the law itself provides no mechanism to enforce physician compliance. Thus, implementation and enactment of the PSDA rests with the institutions and care providers. Explaining to patients and their families the provisions of the law and implications of patient decisions can be a challenging task. The task is made somewhat easier for all if the materials describing advance directives are presented at an elementary (e.g., sixth-grade reading level) rather than an advanced level (Rice, et al., 1997).

[2]   Euthanasia and Professional-assisted Suicide

Finally, there is the question of the patient's right to die, usually taken to mean "with dignity." Two types of euthanasia (literally, "good death") are recognized in the context of health care: passive and active (Bandman and Bandman, 1995). In *passive euthanasia,* the person is allowed to die without medical intervention. *Active euthanasia* involves the administration of a death-facilitating agent (commonly a high dose of morphine). Although neither suicide nor attempted suicide is illegal under state laws, active euthanasia is illegal (Bosek and Jezuit, 1995). Moreover, active euthanasia is not officially supported by either the American Medical Association or the American Nurses Association. The reality, however, regarding both attitudes and behavior, is another matter.

Professional-assisted suicide (PAS), for example, has been brought to prominence by Dr. Jack Kevorkian, dubbed Dr. Death by the media. Dr. Kevorkian has avoided conviction for active euthanasia by providing the means to death (a device that delivers a lethal dose of carbon monoxide) but allowing the patient to self-administer it. To date, the courts have found in favor of the individual's right to request and receive assistance in dying (Rice, et al., 1997). One recent study (Young, et al., 1993) found that 44 percent of oncology nurses favored PAS in selected cases, although most said they would hesitate to administer the lethal agent themselves. In another study done two years later, 60 percent of oncology and dementia care nurses said they not only supported active euthanasia but would be willing to participate (Davis, et al., 1995). In a more recent study (Asch, 1996), 16 percent of critical care nurses interviewed reported that they had engaged in active euthanasia or PAS when they were requested to do so.

The ethical, legal and medical debate over professional-assisted dying is complex and ongoing (see, for example, Beauchamp and Childress, 1995; Husted and Husted, 1995; Bandman and Bandman, 1995). The most common complaint of the elderly—pain—also provides an illustration of the complexities and subtleties of the issue. The desire for relief from intolerable pain appears to be the most common reason patients seek PAS (van Duynhoven, 1995). Many have thoughts of suicide and consider death to be their safety valve and way out if life becomes unbearable. The thought that there is one form of release actually offers a little comfort in providing some sense of control over the situation. On the other hand, it is well recognized that pain management remains inadequate and poorly understood by the majority of health care professionals (van Duynhoven, 1995). Among the many forms of pain mismanagement, for example, is undermedication of pain due to mistaken adherence to the old notion that patients will become addicted to painkillers that are prescribed for too long and in too large a dose. Effective pain management by knowledgeable practitioners may represent an alternative to PAS in this case (van Duynhoven, 1995).

Although it is not clear whether any shift in attitudes has occurred among the medical or nursing professions, those who support PAS tend to cite the precedence of the autonomy of the individual as the rationale for their ethical position. Given that the nursing profession has the largest membership of any health care profession as well as the greatest scope and depth of involvement with the elderly and those with chronic conditions, it has been suggested that nurses should take the lead in setting the future agenda for health policy and research on health care for the aged (Rice, et al., 1997).

17.34 Compliance

An essential component of successful long term care is patient compliance (also called adherence) with prescribed treatment. Unfortunately, poor compliance is a significant problem in all areas of medicine. The severity of the problem is illustrated by the example of patients with hypertension (high blood pressure). One study found that half of this patient population does not comply with treatment at all, and of those who do comply initially, half leave treatment within a year (Kaplan and Sadock, 1994a).

Poor adherence to treatment regimens is more common among psychiatric patients than among medical patients. As a general rule, approximately a third of all patients adhere to prescribed treatment, another third comply with some of their prescription some of the time, and a third never comply (Kaplan and Sadock, 1994a).

In addition to taking prescribed medications properly, compliance includes matters such as completing a course of treatment that has been entered into, keeping scheduled appointments and making recommended dietary, life-style and behavioral changes. A number of factors influencing the rate of compliance have been identified. Factors that have been associated with decreased compliance include the following (Kaplan and Sadock, 1994b):

- overly complicated treatment regimen (e.g., more than three medications per day or more than four daily doses per medication);

- multiple physicians;

- poor doctor-patient relationship;

- resentment or lack of trust in physician or other caregivers; lack of confidence in self;

- slow onset of beneficial effects of treatment;

- early onset and persistence of side effects (especially if not noticed and corrected by the clinician);

- low perceived risk of relapse if treatment is interrupted;

- lack of patient information/education about the treatment plan;

- financial hardship;

- conflicting obligations;

- illiteracy, confusion and/or cognitive deficits (e.g., memory impairment), impaired hearing, impaired vision;

- psychopathology (for example, psychosis, paranoid delusions, personality splitting, anxiety, fear, hopelessness, ambivalence, denial, controlling, passive-aggression, passive dependence, masochism, sociopathy, substance abuse); and

- inevitable human error.

Race, sex, intelligence, marital status, socioeconomic status, educational level and religion have not been clearly associated with rates of adherence to treatment (Kaplan and Sadock, 1994a).

The most important factor influencing compliance is the doctor-patient relationship. Personal qualities of the clinician that increase compliance include mature age; experience; willingness to spend time talking to the patient, during which the clinician displays interest, enthusiasm and permissiveness; and punctuality in keeping the appointment (short waiting room time).

The quality of communication within the doctor-patient relationship is equally important. Compliance is increased when the physician takes the time to discover and understand the patient's priorities, expectations, style of communication and system of beliefs, values and perceptions, and to include the patient as a participant in his or her own health care. This includes making sure that the patient knows the names and effects of each of the medications being taken or procedures being undergone, and the reason, benefits, risks and expected outcomes of the treatment plan.

The patient's subjective feelings are as important as objective medical facts in this regard. A patient must believe that he or she is ill in order to be motivated to comply with treatment; asymptomatic illnesses such as hypertension pose a particular challenge because of this.

Close supervision and effective communication on the part of the clinician satisfy the patient's subjective sense that the physician has met expectations and increases patient compliance. A number of strategies to improve compliance have been suggested. Most fundamentally, to assure that the clinician understands the patient's point of view and to foster rapport, the patient should be asked to answer the following questions: What do you believe is wrong with you? What do you believe should be done about it? What do you believe I believe should be done? What do you believe to be the benefits and risks of following the treatment plan I've recommended?

If possible, no more than three medications per day should be prescribed, and none should have to be taken in more than four daily doses. Information and instructions regarding treatment should be given to the patient in written form, since patients often forget or misunderstand purely verbal instructions. The patient should be asked to read the instructions back; to state explicitly what medications should be taken, in what amounts and when; and to ask any questions he or she might have about the instructions and information. These measures are especially important with elderly patients, who often have impaired hearing or vision that prevents them from receiving the information being communicated. For elderly patients, fine print should be avoided in any written instructions or informational material.

When patients fail to comply deliberately rather than due to error, a patient contract should be negotiated between the patient and the clinician. Deliberate noncompliance is often due to legitimate problems caused by conflicting obligations of time, work or family. The contract allows mutual expectations to be spelled out. It can be renegotiated, and either party can make suggestions regarding how compliance might be improved. In this way, while perfect compliance may not be achieved, better adherence to treatment may be. In the case of an elderly patient with cognitive impairment, the family caregiver must be included in the these discussions and measures.

17.35 Illness Behavior and the Sick Role

The ability to accept the sick role and to engage in appropriate, health-promoting illness behavior is also important to adaptation to long-term care. Models of adaptation,[6] such as the coping skills model, derived from integrative field theories, hold both internal thoughts and feelings and external events (both physical and social) to be important (Rohe, 1993). These models have given rise to the concepts of illness behavior and the sick role.

Illness behavior describes the patient's reactions to being ill. The *sick role* is the role society assigns to a person who is ill. Five stages of illness behavior have been identified (Kaplan and Sadock, 1994a):

1. the experience of symptoms, during which the person realizes that something is wrong;

2. taking on of the sick role, during which the person decides that professional care is needed;

3. contact with providers of medical care, during which medical care is sought;

4. taking on of the dependent-patient role, during which the person decides to relinquish control to the health care provider and to follow prescribed treatment; and

5. recovery or rehabilitation, during which the person decides to give up the patient role.

As with other stage models, these reactions are not universally applicable to all patients; neither will a given patient be likely to progress linearly through the stages. Getting stuck in any of the stages is quite possible and represents a challenge to adaptation and signals a need for intervention. Refusal to relinquish the dependent-patient role, for example, lies at the other end of the spectrum of illness behavior from noncompliance with treatment and is just as problematic. In the case of chronic illness, and particularly among the elderly, appropriate adjustment to the "patient" role can present a difficult challenge, since unlike the patient with an acute illness, the chronically

---

[6] *See* 17.50 *infra.*

ill person will, in fact, always be a patient. What the chronically ill person must be helped to focus on is gaining as much independence as possible and understanding the positive role of health care in helping achieve that.

A number of factors influence the nature of a person's illness behavior and sick role. These include previous experience with illness; personality makeup and personal beliefs about health and disease;[7] and cultural beliefs about health and disease.[8]

17.40 STRATEGIES FOR ADAPTING TO LONG-TERM CARE

Even when the patient's physical condition is one that is not likely to change, especially in a chronic illness, long-term care is not static. Developing strategies, either consciously or unconsciously, to deal with the situation, will either help or hinder, depending on whether these strategies are positive or negative.

17.41 Patient and Family Education and Counseling

Because patients and their families are now expected to administer many aspects of treatment at home, even when complex diseases are involved, a sound understanding of the patient's condition and its treatment on the part of both patient and family caregiver is essential. Patient/family education and counseling programs have been established to meet this demand (Butcher, 1994).

Equally important in this equation is meeting the needs of the family caregivers (Jones and Lester, 1994). Studies have found that those who care for an elderly relative experience significantly more emotional distress (including depression and grief reactions) and more adverse health effects than do matched controls who are not involved in caregiving (Worcester and Hedrick, 1997). In addition to sheer physical and mental exhaustion, these increased negative effects are due to disruption of family and personal routines, forced role changes, assumption of new responsibilities and a diminished sense of control (Milne, et al., 1994).

It is very important to the well-being of both caregivers and those being cared for that these negative effects on caregivers be addressed

---

[7] *See* 17.31 *supra.*

[8] *See* 17.47 *infra.*

and managed. One means for achieving this is respite care, an informal or a formal arrangement in which someone relieves the primary caregiver of his or her responsibilities for a time. Curiously, although family caregivers commonly express the need and desire for respite, and despite the fact that respite providers are increasingly available, caregivers typically request respite too infrequently and too late in the trajectory of the patient's illness to avoid negative effects on caregivers' health (Theis, et al., 1994). The result can be "burnout" of the caregiver, institutionalization of the patient and disruption of the entire family.

The principal reasons cited for not using respite include concerns that respite providers will not understand how to communicate with the patient or the complexities of his or her condition and needs; feelings of imposing on the respite provider; and feeling imposed on by the respite provider. In general, caregivers report finding respite more stressful than beneficial (Worcester and Hedrick, 1997).

Family caregivers must be helped to understand that respite is not a luxury but a necessity (Jackson and Cleary, 1995). Nurses and other health care professionals can assist family caregivers in finding ways to make respite acceptable. Promising approaches currently being investigated include forming a partnership between family caregivers, patients and respite providers in order to match compatibilities; allow the caregiver, patient and respite provider to get to know one another; and assure the caregiver and patient that the patient's needs will be adequately met in the caregiver's absence (Hutchinson and Quartyaro, 1995). Various community organizations also publish informational literature that can aid families in identifying their needs and working with a variety of respite providers (e.g., Task Force on Aging, 1996).

17.42   Attitudes of Caregivers

Individuals with chronic conditions are more likely than acute-care patients to experience negative attitudes from the health care staff, according to a number of studies (Murrow and Oglesby, 1996). Naturally such attitudes are detrimental to the patient's health care and his or her adaptation to it. This issue is particularly critical as concerns the nursing staff, since the chronically ill individual's predominant health care need is for nursing care.

A number of possible explanations for these negative attitudes have been offered. For example, although some acute care nurses find working with the chronically ill to be more challenging and creative than providing acute care, most find chronic care to be discouraging and beneath their level of knowledge and skills. This may be in part because the emphasis nursing schools place on acute care in the hospital setting leaves nurses with less understanding of the nature and demands of chronic illness and thus less prepared to care for these patients.

Providing long-term care for people with chronic illness may also be considered less prestigious than providing acute care, because of the latter's highly technical methods and more dramatic atmosphere. While patients with acute conditions can generally be expected to respond dramatically and predictably to treatment—and be cured—patients with chronic conditions respond unpredictably to treatment, exhibit a downward course overall and generally cannot be expected to be cured. The usual source of satisfaction in administering treatment is thus missing from chronic care. Individuals providing chronic illness care must therefore be taught that satisfaction is to be derived from the act of performing a valuable service for the patient and not from witnessing or contributing to improvement or ultimate cure of the illness.

In addition to the negative attitudes that many hold regarding chronic illness and the people it afflicts, the elderly also face negative attitudes toward aging, death and dying. Health care professionals who work with the elderly should be helped to identify and overcome any problems they may have in this area; otherwise less than optimum patient care, not to mention provider stress, will result.

[1]   Interpersonal Skills ("Bedside Manner")

Good interpersonal skills (commonly known as bedside manner) are a necessity, not a luxury, for providing effective, quality health care. Fortunately, it is now appreciated that such skills can be learned and improved through practice (Twining, 1996). Technology, especially employing videotape, has greatly facilitated the teaching of interpersonal skills. Effective communication, in particular, effective listening, is perhaps the core skill. Although good interpersonal skills are essential for providing effective care to patients of all ages, their application to caring for the elderly is particularly important and challenging.

[2]   Societal Attitudes

The attitudes of society as a whole also tend to be more negative toward people with a chronic condition (Murrow and Oglesby, 1996). This stems from the norms of societal expectations regarding people's appearance, activities, abilities, roles and so on. Anyone who deviates from these expected norms will be labeled as different and may be stigmatized.

The degree of stigmatization varies with the type of chronic condition and the social context as well as the person's gender, race and individual characteristics. For example, conditions that are more threatening or anxiety-provoking in others (e.g., AIDS and cancer) will tend to elicit a stronger stigma.

The results of stigmatization include discrimination, devaluation, social isolation and even threats to safety. The stigmatized person may attempt to escape the harsh realities of prejudice and stereotyping by minimizing or denying his or her condition. This implies ignoring treatment as well, so that the entire adaptive process is undermined. If this situation is carried to the extreme, the person may become socially isolated and withdrawn from all of life, not just the stigma. Unfortunately, the adjustments a person makes in a genuine and healthy effort to adapt and function at maximum potential can also accentuate the appearance and sense of being different, which can in turn exacerbate stigmatization and all the adverse effects it brings with it.

Important changes in societal attitudes have been brought about to some degree by consciousness-raising public education measures and changes in public policy, such as passage of the Americans with Disabilities Act in 1990. Although these measures should continue, the most effective way to help chronically ill individuals cope with and overcome the effects of stigmatization is probably through helping them establish (or recover) a sense of their own intrinsic worth as people. They must be helped to see that they are not their disease; rather, they are unique people who happen to have an additional challenge in their life. This can be done through simple day-to-day support and encouragement from the nursing staff, as well as more formally, through support groups, family counseling, individual therapy and education.

The youth orientation of American culture is legendary. In addition to being recipients of negative societal attitudes toward chronic illness, the elderly are also subject to the stigmas attached to aging, death, and dying. Even when elders attempt to remain socially active, they may find access to mainstream society denied by both physical and social barriers. On the other hand, the older person's perceptions or misperceptions of the attitudes and reactions of society toward them can significantly influence those attitudes and reactions and help determine their level of acceptance. Organizations established to serve the interests of older people, such as the American Association of Retired Persons (AARP), provide valuable support in a variety of ways to elders in society.

One extreme but pervasive manifestation of negative social attitudes toward the aged is elder abuse. This can take the form of physical, sexual, psychological or financial abuse as well as neglect (Kingston and Phillipson, 1994). Elder abuse may occur in any setting—in institutions such as hospitals and nursing homes, within the home care setting and within the family. As with child abuse, all those who work in health care and social services should be aware of the signs of elder abuse and appropriate means of intervention (which may consist of simply knowing the appropriate authorities or health professionals to notify). Abuse and neglect will obviously interfere with and may even destroy a patient's efforts to adapt to a chronic condition and its care. Maladaptive adjustment to the abuse and neglect may also occur, depending on the psychological makeup and the medical status of the individual.

17.43 Institutional Care

Various types of institutions are available for elderly people needing long-term care. These include day-care and community centers, retirement communities, nursing homes, extended care facilities and residential care facilities ("old-age homes" and "board-and-care homes").

Even if family members are willing to care for the person at home, it is highly unlikely that they will be able to cope alone with the patient's demanding around-the-clock needs. Institutions offer the advantage of a comprehensive approach to therapy for mind and body: psychiatrists, psychologists, social workers, occupational therapists, activity therapists, exercise therapists, nutritionists and other specialists are often available as a multidisciplinary team. Individuals who work in these professions must be thoroughly aware of their own attitudes toward aging and the aged, chronic illness and death and dying if they are to provide effective care. The belief that older persons have value and the ability to change is central to working with individuals in the last stages of the life cycle.

Day-care and community centers offer nonresidential places for the elderly to meet, socialize and deal with feelings of anxiety, depression, boredom and loneliness. Retirement communities are residential communities made up of relatively healthy older people who live and work together. This type of facility is relatively new and is actually designed to help many older people avoid institutionalization. Many retirement communities have an associated medical facility. Although most retirement communities are still operated by nonprofit organizations, for-profit corporations are increasingly establishing retirement communities.

Nursing homes are designed for short-term convalescence and rehabilitation to enable individuals to return to home and community. Approximately half of the people who enter nursing homes, however, remain as permanent residents (Kaplan and Sadock, 1994e).

Residential care facilities are designed to accommodate elderly persons in a protective setting for the rest of their lives, without any attempt to prepare them for discharge and return to home or family. They are run by nonprofit organizations. Both nursing homes and residential care facilities now have a substantial population of disorganized and violent patients with dementia. This is due to the fact that state psychiatric hospitals, which used to house these individuals, no longer accept patients with dementia, unless the condition is mild or reversible and the person is not likely to become a permanent resident of the hospital.

17.44   Psychotherapy

The traditional Freudian view has been that persons over 50 years of age lack sufficient plasticity of personality to change and so cannot benefit from insight-oriented psychotherapy. Although mental elasticity does undergo limitation with age, the degree of limitation varies widely among individuals, so that many older persons can indeed benefit from insight-oriented psychotherapy (Kaplan and Sadock, 1994e). Such therapy is contraindicated, however, for those for whom insight would bring only the realization that life has been a failure and they have no opportunity to change this.

In addition to insight-oriented psychotherapy, the aged can benefit from supportive psychotherapy, cognitive therapy, group therapy, family therapy and occupational therapy. Insight-oriented psychotherapy can help elders deal with emotional problems, understand their own behavior and its effect on others, improve interpersonal relationships, increase self-esteem and self-confidence, and decrease feelings of helplessness and anger. In general, psychotherapy improves the quality of the person's life by allowing him or her to deal with and overcome problems that were previously avoided and thus to function more fully within the limitations of their health status.

For those with cognitive impairments, psychotherapy can improve both mental and physical symptoms. One study found, for example, that nearly half of the patients who received insight-oriented psychotherapy showed greater mental alertness, improved memory and better hearing as well as decreased urinary incontinence and improved gait (Kaplan and Sadock, 1994e). Even without delving into the person's psychology in search of insights, the simple fact of having an encouraging, supportive, reassuring listener and adviser in the person of the therapist can increase the patient's self-confidence and general sense of well-being.

Cognitive therapy is aimed at correcting distorted thinking, such as stereotypical negative beliefs about aging and the ability to change, that can become self-fulfilling prophecies of failure and a diminished life. Common beliefs that they are "too old" for sex, sports, acquiring new skills or knowledge, learning a new job or helping others can all be corrected through cognitive therapy. Adaptive coping strategies can also be taught to help older individuals overcome inhibitions and phobic avoidances of situations or activities.

Group therapy provides the mutual support of peers facing common challenges and the opportunity to make new friends and counteract the loss of former ones. The opportunity to help, as well as be helped, increases self-esteem. The group setting also provides stimulation and activity, which helps individuals with dementia stay oriented.

Family therapy is often not only desirable but essential for dealing with the complex network of individual and family issues and conflicts that affect the patient's long-term care.

17.45   Restraints

Physical restraints such as belts and vests are sometimes used to protect older patients from exacerbating existing conditions or sustaining new injuries (e.g., falling out of bed, wheelchair and so on), and to keep them from wandering away from their care facility. Restraints should be used far more judiciously than is presently the case, however; government surveys have found that as many as 40 percent of nursing home patients are routinely subjected to some form of physical restraint (Kaplan and Sadock, 1994e).

Restraint is associated with decreased muscle tone due to limitation or prevention of walking and other exercise, a diminished sense of mastery and independence, and increased rage. Thus restraints should be used only for patients for whom lack of restraint presents a clear risk to their well-being, such as those who repeatedly pull out feeding and oxygen tubes. The majority of patients who require some form of added protection can be managed by alternative methods, such as tilted recliners, safe walking paths and floor alarms (to signal an exit from safe areas).

17.46 Financial Challenges

The economic burden of chronic illness care can be a major source of stress for the patient and family, and the situation is further aggravated in this regard by the current pattern of allocation of health care funds in industrialized societies (Teague, et al., 1993; Miller, 1993). In the United States, for example, 42 percent of the health care dollar spent on the elderly goes to hospital costs, 21 percent to physician services, 20 percent to nursing home care and 4 percent to home health care (Fowles, 1993; Murrow and Oglesby, 1996).

The total cost of nursing home care in the United States is about $38 billion a year, with the average cost of an individual stay being more than $30,000 a year (the range is from $20,000 to $50,000) (Kaplan and Sadock, 1994c; 1994e). These costs are not covered by Medicare, but approximately half of the amount is paid by Medicaid. An increasing proportion is now being covered by private insurance companies through long-term-care insurance policies.

Family caretakers, usually a daughter, spend about $120 per month on expenses such as travel, telephone, special foods and medication (Kaplan and Sadock, 1994c). The nurse can work with the social worker to help the patient and family identify sources of economic assistance and to secure them.

17.47 Cultural Perspectives

Those outside the mainstream of a society, such as ethnic and religious minorities and the poor, face the challenges of discrimination, lack of cultural understanding on the part of health care staff, and limited access to health care, in addition to the challenges presented by advancing age and chronic illness. This can magnify the emotional reactions common to all people, such as anxiety and distress, that occur upon entering the strange hospital world and, combined with linguistic and cultural misunderstandings, can cause conflict with staff over treatment plans. Provision of quality health care to minority populations thus requires staff training in their special needs, as well as certain specialized staff, particularly linguistic and cultural translators and interpreters who can mediate negotiations over appropriate medical care practices (George and Young, 1996).

Specific examples of cultural differences from which problems may arise include the basic requirements of diet, hygiene and religion. For example, what Muslim patients may eat is strictly dictated by the Koran. Most will adhere to a vegetarian diet, since pork and pork products are strictly forbidden, and other meat will not be prepared according to Islamic law *(halal)*. Since alcohol in any form is also forbidden, the content of medications should be checked before prescribing or administering them; if the patient cannot be reassured as to the contents of a medication, he or she may refuse to take it (George and Young, 1996).

With regard to hygiene, many Asian patients will prefer to wash in free-flowing water rather than in a static bath. People from the Indian subcontinent typically use the left hand for washing the private parts of the body and the right hand for eating and other social functions. The right hand should thus be kept as free as possible (e.g., when fixing intravenous lines); food should be placed so it can be reached with the right hand, and objects should be handed to the person so they can be taken with the right hand. Many people, particularly Muslim, Hindu and Sikh women, place a high value on personal modesty, which should be maintained during nursing and treatment procedures. The split-back hospital gowns traditional in the West may not be acceptable to these individuals.

In Asia and in many developing countries, it is customary for the family to take an active role in the patient's health care, and one family member usually remains at the patient's bedside at all times. The usual restrictions on visitation may thus have to be relaxed. On the other hand, illness is often regarded as something to be suffered through, in the sickbed, until a complete cure has occurred. In the case of a chronic condition, therefore, considerable tactful explanation and negotiation may be required in order to gain acceptance of the practice of active, long-term care and limited recovery. Staff may also need to mediate conflicts between traditional family members and younger, more Westernized members with regard to all these traditions.

As described, a variety of cultural differences must be taken into account when caring for people who belong to non-Western or minority cultures, if good care is to be provided. Differences in health-related attitudes, beliefs and behaviors as well as socioeconomic differences can be significant and can have significant implications for health, well-being and longevity. For example, African-Americans, the largest minority population in the United States, continue to have a lower life expectancy in later life (15.5 years at age 65) and to reach old age with a higher prevalence of both chronic and acute medical problems, disability and low utilization of health care resources than Caucasians (Weaver and Gary, 1996). In contrast, Mexican-Americans, who make up 60 percent of the Hispanic population—the second largest minority in the United States—have a favorable health profile that is similar to the Anglo population (Markides and Black, 1996).

Data from which to construct a health profile for Asians and Pacific Islanders is limited. What is known about elderly Korean-Americans, for example, indicates that they practice good health behavior overall, but that smoking cessation is a problem for elderly Korean men, and weight reduction is a problem for elderly Korean women (Wallace, et al., 1996). Community-based organizations are particularly important for promoting healthy behavior among elderly Koreans, because of the limited English-speaking ability and educational level of many. Further research remains to be done on the needs of minority individuals, who make up an increasingly important segment of the chronic care population (George and Young, 1996).

17.50 MODELS OF ADAPTATION AND INTERVENTION

The process of adaptation has been formalized in a number of models over the years. The main types are briefly described in the following sections. It should be kept in mind that these models are formal, generalized conceptualizations of a complex and highly individualistic process; they are designed to aid understanding of the adaptive process, to monitor a patient's progress through that process and to guide intervention; they are not intended to serve as a programmatic mold into which each patient must be made to fit.

Moreover, the models are based on different formal theories of psychological adaptation to chronic illness and disability. These theories are derived from the broader field of general psychological theories, the popularity and acceptance of which have waxed and waned over the years with respect to their explanatory power and validity as applied to adaptation to chronic conditions. In brief, theories and models of adaptation range from mentalistic theories (e.g., stage models), which emphasize internal thoughts and feelings, to behavioral or social theories (e.g., behavioral models), which emphasize external events. In between lie integrative field theories (e.g., the coping skills models), which hold both internal thoughts and feelings and external events (both physical and social) to be important (Rohe, 1993). Family-focused intervention (Butcher, 1994) and trajectory theory (Miller, 1993) are newer theoretic approaches tailored more closely to the nature and practical realities of chronic illness care.

Whatever the theory, model or approach, current opinion is that there is no evidence for a universal response to chronic illness and its consequences, or for an orderly, sequential progression through fixed stages of adjustment. Individual variation in both the nature and sequence of emotional response is the rule, and acceptance and adaptation may never be complete. External physical and social barriers, not the chronic condition or internal events (e.g., motivation), are currently thought to be the major source of adjustment problems (Rohe, 1993).

17.51 Stage Models

Stage models typically identify three to six stages through which a person is presumed to progress as he or she adjusts to chronic illness and long-term care. Common stages include initial shock and psychic numbing; denial; anger and depression; grief and mourning; acceptance and integration; and adaptation. Failure to negotiate these stages successfully is said to result in maladjustment.

17.52 Behavioral Models

Behavioral models focus on external events and observable behavior rather than on internal thoughts and feelings. Four tasks must be accomplished by the patient: remaining in the chronic care environment; eliminating chronic-care-incongruent (inappropriate) behaviors; acquiring chronic-care-congruent (appropriate) behaviors; and maintaining chronic-care-congruent behaviors. Intervention is based on learning theory and involves the application or withdrawal of reinforcers of desired or undesired behavior, respectively (Rohe, 1993).

17.53   Coping Skills Models

The coping skills model, which focuses on both internal and behavioral factors, presents the patient with seven major adaptive tasks and seven major coping skills to master: (1) denying or minimizing the seriousness of a crisis (to promote clear thinking on an emergency basis); (2) seeking relevant information; (3) requesting reassurance and emotional support; (4) learning specific illness related procedures (e.g., skills that minimize functional impairment); (5) setting concrete, limited goals; (6) rehearsing alternative outcomes; and (7) finding a general purpose or pattern of meaning in the situation (e.g., to satisfy the human belief that the world is a meaningful and comprehensible place) (Rohe, 1993).

17.54   Family-focused Interventions

The family-focused intervention approach recognizes that a chronic condition and adaptation to it is a matter that affects the entire family unit (Butcher, 1994). Interventions are aimed at promoting the adjustment and growth of the family unit as a whole, as well as of the patient and other individual family members.

Interventions, mediated by the nurse, include identification and marshaling of relatives, friends and community support groups as additional resources; individual and family counseling; changing negative attitudes; educating the patient and the patient's family about the chronic condition and its care; promoting effective communication and shared values within the family; and establishing effective family decision-making and problem-solving strategies.

17.55   Trajectory Framework

In chronic illness care, the course or prognosis of the condition may be described in terms of a trajectory. More specifically, trajectory theory conceptualizes chronic illness care in terms of a framework that takes into account the variability of the severity of the illness over time and the possibility of its management or technologic stabilization

(Miller, 1993). Commonly recognized trajectory phases include: (1) the diagnostic phase—when the need for care is recognized; (2) the management phase—when resources are identified and utilized; and (3) the stabilization or resolution phase-—when the condition is in remission or controlled.

As with stage models, the patient, family and caregivers (family and professional) should all resist thinking of the patient's trajectory as a tidy, one-way progression through the phases to ultimate and complete recovery in the near future: by definition, the outcome of a chronic condition is uncertain and far away in time, at best; and because of the variable course of chronic conditions over the long term, patients may be expected to move back and forth between the management and stabilization phases.

A disparity in perception with regard to these facts among those involved in the patient's care can cause misunderstandings and disharmony among the team and adversely affect the patient's status. A common disparity between the patient and the family caregiver, for example, involves the extent of care and assistance that will be required and the length of time for which they will be needed. It is the responsibility of the nurse to ascertain the perceptions and expectations of all parties involved as to the course of the illness and the nature of the treatment methods used, and to facilitate bringing these into agreement, if necessary. Cooperative problem solving aimed at generating mutually satisfactory solutions is a key tool here.

17.56 Stages of Change/Readiness

The stages-of-change model categorizes individuals along a five-stage continuum of readiness to change health-related behavior (Prochaska and DiClemente, 1992):

- Stage 1—Precontemplation: no intention of changing health behavior.

- Stage 2—Contemplation: awareness that a problem exists, but still no commitment to take any action.

- Stage 3—Preparation: intention to take action within the next month; the action was also taken, unsuccessfully, within the past year.

- Stage 4—Action: process of changing a health behavior is initiated.

- Stage 5—Maintenance: relapse prevention.

Two characteristics of the stages-of-change model may account for its popularity in the literature: (1) it has a positive focus, and (2) it promises the clinician a relatively precise means of prescribing behavioral change intervention (Haber, 1996). However, the model, in its current stage of development, has two weaknesses that may limit rather than facilitate behavioral change, particularly in older adults: (1) it is difficult to assess a patient's stage of readiness with accuracy, and (2) the implications for how to help during a given stage of readiness are not clear (Haber, 1994).

The practical consequences of the model's shortcomings are that opportunities for intervention and change may be missed by offering strategies appropriate for a specific stage of readiness when, in reality, a given person may not fit neatly into that one stage as defined. For example, a person who is classified as being in the precontemplation stage because of an initial reluctance to move toward a suggested goal may in fact be quite willing to change when offered a more modest goal or a goal in a different but related area of behavior.

Until these weaknesses can be eliminated or minimized by further research and understanding of the variables involved in making changes in behavior, the person should be offered behavior change strategies that will be relevant to most people. These include accurate and readily understandable health education, social support, easily learned behavioral and psychological management skills, and referral to community resources (Haber, 1994).

Finally, many of the problems in the area of behavioral change lie not with the patient or the theoretic models of change, but with health care providers themselves. For example, although an abundance of patient education materials is available, many health care providers are reluctant to distribute it, particularly to the elderly (Haber, 1993). One reason may be that the very abundance of materials contains much that is contradictory, so that with the lack of universal consistency and the enormous task of sifting through the literature, health care providers find it easier simply to discount it all. Also, there appears to be a belief that older adults are less able to change their behavior and have limited time to benefit from the changes, in any case. Many health care providers focus on the technical aspects of providing medical care and limit their educational role to the provision of warnings ("You need to lose some weight," or "You need to stop smoking"); this is likely due to lack of training or reimbursement for educational activities (Haber, 1993). Studies have shown that brief counseling is twice as likely as brief warnings to result in behavioral change in the patient (Haber, 1996).

17.60 SPECIFIC CONDITIONS INVOLVING LONG-TERM CARE

Some specific chronic conditions are cited here as brief illustrations of the foregoing discussion.

17.61 Stroke

Although stroke (cerebrovascular accident; CVA) may occur at any age, it is much more common among the elderly than in other age groups. Stoke provides a comprehensive example of the characteristics of chronic illness and long-term care that produce psychological distress and adaptive difficulties (Hayne and Fisher, 1997; Ozer, et al., 1994). It has a sudden, unanticipated onset and it can lead to marked disability (provoking grief reactions); it has an uncertain prognosis (causing motivational problems); and it can affect not only physical function but mood, behavior, cognitive function and appearance as well. Depression is a common sequela. The fact that the illness has its origin in the brain can be difficult for many patients to cope with.

17.62 Trauma and Orthopedic Conditions

Although orthopedic injuries are often thought of as being routine, they can push the elderly individual from independent functioning to dependency (Twining, 1996). Common adverse effects associated with orthopedic injuries include pain, infection, potential isolation due to infection, and the disorienting effects of hospitalization. Slow, painful recovery can impair motivation, and aggravation of a pre-existing chronic condition (likely to be present in an elderly person) can compound the problem. Depression and anxiety are common and should be treated.

17.63 Parkinson's Disease

Perhaps the most problematic feature of Parkinson's disease is its unique type of uncertainty (Twining, 1996). Although medication will control the symptoms in most patients initially, some will later develop disabling symptoms that the medication cannot control. It is impossible to predict into which group patients will fall, or when. Symptoms such as "freezing" (stiffening up), for example, can fluctuate from hour to hour, disrupting the person's control over his or her life. Although some patients are able to cope with this, others develop "learned helplessness" and depression. Because the person may be functioning fine one minute and disabled the next, many family members, some staff and even the patient may conclude that he or she is simply not trying hard enough during symptomatic episodes. Needless to say, such misperceptions can impede adjustment. Negative attitudes and beliefs about the origin of the disease in the brain are likewise unhelpful to adaptation.

17.64   Cognitive Impairment and Dementia

The level of a person's cognitive functioning is an extremely important determinant of her or his safe and effective independent functioning and thus of adaptive outcome (Twining, 1996). Screening assessments of cognitive function should be done routinely in the elderly, and care should be taken to distinguish between normal and abnormal cognitive changes. The status of a person's insight function is equally important.

17.100   BIBLIOGRAPHY

Text References

Annas, G. J.: The Health Care Proxy and the Living Will. N. Engl. J. Med. 324:1210-1213, 1991.

Asch, D.: The Role of Critical Care Nurses in Euthanasia and Assisted Suicide. N. Engl. J. Med. 334:1374-1379, 1996.

Bandman, E. and Bandman, B.: Nursing Ethics Through the Life Span, 3rd ed. Norwalk, Conn.: Appleton & Lange, 1995.

Barder, L., et al.: Depression and Issues of Control Among Elderly People in Health Care Settings. J. Adv. Nurs. 20:597-604, 1994.

Beauchamp, T. and Childress, J.: Principles of Biomedical Ethics, 4th ed. New York: Oxford, 1995.

Beck, C. and Vogelpohl, T.: Cognitive Impairment and Autonomy. In: Gamroth, L., et al. (Eds.): Enhancing Autonomy in Long-Term Care: Concepts and Strategies. New York: Springer, 1995.

Bosek, M. and Jezuit, D.: The Nurse's Role in Assisted Suicide. Med. Surg. Nurs. 4:373-378, 1995.

Brenneman, S. A.: A Critical Review of Health Care for an Aging Population. Aging 18:10-13, 1995.

Butcher, L.: A Family-Focused Perspective on Chronic Illness. Rehabil. Nurs. 19:70-74, 1994.

Canam, C.: Common Adaptive Tasks Facing Parents of Children with Chronic Conditions. J. Adv. Nursing 18:46-53, 1993.

Clark, P. G.: Ethical Dimensions of Quality of Life in Aging: Autonomy vs. Collectivism in the United States and Canada. Gerontologist 31:631-639, 1991.

Coker, L. and Johns, F.: Guardianship for Elders: Process and Issues. J. Gerontol. Nurs. 21:25-32, 1992.

Davis, A., et al.: Nurses's Attitudes toward Active Euthanasia. Nurs. Outlook 43:174-179, 1995.

Estes, C. L., et al.: The Long-Term Care Crisis: Elders Trapped in the No-Care Zone. Newbury Park, Calif.: Sage, 1993.

Faux, S.: Siblings of Children with Chronic Physical and Cognitive Disabilities. J. Pediatr. Nurs. 8:305-317, 1993.

Fowles, D.: A Profile of Older Americans. Washington, D.C.: American Association of Retired Persons, 1993.

Gamroth, L., et al.: Enhancing Autonomy in Long-Term Care: Concepts and Strategies. New York: Springer, 1995.

George, J. and Young, J.: Rehabilitation and Elderly Ethnic Minorities. In: Squires, A. J. (Ed.): Rehabilitation of Older People, 2nd ed. London: Chapman & Hall, 1996.

Gerety, M.: Health Care Reform from the View of a Geriatrician. Gerontologist 34: 590-597, 1994.

Gibson, F.: Reminiscence and Recall: A Guide to Good Practice. London: Age Concern, 1994.

Haber, D.: Strategies to Promote the Health of Older People: An Alternative to Readiness Stages. Fam. Commun. Health 19:1-10, 1996.

Haber, D.: Health Promotion and Aging. New York: Springer, 1994.

Haber, D.: Guide to Clinical Preventive Services: A Challenge to Physician Resourcefulness. Clin. Gerontol. 12:17-29, 1993.

Hayn, M. A. and Fisher, T. R.: Stroke Rehabilitation. Nursing 97 27:40-46, 1997.

Husted, G. and Husted, J.: Ethical Decision-Making in Nursing, 2nd ed. Boston: Mosby-Year Book, 1995.

Hutchinson, R. R. and Quartyaro, E. G.: High-Risk Vulnerable Populations and Volunteers: A Model of Education and Service Coordination. J. Commun. Health Nurs. 12:111-119, 1995.

Idler, E. L. and Kasl, S. V.: Self-Ratings of Health: Do They Also Predict Change in Functional Ability? J. Gerontol. Soc. Sci. 50B:344-353, 1995.

Jackson, D. G. and Cleary, B. L.: Health Promotion Strategies for Spousal Caregivers of Chronically Ill Elders. Nurse Practitioner Forum 6:10-18, 1995.

Jones, D. and Lester, C.: Hospital Care and Discharge: Patients' and Carers' Opinions. Age and Ageing 23:91-96, 1994.

Kane, R.: Autonomy and Regulation in Long-Term Care: An Odd Couple, an Ambiguous Relationship. In: Gamroth, L., et al. (Eds.): Enhancing Autonomy in Long-Term Care. New York: Springer, 1995.

Kaplan, H. I. and Sadock, B. J.: The Doctor-Patient Relationship and Interviewing Techniques. In: Kaplan, H. I. and Sadock, B. J.: Kaplan and Sadock's Synopsis of Psychiatry: Behavioral Sciences, Clinical Psychiatry, 7th ed. Baltimore: Williams & Wilkins, 1994a.

Kaplan, H. I. and Sadock, B. J.: General Principles of Psychopharmacology. In: Kaplan, H. I. and Sadock, B. J.: Kaplan and Sadock's Synopsis of Psychiatry: Behavioral Sciences, Clinical Psychiatry, 7th ed. Baltimore: Williams & Wilkins, 1994b.

Kaplan, H. I. and Sadock, B. J.: Human Development Throughout the Life Cycle. In: Kaplan, H. I. and Sadock, B. J.: Kaplan and Sadock's Synopsis of Psychiatry: Behavioral Sciences, Clinical Psychiatry, 7th ed. Baltimore: Williams & Wilkins, 1994c.

Kaplan, H. I. and Sadock, B. J.: Contributions of the Psychosocial Sciences to Human Behavior. In: Kaplan, H. I. and Sadock, B. J.: Kaplan and Sadock's Synopsis of Psychiatry: Behavioral Sciences, Clinical Psychiatry, 7th ed. Baltimore: Williams & Wilkins, 1994d.

Kaplan, H. I. and Sadock, B. J.: Geriatric Psychiatry. In: Kaplan, H. I. and Sadock, B. J.: Kaplan and Sadock's Synopsis of Psychiatry:

Behavioral Sciences, Clinical Psychiatry, 7th ed. Baltimore: Williams & Wilkins, 1994e.

Kaufman, J. E.: Persoanl Definitions of Health Among Elderly People: A Link to Effective Health Promotion. Fam. Commun. Health 19:58-68, 1996.

Kelly, K and Maas, M.: Health Care Rationing: Dilemma and Paradox. St. Louis: Mosby-Year Book, 1994.

Kingston, P. and Phillipson, C.: Elder Abuse and Neglect. Br. J. Nurs. 3:1171-1190, 1994.

Kjervik, D. K., et al.: Trigger Events That Indicate the Need for Proxy Decision-Making in Cognitively-Impaired Older Persons. Am. J. Alz. Care Relat. Dis. Res. 3:21-28, 1993.

Markides, K. S. and Black, S. A.: Aging and Health Behaviors in Mexican Americans. Fam. Commun. Health 19:11-18, 1996.

Mezey, M., et al.: The Patient Self-Determination Act: Sources of Concern for Nurses. Nurs. Outlook 42:30-38, 1994.

Miller, C.: Trajectory and Empowerment Theory Applied to Care of Patients with Multiple Sclerosis. J. Neurosci. Nurs. 25:343-348, 1993.

Milne, C., et al.: Correlates of Well-Being Among Caregivers of Cognitively Impaired Elders. Canad. J. Nurs. Res. 26:27-39, 1994.

Mockenhaupt, R.: Self-Care for Older Adults: Taking Care and Taking Charge. Generations 17:5-6, 1993.

Murrow, E. J. and Oglesby, F. M.: Acute and Chronic Illness: Similarities, Differences and Challenges. Orthop. Nurs. 15:47-51, 1996.

Omnibus Budget Reconciliation Act of 1990: Pub. L. No. 101-508[4206, 4751 (codified in scattered sections of 42 USC, especially 1395cc, 139a)] (West suppl. 1991).

Ozer, M., et al.: Management of Persons with Stroke. St. Louis: Mosby-Year Book, 1994.

Parker, M.: Families Caring for Chronically Ill Children with Tuberous Sclerosis Complex. Fam. Commun. Health 19:73-84, 1996.

Pinch, W. and Parsons, M.: The Patient Self-Determination Act: The Ethical Dimensions. Nurs. Pract. Forum 3:16-22, 1992.

Prochaska, J, and DiClemente, C.: Stages of Change in the Modification of Problem Behaviors. In: Herson, M. (Ed.): Progress in Behavior Modification. Newbury Park, Calif.: Sage, 1992.

Ray, L. D. and Ritchie, J. A.: Caring for Chronically Ill Children at Home: Factors That Influence Parents' Coping. J. Pediatr. Nurs. 8:217-225, 1993.

Reinhardy, J. R.: Relocation to a New Environment: Decisional Control and the Move to a Nursing Home. Health Soc. Work 20:31-38, 1995.

Rice, V. H., et al.: Ethical Issues Relative to Autonomy and Personal Control in Independent and Cognitively Impaired Elders. Nurs. Outlook 45:27-34, 1997.

Rodin, J. and Tribo, C.: Sense of Control, Aging, and Health. In: Ory, M. G., et al. (Eds.): Aging, Health, and Behavior. Newbury Park, Calif.: Sage, 1992.

Rohe, D. E.: Psychological Aspects of Rehabilitation. In: DeLisa, J. A., et al., (Eds.): Rehabilitation Medicine: Principles and Practice, 2nd ed. Philadelphia: Lippincott, 1993.

Salsberry, P.: Assuming Responsibility for One's Health: An Analysis of a Key Assumption in Nursing's Agenda for Health Care Reform. Nurs. Outlook 41:212-216, 1993.

Task Force on Aging: Reclaiming Time: Caregiver Relief and Renewal. Seattle: Church Council of Greater Seattle, 1996.

Teague, B., et al.: Hightech Homecare for Children with Chronic Health Conditions. A Pilot Study. J. Pediatr. Nurs. 8:226-232, 1993.

Theis, S., et al.: Respite for Caregivers: An Evaluation Study. J. Commun. Health Nurs. 11:31-44, 1994.

Twining, C.: Psychological Approaches with Older People. In: Squires, A. J. (Ed.): Rehabilitation of Older People, 2nd ed. London: Chapman & Hall, 1996.

van Duynhoven, U.: Patients Need Compassionate Pain Control: An Alternative to Physician-Assisted Suicide. Oregon Nurs. 59:11-12, 1995.

Viney, L. L.: Life Stories: Personal Construct Therapy with the Elderly. Chichester, England: Wiley, 1993.

Vogelpohl, T., et al.: "I Can Do It" Dressing: Promoting Independence through Individual Strategies. J. Gerontol. Nurs. 23:39-42, 1996.

Wallace, S. P., et al.: Health Practices of Korean Elderly People: National Health Promotion Priorities and Minority Community Needs. Fam. Commun. Health 19:29-42, 1996.

Walters, J. W. (ed.): Choosing Who's to Live: Ethics and Aging. Urbana: University of Illinois Press, 1996.

Weaver, G. D. and Gary, L. E.: Correlates of Health-Related Behaviors in Older African American Adults: Implications for Health Promotion. Fam. Commun. Health 19:43-57, 1996.

Winslade, T.: Legal Regulation of Terminal Care: Options and Obstacles. Tex. Med. 87:70-75, 1991.

Worcester, M. and Hedrick, S.: Dilemmas in Using Respite for Family Caregivers of Frail Elders. Fam. Commun. Health 19:31-48, 1996.

Young, A., et al.: Oncology Nurses' Attitudes Regarding Voluntary Physician-Assisted Dying for Competent Terminally-Ill Patients. Oncol. Nurse Forum 20:445-451, 1993.

Additional References

Beining, K. and Whitaker, J.: Communication Problems of Older People. In: Squires, A. J. (Ed.): Rehabilitation of Older People, 2nd ed. London: Chapman & Hall, 1996.

Butler, R. and Lewis, M.: Late-Life Depression: When and How to Intervene. Geriatrics 50:44-55, 1995.

Fabacher, D., et al.: An In-home Preventive Assessment Program for Independent Older Adults. J. Am. Geriatr. Soc. 42:630-638, 1994.

Homer, A. C. and Gilleard, C.: The Effect of Inpatient Respite Care on Elderly Patients and Their Carers. Age and Ageing 23:274-276, 1994.

Jones, D. A. and Vetter, N. J.: A Survey of Those Who Care for the Elderly at Home: Their Problems and Their Needs. Soc. Sci. Med. 19:511-514, 1994.

Karlowicz, K. (Ed.): Urologic Nursing: Principles and Practice. Philadelphia: Saunders, 1995.

Leonard, K. M., et al.: Prolonged Cancer Death. A Family Affair. Cancer Nurs. 18:222-227, 1995.

Spiegel, D.: Cancer and Depression. Br. J. Psychiatry Suppl.:109-116, June 1996.

Swift, C. G.: Disease and Disability in Older People—Prospects for Intervention. In: Squires, A. J. (Ed.): Rehabilitation of Older People, 2nd ed. London: Chapman & Hall, 1996.

INDEX

A

ADENOCARCINOMA OF THE PROSTATE (See PROSTATE CANCER)

AGING, ADAPTATION TO
Generally . . . 25-26
Advance directives regarding treatment . . 772-73
Agoraphobia, coping with . . . 766
Anxiety, coping with . . . 766
Autonomy, personal
    Generally . . . 768-70
    Cognitive impairment affecting 770
    Impediments to . . . 770-71
Challenges of . . . 759-62
Chronic illness
    Challenges posed by . . . 762-67
    Reaction to, factors determining . . . 767-79
Cognitive changes . . . 760-61; 770
Decisions on death and dying
    Generally . . . 771-72
    Advance directives . . . 772-73
    Euthanasia . . . 774-75
    Professional-assisted suicide 774-75
Depression, coping with . . . 766-67
Designation of proxy directives . . 772-73
Durable power of attorney, granting of . . 773
Emotional changes . . . 761-62
Euthanasia, decisions regarding . . 774-75
Function, coping with loss of . . . 764
Grief and loss, coping with (See subhead: Loss, coping with)
Information processing, changes in speed of . . . 761
Language ability, changes in . . . 761
Living wills regarding treatment . . . 772
Long-term care, adaptation to (See LONG-TERM CARE)
Loss, coping with
    Generally . . . 762
    Function, loss of . . . 764
    Loved one, loss of . . . 763
    Lowered expectations, coping with . . . 764-65
    Reminiscence, role of . . . 765-66

AGING, ADAPTATION TO—Cont.
Loss, coping with—Cont.
    Self-concept, changing . . . 765
Loved ones, coping with loss of . . . 763
Lowered expectations, coping with 764-65
Memory changes . . . 760-61
Natural death acts . . . 772
Patient Self-Determination Act . . . 773
Patient-specified treatment instructions . . . 772
Perceptions about health, role of . . . 768
Personality changes . . . 761-62
Professional-assisted suicide, decisions regarding . . . 774-75
Psychological challenges . . . 25; 760-62
Reminiscence, role of . . . 765-66
Suicidal intent, dealing with . . . 767

ALZHEIMER'S DISEASE
Generally . . . 15; 684-85
Active Daily Living scales to diagnose . . 711
Age, related to . . . 688
Agnosia
    Management of . . . 716
    Symptom, as . . . 691
Agraphia as symptom . . . 691
Aluminum exposure as cause . . . 698-700
Antemortem examination to diagnose . . . 709-10
Aphasia
    Management of . . . 716
    Symptom, as . . . 691
Apraxia, management of . . . 716-17
Behavioral changes as symptoms 692-93
Categories of . . . 703-4
Chelators, treatment with . . . 714
Chemical imbalance as cause . . . 698
Clinical Dementia Rating scale to diagnose . . . 711
Cognitive deterioration as symptom 690-92
Computed tomography to diagnose 707-9
Confirmation, neuropathological . . 693-94
Delay of onset, estrogen replacement therapy for . . . 4
Delusions as symptom . . . 692-93

G

SENSORY DISORDERS—Cont.
Glaucoma (See GLAUCOMA)
Hearing loss (See HEARING LOSS)
Olfactory sense, loss of
    Generally . . . 19
    Risks associated with . . . 19
Vision impairment (See VISION IMPAIR-MENT)

SICKLE CELL ANEMIA
Stroke, symptoms similar to . . . 367

SKIN DISEASES AND DISORDERS
Diabetes mellitus, complication of . . 433
Hip surgery, skin compromise as complication of . . . 59
Rheumatoid arthritis, skin changes as symptom of . . . 198
Stroke, complications of . . . 373

SKULL
Paget's disease of . . . 170-71

SMOKING
Heart diseases, as risk factor for 246-47
Osteoporosis, as risk factor for . . . 143

SPINAL CORD INJURIES
Urinary incontinence, related to . . . 619

SPINAL FRACTURES
Generally . . . 3; 8
Kyphosis . . . 3; 8
Osteoporotic . . . 157-58, 159: Fig. 4-7

SPINAL TAP
Stroke, diagnosis of . . . 356

SPINE
Fractures (See SPINAL FRACTURES)
Osteoporosis (See OSTEOPOROSIS)
Paget's disease . . . 171; 178
Stenosis, Paget's disease causing . . . 171; 178

STROKE
Generally . . . 336
Anatomy and physiology
    Generally . . . 320-21: Fig. 8-1
    Arachnoid membrane . . . . 321, 325: Fig. 8-5
    Blood vessel walls . . . 321, 322: Fig. 8-2
    Brain stem . . . 321, 324: Fig. 8-4

STROKE—Cont.
Anatomy and physiology—Cont.
    Carotid arteries . . . 322, 326: Fig. 8-6
    Central nervous system . . 321, 323: Fig. 8-3
    Cerebellum . . . 321, 324: Fig. 8-4
    Cerebral lobes . . . 321, 324: Fig. 8-4
    Cerebrospinal fluid . . . 321, 325: Fig. 8-5
    Circle of Willis . . . 322, 327: Fig. 8-7
    Dura mater . . . 321, 325: Fig. 8-5
    Meninges . . . 321, 325: Fig. 8-5
    Pia mater . . . 321, 325: Fig. 8-5
    Vertebral arteries . . 322, 326: Fig. 8-6
Aneurysm, caused by
    False aneurysm . . . 330-31: Fig. 8-8
    Spontaneous intraparenchymal hemorrhage . . . 346
    Spontaneous subarachnoid hemorrhage . . . 336-38
    Traumatic aneurysm . . . 330
Angiomas, spontaneous subarachnoid hemorrhage caused by . . . 338
Anticoagulants, treatment with
    Cardiac embolic ischemic brain infarction . . . 365-66
    Thrombotic ischemic brain infarction . . . 357-58
Antihypertensives, treatment with
    Cardiac embolic ischemic brain infarction . . . 365
    Thrombotic ischemic brain infarction . . . 357
Arterial contusion and thrombosis, role of . . . 329-30; 350
Arterial laceration and transection, caused by . . . 329
Arteriography, diagnosis with
    Generally . . . 325
    Spontaneous subarachnoid hemorrhage . . . 342
Arteriovenous malformation, caused by
    Generally . . . 345-46
    Fistula . . . 331-32: Fig. 8-9
Arteritis presenting as . . . 367-68
Atherosclerosis
    Caused by . . . 10; 349
    Risk factors, reduction of . . 359-60
Bacterial endocarditis presenting as 369-70